Health Psychology

Now in its fourth edition, *Health Psychology* takes a truly interdisciplinary approach to studying health psychology, and offers a comprehensive overview of the subareas within this fascinating subject.

Fully revised to reflect current research and studies, and now in full color, the book includes new content on the impact of COVID-19 and greater coverage of health diversity. It unpacks the issue of social inequities in health by addressing how race and social economies have been traditionally confounded. The author achieves this by focusing on five systems that affect individual health outcomes: individual, family/community, social/physical environment, health care systems, and health policy. The social ecological perspective on health psychology creates a depth of understanding of the diverse facets of health, and examines health from a global perspective by exploring the impact of infectious and chronic illnesses both regionally and globally. This new edition has been packed with updated statistics and references, as well as helpful video links infused throughout, to actively engage readers in each topic.

While grounded in psychology, the book incorporates perspectives from anthropology, biology, economics, environmental studies, medicine, public health, and sociology, and will be of particular interest to undergraduate students in health psychology and public health and for masters' students of health psychology.

For additional instructor resources, please visit www.routledge.com/9781032292557, which includes lecture slides, an instructor manual, and test bank.

Deborah Fish Ragin is Professor Emerita of Psychology at Montclair State University, New Jersey. She served as Assistant Professor on the faculties of Hunter College, City University of New York, and as Associate Research Professor at the Mount Sinai School of Medicine (now the Icahn School of Medicine) before joining Montclair State. She also served as an American Psychological Association Representative to the United Nations, focusing on the psychosocial impact of HIV/AIDS.

"There is no better health psychology book on the market with an ecological perspective."
—**Ellen Langer**, *Harvard University*, USA.

'Capturing the field of Health Psychology in a single textbook can be quite challenging – the field's expansive research across multiple fields of study must be balanced with accessible content and student engagement. Dr. Debby Ragin meets this challenge in her newly revised 'Health Psychology: An Interdisciplinary Approach'. This textbook is a perfect blend of theory, concepts and contributions from multiple fields (e.g., Epidemiology), and data-driven examples. Perhaps most importantly, theories and concepts are applied in the form of stories throughout, as well as beginning each chapter with an "Opening Story" and closing with a "Personal Postscript". This approach is engaging and memorable, moving well beyond the "data dump" found in some textbooks, and helping students find the relevance of this material to their lives.'
—**Brooks B. Gump**, PhD, MPH;
Falk Endowed Professor of Public Health, *Syracuse University*, USA.

'This new edition caters for the decolonisation of health for illness care and management. The focus on holistic healthcare and diversity, with interesting case studies, puts forward excellent practical integration to theoretical contexts- an ideal for students from various disciplines. The importance of spiritual, emotional, religious, environmental, and cultural contexts for health and wellbeing, emphasises how useful this book is, to understand healthcare behaviours in different global community contexts.'
—**Sabihah Moola**, *University of South Africa* (UNISA), South Africa.

Praise for the previous edition:
'Within the pages of Ragin's Health Psychology: An Interdisciplinary Approach, the fascinating complexity of human health is depicted through a social ecological framework that seamlessly integrates the many individual, social, institutional, and structural factors influencing the health of individuals and populations, artfully rendered through accessible coverage of judiciously selected research and illuminating real-world examples, including both historical and current events from across the globe.'
—**Susan E. Walch**, *The University of West Florida*, USA.

Health Psychology

An Interdisciplinary Approach

Fourth Edition

Deborah Fish Ragin

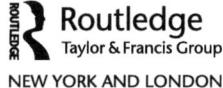

Routledge
Taylor & Francis Group

NEW YORK AND LONDON

Cover Image: Mathisworks via Getty Images

Fourth edition published 2025
by Routledge
605 Third Avenue, New York, NY 10158

and by Routledge
4 Park Square, Milton Park, Abingdon, Oxon, OX14 4RN

Routledge is an imprint of the Taylor & Francis Group, an informa business

First edition published by Pearson 2010

Second edition published by Routledge 2013

Third edition published by Routledge 2017

ISBN: 978-1-032-29254-0 (hbk)
ISBN: 978-1-032-29255-7 (pbk)
ISBN: 978-1-003-30067-0 (ebk)
ISBN: 978-1-032-84972-0 (eBook+)

DOI: 10.4324/9781003300670

Typeset in Sabon
by Apex CoVantage, LLC

Access the Instructor and Student Resources: www.routledge.com/9781032292557

Brief Contents

Contents

Video links have been included within the text to enhance the readers' understanding, and will send the user directly to the video's webpage when clicked. These videos are designed to engage readers, simplify complex concepts and provide key further information on each topic.

PREFACE

A lot has happened since the publication of the third edition of this textbook in 2018: the worst pandemic in over 100 years, alarming increases in the use of opioids in developed countries, a marked increase in alcohol consumption among older adults, and a disturbing decrease in the quality of mental health, especially among adolescents. That weighty list would be depressing if we stopped there. But health psychologists, along with health professionals in other fields, have discovered more opportunities for interdisciplinary work to not only address these new challenges but also to work towards improvements in the overall well-being of individuals and communities.

Health psychologists have come to view health as a dynamic process that involves the interaction of physiology, human behavior, physical and social environments, health systems, and health policy. Perhaps one good example of this claim is found in Flint, Michigan.

In 2014 local government officials decided to change the source of Flint, Michigan's drinking water from Lake Huron to the Flint River. But the water from the Flint River was not treated with an anti-corrosive agent so that it did not corrode the pipes, as required by federal law. The result? The untreated water caused lead to leach from the pipes into the water supply. Families in Flint who relied on this water were ingesting lead with each glassful of water. Now, health care providers are carefully monitoring Flint's children for signs of lead poisoning that may have a lasting and irreversible impact on children including impaired cognitive processes, behavioral disorders, and developmental delays.

This example and scores of others illustrate the complex relationship between physical environments, health policies, and individual health outcomes. It illustrates also why, as health psychologists, we must look at the role of external factors as well as individual, internal determinants when attempting to explain and improve health outcomes.

Health Psychology: An Interdisciplinary Approach presents a social ecological perspective, an approach, that in addition to being consistent with the changes and developments in the field also examines the impact of physiological, cultural, environmental, spiritual, and systems factors on health and health outcomes. This expanded perspective encourages, and in fact requires, that we consider the role of related disciplines such as anthropology, biology, economics, environmental studies, medicine, public health, and sociology on health outcomes. Many health psychologists contend that it is only through the lens of such an interdisciplinary approach that we come to understand how health affects the individual on a mental and emotional level, and how the individual responds to these challenges.

Consistent with this interdisciplinary approach to health, we introduce several topics in this text not typically covered in health psychology. For example, we introduce and explore in greater detail than many texts the global nature of health. Comparing the health outcomes of people with the same illness in different countries allows us to see the impact of an individual's socioeconomic status, a country's gross national income, built environments, health systems, and health policy on health status. Unlike other health psychology textbooks, we also devote a full chapter to psychoneuroimmunology, an integral component to our understanding of the relationship between psychological, neurological, and immunologic health.

Departing from the format of some health psychology textbooks, this text does not include a separate chapter on biological systems. Rather, where appropriate, we incorporate in each chapter a section on the physiological systems relevant to that issue. For example, when discussing emotional health and well-being, we devote a section of the chapter to a discussion of the biological systems and neurotransmitters that are essential to understanding the body's response to emotions. Likewise, in the chapter on cardiovascular health, we review the heart and its components as well as the circulatory system prior to discussing specific cardiovascular diseases or their treatments. And, in the chapter on chronic pain management and arthritis, we explore the physiology of pain in some detail.

Several features are included in this text to underscore the point that health is an integral part of our lives. First, each chapter begins with an *opening story* that poses a scenario or problem for consideration. The opening stories highlight a central concept in the chapter and draw readers into the main topic. Stories summarize current events that pertain to or impact health or the work of health psychologists, and allow the reader to apply the concepts in the chapter to real life situations. For example, Chapter 5, Risky Health Behaviors, Part I, begins with a real story about a teenager who developed the lungs of a 70-year-old person as a result of his vaping habit.

Second, each chapter ends with a *personal postscript* that encourages students to reflect on the main concepts of the chapter and to apply them to actual or likely life events. Personal postscripts are designed especially for a college-aged audience. They propose situations and offer advice or solutions to situations commonly encountered by college students that pertain to health. Finally, the postscripts bring the chapters full circle, allowing students to reflect again on the applied aspects of the health issues presented in the chapter.

Following the personal postscript are *questions to consider* and *true or false questions*, prompts that encourage the students to reflect on what they read and apply their new knowledge to broader issues.

Fourth, the chapters include special *boxes* that explore selected material in depth without disrupting the flow of the text. These are ideal for students and instructors who seek more details about topics introduced in the text. At the same time, the information in boxes can be omitted by readers who are less interested in the details.

Fifth, and central to the social ecological model, one chapter is dedicated to the role of health systems and also identifies career opportunities in health policy. Students are presented with various ways in which health psychologists can participate in research and/or direct service to individuals and health policy institutions that impact the health of individuals, communities, regions, and countries.

Sixth, the chapters conclude with *important terms*, concepts, and procedures common in health and health related fields. These terms are highlighted and defined in text and itemized at the end of each chapter to remind students of the important concepts to remember in each chapter.

NEW TO THIS EDITION

New innovations in health seem like a daily occurrence. Along with these innovations come discoveries of new factors that affect individual well-being and improved treatment regimens. In light of these changes, any textbook in the field of health psychology will need to be updated regularly. *Health Psychology: An*

Interdisciplinary Approach is no exception. Several major changes and additions have been made for the fourth edition based on feedback from adopters and reviewers.

1. **E-book features** – Two new features were added to enhance this book visually. First, most chapters contain links to brief video segments that explain concepts or methodologies introduced in the text. Second, hyperlinks are included in each chapter that allow students to access articles from popular but reliable news sources or professional organizations that provide additional, in-depth information about topics or concepts mentioned in the text but cannot be fully explored within the textbook. Welcome to the field of Health Psychology.

2. **Three major changes** were implemented in each chapter:

   a. *Updated statistics* – Data on vital global health statistics and statistics for specific countries, where applicable, have been updated using a number of trusted sources, including the American Psychological Association, the Centers for Disease Control and Prevention, the World Health Organization, the World Bank, and other expert national, global, nonprofit, and professional organizations.

   b. *Updated references* – As noted previously, cutting-edge research in health is occurring daily. We have updated the research findings and references throughout the text, paying particular attention to findings that challenge previously held beliefs.

   c. *Global Health* – This text includes many more references to and examples of global health outcomes, programs, and policies to emphasize the need to examine health outcomes in many different contexts if we are to truly understand this issue.

2. **Changed chapter order** – Chapter 4, Theories and Models of Health Behavior Change, has been renumbered. It is now Chapter 3 and follows immediately after the chapter on Research Methods (Chapter 2). With this change, the first three chapters of this textbook constitute core chapters that provide a foundation for the information and discussions presented in subsequent chapters.

3. **Significant changes were made to specific chapters**. They include:

   - **Chapter 2** – As we noted earlier in this section, SARS-CoV-2 was a major global event. There is much to learn from this pandemic as it informed and continues to inform our response to major crises and our understanding of the impact of these crises on global health and well-being. It even informs our data collection and analysis process! As such, we include it in the chapter on Research Methods when explaining a number of key health statistics, specifically **relative risk**, a concept that came to be well understood even among the lay population. SARS-CoV-2 examples can be found throughout the book where appropriate.

   - **Chapter 4** – Using both SARS-CoV-2 and the more recent human papillomavirus vaccine (HPV) as examples, we introduce the issue of vaccine hesitancy and vaccine refusal here and also in Chapter 11, Cancer. Global statistics show, overall, a decline in vaccine acceptance for some vaccines, a factor that holds implications for the general health and well-being of many populations, but especially for children. As this trend continues to grow, health psychologists will find that they may be called upon to assist with messaging and motivating people to reconsider their reluctance.

- **Chapter 5** – We tried to cover a host of risky health behaviors and their consequences in one chapter. It did not work! Therefore, this topic is now covered in two parts of one chapter. Chapter 5, Risky Health Behaviors, Part I addresses only substance use/abuse and risky sexual behaviors. Included here is a full discussion and updated research and statistics on the use of cigarettes, e-cigarettes, vape products, marijuana, and various opioids including fentanyl. In this part of the chapter, we pay particular attention to those substances for which data show a marked increase in use over past years. Highlighted also is the concerning research on the effects of frequent vaping on adolescent health. The opening story for this chapter, "70-Year-Old Lungs in a Teenage Wrestler: Is Vaping the Cause?" was chosen to reflect current substance use trends among adolescents and to prompt a discussion about this little-understood product. Finally, we include risky sexual behaviors in this chapter for reasons that may be quite obvious. Reports of risky sexual encounters are frequently associated with substance use/abuse.

  Chapter 5, Risky Health Behaviors, Part II is devoted to a discussion of unintentional injuries, including homicides (with a special focus on gun violence), domestic and dating violence, suicide, and eating disorders. While this might seem like an unusual pairing, we contend that each of these topics entails unintentional injury to either the victim, family members, or the immediate community. In addition, the escalating rates of gun violence, primarily in the U.S. and nominally elsewhere, elevates this issue as a topic of concern. While we contend that eating disorders are forms of self-harm that are rooted in a number of causal factors, we take this opportunity to include new research on possible physiological factors that contribute to obesity. Specifically, we examine research on glucagon-like-peptide-1 (GLP-1), a medication that interacts with the body's brain circuitry to reduce cravings and result in significant weight loss.

- **Chapter 8**, Psychoneuroimmunology is not new, but the research in psychoneuroimmunology is proceeding at a fast pace. Therefore, we updated this chapter to include recent findings on the role of *cytokines* including *interleukin-1B (IL-1B), interleukin-2 (IL-2), interleukin-4 (IL-4), interleukin-6 (IL-6)* and *interleukin-10 (IL-10)* on the immune system. Included is an expanded discussion of a timely topic: the possible relationship between cyber networks, psychological factors, and immune response. Specifically, we explore the relationship between loneliness, cyber networks, and immune response.

- **Chapter 12** – This chapter continues to update the changing landscape of the effects of access to health care on health outcomes. Updated research and statistics show that access to care continues to negatively impact health outcomes globally. In the developed countries, the U.S. offers the best example of this negative effect. We retain the extensive review of the **Affordable Care Act**, the most significant piece of legislation on health policy in the United States in over 60 years, in this fourth edition, and update data on the impact of this new program now almost 15 years after its adoption.

SUPPLEMENTS

Please visit the Instructor and Student Resources at www.routledge.com/9781032292557

ACKNOWLEDGMENTS

If it takes a village to raise a child, it also takes one to create a textbook. The fourth edition of this text involved a new production team at Routledge who have been immensely helpful in too many ways to enumerate. A number of people also have given generously of their time, talents, and knowledge and they, too, must be acknowledged. My sincerest thanks to the outstanding editorial staff at Routledge, under the fantastic direction of Lucy Kennedy, which includes Maddie Gray, Simran Kaur, Gaba Lakshay, Yashika Tanwar, and Georgette Enriquez, and the immensely helpful production staff, led by Christopher Mathews.

I owe a great debt of gratitude to two research assistants, Sabina Rodriguez and Dellian Sehra, who invested many hours searching for the right videos for the e-book version and for painstaking editorial reviews. I could not have completed this work without you.

I wish to thank the adopters and reviewers of previous editions of this text for their suggested improvements for this edition. Their comments contributed to an enhanced fourth edition and to significant changes to several chapters.

I also wish to thank the many reviewers of this edition and earlier editions for their valuable comments and suggestions during the preparation of those versions, which continue to be instructive. Included in this list are Todd Doyle, Karla Felix, Caren Ferrante, Brooks B. Gump, Timothy Hedman, Dave Holson, Michelle Loudermilk, Rafaela Machado, Cruz Medina, Meg Milligan, Sabihah Moola, Christina J. Ragin, Luther M. Ragin Jr., Renee Michelle Ragin, Sarah Riddick, Sangeeta Singg, Guido G. Urizar, Eboni Winford, and Gary Winkel. Special thanks go to Lynne D. Richardson, the late Shelly Jacobson, and my colleagues at the Mount Sinai School of Medicine, Department of Emergency Medicine, for their support and assistance in our research on health care, which shaped my current perspectives of health.

Finally, my greatest debt is to my husband, Luther M. Ragin Jr., and our two daughters, Renee Michelle and Christina, without whose support and assistance I could not have written this text.

Deborah Fish Ragin

ABOUT THE AUTHOR

Deborah Fish Ragin is Professor Emerita of Psychology, Montclair State University. She is a graduate of Vassar College, where she earned an A.B. in psychology and Hispanic studies in 1978. She continued her studies of psychology at Harvard University, where she earned her M.A. in 1984 and her Ph.D. in experimental psychology in 1985. Dr. Ragin served on the faculty of Hunter College at the City University of New York, and on the faculty of the Mount Sinai School of Medicine, Department of Emergency Medicine (now the Icahn School of Medicine, New York City).

Dr. Ragin's professional service includes a five-year appointment as an American Psychological Association (APA) representative to the United Nations, where she focused on global efforts to address the psychosocial impact of HIV/AIDS. She completed a three-year term as President of the APA's Society for the Study of Peace, Conflict and Violence (Division 48 Peace Psychology) in 2009; is a member of the Health Research Council of the Health Psychology Division (Division 38) of the American Psychological Association; and held a four-year appointment as a Society for the Study of Psychological Issues (SPSSI) representative to the United Nations.

Dr. Ragin's research focuses on health systems and health policy, particularly as it impacts disparities in health care. She is the author of numerous articles on HIV/AIDS, domestic violence, health care disparities, healthy communities, and research ethics.

An Interdisciplinary View of Health

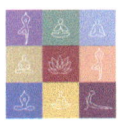

Source: 3xy/ Shutterstock.

Chapter Objectives

After studying this chapter, you will be able to:

1. Identify three ancient cultures that contributed to our current concept of determinants of health.

2. Identify Hippocrates and explain the mind–body connection in health.

3. Identify the role of health policy as a determinant of health in three civilizations.

4. Describe how religion influenced beliefs about health and illness.

5. Identify the four domains of health as defined by the American Psychological Association Division of Health Psychology.

6. Identify and describe four current models of health.

OPENING STORY: HOW WOULD YOU DESCRIBE WINSTON'S HEALTH?

Winston describes himself as an "average high school senior." He is the captain of his school's varsity baseball team, he helps coach his younger sister's Little League softball team, he writes for his school newspaper, and he is applying to college. Yet most people who know him think Winston

DOI: 10.4324/9781003300670-1

is exceptional. He performs all of his academic and extracurricular activities well while managing health flare-ups caused by multiple sclerosis.

*   **Multiple sclerosis** (MS) is a persistent neurological disease that occurs when a person's immune system attacks their brain and spinal cord (World Health Organization, 2023a), causing damage to the tissues of the central nervous system (Hauser & Cree, 2020; See Chapter 6, Emotional Health and Well-Being). The damage disrupts normal neurological functions and can cause a variety of symptoms, including fatigue, vision problems, numbness of arms or legs, and difficulty walking and maintaining balance (World Health Organization, 2023a). Some people with MS also report mental and emotional problems, including mood swings or depression.*

*   Winston was diagnosed with MS at age 16, after numerous episodes of fatigue, blurred vision, and weakness in his arms and fingers. Now, at age 18, Winston says he has learned to manage his disease. He takes medication to control the symptoms but can have occasional flare-ups. Still, Winston does not let his condition stop him from participating in the activities he enjoys. He attends every varsity baseball practice and game. When he feels unable to play, he asks the team's designated hitter to take his place. And, when fatigued, he still cheers loudly from the dugout.*

*   He even manages to maintain his sense of humor about his illness. Once, while warming up before a game, Winston noticed his vision was blurry. His coach insisted he rest for the first several innings. Eventually, Winston convinced the coach he was ready to return to the game. But, as he walked to the plate, he turned and jokingly asked, "Coach, which pitcher should I focus on, the one on the left or the one on the right?"*

*   In spite of the difficulties, when asked about his health, Winston always responds the same: "I'm great. I'm doing well, and my health is excellent."*

*   Would you agree?*   ■

Not everyone would agree with Winston's characterization of his health. For some, having a disease or illness is, by definition, inconsistent with being in "excellent health." Others might label Winston's health status as "fair" because he takes medicine for his illness and, at times, is unable to perform specific activities. Finally, people who consider Winston to be in "good health" may contend that even though he has a **chronic illness**, here meaning an illness that is persistent and lasts over time (see Chapter 4, Global, Communicable, and Chronic Disease), he appears to manage well with the help of medication. In addition, he appears to be coping well emotionally. Winston's positive attitude and his efforts to remain active would suggest, to some people, overall good health.

What explains the diverse opinions about Winston's health? Different theories about what constitutes health, which are shaped in part by historical and cultural factors, is one explanation. We introduce some of these theories in this chapter and return to them throughout the book. But briefly, some people believe that health is determined by a person's **physiological state**, here meaning a person's ability to physically perform his or her daily functions without limitations, restrictions, or impediments. Such beliefs may derive from theories that propose that an individual's health is defined by the presence or absence of disease, dysfunction, or other abnormal biological changes in the body (see Chapter 6, Emotional Health and Well-Being; Wade & Halligan, 2004). Others believe that health is defined not only by a person's physical functional status but also by that person's attitude about the illness and their overall mental and emotional state. For these people, health is a holistic concept. We define *holistic health* as a state of being influenced by physiological, psychological, emotional, and social factors. *Hippocrates*, a Greek physician and philosopher, is often credited as the first to acknowledge the connection between emotions and health (Salovey, Rothman, Detweiler, & Steward, 2000; Schneiderman & Siegel, 2012). Yet, we will see here and in Chapter 6 (Emotional Health and Well-Being) that many other cultures also believed that physical health was integrally linked to emotional and mental health. In fact, a review of the history of health will reveal that health is an evolving concept that has been shaped over time by science, culture, and history (Boddington, 2009; Huber et al., 2011).

VIDEO #1/60

Chapter 1: An Interdisciplinary View of Health
- *Hippocrates: Who was Hippocrates?*
- *Website: https://www.youtube.com/watch?reload=9&v=j1fywohyeew*
- **The WHO YouTube videos are made for educational purposes and are accessible and free to the public.**

Winston's characterization of his own health is consistent with the holistic definition. When describing his health, he considers his physiological condition, including his ability to perform tasks (especially favorite activities such as baseball), his psychological and emotional state, and his level of satisfaction with his life. Using this holistic definition, it may be easy to see why Winston describes his health as excellent.

History shows that for centuries scholars have identified a host of different primary or contributing factors that influence health outcomes. We call these factors *determinants of health*. We will see that some determinants are universal, while others are specific to a culture or time.

Psychologists who adhere to a holistic model identify four health determinants: physiological, psychological, emotional, and social. There are, however, more. We will see in this chapter that proponents of the social ecological model, derived in part from Bronfenbrenner's ecological model of human development (Bronfenbrenner, 1977, 1986), propose that a person's health outcomes are a product of five determinants which, individually and through their interaction, impact health (Eriksson, Ghazinour, & Hammarström, 2018; Stokols, 1996). Specifically, the social ecological model states that an individual's physiology and behaviors (such as diet, exercise, and use of alcohol), family and cultural traditions (diet, social customs, and belief systems), physical environmental conditions (such as clean water and safe neighborhoods), health systems (health care delivery organizations), and health policies (regulations that promote or protect the health of communities; Stokols, 1996) all contribute to health outcomes. It is important to note that like Bronfenbrenner's model, the social ecological model stresses that the interaction between and within these levels contributes significantly to health outcomes.

Some social ecological models even include a sixth determinant: spiritual well-being. Although we explore the social ecological model later in the chapter, for the moment, it is important to note that these are, perhaps, the only models that specifically name health systems and health policy as health determinants, factors that were also introduced by earlier civilizations as important to health outcomes.

Which model best characterizes Winston's views? Recall that in the opening story, we noted that Winston's concept of health was consistent with a holistic health perspective. He assessed his physical, psychological, emotional, and social well-being, all of which he believed were excellent.

In this chapter, we will begin our overview of health and well-being in Section I by exploring health determinants identified in earlier civilizations, such as those in the Indus Valley, ancient China, Egypt, and Greece. As we progress forward in time, we will compare these early beliefs with the healing practices of Native American and southern African cultures in which *botany*, here meaning the study of plants and plant life, were important to their health practices. We conclude this limited historical review by examining the impact of spiritual beliefs on health in Western Europe during the Middle Ages and afterward during the Renaissance.

In Section II, we review three models often used by health psychologists: the biopsychosocial model, the wellness model, and the social ecological model. All three and others are explored in greater depth in Chapter 6, Emotional Health and Well-Being. Here, however, we focus on these three models to complete an abbreviated historical timeline of the definitions and determinants of health.

Finally, in Section III, we review current research that explores the role of biological (physiological), social (including family and community), and environmental factors, as well as health systems and health policies on individual health outcomes. In other words, we review the research that lends credence to the social ecological model. We then explore the contributions of health psychologists in explaining and changing individual health outcomes.

After reading this chapter, you will be able to summarize the changes over time and across cultures in the concepts and determinants of health. You also will be able to compare and contrast the earlier views of health with current and modern concepts and to describe the research that supports or refutes the current perspectives.

SECTION I. A BRIEF HISTORY OF HEALTH

It is tempting to think that our current beliefs about health reflect new knowledge based partly on new research findings. But history shows us that early civilizations, beginning in the third century BCE (Before Common Era), pioneered some of the "modern" concepts of health that we embrace today. From written records, public works (infrastructure), and even art, we can glimpse the health beliefs and practices of these civilizations and link them to the health outcomes of their populations.

Health Practices in Early Civilizations
UNDERSTANDING HEALTH THROUGH HEALTH POLICY There are many health behaviors that we take for granted. For example, most people today accept that clean water and sanitation are essential to prevent illness and to maintain good physiological health. But did you know that early Egyptian and Indian civilizations also considered clean water and sanitation important health determinants? The notions of health in these civilizations may differ, but both cultures established and maintained public water delivery systems that enhanced the health of their populations.

For example, archeological records from the Indus Valley region in the second millennium Before Common Era (2000 BCE) revealed evidence of bathrooms and sophisticated public and private drainage systems, as shown in Figure 1.1. Located in an area known presently as Pakistan, the Indus Valley civilization consisted of more than 100 well-ordered and structured towns and villages that appeared to be administered by a centralized form of government. The ruins from the largest cities in the Indus Valley, Harappa, and Mohenjo-Daro also revealed large water reservoirs constructed on the outskirts of the communities to collect and store clean water for personal consumption (Misra, 2001). Ancient Greek aqueducts that transported water show that this culture also understood the health implications of clean water.

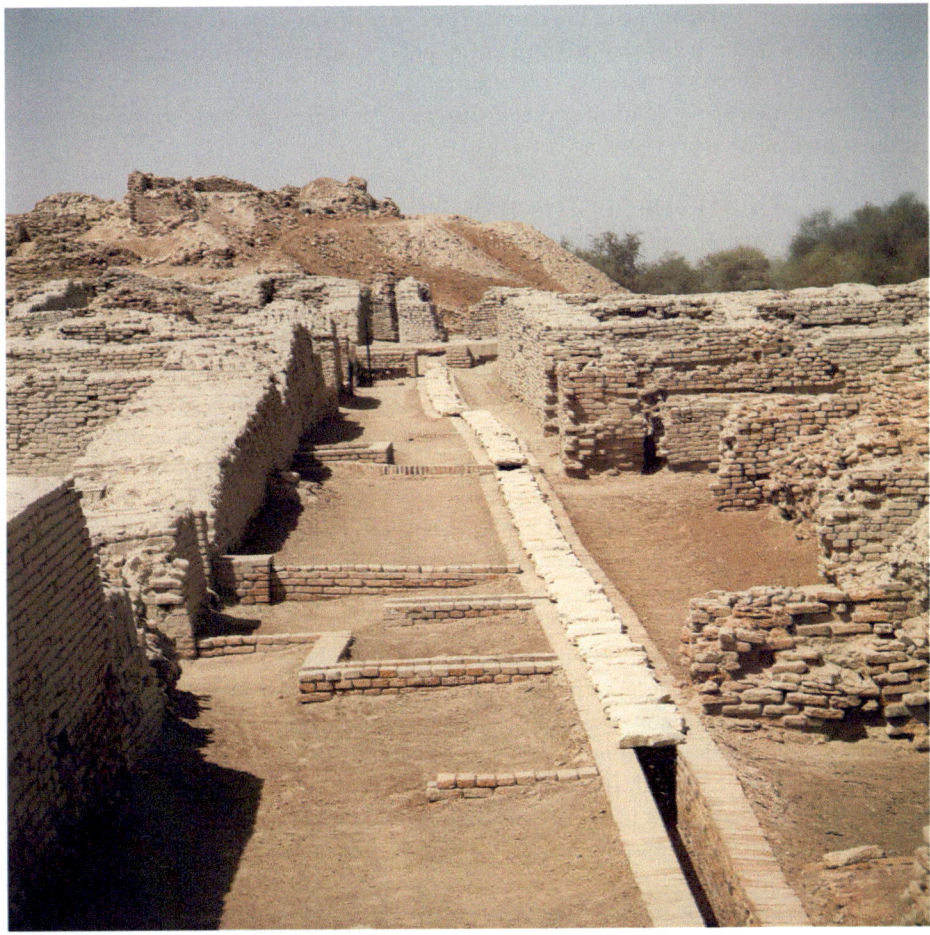

FIGURE 1.1 An archeological site in present day Pakistan reveals brick foundations and walls of private homes, four to six feet in height, and an external drainage system connected to each home.

Source: Robert Harding Picture Library Ltd/Alamy.

What is more, similar aqueducts were also discovered in Jerusalem and Bethlehem in the second and first centuries BCE, as well as throughout the Roman Empire (Franco & Williams, 2000).

Water, drainage, and sewer systems are examples of infrastructure constructed usually as a result of policies issued by a ruler or other governing authorities charged with protecting the water supply for its citizens. For example, health policies that provided access to clean water ensured that civilizations as diverse as the Indus Valley and ancient Greece and Rome would have less exposure to contaminants that could cause illnesses. The policies were a determinant of health in these civilizations.

To put the early policy works into perspective, consider this: The aqueducts and drainage systems of earlier civilizations are similar to the extensive sewer, drainage, and water supply systems we find in many western cities today. Centuries from now, the remnants of our current systems may be interpreted by later civilizations as evidence of our belief that the structures and policies that provide access to clean water to inhabitants are two important determinants of health.

In essence, artifacts such as the ruins of earlier civilizations are one way we learn about health beliefs and practices that predate modern views.

UNDERSTANDING HEALTH THROUGH PHILOSOPHY AND MEDICINE Many people credit Hippocrates, a Greek physician, with proposing an association between the mind and the body that affects health. His views about the mind–body connection are represented in his *humoral theory*, a topic we discuss more fully in Chapter 6, Emotional Health and Well-Being.

But Hippocrates was not the first to link emotional and physiological health. For example, researchers have often noted that the mummification process and rituals used by the Egyptians in the third millennium BCE revealed a sophisticated knowledge of the body and the circulatory system (Greydanus & Merrick, 2020; Nunn, 1996; Shuhata et al., 2023). In Egyptian culture, a person's health was influenced not only by anatomical systems but by scientific and spiritual beliefs as well. And *Daoist philosophy* (developed by ancient Chinese civilizations) determined that the harmonic balance of yin and yang, the environment, and the energy or life force, called *Qi* (pronounced "chi"), were essential determinants of health. As we will see in Chapter 6, Emotional Health and Well-Being, Daoist philosophy greatly influenced Chinese traditional medicine, a form of medicine that is practiced by many today as complementary to or in lieu of Western medicine.

Hippocrates' theory of a mind–body connection that influenced health was challenged by other Greek philosophers. For example, in 500 BCE, some Greek philosophers proposed the *Aesculapian theory*, which held that illnesses had spiritual origins and required spiritual intervention, ritual cures, and mediation by priests. Still others supported the *Cnidian theory*, which stated that illnesses were associated with physical diseases and were unrelated to mental, spiritual, or emotional well-being (Chambers, 2001; Greydanus & Merrick, 2020). Table 1.1 provides a brief timeline of these and other changing concepts of health.

What is interesting is that concepts of health, like the three proposed by Greek philosophers, reappear over time and in other cultures. For example, like the Cnidians, Galen, a noted philosopher and physician in Rome in 200 CE, and Descartes, a philosopher and mathematician in France in 1600 CE, proposed that a disease affected only the body, disassociating the body from influences of the mind or emotion. But, like Hippocrates, Galen also believed that humors could cause illnesses. According to Galen, the diseases that caused imbalance were located in the organs and not, as Hippocrates suggested, in the body fluids. Clearly, Galen's view was more consistent with a physiologically based concept of health and illness.

In comparison, other civilizations, such as the pre-Columbian cultures that include the Mayans and Aztecs (1400 CE), the more than 1,000 Native American cultures in North America (1300 CE), and African cultures such as the Khoisan (southern Africa) and the Yoruba and Dahomey (western Africa, 1500–1600 CE), linked the spiritual health of individuals with their physiological health. These cultures treated health ailments with both natural herbs and plants from their environments (Ajima & Ubana, 2018; Bojuwoye & Moletsane-Kekae, 2018; Bucko & Cloud, 2008).

We explore Native American, southern and western African, and other traditional health practices in Chapter 6, Emotional Health and Well-Being. The important point here is that prior to the 16th century there were a variety of concepts about health. Some, like Galen, believed health to be affected largely by

TABLE 1.1 Concepts of Health

Era	Year	Culture	Concept of Health
Before Common Era (BCE)	2600	Egypt, Old Kingdom	Health influenced by anatomical, scientific, and spiritual beliefs. Sophisticated knowledge of body's circulatory system.
	500	Greece	Three views of health: 1. *Aesculapian theory*: Illness required spiritual intervention and ritual cures. 2. *Cnidian theory*: Illness linked to physical disease. 3. Hippocrates' *humoral theory*: Connection between mind and body shapes health.
	250	Ancient China	Three determinants work together: 1. harmonic balance of forces 2. nature's five elements 3. an energy or life force
Common Era (CE)	200	Rome (Galen)	Health rooted in diseases caused by bad air or body fluids that impair bodily activities.
	500–1400	Middle Ages, Europe	Disease as God's punishment.
	750–1260	Islamic cultures	Holistic approach to health integrating anatomy, spirituality, and culture.
	1400	Pre-Columbian civilizations	Health determined by spiritual forces, but could be remedied by herbal or physical treatments.
	1600	Descartes (France)	Separation of mind and body: diseases affected body.
	1880	Koch (Germany)	Bacteria cause disease.
	1890	Freud	Health influenced by emotions and mind.
	1930s	Flanders and Dunbar	Psychosomatic medicine linking biological, behavioral, psychological, and social contributors to health.
	1948	World Health Organization (WHO)	A state of complete physical, mental, and social well-being and not merely the absence of diseases or infirmity.

physiological states. Others, like the ancient Egyptian, Indian, Chinese, Native American, and African cultures, examined the roles of emotional, spiritual, or environmental determinants as contributors to individual health status. We will see shortly that some Western concepts of health include many of the same determinants.

UNDERSTANDING HEALTH THROUGH PHARMACOLOGY Early and later civilizations also demonstrated knowledge of health through botany, the study of plants and plant life. For example, artifacts from the Zulu and the Khoisan of southern Africa (van Wyk, 2008) and the Chinese and Indian cultures in Asia, as well as the Native American and pre-Columbian cultures we referred to previously, demonstrate extensive knowledge of the ***materia medica***, the medicinal properties of plants (Redvers & Blondin, 2020; Yuan, Ma, Ye, & Piao, 2016). Plants provided the tools to address the physical, mental, emotional, and spiritual health of members of these cultures. Consider this: Moerman (1998), studying the medical practices of Native American cultures, found that many tribes used over 4,000 plants to treat in excess of

25,000 different medical – here meaning physiological – illnesses. Yet, the same plants also addressed over 15,000 spiritual and emotional health ailments as well. Similar discoveries of the use of *materia medica* were found in Mesoamerican cultures, including the Mayan and Aztec cultures (Cruz-Coke, 2007; Geck et al., 2020).

How do we know that plants were used as health aids? You may remember that at the beginning of the section, we stated that some cultures maintained written records of their health beliefs and practices while others recorded their practices in art or other artifacts. Specifically, some accounts of the use of medicinal herbs have been maintained in written records in China and India (Jaiswal, Liang, & Zhao, 2016). But the use of medicinal herbs in other cultures, which traditionally were passed on orally from one generation to the next (Mahwasane, Middleton, & Boaduo, 2013), is documented in artwork, such as sculptures, paintings, and other artifacts (see Box 1.1 and Figure 1.2). For example, historians have identified and decoded many depictions of medical practices and health remedies in sub-Saharan African art found in Ghana, Nigeria, the Democratic Republic of Congo, and Burkina Faso, to name a few (De Smet, 1998). In some cases, the art depicts health procedures such as craniotomies (a cut into the skull, usually to gain access to the brain). In others, the works depict a process such as extracting bark from a tree. In some cultures, tree bark is used to prevent the growth of bacteria or to ease pain.

Box 1.1 Artifacts: A Roadmap to Health Practices When Written Records Are Not Available

What happens to the knowledge possessed by earlier cultures when there are no written records? Fortunately, historians interested in the health practices and behaviors of earlier civilizations have found a way to extract information about the health beliefs in such cultures through art.

Take, for example, African art objects. Carvings and other works of art produced by some African cultures are interesting because of the level of detail depicted in the work, the artist's skill in reproducing images or people, and the material used to create the piece. Over the past 40 years, **ethnopharmacologists**, researchers who study the medicinal practices of different cultures, have discovered an added benefit of the works. The artwork also contains a wealth of information about health practices and medicines used at the time. The discovery helps health researchers expand their understanding of the concepts of health in different cultures.

One example of the health practices evident in art is seen in the pendant displayed in Figure 1.2. At first, the pendant appears to be an ornamental piece of jewelry. But ethnopharmacologists discovered the pendant serves two purposes. True, they are decorative and ornamental pieces, but in certain African societies, they are also functional: They are ear cleaners! Without knowledge of a culture or its past medical practices, it is easy to mistake the pendant for ornamental jewelry with little functional value.

Current research also suggests that some African art depicts procedures such as extraction of teeth, cesarean sections, or craniotomies. Others depict activities such as removal of tree bark or cassava root, two ingredients used in some medicines.

Through research, we are learning that the artistic record is yet another way that earlier civilizations recorded health practices and reflected their concept of health.

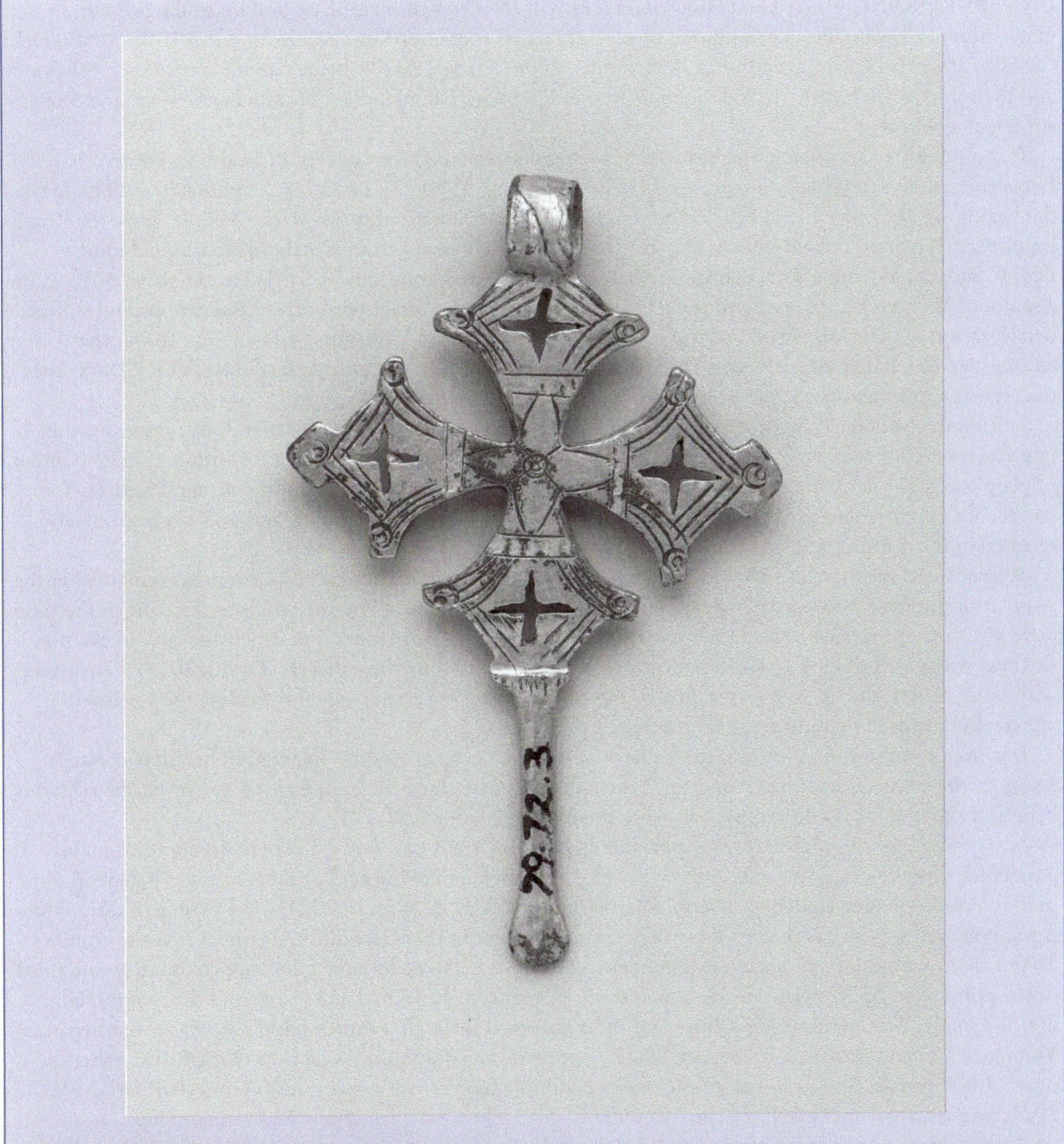

FIGURE 1.2 This cross-shaped pendant serves two purposes: decorative jewelry and practical medicinal use. Each end of the cross is shaped as a diamond. The southern end of the cross narrows to serve as an ear cleaner.

Source: Pendant Cross, Amhara (silver), Ethiopian/Brooklyn Museum of Art, New York, USA/Gift of George V. Corinaldi Jr./The Bridgeman Art Library.

UNDERSTANDING HEALTH THROUGH RELIGION   Over the centuries, and up to the present, in many cultures, spirituality has been one of several factors that contribute to health (Cruz-Coke, 2007; Del Castillo, 2021; Falagas, Zarkadoulia, & Samonis, 2006; Fardin, 2020). Beliefs about spirituality, religion, and their impact on health are well documented in Egyptian, Islamic, pre-Columbian, African, and North American cultures.

It should not be surprising, therefore, that religion also shaped the concept of health in Western European cultures, especially during the Middle Ages (500–1500 CE). Briefly, approximately 500 CE marked the beginning of the decline of the Roman Empire. We must note that, prior to the Middle Ages, the Roman Empire actively participated in extensive trade with other civilizations in Northern Africa (including Egypt), India, and China. Through trade, these cultures shared goods and knowledge. At about 500 CE, the peoples of Western Europe reduced their trade, exchange, and contact with other civilizations and suffered deterioration in their infrastructure and a weakened economy. The self-imposed isolation from other cultures led to what some historians characterize as a cultural decline (once referred to as the "Dark Ages") that lasted approximately 1,000 years.

During the Middle Ages, Rome also experienced a significant loss of population. One reason for the population decline was a successive wave of *pandemics*, communicable diseases that affected large numbers of people across a geographic region (see Chapter 4, Global, Communicable, and Chronic Disease). Two pandemics in particular, the first and second *plagues of Justinian* (541–542 CE and 588 CE, respectively), resulted in the death of millions of inhabitants.

What caused the plagues? We now attribute them to a recurrent bacterial infection that remained in the population for over 200 years (Little, 2007; Walloe, 2008). Influenced by the religious doctrine of the time, however, many people embraced the view that demons caused the plagues and other diseases. In essence, sickness was a sign of God's punishment for the sins committed by the sufferers (Orent, 2013). Consistent with these beliefs, the Church – specifically, the priests – became responsible for healing the spiritual afflictions that were thought to be the source of the disease.

It is important to point out that the belief that illnesses were caused by spiritual ill health is common. Many of the cultures described earlier in this chapter held similar beliefs. In Europe, however, the religious beliefs of the time stressed that diseases were punishments from God.

Near the end of the Middle Ages (approximately 1346–1353 CE), Europe experienced a third major pandemic, often referred to as the "Black Death." Researchers now note that this term was a general term used to refer to plague epidemics overall (Barbieri, Drancourt, & Raoult, 2021). The plague of the Middle Ages, however, was by far the deadliest. It accounted for more than 25 million deaths across the continent. To put that number into perspective, the plague of 1346 is believed to have killed approximately one-third of the population of Western Europe in just seven years, from 1346 to 1353 (Gowland & Chamberlain, 2005). Finally, Asia, particularly China and India, suffered through a fourth pandemic wave that began in Yunnan, a Chinese province, in the late 1800s. It spread both south and west into Hong Kong, affecting over 24,000 people, and to India, killing over 12 million people over a span of 20 years (Barbieri et al., 2021; Science Museum Group, 2019).

Any illness responsible for more than 12 million deaths is an important event when examining historical health records. Yet the plague of 1346 is also significant because of the change in health beliefs that occurred at approximately the same time. The plague struck just as Western Europe was about to experience a *Renaissance*, a cultural rebirth. The Renaissance prompted a move away from the belief that illnesses were a punishment for evil. In Europe, it marked a return to the scientific exploration of the human body.

Consistent with this revised theory, scholars and physicians during the Renaissance suggested that some diseases were the result of environmental, not spiritual, factors. Thus, to help control the plague, local municipalities in Western Europe instituted a number of policies to stem the outbreak. For example, local administrators isolated and quarantined many people diagnosed with the disease. In addition, buildings and houses were fumigated, and entire towns were burned in an effort to kill the germs and the animals, especially rodents, assumed to carry the disease (Christensen, 2003; Duncan & Scott, 2005).

Isolations, quarantines, fumigation of communities, and sophisticated water disposal and water collection systems show, once again, the role of health policies – regulations designed to protect the health of the community and thereby of individuals, in improving outcomes. Sometimes the policies protect individuals from initial contact with the diseases. Other times, the policies that helped contain diseases minimize their impact on the population. Using health policy and environmental controls to reduce health risks is evidence that by the early 1500s CE, Western Europe embraced the belief that better controls on environmental conditions and the enforcement of health policy would have a positive impact on health outcomes.

Health Practices in the United States

The Renaissance also introduced a period of maritime exploration. Voyagers set out from Europe to colonize "new worlds." In the process, however, they brought with them contagious diseases that had deadly consequences for both the carriers and those who came in contact with them.

As in the case of the pandemics in Europe and Asia, some contagious diseases could decimate the entire population of a region. For the colonizers of new territories like the Americas, outbreaks of yellow fever, smallpox, and other contagious ailments were particularly problematic because they could threaten the viability of new colonies. For this reason, by the early 1800s, shortly after the founding of the new United States of America, major cities such as Philadelphia, New York, Boston, and Washington adopted public health policies to protect their citizens and the new nation (Harvard University Library Open Collections Program, 2008). Once again, health policies became important determinants of health outcomes for individuals as well as entire communities.

Summary

What can we learn about health from a brief review of ancient concepts and the history of health practices? We realize that many cultures established systems, built infrastructures, and made use of their natural resources, such as herbs and plants, to protect and preserve the health of their citizens. By examining diverse cultures, we also see the range of beliefs about health. While some cultures treated health holistically or ecologically, others chose to focus almost exclusively on only one or two factors. We see that discoveries in the medical sciences, specifically anatomy and biology, built on existing knowledge and furthered our understanding of epidemiology, the study of the origins and spread of disease. Such discoveries contributed to the development of the health models that are used by psychologists today.

Finally, we learned that throughout history, health policies have played a critical role in changing the environmental conditions that affect individual health status. By reviewing history, we see that the five determinants of health as identified in the social ecological model – individual physiology and behaviors, social environments (family, communities, and cultures), physical environments, health systems, and health policies – have defined health throughout the centuries.

SECTION II. DEFINING HEALTH TODAY

Early Holistic Concepts

MIND–BODY CONNECTION AND HEALTH Current concepts of health have much in common with the holistic perspectives suggested by earlier cultures. Not surprisingly, psychologists have contributed to the evolution in the definition of health. One well-known contributor is Sigmund Freud, the "father of psychoanalytic psychology."

Some may think it odd to see a reference to Freud in a book on health psychology. But when Freud proposed that physiological illnesses can have psychological causes, he reintroduced the relationship between the mind and body and its effects on health outcomes to Western cultures. This time, however, research on the mind–body association and health resulted in the development of a new field: *psychosomatic medicine*. Like the concepts of health espoused centuries before, psychosomatic medicine examines the relationships among the physiological, psychological, social, and behavioral influences on an individual's health status. In other words, the determinants of health that define psychosomatic medicine include all but two of the factors thought to be influential centuries ago: environment and spiritual forces.

Freud's research on psychosomatic causes of illnesses was largely nonreplicable because he based his theories on his clinical work and intuitions. Fortunately, empirical studies by other pioneers in the field, including Cannon and Washburn as well as Dunbar (Dunbar, 1943; Kimball, 1981), which suggested an association between personality types and disease, supported the link between the mind–body connection and health (Kimball, 1981).

In spite of some empirical support, psychosomatic diseases increasingly were viewed as invalid or false. They became associated with chronic complaints that were more psychological than physiological. The increasing emphasis on physiological causes of illness in the 20th century, together with the prevailing popular view that psychosomatic illnesses were contrived, led to a decline in support for the mind–body connection and health.

WORLD HEALTH ORGANIZATION MODEL OF HEALTH In 1948, the World Health Organization (WHO) introduced another definition of health, one that integrates the physical, emotional, psychological, and social determinants. According to WHO, health is "a state of complete, physical, mental and social well-being and not merely the absence of disease and infirmity" (WHO Basic Documents, 2006, p. 1). In other words, health is more than just a disease. It includes a person's functional ability, psychological well-being, physiological status, and social health. Does this sound familiar? Although not identical to the concepts of health espoused by the earlier civilizations, WHO's definition includes emotional and mental health as factors in overall well-being. Some of these determinants were noted in the opening story as well.

Building on WHO's definition are three additional models that also explore the physiological, psychological, sociological, and, for some, environmental determinants of health. They include the *biopsychosocial model*, the *wellness model*, and the *social ecological model* (sometimes referred to simply as the *ecological model*) of health. We briefly review each model to provide the foundation for the theoretical framework of the field of health psychology.

We begin, however, with the *biomedical model*, a model that is central to the practice of medicine in Western cultures and, according to some, a core component of some holistic health models as well.

Models of Health and Well-Being

BIOMEDICAL MODEL The late 19th century (1880s) marked a return to the theory that germs, rather than sins or spiritual forces, caused diseases. Research by Robert Koch, a German scientist who was the first person credited with discovering that specific bacteria can be linked to specific diseases, supported this renewed belief. Koch's work led to the development of the biomedical model of health, which purported that illness is defined as a dysfunction of the body caused by microorganisms that results in illness or disability (Engel, 1977). The clear association between bacteria and disease once again placed a greater emphasis on physiological factors as the principal determinant of health. While few would challenge the theory that microorganisms can cause diseases, the more relevant question is whether microorganisms can also explain non-physiological causes of illnesses. Most health researchers now agree that the biomedical model's emphasis on physical causes of illnesses overlooks the critical contributions of emotional, social, and environmental factors on health. As we will see in later chapters, newer health theories account for some if not all of these factors.

BIOPSYCHOSOCIAL MODEL An odd-sounding name to be sure, the biopsychosocial model was one of the first 20th-century models to reintroduce a holistic theory of health in which multiple factors, not just physiology, explained health outcomes.

Engel (1977) proposed the biopsychosocial model in 1972 to explain outcomes not adequately accounted for by biological factors alone. Engel suggests that biological factors (*bio*) in addition to psychological influences (*psycho*), including emotions and personality traits (Folkman & Greer, 2002; Ryan & Deci, 2000), as well as sociological (*social*) factors, such as family, culture, community, and social support, also strongly affect overall well-being and health outcomes.

Can emotions really affect our physical health? Research on the relationship between stress and illness offers some of the clearest evidence of the association between emotional (stress) factors and adverse physiological outcomes (e.g., see Chapter 7, Stress and Coping, and specifically Dhabhar, 2014; Khan & Obhi, 2021). For example, earlier research by Dhabhar (2014) suggests that emotions such as stress have an impact on physiological health by affecting the immune system and by influencing health behaviors. Recent studies also report an association between other emotions, such as depression, and illnesses, such as heart disease. Interestingly, some researchers even draw connections among depression, heart disease, and death (Schulz, Martire, Beach, & Scheier, 2005). We explore and update the research on the relationship between stress and physical health in greater depth in Chapter 7, Stress and Coping. Additionally, we examine in greater detail the association between physiological health, psychological states, and immune system response in Chapter 8, Psychoneuroimmunology. For now, just remember that current research supports the link between the mind (emotions) and body that was suggested by earlier civilizations and by individuals such as Hippocrates and Freud. Yet we know, even from our limited review thus far, that health is a complex state influenced by more than just the mind and the body.

CHALLENGES TO THE BIOPSYCHOSOCIAL MODEL In spite of its broader focus, some health psychologists criticize the biopsychosocial model for being too "biocentered." According to these critics, the model places biological determinants at the core of the concept of health. Specifically, Armstrong (2002) notes that in this model, psychological and sociological factors are "add-ons" to explain outcomes that cannot be explained using physiological factors alone. Thus, rather than offering a balanced perspective that gives equal weight to biological, psychological, and sociological determinants of health, the biopsychosocial model is criticized for being a biological model at its core.

A second critique suggests that the model overlooks environmental factors known to influence well-being. Part of the problem here may be the definition of *environmental*. For some, social environmental variables such as family, community, and culture represent environmental determinants of health. For others, however, they do not. For example, some researchers who study the effects of environments on health focus on air and water quality, toxic waste sites, or other pollutants as the principal physical environmental determinants of health status. Indeed, many would agree that poor air quality can cause breathing and other respiratory problems that may result in adverse health outcomes (see Chapter 3, Theories and Models of Health Behavior Change). The point here is that for many researchers, environmental determinants of health refer to the physical, not the social environment, and the biopsychosocial model does not address physical environmental determinants.

Finally, the biopsychosocial model does not account for the effects of perceived quality of life or spirituality on health status. (In truth, very few models include these factors.) As we will see in the following section on the wellness model, some research suggests that quality of life and spirituality are important psychological and emotional factors that also affect health outcomes.

WELLNESS MODEL Not to be confused with ***well-being***, which is defined as one's overall state of health, the wellness model adds two health determinants not commonly found in other models: ***spirituality*** and ***quality of life***. Recall the concepts of health in earlier civilizations that included spirituality as a core determinant. In some respects, the wellness model is suggestive of those earlier beliefs with one caveat. In the wellness model, spirituality refers to an individual's perspective on the meaning of life and the impact of their values on their overall well-being (de Jager Meezenbroek et al., 2012). It is not intended to have religious connotations identified with specific religious groups.

An example of spirituality's contribution to health and well-being in the wellness model is evident in research that suggests that spirituality may enable one to experience peace and tranquility even during stressful events. In other words, it helps to abate stress. Consider this: Research suggests that reducing stress is important for maintaining good physiological health. If spirituality serves to reduce stress and create peaceful environments for some, then we may reason that spirituality abates stress for those individuals, thereby directly contributing to their overall well-being (Bosswell, Kahana, & Dilworth-Anderson, 2006; Lima et al., 2020; Reid & Smalls, 2004; Shattuck & Muehlenbein, 2020).

One additional point should be made regarding spirituality and stress. Some spiritual beliefs encourage individuals to adopt behaviors that lead to healthier outcomes. For example, an individual may refrain from drinking alcohol or smoking cigarettes because of spiritual beliefs. Avoiding alcohol and cigarettes are, themselves, ***health-enhancing behaviors***, that is, behaviors that will increase one's positive health status (Poage, Kitzenberger, & Olsen, 2004; Reid & Smalls, 2004). Thus, in this way, spirituality can lead to *health-enhancing behaviors*, restricting behaviors that negatively affect health. We explore the role of health-enhancing behaviors more fully in Chapter 5, Risky Health Behaviors.

Other contemporary examples of spiritual beliefs that are integral to health are found in the traditional medical practices of many Native American tribes, in ***curanderismo*** – a religious and cultural belief system that informs health and wellness among many Central and South American cultures, and also among the Suku, a group in the Democratic Republic of the Congo in Africa. When addressing a physiological health concern, it would not be uncommon in these cultures for the healer to attend to the emotional and spiritual health of his or her "patient." All three cultures as well as others consider spirituality to be a core component of health (Chaves et al., 2015; Fardin, 2020; VanderWeele et al., 2017). We review this concept more fully in Chapter 6, Emotional Health and Well-Being.

Finally, the wellness model is the only model that includes the psychological concept of quality of life as a determinant of health. In the wellness approach, an individual's perceived satisfaction with life will affect his or her overall well-being. Satisfaction is influenced by psychological as well as physiological states. Remember Winston from our opening story? Most likely, Winston believes he has a very good quality of life. Although he has MS, Winston's positive psychological state undoubtedly helps him cope with his physical limitations.

Not everyone enjoys a good quality of life, however. Consider a different scenario. A young man has been a star athlete in basketball since his junior varsity days in middle school. As a college student, he was widely recognized as an outstanding player who was destined for a career as a professional basketball player. A sudden accident permanently damaged his spinal column, paralyzing him from the hips down. The accident ended his dreams of playing professional basketball, confining him to a wheelchair. For weeks after the accident, he was depressed and despondent. While he has learned to be largely self-reliant with respect to his daily functions, he never speaks of basketball and forbids others to raise the subject with him. How would you rate this former athlete's quality of life?

The biopsychosocial model and the wellness model identify specific psychological, sociological, and for the wellness model, spiritual factors that, researchers suggest, influence health outcomes. Yet according to some researchers, there are still other critical determinants of health.

SOCIAL ECOLOGICAL MODEL We traced the evolution of the definition of health through a total of four models. In the process, we found that, with the exception of the biomedical model, most definitions of health included both physiological and non-physiological determinants, including biology, emotions, psychological states, social factors, quality of life, and spirituality. Can there be anything else? There is, according to the social ecological or ecological model.

As depicted in Figure 1.3, the ecological model includes five major determinants of health. The individual (biology and behavior) and the social environment created by family, community, and cultural practices are the first two. Uniquely, the ecological model includes three new dimensions. First is the *physical environment*, which includes factors such as housing conditions, neighborhood sanitation, cleanliness, safety, and a physical space free of toxicity or pollutants. Second is *health systems*, defined here as the health care delivery organizations that provide access to care. Last is *health policy*, which, as we saw earlier in the chapter, is made up of the regulations that promote or protect the health of individuals in the community.

The social ecological model suggests that an individual's physical setting can contribute to or inhibit good health outcomes. For example, waste products from manufacturing plants and automobile exhaust can affect a community's air and water quality, essential elements for life. The role of the physical environment on health may be easy to grasp when considering environmental pollutants. However, the model also addresses the physiological and psychological consequences of negative environmental factors such as crime and violence. Consider this: Is there a relationship between a neighborhood's high rates of crime and obesity? Researchers seem to think so. Several studies have shown that children and adults living in neighborhoods perceived to be unsafe due to crime and violence are at greater risk for obesity than those in "safer" environments (Singleton, Winata, Parab, Adeyeme, & Aguiñaga, 2023; Stolzenberg, D'Alessio, & Flexon, 2019; Tung et al., 2018). The cause? Safety concerns make parents or other caregivers less likely to allow children outdoors, limiting opportunities for physical activity. What is more, by remaining inside, children also increase their likelihood of consuming high-calorie, high-fat foods, further compounding problems of weight gain and obesity. A fuller discussion of the effects of physical environments on health

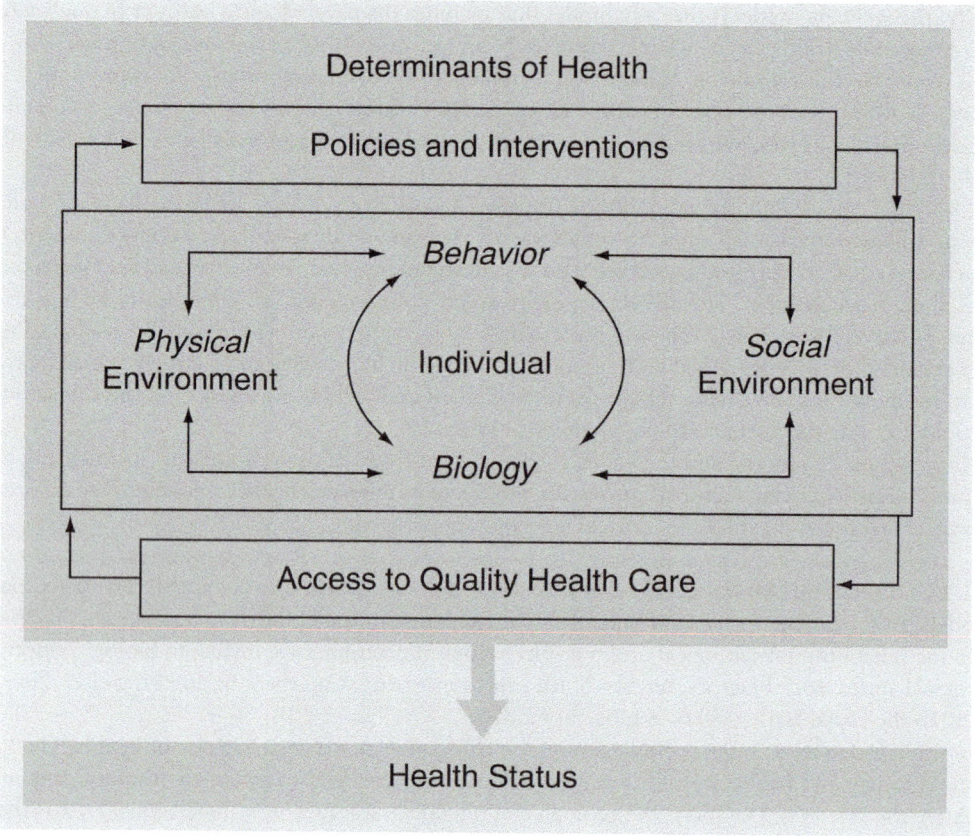

FIGURE 1.3 The model identifies, in words, the five factors: individual, physical environment, social environment, access to quality health care, and health policies. The individual is at the center of this model, with reciprocal interactions with the physical environment (left), the social environment (right), access to quality health care (bottom), and health policies and interventions (top).

is presented in Chapter 3, Theories and Models of Health Behavior Change, and Chapter 5, Risky Health Behaviors, Part II.

Finally, the ecological model is perhaps the only model that proposes that health systems and health policy also influence health. Let's examine this by way of another example. An individual's ability to obtain timely medical attention and to receive needed medical care may determine whether that person's health concern will be resolved quickly with minimal long-term impact or become a protracted problem requiring longer-term treatment. Yet, as we will see in Chapter 12, Health Care Systems and Health Policy, health systems and policies may contribute to a delay in access to care or limit one's ability to obtain the full spectrum of care to resolve the problem. The social ecological model proposes that any system that controls access to care or that prescribes the type of care available will, by definition, determine an individual's health outcomes.

Defined in this way, it is apparent why health systems and health policy should be included in a discussion of the determinants of health, yet they are absent in most other models.

APPLYING THE SOCIAL ECOLOGICAL MODEL TO HEALTH PSYCHOLOGY With four models and at least five different determinants, how do we decide which model(s) best characterizes health?

Remember, in psychology, there are often multiple theories that explain a phenomenon. The same is true for the discipline of health psychology. Yet new directions in the field may help determine which models are most applicable to our current concepts of health. In 2002, the American Psychological Association's Division of Health Psychology redefined the field, acknowledging the central role of health systems and policy on health status. Now, when characterizing health psychology, the division describes the field using four principal domains: the individual, the family/community, health systems, and health policy. The new definition is consistent with Joseph Matarazzo's reconceptualization of the field in 1980, in which he describes health psychology as:

> the aggregate of the specific educational, scientific, and professional contributions of the discipline of psychology to the promotion and maintenance of health, the prevention and treatment of illnesses, and the identification of etiologic and diagnostic correlates of health, illness, and related dysfunction, and to the analysis and improvements of the health care system and health policy formation.
>
> (Matarazzo, 1980, pp. 807–817)

Put simply, Matarazzo acknowledges the traditional role of health psychologists as professionals who focus on health promotion, disease prevention, and health maintenance at the individual and the family/community levels. But he sees two additional functions. First, he identifies an investigative role for health psychology, exploring the causes (*etiology*) and the related consequences of illnesses. Second, Matarazzo sees health psychologists as analysts, capable of identifying problems and recommending solutions that help improve the health care system and health policy.

What is more, Matarazzo and the APA's revised description lends support to the social ecological model of health because both include individuals, society, health systems, and health policy as determinants of health. Furthermore, Matarazzo's definition may also include environmental determinants because the environment is often an etiology of health outcomes.

Again, we caution that the study of any field of psychology rarely contains only one explanatory theory. Thus, the social ecological model remains one of several currently in use.

SECTION III. CURRENT VIEWS ON DETERMINANTS OF HEALTH: A HEALTH PSYCHOLOGY PERSPECTIVE

The models used by health psychologists highlight the role of some determinants on health outcomes. But as we indicated, "individual determinants" or "environmental determinants" can mean many things. In this section, we identify the specific components of health determinants from a health psychology perspective. We will explore their contributions to health status and suggest ways in which psychologists can modify determinants in order to improve outcomes.

Individual/Demographic Influences

We return to Winston and the opening story to illustrate the role of individual/demographic influences on health. We noted in the story that Winston plays baseball for his high school. We did not mention that he joined the team in his sophomore year in high school. In the first week of practice, Winston collided with another teammate while running to home plate. He fell and hit his head on the field. Winston complained of dizziness and fatigue several hours after the incident. When Winston complained again several weeks later about dizziness and fatigue, his coaches thought the symptoms were related to his accident.

Health psychologists interested in understanding what factors contribute to an individual's health outcome may review Winston's story and ask whether his health condition is due to his accident, or whether it is due to genetic makeup, that is, familial (inherited) factors or even environmental factors. Like his coaches, health psychologists may be tempted to conclude initially that his recurrent symptoms were due to his behavior – a collision with a teammate. Although unintentional injuries such as a collision or head injury can cause short- or long-term health consequences (see Chapter 5, Risky Health Behaviors, Part II), we know from the opening story that Winston's problems were not due to the injury. Rather, the determinants of Winston's health problem appear to be genetic.

We noted in the opening story that MS results from damage to the body's nerve fibers. We review the function of the body's nerve fibers in Chapter 6, Emotional Health and Well-Being. For the moment, it is sufficient to know that nerve fibers transmit neurochemical messages throughout the body. The fibers are encased in a *myelin sheath*, a coating that protects the fibers from damage and helps speed message transmission. Damage to the myelin sheath increases the risk of damage to the fibers, which could slow or impede message transmission. The interruption of message signals to or from the spinal column or to the brain could result in an impairment of motor movements or other body functions and result in the symptoms Winston reported. One cause of erosion to the myelin sheath is genetic. Researchers have established that multiple sclerosis is a complex trait whose onset is due, in part, to the interaction of several genes (Handel, Handrennetthi, Giovannoni, Ebers, & Ramagopalan, 2010; Jacobs et al., 2021).

In addition to genetic factors, demographic characteristics also help determine when a person is most likely to be affected by the disease. You may have seen the term *demographic variables* in a statistics or research methods class. Demographics may be fixed characteristics, such as gender or race/ethnicity. But demographics can also be characteristics that are subject to change, such as age, socioeconomic class, level of education, and occupation. Consider again MS, the most common neurological disease affecting young adults (Ramagopalan, Knight, & Ebers, 2009). The usual onset for MS is between 20 and 40 years of age. In addition, women are somewhat more likely to be affected by the disease than men (World Health Organization, 2023a). Can an individual's demographic characteristics really influence his or her health outcomes? In the following chapters we explore this question more fully when examining chronic illnesses such as cardiovascular disease, arthritis, and cancer. We will see that, in fact, diseases such as cancer or cardiovascular disease can affect people differently based on some characteristics, including genetic makeup, gender, and sometimes race or ethnicity.

What does this mean for Winston? First, study findings suggest that Winston's health problem may be rooted in a genetic abnormality. In other words, Winston's genetic composition may make him susceptible to MS. We also note that the fact that MS is associated with young adults increases the likelihood that, with a prior susceptibility to the disease, Winston, at 16, could show signs of the illness. Admittedly, he is on the younger end of the estimated age of onset. Yet, estimated age at onset of an illness is just that: an estimate. The illness can occur at slightly earlier or slightly later ages. Table 1.2 includes a sample of factors that can determine health outcomes.

Family/Cultural Influences

We inherit many observable traits from family members: eye color, hair color, facial features, and even handedness. Is it likely, therefore, that we might also inherit a susceptibility to specific illnesses? Scientists seem to think so. As we noted earlier, current research on MS points conclusively to a familial link to the illness. Research by Eskandarieh, Sahraiain, Molazadeh, and Moghadasi (2019) established that individuals with *first-degree relatives*, here meaning parents, or siblings, or *second-degree relatives*, which includes grandparents, aunts, uncles, with MS were more likely to develop MS than were individuals without such a family history.

TABLE 1.2 Factors That Influence Health in an Ecological Model

Determinant of Health	Factors
Biological	Genetics Immune system Nutrition Physiology Gender Age
Psychological	Coping strategies Personality Pessimism/optimism Risk-taking behaviors Response to stress
Sociological	Cultural beliefs Diet Ethnicity Socioeconomic class Social support networks Concept of health Spiritual beliefs
Environmental	Air/water quality Neighborhood safety Neighborhood cleanliness
Health systems	Accessible health facilities Health insurance Medical specialists Emergency care options Affordable care Treatment options Long-term care options Mental health care providers
Health policy	Mandated health plan Water/sewage disposal systems Safety legislations Workplace safety regulations Air and water quality

Genes also have been found to play a role in the transmission of many other diseases. For example, asthma and some forms of coronary artery disease, sometimes referred to as heart disease, tend to run in families. Genetics, therefore, can also be a *familial determinant of health*.

Other familial determinants of illnesses may be rooted in our behaviors. Just as there are genetic factors that occur in families, there are also health behaviors or practices that are common to family members. Consider this: In past generations, it was not uncommon to find several smokers within one family. In fact, smoking could be thought of as an activity in itself or something done in conjunction with other activities such as bowling, card games, or even fishing. Researchers studying MS now suggest that smoking behaviors may be another factor that increases susceptibility to the disease (World Health Organization, 2023a). In this instance, a health behavior practiced by many family members may increase the risk of a disease that also has a genetic determinant. As we will see in later chapters, there are a number of health behaviors that increase the risk of illnesses. For example, eating high-fat, high-calorie foods increases the risk of cardiovascular disease (see Chapter 9, Cardiovascular Disease), obesity, and Type 2 diabetes (see Chapter 4, Global, Communicable, and Chronic Disease). Some of these behaviors are attributed to individual lifestyles, whereas others, such as dietary practices, may also be associated with family practices, much like smoking.

Thus, to effectively change behaviors that contribute to health problems, psychologists may need to be mindful of and address familial and cultural health beliefs and practices that shape behaviors. In other words, people in the profession may need to borrow some techniques from medical anthropologists and explore the behaviors and culture of their target populations before attempting to change behaviors. As Hippocrates noted:

> Whoever wishes to investigate medicine properly, should proceed thus . . . the mode in which the inhabitants live, and what are their pursuits, whether they are fond of drinking and eating to excess, and given to indolence, and are fond of exercise and labor, and not given to excess in eating and drinking.
>
> (Hippocrates, ca. 400 BCE)

Are familial risk factors another possible determinant of Winston's condition? It is impossible to determine just from the information presented in the opening story. Additionally, while research suggests that a family history of MS may increase susceptibility to the illness, we have no information to suggest that any of Winston's *first-degree relatives* have the disease.

Physical Environmental Influences on Health

We noted earlier that the term *environmental determinants* can have more than one meaning. It can refer to physical entities such as air, water, land, or neighborhood. Yet it can also imply social conditions, as in a "hostile environment," a "threatening environment," or a "friendly environment."

The physical environmental conditions that could impair or enhance health outcomes are readily identifiable in many communities. For example, it is easy to detect the strong odors produced from water treatment plants or the smell of exhaust from a bus depot that houses a fleet of public buses. Physical environmental determinants of health are important contributors to an individual's well-being because they may introduce contaminants that compromise health. Yet, they may pose greater problems for health psychologists attempting to improve the outcomes of an individual or a community. When the cause of a health condition is rooted in environmental determinants of a physical nature, psychologists may resort to health policy interventions rather than just individual behavior changes to improve outcomes.

Think about this: We now know that secondhand smoke presents a hazard to all people, including nonsmokers. Many people attempt to reduce their exposure to such smoke. An impractical strategy for avoiding secondhand smoke is to teach individuals to leave an environment in which people are smoking. This is impractical for two reasons. First, it may be impossible for an individual to leave the site. For example, if smoking is permitted in the workplace, it may not be feasible for an employee to leave the worksite to avoid inhaling secondhand smoke. Second, such a strategy encourages smokers to continue their behavior with the expectation that people who do not like the unhealthy habit will accommodate the smoker at their own expense.

Instead, health policy regulations put in place by local and national policy regulators (thanks in no small part to studies on secondhand smoke conducted by many health researchers) ban smoking in many public places. We explore the issue of health policy and smoking more thoroughly in Chapter 13, The Health Psychologist's Role: Research, Application, and Advocacy. For now, it is important to note that in such instances, health psychologists' work on environmental determinants has focused on policy initiatives that benefit large populations rather than selected individuals or targeted groups.

Returning to our example of Winston and MS, here, too, researchers have found a possible environmental link to MS. Several studies confirm that insufficient exposure to ultraviolet (UV) light may increase risks of susceptibility to MS (Gallagher et al., 2019; Handel et al., 2010; van der Mei et al., 2003). Specifically, studies that examine population occurrences of MS suggest that this disease is more prevalent in people who live farthest from the equator. In other words, in geographic regions in which exposure to UV light is reduced, researchers found higher incidences of MS. When interpreted together, the results of these MS studies suggest that genetic factors (individual or familial determinants), smoking behaviors (individual/behavioral determinant), and physical environmental conditions (UV light) account for 75% of the prevalence of MS cases in European study samples (Handel et al., 2010).

What do these studies suggest about a possible environmental determinant of MS for Winston? We cannot tell. Not knowing where Winston lives, and without additional studies to corroborate such findings, we can only note that environmental factors such as UV light may contribute to susceptibility to MS.

Social Environmental Influences on Health

Social conditions in the environment that affect health are more challenging to identify and address because they depend, in part, on an individual's perceptions of an environment. We have no research to suggest that social environmental factors may contribute to the development of MS; therefore, we will examine the impact of social environmental determinants on other health issues.

Take this example: When walking in an unfamiliar neighborhood in which the residents are of a different ethnic group, one individual may perceive the residents of the community as hostile, whereas another may not. Some researchers have explored the perception of racism or of a racist environment on health outcomes. Several studies suggest that environments that are perceived to be racist can foster high stress levels in some individuals that result in adverse health conditions, such as high blood pressure and other heart conditions (Albert et al., 2008; Barksdale, Farrug, & Harkness, 2009; Cooper, Mills, Bardwell, Ziegler, & Dimsdale, 2009). Additionally, new research suggests that the effects of perceived racism may persist across generations. A study by Snyder, Ribeiro Santiago, Sawyer, and Jamieson (2023) explored the effects of perceived racism by Aboriginal Australian mothers on their children. They surveyed pregnant Aboriginal women's experiences with indigenous racism and followed up with another survey after five years. Their results showed that children five years of age or younger had a higher risk of social and/or emotional difficulties if their mothers experienced perceived racism at least once during their pregnancy.

However, individual differences in perception may mean that some may not interpret the same environment as stressful. As such, it will not evoke a negative psychological response. In spite of these individual differences, if an environmental stressor causes an adverse physiological response for a significant minority of persons, psychologists may turn to health policy to address the multiple causes of the problem. We explore social environmental determinants more fully in Chapter 5, Risky Health Behaviors, and Chapter 9, Cardiovascular Disease.

Health Systems/Health Policies Influences

Lately, health psychologists have come to recognize the role of health systems in enhancing or inhibiting good outcomes. We explained earlier that, by definition, any system that regulates an individual's access to medical care also regulates that person's outcomes. As such, it is a determinant of health.

We explore more fully the effects of health systems on an individual's status in Chapter 12, Health Care Systems and Health Policy. Here, we just emphasize two points. Access to timely, quality health care appears to be a significant contributor to good outcomes, but it appears that both individual and systems factors affect access to health care. Thus, our first point is that factors such as employment status, income, and sometimes age or gender may influence an individual's likelihood of seeking health care or of securing the means of access to care. In the United States, prior to the Affordable Care Act, employment status was a significant impediment to access to health care for many. In comparison, in some European countries, age may limit access to more aggressive treatment for illnesses such as heart disease (Veenis et al., 2019). In such instances, a health psychologist may work specifically with individuals to improve access to care and to change beliefs about the need for care.

Second, research comparing health policies suggests that universal health care, a system that provides free or greatly subsidized care, ensures better overall access to care and results in improved long-term outcomes (Bermejo et al., 2021; National Health & Hospitals Reform Commission, 2009; Siddiqi, Zuberi, & Nguyen, 2009; Young, Alharthy, & Hosler, 2021). We explore the concept of universal health care in Chapter 12, Health Care Systems and Health Policy. For the moment, it is important to note that, while there are many different types of universal systems of care in the world, all share one common element: The systems ensure that all persons seeking medical or mental health services will receive care without regard to their employment status, income, or economic status. The important part is that this care is funded by one provider – usually the government. The benefits of universal access to care became a major political and policy issue once again in the United States beginning in 2009, just as they were in 1994, 1968, and even earlier. We explore current changes to the health care system in the United States in Chapter 12, Health Care Systems and Health Policy.

Again, we return to Winston and ask: How could access to health care, health care systems, or health policy affect Winston's status? It is simple. Without access to health care, Winston's condition could have been untreated or misdiagnosed. Either outcome could have resulted in health limitations that could have affected Winston's ability to play baseball or to pursue his studies. In other words, untreated or misdiagnosed illnesses can limit an individual's ability to perform his or her usual daily or preferred activities. Winston was able to obtain the needed health care to identify the problem and to adopt behaviors that allow him to manage his disease while enjoying his favorite activities, maintaining what he would probably consider a good quality of life. Without such care, baseball could have been just a dream.

Summary

This is an exciting time to study the field of health psychology. Evolutions in the concept of health, new developments in science and medicine that explain pathways to disease and illness, changes in health policy that will change access to care and health outcomes, and the work of health psychologists on the many determinants we have discussed suggest that there is still much to learn about the factors that affect and shape our health. This growing field offers individuals interested in health psychology opportunities to work in many different and interdisciplinary settings on a wide array of issues.

Health psychologists can be found in research settings in hospitals, medical laboratories, academia, pharmaceutical companies, and a host of other research-related environments. If one is interested in applying research to help individuals change behaviors and improve health status, health psychologists can fit easily into community-based health centers, medical centers with outpatient health programs, and even private physician's offices in which allied health services are offered. Health psychologists interested in specific populations are often found in school settings, senior citizen centers, and nursing homes, in which attention to health and health behaviors is an ongoing concern.

Finally, if one is interested in the health issues of a community or larger populations, psychologists can and do contribute to health policy work through local and national departments of health, as well as international organizations, responsible for creating, monitoring, and maintaining policy, as well as address global health problems.

Personal Postscript

After reading the chapter, how would you describe your health? Maybe the following scale can help. While rating yourself, see how many determinants of health you can identify in the scale.

ASSESSING YOUR HEALTH

1. In general, would you say your health is:
    Excellent
    Very good
    Good
    Fair
    Poor
2. For how long (if at all) has your health limited you in each of the following activities?

Activity	Limited >3 Months	Limited <3 Months	Not Limited at All
The kinds or amounts of vigorous activities you can do, like lifting heavy objects, running, or participating in strenuous sports			
The kinds or amounts of moderate activities you can do, like moving a table, carrying groceries, or bowling			
Walking uphill or climbing a few flights of stairs			
Bending, lifting, or stooping			
Walking one block			
Eating, dressing, bathing, or using the toilet			

3. What level of bodily pain have you had during the past four weeks?
    None
    Very mild
    Mild
    Moderate
    Severe
    Very severe
4. Does your health keep you from working at a job, doing work around the house, or going to school?
    Yes, for more than three months.
    Yes, for three months or less.
    No

5. Have you been unable to do certain kinds or amounts of work, housework, or schoolwork because of your health?
    Yes, for more than three months.
    Yes, for three months or less.
    No

6. For each of the following questions, please check the box for the one answer that comes closest to the way you have been feeling during the past month.

Activities	All of the Time	Most of the Time	A Good Bit of the Time	Some of the Time	A Little of the Time	None of the Time
How much of the time, during the past month, has your health limited your social activities (like visiting with friends or close relatives)?						
How much of the time, during the past month, have you been a very nervous person?						
During the past month, how much of the time have you felt calm and peaceful?						
How much of the time, during the past month, have you felt downhearted and blue?						
During the past month, how much of the time have you been a happy person?						
How often, during the past month, have you felt so down in the dumps that nothing could cheer you up?						

7. Please check the box that best describes whether each of the following statements is true or false for you.

Description	Definitely True	Mostly True	Not Sure	Mostly False	Definitely False
I am somewhat ill.					
I am as healthy as anybody I know.					
My health is excellent.					
I have been feeling bad lately.					

Source: Adapted from Ware and Sherbourne (1992).

Questions to Consider

1. Are there other ancient or modern beliefs that influenced the health behaviors of their communities in their time?

2. Pioneering research in medicine suggests that we may be able to identify future health issues by mapping a person's DNA. If true, could such a discovery negate the role of the biopsychosocial or social ecological model in explaining health outcomes?
3. The interest in traditional and alternative medicines has increased in the United States in the past 40 years. How might these changing trends affect theories and practices in health psychology?

True or False Questions

1. The humoral theory is widely regarded as accurate today. True or False.
2. Public health programs in the U.S. date back to the early 1800s. True or False.
3. The World Health Organization's model of health is most closely aligned with the biopsychosocial model. True or False.
4. The wellness model of health accounts for health systems and policy. True or False.
5. Environmental determinants of health include an individual's perceptions about their environment. True or False.

Important Terms

Aesculapian theory   6
biomedical model   12
biopsychosocial model   12
botany   4
chronic illness   2
Cnidian theory   6
curanderismo   14
Daoist philosophy   6
determinants of health   3
ecological model   12
ethnopharmacologists   8
etiology   17
familial determinant of health   19
first-degree relatives   18
health-enhancing behaviors   14
health policy   15
health systems   15
Hippocrates   3
holistic health   3

Research Methods

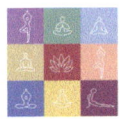

Source: 3xy/
Shutterstock.

Chapter Objectives

After studying this chapter, you will be able to:

1. Identify and describe the five classic indicators of health.
2. Explain proximal and distal causes.
3. Identify and describe nonexperimental research designs.
4. Explain the relevance of nonexperimental designs for health research.
5. Identify and describe experimental designs.
6. Explain the relevance of experimental designs for health research.
7. Describe intervention studies.
8. Explain the relevance of intervention studies for health research.
9. Identify historical events leading to the establishment of the Nuremberg Code of Conduct, the Declaration of Helsinki, and the U.S. National Research Act.
10. Describe IRBs, their role, and their function.
11. Identify and explain two principal violations of research ethics in the Tuskegee study.

DOI: 10.4324/9781003300670-2

12. Identify and explain the psychological harm to participants in the Stanford prison experiment.

13. Explain the concept of "research without informed consent."

OPENING STORY: DEATH BY RESEARCH STUDY?

Dr. Bret Rutherford was an outstanding researcher. An associate professor at Columbia University, Dr. Rutherford was awarded 32 grants from the National Institute of Mental Health and is the author of a number of articles in his field. But it all came to an abrupt halt on June 1, 2023. Tragically, a study participant in one of Dr. Rutherford's studies committed suicide.

What happened? Dr. Rutherford was conducting a study to examine the potential benefits of **levodopa,** *a psychiatric drug which he believed would help reduce late-life depression and increase mobility in older persons who suffered from* **Parkinson's** *disease. Parkinson's is a brain disorder that results in a host of symptoms, including unintentional or uncontrollable tremors in the hands, arms, legs or head, stiffness, and difficulty with balance and coordination. Over time, it may include difficulty talking, sleeping, and even depression (National Institute on Aging, 2022).*

So why did the person commit suicide? The details are unavailable, but an investigation into the study revealed methodological errors in the study protocol that may provide clues. Because this study involved the use of a psychiatric drug, study participants are required to "wash out" or suspend taking their regular antidepressant medication 28 days before participating in the new drug trial. This allows the researchers to test the effectiveness of the new drug while minimizing possible drug interactions (Hoffman, Schiller, Greenblatt, & Iosifescu, 2011). Research records show that Dr. Rutherford's study did not follow this procedure. Of the 31 study participants, only eight "washed out" and only for, on average, 10 days before beginning the new study drug. Reportedly, one participant stopped taking their regular medication only one day before joining the study.

Emily Roberts, a research assistant to Dr. Rutherford, told reporters that recruiting subjects for this study had been difficult. They were only able to recruit one-third of the targeted number of participants, so they relaxed some of the criteria to get participants. But she became so disillusioned with the lack of rigor with the study protocol that she left this field of work altogether (Barry, 2023).

Ms. Robert's unease with the study methodology was shared by experts in the field. In fact, two scientific journals, the Journal of Affective Disorders *and* Biological Psychiatry, *retracted several papers published by Dr. Rutherford and his colleagues that reported this study's preliminary findings. The journal editors cited newly detected evidence of errors, omissions, irregularities, and deviations from approved protocol (Borrell, 2023).*

What happened next? The **Office of Human Research Protections** *(OHRP), the federal agency in the U.S. responsible for protecting the rights, welfare, and well-being of human subjects participating in research funded by the agency, suspended Dr. Rutherford's study in January 2022, and terminated it in May of 2023. And even though the New York State Psychiatric Institute itself voluntarily suspended all studies involving human subjects, the OHRP reinforced this decision by requiring a suspension of* **all** *studies involving human subjects at the Institute until the OHRP fully investigated the safety protocols for human subjects at the Institute (Barry, 2023).* ■

Few people think that participating in a research study can be hazardous to their health. Unfortunately, in rare cases it is. In an earlier edition of this textbook, we relayed the story of Ellen Roche, an employee at Johns Hopkins University, and a healthy volunteer who agreed to participate in a study to test the effectiveness of a new asthma medication. Something went wrong in that study, and Ellen, the 24-year-old volunteer, died. After her death, the *Office for Human Research Protection (OHRP)* suspended all federally funded medical research involving human subjects at Johns Hopkins University pending an investigation, exactly what they did at the New York State Psychiatric Institute (Savulescu & Spriggs, 2002). These two studies illustrate the OHRP's response to the death, injury, or illness of study participants, as a result of their involvement in an approved research study. Such outcomes are called *adverse events*, requiring investigation.

Research that aims to identify new and better medications for people with asthma, Parkinson's, or other illnesses is important. But, when researchers commit methodological errors, they can put at risk the lives of their participants while also jeopardizing future studies on these and other health issues.

All research involving human subjects must balance the potential benefits of the study with the potential harm to participants. For this reason, studies that involve human subjects must be reviewed, approved, and monitored by local and/or national research review boards. The job of the review boards is to protect the health and welfare of human subjects and to ensure that investigators comply with the code of conduct for research with human subjects.

We do need to point out one fact. The overwhelming majority of studies conducted, including those in health psychology, are safe. The research review boards help to ensure participants' safety. Yet accidents do happen. Later in this chapter, we highlight four historical studies or events that are often cited to demonstrate the adverse consequences that can occur when the health and welfare of study participants are overlooked, intentionally or unintentionally. The Johns Hopkins and the New York State Psychiatric Institute studies are just recent and notable examples.

In Section I of this chapter, we begin with a review of research terms. The review will introduce, or reintroduce for some, research methodology and concepts needed for our discussion of research ethics later in the chapter. It will also serve as a guide to the methodologies used in other studies presented throughout the text. We then continue in Section II with a discussion of some of the research methods used often by health psychologists. By the end of Sections I and II, you will be able to identify and define the five classic measures used to describe the health of a population, explain distal and proximal causes of illnesses, and describe nonexperimental, experimental, and quasi-experimental study designs and their relevance for health psychology research.

Finally, in Section III, we examine rules regarding the ethical conduct of research involving human subjects. Using the research terms and methods that we learned in Sections I and II, we examine two classic and often referenced studies in detail, the Tuskegee Syphilis Study and Philip Zimbardo's Stanford prison experiment, and discuss the research methods and ethics violations in each case.

SECTION I. MEASURING HEALTH

Borrowing from Epidemiology

Health psychology borrows some concepts from the field of epidemiology. *Epidemiologists* study factors or determinants of health status among population groups. They examine the distribution, frequency, and patterns of health events in a population, and then use that knowledge to help control the spread of health problems in the population (Centers for Disease Control [CDC], 2012). The word *epidemiology* derives from three Greek words: *epi*, meaning "among"; *demos*, meaning "people"; and *logos*, referring to a scholarly discipline or study.

Epidemiologists are like detectives. In fact, they can be thought of as "medical detectives." When studying the causes of a health problem, epidemiologists attempt to determine the origins of a disease by identifying and examining the first or earliest known human infected as well as the agent that caused the infection. A crucial second component of their work is determining the risk posed by the disease to current and future populations. Thus, one application of epidemiological research is to inform us about the origins of a disease, its impact on prior generations, and its potential risk to people at present and in the near future.

MORTALITY VERSUS MORBIDITY Two measures that describe the health of a population are mortality and morbidity. *Mortality* refers to death. For example, mortality data on the number of deaths due to heart disease could be used to describe the cardiovascular health of people over 65 years of age in a specific geographic area. On the other hand, *morbidity* refers to diseases that may contribute to death. Take diabetes, for example. Diabetes is a disease that will not cause death but can cause a number of health problems that lead to death. The number of people with diabetes, therefore, could be a morbidity statistic that also describes the health of a population.

Epidemiologists and other health researchers use two types of data when reporting mortality and morbidity statistics: *raw data* and *rates*. When measuring mortality, the raw data are the total number of deaths for a defined population. For example, Figure 2.1a-c shows infant mortality data for low-middle, upper-middle, and high-income countries, as defined by the World Bank for 2020–2021 (World Bank, 2022). A discussion of the World Bank classification system is beyond the scope of this book. But briefly, low-income countries are defined as countries with an annual average or *gross national income (GNI) per capita* – a Latin term meaning per person or individual – of less than $1,046. For low-middle income countries, that amount is a range from $1,046 to $4,095. Upper-middle income countries have

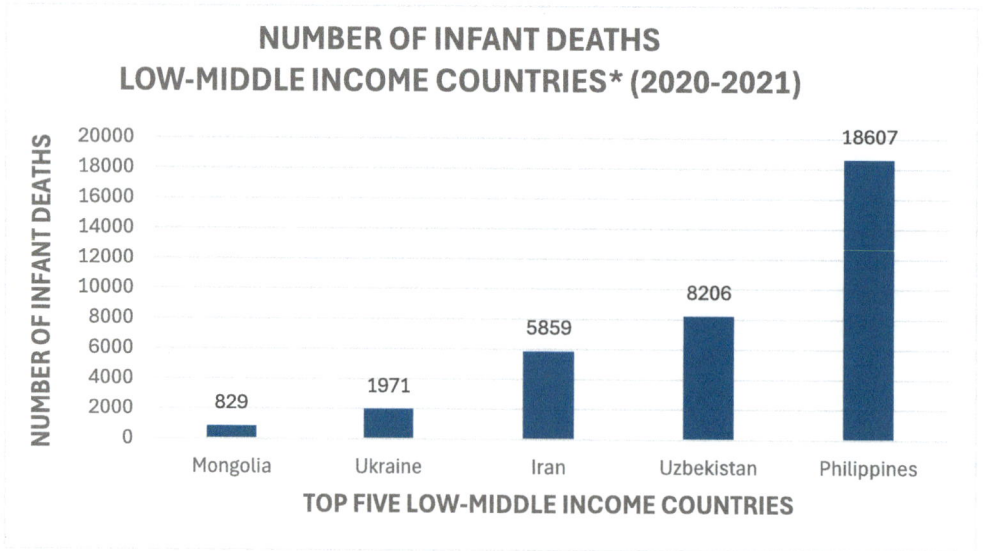

FIGURE 2.1a A bar chart shows the top five low-middle-income countries with the highest number of infant deaths. Philippines ranks first with 18,607 deaths, Uzbekistan second, 8206 deaths, Iran third, 5859 deaths, Ukraine fourth, 1971 deaths, Mongolia fifth, 829 deaths.

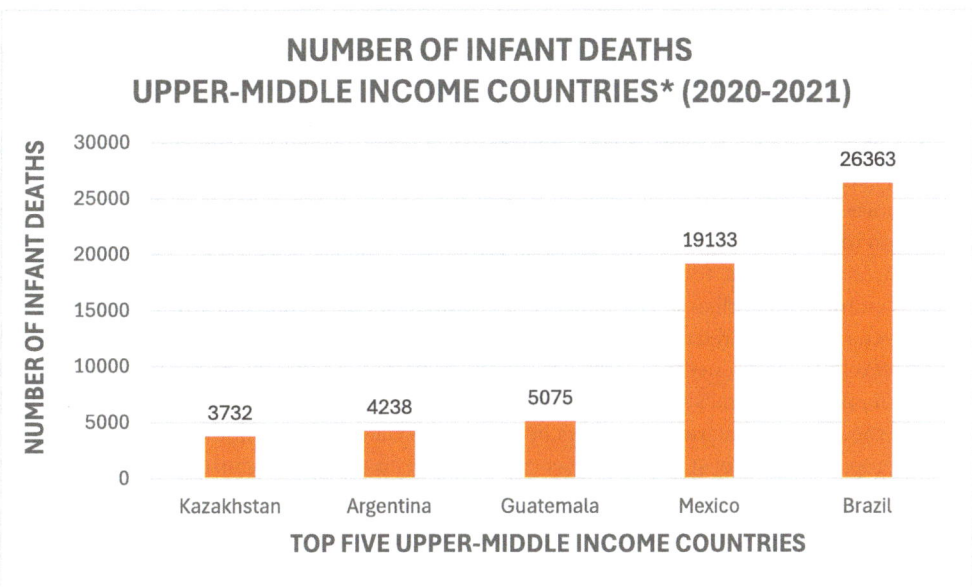

FIGURE 2.1b A bar chart shows the top five upper-middle-income countries with the highest number of infant deaths. Brazil ranks first, followed by Mexico second, 19,133 deaths, Guatelmala third, Argentina fourth, and Kazakhstan fifth.

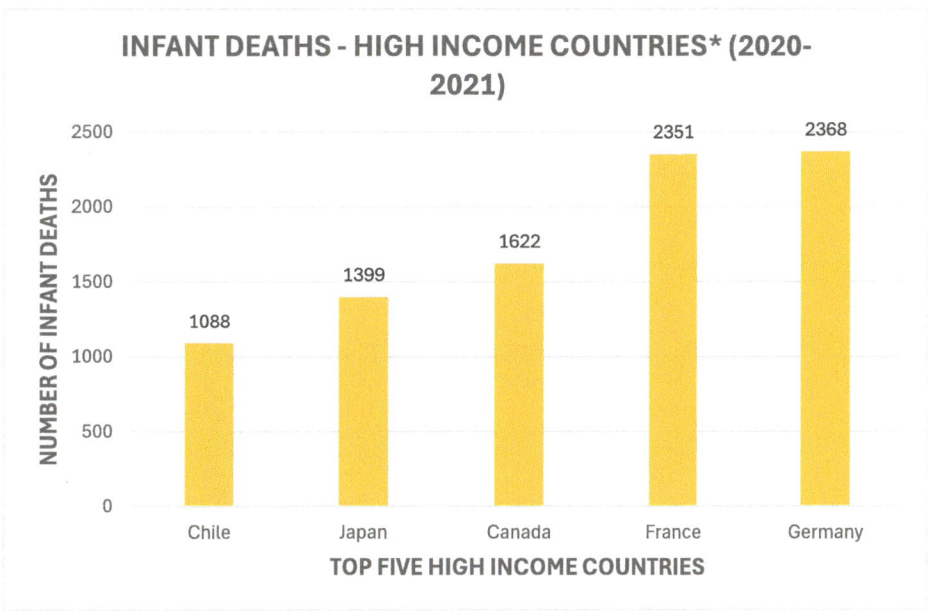

FIGURE 2.1c A bar chart shows the top five high-income countries with the highest number of infant deaths. Germany is ranked first with 2368 deaths, followed closely by France, 2351 deaths, third is Canada, 1622 deaths, fourth is Japan 1399 deaths, fifth is Chile, 1088 deaths.

an average annual *GNI* of \$4,096–\$12,695, and the annual *GNIs* in high-income countries is \$12,695 or higher (Hamadeh, van Rompaey, Metreau, & Eapen, 2022). The raw data in Figure 2.1a-c shows the five countries with the highest number of infant deaths in the low-middle, upper-middle, and high-income categories for 2020 or 2021, the most recent years for which full statistics are available.

Using raw data to compare the infant mortality statistics of, for example, low-middle, upper-middle and high-income countries is a little like comparing apples and oranges. In addition to the effects of income on health outcomes, comparing the raw data of different countries does not adjust for the size of the infant population in each country. Consider this: Using just the raw data presented in Figure 2.1b for upper-middle-income countries, for example, we would conclude that Brazil reported five times more infant deaths (26,363 infant deaths) than Guatemala (5,075 deaths), six times more deaths than Argentina (4,238 deaths), and seven times more deaths than Kazakhstan (3,732 deaths; see Figure 2.1b). Does this mean that Brazilian infants are five times more likely to die than infants in Guatemala, six times more likely to die than Argentinian babies, and seven times more likely to die than infants in Kazakhstan? Not really. It just means that the larger population of infants in Brazil also yields a larger number of infant deaths. To meaningfully compare mortality statistics across two or more countries, we must adjust for the difference in the size of the populations. For this type of comparison, we use rates.

We can compute *mortality rates* using the following formula: (total number of infant deaths in a given period of time for a specific population/total population of infants for the same time period × 1,000). This formula allows us to convert the raw data on infant mortality in Figure 2.1a-c to *infant mortality rates* for these countries by income groups (see Figure 2.2a-c). The rates express infant deaths for every 1,000 infants born in the country.

Using death rates for the same groups of countries, we now see that although Brazil had the highest number of infant deaths among upper-middle-income countries, it ranks third highest in the rates of

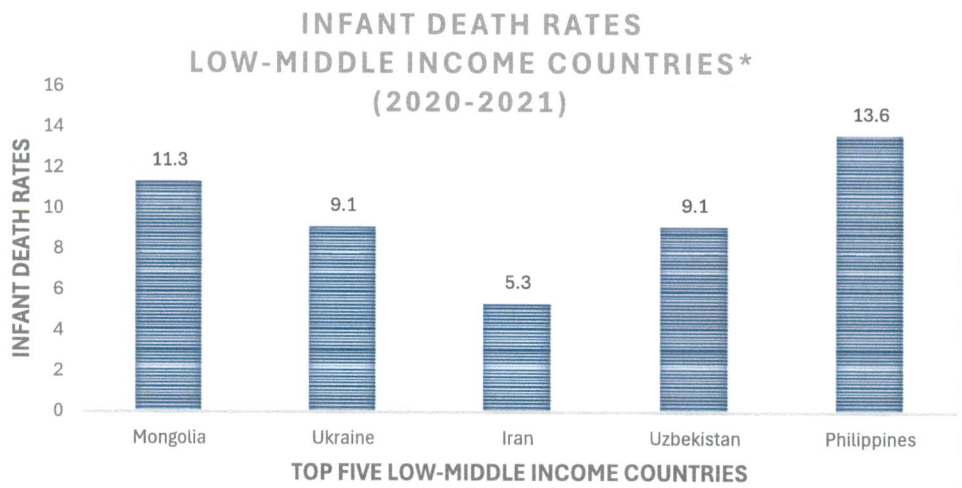

FIGURE 2.2a A bar chart shows the top five low-middle-income countries with the highest infant death rates. The Philippines still ranks first in infant deaths when using rates (13.6). Mongolia ranks second, 11.3, Ukraine and Uzbekistan tie for third, 9.1, and Iran is fifth, 5.3.

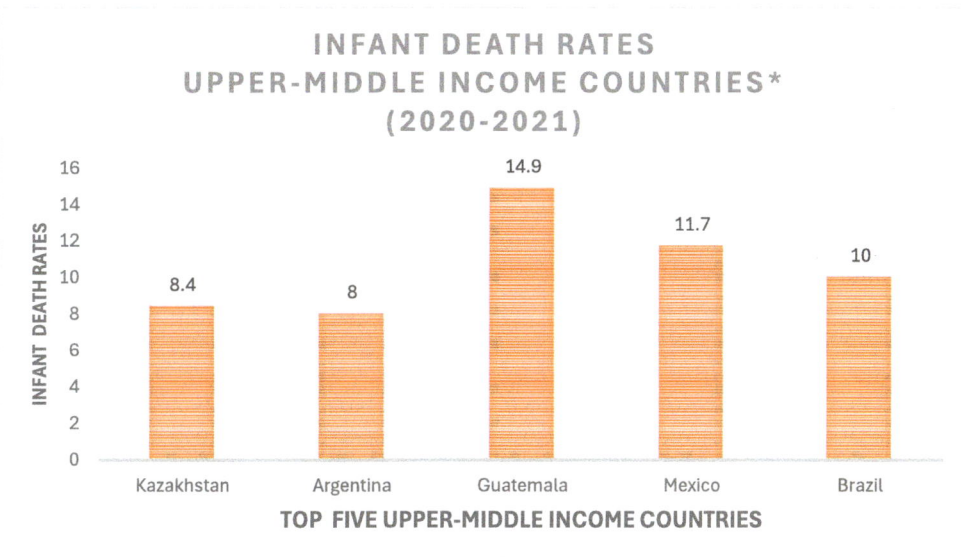

FIGURE 2.2b A bar chart shows the top five upper-middle-income countries with the highest infant death rates. Here, Guatemala is highest, 14.9, followed by Mexico,11.7, Brazil, 10.0, Kazakhstan, 8.4, and Argentina, 8.

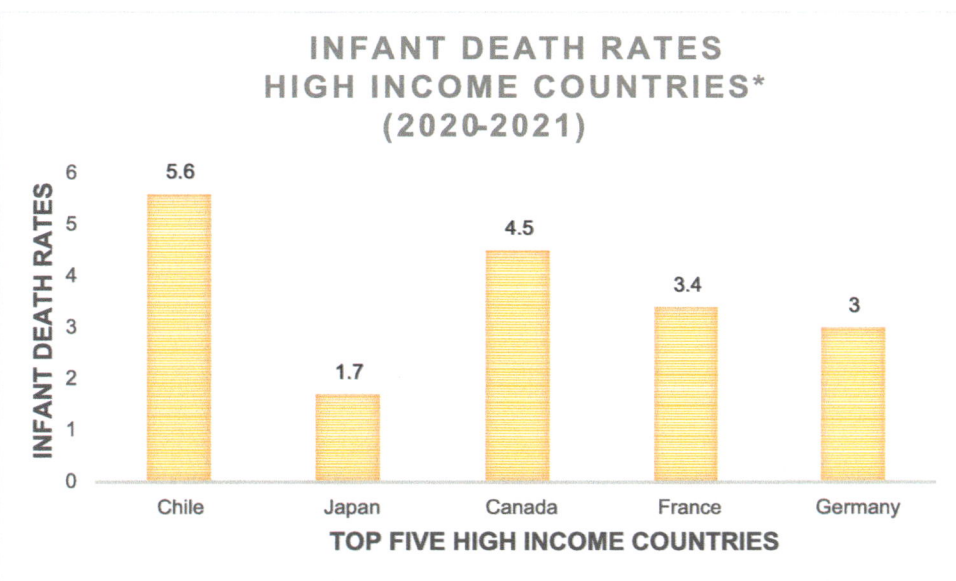

FIGURE 2.2c A bar chars shows the top five high-income countries with the highest infant death rates. Here Chile, not Germany or France, is ranked highest, 5.6, followed by Canada, 4.5, France, 3.4, Germany, 3.0, and last, Japan, 1.7.

Source: United Nations (2023). Population and Vital Statistics Report. Technical Note, Table 3: Live Births, Deaths, and Infant Death Rates, Latest Year Available Year (2007–2021). https://unstats.un.org/unsd/demographic-social/products/vitstats/seratab3.pdf

infant deaths (10 per 100,000) among this group, after Mexico (11.7 per 100,000), which is now ranked second highest, and Guatemala (14.9 per 100,000) with the highest rate of infant deaths. And, what about Argentina and Kazakhstan? That order has changed also. In this group of upper-middle-income countries, Argentina has the lowest rate of infant deaths at 8 per 100,000, lower than Kazakhstan at 8.4 per 100,000. In essence, converting these data to infant death rates completely reversed the ranking of these countries with respect to infant mortality rates. In Table 2.1, you will find the basic formulas for calculating mortality, morbidity, incidence, prevalence, and relative risk, using a sample of other health or health-related concerns.

To summarize, the raw infant mortality statistics present the total number of infant deaths. But, if we want to understand the magnitude of a health problem – here meaning infant deaths – or to compare infant deaths between countries, we must use mortality rates rather than the raw data.

In some instances, the infant mortality statistics also provide information on the health of other members in the community. Think about this fact: In 2020, the four leading causes of death for infants in the U.S. were congenital anomalies (birth defects), short gestations (disorders related to premature births), maternal complications during pregnancy, and sudden infant death syndrome (SIDS; Centers for Disease Control, 2020a). But researchers note that two of the principal causes of birth defects result from a lack of prenatal care for the mother or the mother's use of substances (cigarettes, alcohol, or illegal drugs) while pregnant. Because two of the main causes of infant deaths can be linked to maternal health factors, infant death rates may be indicators of maternal health as well as the overall health of the infant (Ebrahim & Atrash, 2006).

TABLE 2.1 Calculating Rates

Rate	Definition	Sample Calculation
Mortality	Number of deaths (cause specific or general) in a total population for a specific period	$\dfrac{\text{Automobile fatalities in 2020}}{\text{U. S. Population in 2020}} \times 100,000^{a}$
Morbidity	Specific illnesses that may contribute to death in total population for a specific time period	$\dfrac{\text{Hypertension in 2020}}{\text{U. S. Population in 2020}} \times 100,000^{b}$
Incidence	The number of new cases of a disease in the population for a specific time period	$\dfrac{\text{New U.S. COVID}-19\text{ Cases in 2020}}{\text{U. S. Population in 2020}} \times 100,000^{c}$
Prevalence	The number of all current cases of disease in the population for a specific time period	$\dfrac{\text{All U.S. Covid}-19\text{ Cases in 2020}}{\text{U.S. Population in 2020}} \times 100,000^{d}$
Relative risk	The ratio of deaths due to COVID in one group compared to the deaths due to COVID in another group	Risk of death in group of interest (A) Risk of death in comparison group (B) Risk ratio of group A (RR^A) = Group A Deaths/ Total Population Group A Risk ratio of group B (RR^B) = Group B Deaths/ Total Population Group B Relative Risk: Group A compared with Group B = RR^A/RR^B

Notes: [a] Expressed as automobile fatality rate in the U.S. per 100,000 people in 2020.
[b] Expressed as hypertension rate in U.S. per 100,000 people in 2020.
[c] Expressed as incidence rate of COVID-19 in U.S. per 100,000 people in 2020.
[d] Expressed as prevalence of COVID-19 in U.S. per 100,000 people in 2020.
[e] Expressed as relative risk of COVID-19 in high-risk group when compared with a non-high-risk group in U.S. per 100,000 people in 2020.

Furthermore, maternal health is affected, in part, by the income status of a country; hence, another reason why it is important to consider the income status or *GNI* of countries when comparing health outcomes across countries.

INCIDENCE, PREVALENCE, AND RELATIVE RISKS Incidence Three additional statistics provide a gross measure of the health status of a population: incidence, prevalence, and relative risk. *Incidence* refers to the number of new cases of a disease in a specific population for a given time period. We can examine how quickly a disease is spreading through a population by examining the number of new cases, or incidence, of a disease. Take, for example, the SARS-CoV-2 (COVID-19) pandemic. We discuss this global pandemic in detail in Chapter 4, Global, Communicable, and Chronic Disease. Here, we note that this disease, which most experts agree began in Wuhan, China, spread quickly to all parts of the world and resulted in millions of infections and millions of deaths.

Incidence data on SARS-CoV-2 (COVID-19) in China, specifically from Wuhan, would be ideal to understand how and how quickly this disease and its variants moved through the population. However, reliable data from China is difficult to obtain. Therefore, we look to other countries to obtain epidemiological data on this illness. South Africa, one of many countries hard hit by this illness, maintained excellent statistical data, so we look at their data to illustrate this concept.

South Africa reported no cases of COVID-19 before March 2020. Even then, initially the number of new cases of COVID-19 were few: two incidences on March 2, 2020, growing to 745 incidences, or new cases, on March 23, just three weeks later (see Figure 2.3). By May 2020, however, the number of new cases each week numbered in the thousands. On May 4, South African health authorities reported 1,109 incidences of COVID-19, but more than two times that number (2,636) the week of May 25 (World Health Organization, 2023b; see again Figure 2.3). From these data, we can see that the incidences of COVID-19

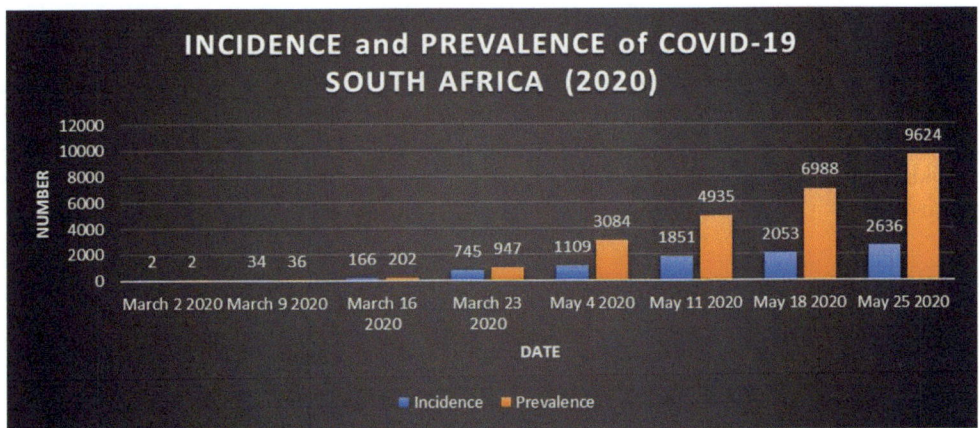

FIGURE 2.3 A bar chart presents incidence and prevalence of COVID-19 cases in South Africa in 2020. March 2, incidence and prevalence were both 2. March 9, 34 incidences, prevalence 36; March 16, 166 incidences, prevalence 202; March 23, shows a 4 fold jump in incidences and prevalences, 745 incidences, prevalence 947. Afterwards a steady increase in incidences and significant jumps in prevalence in just one month: May 4, 1109 incidences, prevalence 3084, May 11, 1851 incidences, prevalence 4935; May 18, 2053 incidences, prevalence 6988; and May 25, 2636 incidences, prevalence 9624.

Source: Adapted from World Health Organization Health Emergency Dashboard: Global South Africa. https://covid19.who.int/region/afro/country/za

were increasing and spreading rapidly throughout South Africa, a phenomenon experienced globally, and at the same time. There is good news, however. For the week of December 8, 2022, South African health authorities reported 1,761 incidences of COVID-19, a decrease from the previous months that has remained relatively stable ever since (Republic of South Africa, Department of Health, 2022).

Prevalence In comparison, *prevalence* is the *total* number of cases (old and new) of a specific disease in a population, also for a given time period. This time, look at the data on the prevalence of COVID-19 in Figure 2.3. These data show that the prevalence, or *total* number of cases in South Africa, was also growing at an alarming rate. A total of 36 cases were reported in all of South Africa the week of March 9, 2020. Just 10 weeks later, more than 9,600 total COVID-19 cases were recorded. As of December 8, 2022, the prevalence of COVID-19 cases was a staggering 4,042,912 (Republic of South Africa, Department of Health, 2022). Remember, here we are looking at the total number of cases, not just new cases. The total prevalence of 4,042,912 as of 2022 measures the impact of COVID-19 on the South African population using the actual number of cases.

As with the raw infant mortality data, the raw data on incidence and prevalence of COVID-19 in South Africa are useful when describing the spread of the disease within a country. But to make meaningful comparisons between South Africa and other countries, we must convert the raw data to *incidence rates* and *prevalence rates*.

As of 2023, South Africa's COVID-19 prevalence rate was 6,866.67 per 100,000 people. The death rate was 172.99 per 100,000 people. On their own, those numbers seem quite high. But compare them to the prevalence and death rates of six other countries similarly affected by COVID-19, as shown in Table 2.2. Israel, the U.K., the U.S., Brazil, Canada, and Egypt all report considerably higher prevalence rates than South Africa. In fact, compared with these countries, South Africa ranks sixth in the prevalence rate of COVID-19 and fourth in death rates. By comparing prevalence and death rates, we see that South Africa's COVID-19 prevalence and death rates were high, but certainly not the highest when compared with other countries.

Relative Risk The basic formula for computing *relative risk* was presented earlier when examining data on infant deaths (see again Table 2.1). But a more specific example with actual data may help. Here, we compute the relative risk to older individuals of dying of COVID-19 when compared to all other age groups. Specifically, we will calculate the risk of older persons, say those 65 years of age or older, dying of COVID-19 relative to persons younger than 65 dying of the same illness. This was and remains an issue for health providers because one of the groups most at risk of dying from the earliest variant of COVID-19 was older persons.

TABLE 2.2 Comparing COVID-19 Prevalence and Death Rates in Seven Countries

Country	Prevalence per 100,000	Deaths per 100,000
Israel	55,788.17	145.16
U.K.	36,291.19	335.16
U.S.	31,249.55	340.53
Brazil	17,715.54	331.07
Canada	12,423.32	140.06
South Africa	6,866.67	172.99
Egypt	504.25	24.26

Source: Adapted from World Health Organization (2023). Health Emergency Dashboard.

To assist us in this analysis, we draw on the research by Yanez, Weiss, Romand, and Treggiari (2020), who examined the age-specific rates of COVID-19 mortality for 16 countries for six weeks during the early stages of the pandemic, specifically March and April of 2020. We will use their data to compute the relative risk of death for persons over 65 years of age in two countries hit hard by the pandemic: Brazil and the U.S.

Brazil's estimated population of persons 65 years of age or older (65+ years) is 19.5 million. Of that population, 5,840 persons died over the six-week period captured in the study by Yanez and colleagues (2020). Thus, the relative risk (RR) of people 65+ years dying of COVID-19 in Brazil for that six-week period is 5,840/19,500,000 = .000299 or .0299% (see Box 2.1 and Table 2.3). In comparison, the estimated

---

Box 2.1 Computing Relative Risk

The risk of dying of COVID-19 can serve as an excellent and timely example of how to compute relative risk. You may recall that, particularly in the early stages of this illness, older persons (that is, those older than 65 years of age) and people with chronic health conditions (such as diabetes, heart disease, cancer, and obesity) were at higher risk of death of contracting the early Omicron strain of this virus. But how did scientists determine that this was the case?

Using the example of relative risk based on age, researchers computed the rates of death from COVID-19 for people over 65 years of age and the rates of those younger than 65 years and then compared the two to determine if, in fact, older persons were at higher risk for death. This comparison helped inform the policy decision that those over 65 years and those with specific chronic health conditions should be prioritized when distributing the free but initially limited supply of vaccines.

TABLE 2.3 Calculating Relative Risk

Procedure	Example: Brazil	Example: U.S.
Step #1 Divide the number of COVID deaths for persons over 65 years for a specified time period in a specific location by the total population of persons older than 65 for the same time period and location. Stated another way: $$\text{Relative Risk} > 65 = \frac{\#\text{of Covid deaths for} > 65 \text{ year olds}}{\text{population of} > 65 \text{ (place / time specific)}}$$	$\dfrac{5,840}{19,500,000} = .000299$	$\dfrac{40,673}{56,000,000} = .000726$
Step #2 Compute the same for persons younger than 65. $$\text{Relative Risk} < 65 = \frac{\#\text{of Covid deaths for} < 65 \text{ year old}}{\text{population of} < 65 \text{ (place / time specific)}}$$	$\dfrac{2,039}{192,500,000} = .0000105$	$\dfrac{10,762}{277,000,000} \times .0000388$
Step #3 Finally, divide the relative risk (RR) calculated for persons >65 by the relative risk (RR) for persons <65, $$\text{Relative Risk: Deaths by age} = \frac{RR > 65}{RR < 65}$$	$\dfrac{.000299}{.0000105} = \mathbf{28.47}$	$\dfrac{.000726}{.0000388} \times \mathbf{18.7}$

population of persons younger than 65 years of age in Brazil is 192.5 million, of which 2,039 died of COVID-19 in the six weeks sampled. Therefore, the RR of people under 65 years of age dying of COVID-19 in Brazil during the same time period is 2,039/192,500,000 = .0000105 or .00105%. Now, we can calculate the (RR) of older persons dying of this disease during these six weeks in Brazil as opposed to all other age groups. Here we compute .000299 (RR 65+)/ .0000105 (RR < 65) = 28.47. Translated, this means that persons 65+ years of age in Brazil were 28.47 or almost 28 times as likely to die of COVID-19 during the six weeks sampled by Yanez and colleagues (2020).

Sounds incredible? Perhaps. But when compared with other countries, like the U.S., maybe not. Using the same procedure, we can compute the relative risk of older persons dying of COVID-19 in the U.S. during the same time period when compared with all other age groups (see again Table 2.3). Fully 40,673 of the 56 million persons 65+ in the U.S. died of COVID-19 during this period, yielding a relative risk of .000726 or .0726%. In comparison, only 10,762 of the 277 million persons <65 years of age died during the same period in the U.S., for a relative risk of .0000388 or .00388%. When comparing the two groups we get an RR of 18.7! That means that in the U.S., persons 65 years of age or older were 18.7 times more likely to die of COVID-19 than those <65 years of age. From these calculations, we can see that persons 65+ in the U.S. had a much lower relative risk of dying of COVID-19 in March and April of 2020 than did the same age group in Brazil.

In sum, measures of mortality, morbidity, incidence, prevalence, and relative risk are five classic measures of the health of a population. They are, however, only gross measures of the community's health. For a more in-depth description of the health status of individuals or of a community, we turn to more specific measures.

PROXIMAL VERSUS DISTAL CAUSES OF ILLNESS Proximal Two measures that help explain individual or community health problems are *proximal* (or *precipitating*) and *distal* (or *predisposing*) causes of health and illness. Proximal and distal causes may include individual, situational, or environmental factors. Consider this example: In December 2006, 71 people in five states in the U.S. (Delaware, New Jersey, New York, Pennsylvania, and South Carolina) reported gastrointestinal problems (diarrhea, bloating, or nausea due to problems in the stomach or intestines) shortly after eating at a Taco Bell restaurant in four of the five states listed earlier. Epidemiologists and health officials found that the proximal cause for the gastrointestinal problems of the 71 patients was the *E. coli O157:H7 bacterium*. It appears that several shipments of shredded lettuce from a food manufacturing plant were accidentally contaminated with *E. coli*. The lettuce was shipped to the Taco Bell restaurants in Delaware, New Jersey, New York, and Pennsylvania and was consumed by the customers who became ill (Centers for Disease Control, 2006c). After further investigation, the CDC determined that the contamination resulted from poor hygiene or poor food preparation procedures at the processing plant that supplied lettuce to the Taco Bell restaurants in the four states.

You will notice, however, that the fifth state, South Carolina, was not included in the delivery. If the contaminated lettuce, the proximal factor, was not delivered to South Carolina, why was a related case of *E. coli* discovered there? In one word: travel. A resident of South Carolina dined at a Taco Bell restaurant in one of the four affected states before returning home. The "medical detective" work of the epidemiologists helped to tie the incident of *E. coli* in South Carolina to the proximal environmental cause in the other 70 cases by probing into the recent travels of the South Carolina resident.

Distal To explain distal causes of an illness, researchers may need to examine factors or events that predate the illness by months or perhaps years. For example, heart disease in adults is an illness that could have several distal causes. One cause could be a congenital problem, or a problem present at birth, such as an *atrial septal defect*. Sometimes called a hole in the wall of the heart, atrial septal defect often is undetected at birth. And, if left undetected, the defect may develop into *hypertension* (high blood pressure) in adolescence or adulthood. Thus, a child born with an atrial septal defect may be predisposed to developing heart-related problems such as hypertension (see Chapter 9, Cardiovascular Disease) as an adolescent or adult. For this reason, atrial septal defect could be considered a distal factor that could cause heart disease in later years.

Summary

Five classic measures – mortality, morbidity, incidence, prevalence, and relative risk – enable health researchers to describe the health status of a population in gross terms. Proximal (or precipitating) and distal (or predisposing) factors help explain the timing of an illness as well as the probable cause. In Section II, we review some of the research methods used by health psychologists to analyze the causes of diseases and to predict their future occurrences.

SECTION II. METHODOLOGY

We sometimes refer to methodology as the research design segment of a study. The word *design* suggests a creative process. Here, researchers can use their creativity to craft interesting and unique studies that test research hypotheses. There is just one caveat: A creative study must adhere to a few fundamental principles of research design.

In this section, we will briefly review selected, basic research designs to illustrate the methods used most often by health psychologists. In the process, you will see how the health concepts used by epidemiologists are married to the research techniques and methods used in psychology to produce studies of interest to both epidemiologists and health psychologists. You may want to return to this section as a reference guide when reading about research studies in this and subsequent chapters.

There are two general types of research methods in psychology: *nonexperimental* and *experimental studies*. We will begin with an overview of two types of nonexperimental studies used frequently by health psychologists, qualitative and correlational studies (see Table 2.4). Afterwards, we will review experimental studies including quasi-experimental methods. By the end of this section, you will be able to distinguish among nonexperimental, experimental, and quasi-experimental studies; define qualitative, correlational, intervention, pre-posttest, and clinical trial studies; and describe the types of research questions that each of these methods addresses.

Qualitative Studies

One factor researchers consider when designing a study is the type of data to be collected. In Section I, we described morbidity, mortality, incidence, prevalence, and relative risks: examples of *quantitative data* that characterize numerically the health status of a community. In comparison, proximal and distal data yield contextual rather than numeric information. They provide explanations about an outcome, not just numbers. The purpose of proximal and distal data is to explain the occurrence of the problem rather than to count the number of occurrences.

TABLE 2.4 Sample Research Methods for Health Psychology Research

Design	Purpose	Statistic	Pros (P) and Cons (C)
Nonexperimental			
Qualitative	Explore phenomenon in context	Minimal or no statistical data Analyze content of responses	(P) In-depth analysis of response (C) Cannot examine cause–effect relationships
Case	In-depth exploration of person, place, situation	Minimal or no statistical data Analyze content of responses	(P) In-depth exploration of rare/unique events (C) Cannot examine cause–effect relationships
Focus groups	Gather information Generate insight Explore decision-making Encourage interactions	Minimal use of descriptive data Analyze content of responses	(P) Generate new information, insights (P) Interactive approach (C) Cannot examine cause–effect relationships
Correlational studies	Describe relationship between two variables	Pearson correlation coefficient (r) Range = −1.00 to +1.00	(P) Identifies relationship between two variables (C) Cannot determine causal relationship
Experimental			
Experimental studies	Detect cause–effect relationship between variables	Central tendency (mean, median, mode) Student's t Analysis of variance (ANOVA) Multiple analysis of variance (MANOVA) Linear, multiple, or logistic regression (R^2)	(P) Causal explanation of effects of one or more variables on outcomes (P) Direct control of causal variables (C) Not suitable for all studies (C) No in-depth analysis
Intervention studies	Measure effect of intervention, usually with pre-posttest format	Central tendency (mean, median, mode) Student's t Analysis of variance (ANOVA) Multiple analysis of variance (MANOVA) Linear, multiple, or logistic regression (R^2)	(P) Direct measure of effectiveness of intervention (P) Causal explanation of effects (C) Not suitable for all studies (C) No in-depth analysis
Quasi-experimental			
Quasi-Experimental	Detect cause–effect relationship between two variables with limitations	Central tendency (mean, median, mode) Student's t Analysis of variance (ANOVA) Multiple analysis of variance (MANOVA) Linear, multiple, or logistic regression (R^2)	(P) Limited cause–effect relationship (P) Control of some causal variables (C) Pre-existing conditions may not be controlled
Intervention studies	Measure effect of intervention usually with pre-posttest format	Central tendency (mean, median, mode) Student's t Analysis of variance (ANOVA) Multiple analysis of variance (MANOVA)	(P) Measure intervention effect on single group (P) Limited subject variance (C) Limited inference of causality without control groups

Qualitative studies, like qualitative data, are used when the goal of the researcher is to gather largely non-statistical data that help to explain a behavior or outcome in the environment in which it occurs (Salkind, 2006). Qualitative studies in health psychology, therefore, provide rich, contextual data that allows for an in-depth exploration and analysis of the health issue. But, as we will see shortly, there are benefits and drawbacks to qualitative studies.

In qualitative studies, researchers use the context in which the health event occurred to explore a phenomenon and to identify factors that contribute to an outcome. Consider this: When exploring the proximal causes of the gastrointestinal problems of the 71 Taco Bell customers discussed in Section I, researchers collected information from the customers about their behaviors immediately preceding the illness. Here the critical information came in the form of a brief history of customers' recent travels and eating behaviors – that is, non-statistical data. For example, researchers may have asked the 71 customers what they ate for breakfast or where they ate before going to a Taco Bell. They may have asked also whether they went to Taco Bell with friends or family and whether their friends and family also became ill. Using the customers' histories, the researchers then analyzed the responses, searching for common factors that linked all 71 *E. coli* sufferers. In this case, there were two commonalities: All 71 customers ate at Taco Bell, and all ate shredded lettuce as part of their meal. Undoubtedly, some of the data obtained in the investigation were numerical. But other information, such as what was consumed and other related behaviors, was qualitative.

CASE STUDIES Researchers in the Taco Bell investigation most likely used a qualitative research design called a *case study* to obtain data. Consistent with other forms of qualitative research, case studies allow for an in-depth analysis of rare or unique events. Consider another example: Case study methods are used often by epidemiologists when investigating new outbreaks of diseases. The West Nile virus outbreak in the U.S. is one example in which a case study approach was used to investigate the occurrence of a new health problem that affected many communities.

The first case of West Nile virus in the U.S. occurred in 1999. Some of the people infected with the virus showed symptoms of *encephalitis*, a severe inflammation of the spinal cord and the brain. Epidemiologists used the diagnosis of encephalitis, other medical tests, and descriptions obtained from patients about the events leading up to their illnesses to build a case study of each infected patient. For patients who were unconscious or too ill to respond, family and friends provided the needed information. Researchers then compared the case studies of patients with similar symptoms to identify commonalities and to link the common symptoms to a likely cause. Using medical records, researchers were able to diagnose the then unknown virus as the West Nile virus, a disease that was first reported in Egypt and France in the 1950s and 1960s (Sayed-Ahmed, 2016).

FOCUS GROUPS Another type of qualitative study commonly used by health researchers is a *focus group*. Focus groups serve four main functions: to gather information, to generate insight, to explore a decision-making process, and finally, to encourage interactions between focus group participants that create new insights (Salkind, 2006). The groups are facilitated by a moderator. The job of the moderator is to pose questions for discussion and to ensure that all participants are able and encouraged to contribute.

Participants in a focus group usually have one or more characteristics in common, characteristics that are central to the research question or topic. For example, researchers could convene a focus group of first-year college students to explore new students' perceptions of stress during their first semester. Not all first-semester college students experience stress. But in focus groups, a researcher can obtain information from the students who do as well as those who do not report feelings of stress in order to generate insight into the factors that contribute to stress.

The in-depth information obtained from focus groups may identify new causes of stress that are unknown to the investigator. Additionally, the group format can provide a forum for an exchange of ideas or experiences that may also generate new insight into the causes of stress. Thus, unlike case studies, focus groups yield in-depth information from a group of people simultaneously rather than from people individually.

INTERVIEWS Finally, some research requires structured and unstructured responses to specific questions. For example, the *one-on-one interview* is a data collection technique that allows for a range of responses according to the type of questions posed. Using *closed-ended questions*, here meaning those questions offering a restricted range of responses, such as "yes" or "no," researchers can obtain succinct responses to specific questions. One-on-one interviews may also contain *open-ended questions*, here meaning questions yielding descriptive responses that allow study participants to provide additional information that may offer important details about the person's health behaviors. Open-ended questions also allow respondents to construct and deliver their own answers without regard to the length or format of their responses.

An example of an open-ended question is: What is the reason for your visit to the doctor's office today? Answers to this question may vary based on the participants' reasons for seeking medical care, the choice of words used to describe their illness or injury, and the level of detail they provide when responding.

In essence, qualitative studies often use non-statistical research tools to obtain information about an event in context. But sometimes a researcher requires a more quantitative answer to questions. In such cases, we turn to analytical research methods that use quantitative statistics.

Correlational Studies

We identified methods for describing the health status of a population using, for example, mortality and morbidity data. We also identified methods for explaining a health event using qualitative data. But when researchers want to do more than simply describe a health status or an event, they use analytical research methods. For example, researchers may want to examine the relationship between two variables that affect health outcomes, such as diet and exercise. By "relationship," we mean simply determining whether two variables share something in common. If they do, they may be correlated (Salkind, 2006). Hence, one way to examine the relationship between two variables is through correlation research.

Correlational studies often use the *Pearson correlation coefficient (r)*, a statistic that describes the strength of the relationship between two variables. The correlation coefficient is expressed numerically as a value ranging from +1.00 to –1.00. Correlations can be strongly positive ($r = +1.00$), strongly negative ($r = -1.00$), or totally unrelated, thereby showing no correlation ($r = 0.00$).

Examples of correlations related to health can be found in a study by Bourne (2009). Bourne examined two relationships: one between health-seeking behavior and health insurance and a second between poverty and health insurance. Bourne conducted a *retrospective analysis*, here meaning analyzing data from an existing database, using statistics on health behaviors in Jamaica over 19 years between 1988 and 2007. Bourne found a significant *positive correlation* between health-seeking behaviors and ownership of health insurance. In other words, in the record data from Jamaica during the 19-year period captured, people with health insurance were significantly more likely to seek health care when needed. In this instance, a positive correlation was reported because an increase in the percentage of people with health insurance was associated with an increase in the percentage of people seeking health care. Note, however, that a positive correlation could result if, as one variable goes down, the second variable also decreases in value. Put another way: To demonstrate a positive correlation, both variables must move in the same direction, either both increasing in value or both decreasing in value.

An interesting additional result in the same study indicated that health insurance ownership was related to poverty. Bourne demonstrated that the greater the prevalence of poverty among the population, the less likely they are to have health insurance. In essence, as the prevalence of poverty increases over years, the likelihood of health insurance ownership decreases. This *negative correlation* demonstrates that as one variable increases in value the other decreases.

When using correlation data, the strength of the relationship between the variables is expressed by the correlation coefficient *(r)*. Although the strength of a correlation between two variables is expressed also by the *p*-value of the statistic, here meaning its probability of occurrence in the population, researchers often use the following guidelines to help identify potentially weak, average, or strong correlations. As a general rule of thumb, coefficients between $r = 0.21$ and $r = 0.39$ represent a weak correlation. Coefficients between $r = 0.40$ and $r = 0.59$ suggest moderate correlations, and coefficient values of $r = 0.60$ and above usually are considered high or strong correlations. Values between $r = 0.00$ and $r = 0.20$ indicate no correlation.

One correlation used often as a gross measure of health status is the relationship between a person's height and weight. Using a growth chart, shown in Figure 2.4, physicians examine the relationship between height and weight for boys to determine whether a child's growth in feet and inches corresponds to an increase in weight that is appropriate given their height (Adams et al., 2007). In other words, physicians expect to see a positive correlation between a boy's weight gain and their growth in height. A negative correlation, one in which height increases but weight does not, could suggest health problems such as malnourishment or other physiological problems that threaten the infant's chances of survival. For infants, therefore, the correlation between height and weight is a gross measure of good health status. Note that although this chart applies to boys, a similar trajectory for weight gain and growth in height would be expected for infant girls as well.

We must mention one major limitation with this elegantly simple form of descriptive data. You may remember from your statistics class that correlation does not imply causality. For example, height and weight may be correlated, but we cannot conclude that an increase in height causes an increase in weight or vice versa. Thus, one limitation of correlational studies is the inability to demonstrate a *cause-and-effect relationship* between the variables. Researchers who want to explore causal relationships between variables often turn to experimental research methods.

Experimental Studies

When researchers want to explore whether there exists a cause-and-effect relationship between two variables, they construct an experimental research study. For example, a researcher may ask, "Does exercise affect stress levels?" To determine whether there is a relationship between exercise and stress, a researcher first restates the question as a null hypothesis or as a research hypothesis. A *null hypothesis* is an objective extension of the question that assumes no relationship between exercise and stress. In this case, the null hypothesis would be: There is no effect of exercise on stress.

We must point out, however, that in most published research studies, it is more common to see a *research hypothesis:* an objective extension of the question but one that assumes a relationship between the two variables. Using the same example of exercise and stress, the research hypothesis would be: There is a relationship between exercise and stress. In experimental studies, the researcher poses the null or the research hypothesis to determine whether and how changes in one variable, in this case exercise (the cause), affects the outcome of another variable, stress (the effect).

There are a number of key concepts in an experimental design. Experimental psychology textbooks discuss many of them in great detail. For our purposes, however, we limit our discussion to just four concepts: independent versus dependent variables, experimental versus control groups, random sampling, and longitudinal versus cross-sectional studies.

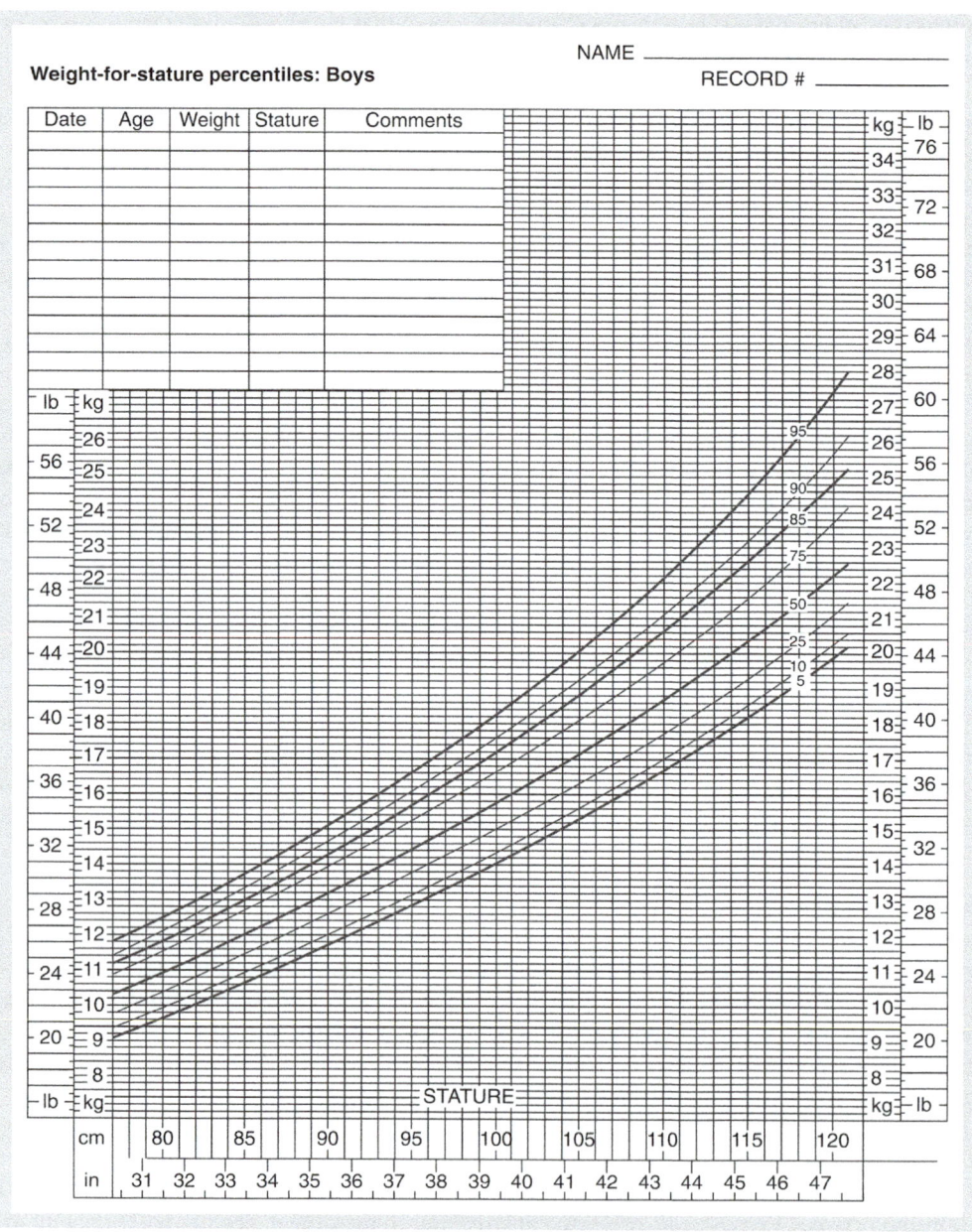

FIGURE 2.4 Boys' growth chart: Weight versus height. This chart is a grid mapping the growth trajectory for boys, infants to 24 months of age. Weight-for-Age is plotted on the X-axis in kilograms and pounds. Length-for-Age is plotted on the Y-axis in centimeters and inches. Centers for Disease Control (2000). published May 30, 2000 (modified November 21, 2000).

Source: Developed by the National Center for Health Statistics in collaboration with the National Center for Chronic Disease Prevention and Health Promotion (2000). www.cdc.gov/growthcharts

INDEPENDENT VERSUS DEPENDENT VARIABLES One advantage of experimental research designs is that the investigator can limit or control many of the variables to be studied. The variable that the investigator manipulates, or controls is called the *independent variable*. In our example of the effects of exercise on stress, the independent variable is exercise. By carefully selecting the independent variables to include in a study, researchers can examine the effect of each variable on the study's outcome. Experimental studies may have multiple independent variables. For simplicity, however, our example has just one independent variable, exercise. Note, however, when designing a study on the effects of exercise on stress, researchers must define the type or types of exercise they include in the study.

A study's outcome variable is called the *dependent variable*. Returning to our example of the relationship between exercise and stress, the dependent variable in this case is stress because the amount of stress experienced is assumed to be influenced by the amount of exercise (independent variable). After the variables have been identified and defined, researchers must develop a method for measuring a participant's level of stress after performing the exercises.

EXPERIMENTAL VERSUS CONTROL GROUPS Experimental research includes at least two groups of study participants: one control group and at least one experimental group. The *experimental group* is the test group. They receive a special treatment or condition. Again, referring to our example of exercise and stress, an experimental group's treatment could consist of 30 minutes of free swimming three times a week. The *control group*, however, would not receive the special condition or treatment. They may receive some form of treatment but nothing that would affect the dependent variable, stress. For example, participants in the control group might be placed in a room for 30 minutes with reading materials about swimming.

RANDOM SAMPLING One goal of psychology researchers is to explain human behavior. Specifically, a goal of health psychology researchers is to explain the health behaviors or health outcomes of individuals or groups. Therefore, even though researchers conduct studies on small samples of people, the real goal is to generalize the results of their study to other similar groups in an effort to explain human behavior.

It is rarely possible to test a research hypothesis or question on an entire population. Consider this: If a researcher were interested in examining the frequency of accidents and injury to left-handed people, would the researcher be able to test the entire population of left-handed individuals? Clearly not. Consequently, research studies test hypotheses using a subset of a population rather than the full population.

When experimenters select a sample of participants from a population they wish to study, they must ensure that all eligible subjects have an equal and independent chance of participating. In addition, they must ensure that they are choosing a sample that is representative of the population. Consider this: If a study on exercise and stress among college students were conducted at your college, researchers would need to advertise the study in such a way that all eligible students at your college would have an equal chance of participating in the study if they so desired. What methods could a researcher use to notify all eligible students? In some colleges, the campus newspaper is one way to disseminate information. For others, campus-wide e-mails, text messages, or social media sites such as Instagram, Facebook (now Meta), Snapchat, TikTok, or even Twitter (now X) updates would provide all students with an opportunity to participate.

When all eligible persons have an equal chance of participating, researchers can be reasonably assured that their recruitment procedures sought and most likely obtained a representative sample of the population. For that reason, researchers emphasize the importance of choosing a *random sample:* a group of people, all of whom have an equal chance of participating in the study and who will be representative of the population to be studied. A truly random sample minimizes the possibility that the individuals chosen for the study reflect the preferences or biases of the experimenter.

Another issue pertaining to random selection is the ***random assignment*** of participants to treatment conditions. We mentioned that experimental studies have at least one experimental group and one control group. The experimenter must randomly assign participants to either group. Here, too, the experimenter must choose a process that allows each volunteer to have an equal chance of being assigned to either condition. Ensuring a random selection of participants and a random assignment of participants to study conditions gives the researcher greater confidence that the results are likely to be unbiased with respect to sample selection and assignment of conditions.

LONGITUDINAL VERSUS CROSS-SECTIONAL DESIGN In this and the subsequent sections we illustrate concepts using well-known, and in some cases, classic studies. Thus, this section may feel more like a history lesson embedded in a methodology section. *Mea Culpa!* The studies presented here are not only good examples of methodological and ethical issues. They are studies that should never be forgotten. Hence, we will just refer to this as a methodology-history lesson. Now, let's begin.

Longitudinal The last of the key concepts in experimental design that we will address is longitudinal versus cross-sectional studies. In *longitudinal study designs*, researchers study a phenomenon over an extended period of time using the same participants. This is a useful design when studying health problems such as stress, because stress is affected by a host of individual and environmental variables that contribute to the condition over time (see Chapter 7, Stress and Coping). A longitudinal study can reveal a pattern of stress that is more reliable and less influenced by episodic changes caused by a specific event. Using the same people over time also helps control variability in the results due to subject factors such as age, ethnicity, or gender.

The disadvantages to using longitudinal studies are that they are time-consuming and can be costly. Another factor, attrition, may negatively affect longitudinal studies because participants are "lost" over time or discontinue participation due to lack of interest, inconvenience, or other reasons.

A classic and often cited example of a longitudinal health study is the ***Framingham Heart Study*** (see Box 2.2). This study, which began in 1948 in Framingham, Massachusetts, was designed as a detailed epidemiological study of heart disease. Its goal was to investigate the possible factors related to the development of various forms of coronary heart disease and hypertension (Dawber & Kannel, 1966). Within the first four years of the study, researchers were able to identify a number of personal and environmental characteristics associated with heart disease. And, equally as important, the Framingham study demonstrated that a longitudinal study of a health problem provided valuable information about previously unknown factors that contributed to the disease. As incredible as it might sound, this longitudinal study continues even today, some 76 years after its inception. Why? By continuing the study, researchers can examine several generations of offspring of the original Framingham study sample, this time to look for genetic as well as individual and environmental factors that contribute to heart disease.

Box 2.2 The Framingham Heart Study: A Longitudinal Design

Would you be willing to participate in a longitudinal study that followed you for life for the benefit of science?

It may sound like an unusual proposition, but in 1948, 5,209 men and women, ages 30 to 62, agreed to become the first **cohort**, or group, of people to participate in the Framingham Heart Study. Researchers decided to choose Framingham, Massachusetts – hence the name of the study – for two reasons. First, Framingham was the site of a previous, and successful, community-based study. Second, Framingham was close to several major medical research centers (Splansky et al., 2007).

The researchers were primarily interested in identifying the personal habits and traits that contributed to the development of coronary heart disease (see Chapter 9, Cardiovascular Disease). Therefore, when recruiting the sample of eligible participants, researchers obtained *baseline*, or initial, health measures on each person. Only individuals with no prior history of heart disease were eligible for the study. This was a key **eligibility criterion**. Researchers wanted to ensure that heart disease was not a pre-existing condition of any of the participants. After enrolling in the study, each participant was reassessed every two years for the duration of the study. During the first 20-year reassessment period, a number of study participants developed heart disease.

Although important, the fact that some of the over 5,000 individuals developed heart disease was not the most significant finding. Rather, the important discovery was that, for the first time, researchers were able to demonstrate an association between coronary artery disease and individual as well as environmental causes. Specifically, researchers demonstrated that high blood pressure, excessive body weight, high cholesterol (related in part to dietary habits), lack of physical activity, smoking, and diabetes, among other factors, significantly increased the chances of heart disease. Individuals who had two or more of the associated characteristics were at a higher risk of heart disease than those who only reported one such factor (Anderson, Odell, Wilson, & Kannel, 1991; Dawber & Kannel, 1966; Kannel, Dawber, Friedman, Glennon, & McNamara, 1964).

These findings may not seem surprising to us today, because many of the individual and environmental causes of heart disease are well known. However, one reason we know the risk factors for heart disease is because of the Framingham study. Remember, the Framingham study began in the late 1940s. The first results were published in the 1950s, when little was known about the risk factors for coronary heart disease.

The Framingham study continues even today (Nayor et al., 2021; Vasan et al., 2022). It monitors some participants from the original cohort and now includes second- and even third-generation offspring of the original group. The information about the heart histories of relatives of the original cohort, including individuals who did and did not develop heart disease, will provide additional data about genetic as well as individual and environmental factors that contribute to heart disease (Splansky et al., 2007). More important, however, the results of this study have provided valuable information to medical doctors.

Finally, in recognition of the need to capture Framingham's more diverse population and the risk of heart disease among other ethnic groups, in 1994 the study added the "Omni Cohort" which included 507 participants of African American, Hispanic, Native American, Asian and Pacific Islander backgrounds. A second Omni cohort was added in 2003 (NHLBI, n.d.). The addition of these new cohorts will enable researchers to apply these findings to a more diverse population and to assist doctors in better understanding their patients' risk of developing heart disease – something they could not do without such a detailed, longitudinal study.

The *Stanford Three Community Study* (see Box 2.3) is a second, somewhat shorter classic longitudinal study that also sought to test factors related to heart disease. One major difference between this study and the Framingham Heart Study is that the Stanford study examined the role of three educational interventions – mass media, individual instruction, or no instruction – on heart disease. The results clearly show the more intervention, the better! Those participants who received the most information – here meaning individual instruction and mass-media sources – reported the best health outcomes.

Box 2.3 The Stanford Three Community Study: An Intervention Study with Three Communities

The Stanford Three Community Study is another example of an intervention study, although shorter in duration than the Framingham project. The Stanford study also examined heart disease; however, its goal was to examine the effect of several types of interventions on risk reduction for heart disease (Meyer, Nash, McAlister, Maccoby, & Farquhar, 1980). Specifically, Meyer and coauthors wanted to determine whether mass-media campaigns and intensive individualized instruction reduced individuals' risk of heart disease.

To test their hypotheses, the researchers chose three communities in California – Watsonville, Gilroy, and Tracy – that fulfilled the study's eligibility criteria. Study researchers determined that the participants from the three communities should be comparable on three demographic categories: age, ethnicity, and socioeconomic status. Yet the communities needed to meet additional *eligibility criteria*. Specifically, all three communities also needed to have community media (television and newspaper), be near Stanford University (the host site for the study), and have no community-based health education programs.

In the study, researchers obtained baseline information on each participant's health status, health habits, and risk factors for cardiovascular diseases. One community in the study, Tracy, served as the control site. Residents of Tracy received no intervention, here meaning no mass-media campaign and no individualized instruction on cardiovascular health. Residents of Watsonville were assigned to an experimental condition that included both the media campaign and individualized instruction. Gilroy residents, the second experimental group, received only the mass-media communication intervention. The Stanford Three Community Study demonstrated the effectiveness of mass media in changing health behaviors and reducing the risk of health disease. By using both experimental and control groups, researchers demonstrated that mass-media campaigns, as opposed to just individualized instruction or no intervention at all, helped reduce the risks of heart disease.

In addition, this study demonstrated that researchers could conduct a longitudinal, *community-based study*, similar in design to the Framingham Heart Study, to understand the health behaviors that increase the risks of heart disease. Studies like the Stanford study are referred to as community-based studies because they measure the impact of an intervention in the participants' natural environment rather than in a laboratory or other environments constructed for the study.

Cross-Sectional A *cross-sectional research design* is used to study a phenomenon across a wide group of participants. Unlike longitudinal studies, cross-sectional designs require less time because they measure each participant or group of participants only once, rather than taking multiple measures from the same participants over time. If conducting a cross-sectional version of the Framingham study, for example, researchers would obtain measures of the occurrence of heart disease from many groups of men and women of different ages, but they would measure each participant only once.

The advantages of a cross-sectional design are shorter duration and lower cost. The disadvantage, however, is the use of multiple subject groups, which introduces more variability in the results due to possible individual or subject differences.

Intervention Studies

Intervention studies occupy a unique position in research design. They can be either experimental or quasi-experimental, depending on the study question. We will examine experimental intervention studies first and discuss quasi-experimental intervention studies in the following section on quasi-experimental design.

Intervention studies are used often in research on health issues because they test the extent to which an intervention (a special program, therapeutic treatment, or training) improves health outcomes. Here, improvements can be defined as enhancements in knowledge, attitudes, or behaviors, or measurable changes in physical or mental health.

In intervention studies, all participants are given a ***pretest*** or ***baseline measure*** to assess their knowledge, performance, or physical or mental status before introducing the treatment. The study group is then given an intervention followed by a second assessment that is identical to or much like the first. The experimental group's performance on the first (pre) and second (post) assessments are compared to determine the effects, if any, of the intervention on the dependent variable specified for the study. Studies that include a pretest followed by an intervention and conclude with a ***posttest*** are also known as ***pretest-posttest studies***, or ***pre-posttest*** for short (see Table 2.5).

One important consideration for researchers when designing intervention studies is whether to use a control group. We introduced the term *control group* in the preceding section on experimental versus control groups (page 49). Control groups allow the researchers to determine whether the performance of study participants, as measured by the dependent variable, is influenced by the experimental treatment (the intervention). Thus, an intervention study in health psychology that uses an experimental and a control group would enable researchers to determine the effectiveness of the health intervention on participants' health outcomes. As we will see shortly, intervention studies that do not include control groups limit researchers' ability to determine the true effectiveness of the intervention.

Ethical Considerations in Experimental Design

Pre-posttest intervention designs are used also in randomized clinical trial studies. ***Randomized clinical trials*** use one control and at least one experimental group to test the effects of a new medication, a therapeutic approach, or an apparatus as a treatment for a medical or mental illness. They are called randomized because participants are assigned at random to either the control or the experimental group(s). Dr. Rutherford's study at the New York State Psychiatric Institute, discussed in the opening story, was designed as a randomized clinical trial. The research participant who died was assigned to the control group.

TABLE 2.5 Sample Pre-Posttest Design

Participants	Phase I	Phase II	Phase III
Experimental group	Pretest	Intervention	Posttest
Control group	Pretest	No intervention	Posttest

One caveat to randomized clinical trials should be noted, especially for health psychology research. As we saw in the opening story, research studies that test the efficacy of new drugs pose clear risks to participants. For this reason, the FDA requires that new drugs undergo several stages of testing, beginning with laboratory tests, followed by tests on laboratory animals, and moving on to tests on people only in the later stages of development. The process can take years.

Because of the lengthy process, some researchers and health advocates argue for a modified experimental design to evaluate the benefits of new and potentially lifesaving drugs or vaccines (Bright, Mills, Bradford, & Stewart, 2023; U.S. Food and Drug Administration, 2007). Their arguments are based, in part, on ethical concerns. For example, some health advocates who challenged the use of control groups in pre-posttest studies of the new COVID-19 vaccine contend that control group participants experience a delay in receiving a potentially lifesaving vaccine, if they receive the drug at all. They claim that the additional time needed to confirm the drug's effectiveness delays the potential benefits for people who need the new drug (Raus, Mortier, & Eeckloo, 2021; Rubin, 2021). The ethical arguments pose problems for randomized clinical trial designs. On the one hand, researchers must ensure that the new vaccines are effective, safe, and do not cause life-threatening complications. Such testing takes time. On the other hand, the time needed to complete all testing procedures delays the distribution of potentially lifesaving vaccines. What would you suggest to researchers evaluating a potentially lifesaving vaccine for COVID-19?

One way to address the ethical dilemma is through a ***pre-post-post-test design***. In this design, both the experimental and control groups would receive the actual treatment, although not at the same time. For example, when testing a potentially lifesaving or life-prolonging vaccine for COVID-19, the pre-post-post-test design for one control and one experimental group could be administered as shown in Table 2.6.

Essentially, the experimental and control groups both get the vaccine, referred to here as the intervention. The only difference is the timing of the intervention. Here, the experimental (A) and the control (B) groups get the pretest at the same time. The experimental group gets the intervention vaccine first, and the control group's intervention is delayed. Control group members will receive the intervention only after receiving a pretest and the first posttest. A second posttest is administered after the delayed intervention.

How does the pre-post-post-test design address the ethical concerns while also addressing the need for carefully controlled experimental studies? Using this design, researchers ensure that both groups (experimental and control) get the vaccine. With a minimal delay in administering the vaccine to the control group, researchers can still conduct a vaccine versus no vaccine comparison to test the vaccine's safety and effectiveness.

An additional strategy, proposed by Raus et al. (2022), is the "non-inferiority" study. In this design, the new vaccine would be compared to the best available alternative vaccine rather than a placebo. While this would not enable everyone to obtain the vaccine designed for the new illness at the same time, it would allow for some medical intervention. The problem is the available alternative intervention may be ineffective in treating or minimizing the full effects of the new illness.

TABLE 2.6 Sample Pre-Post-Post-Test Design

Participants	Pretest	First Intervention	Posttest	Second Intervention	Post-Post-Test
Experimental group (A)	A	A	A	–	A
Control group (B)	B	–	B	B	B

Quasi-experimental Intervention Studies

Up to this point, our discussion on research design included independent variables that could be controlled by the experimenter. But, in truth, health researchers cannot control many of the factors that affect the health conditions they wish to study. Variables such as gender, age, or ethnicity are not subject to complete experimenter control. That is to say, an experimenter cannot randomly assign a person to an ethnicity or age group ignoring the demographics that the subject brings to the experiment. Thus, when conducting research, health researchers must design studies that take into consideration their lack of full control over the independent variables. The solution is to use a modified methodological approach known as a *quasi-experimental design*.

Although a quasi-experimental design adjusts for the fact that researchers cannot always control each independent variable, the adjustment comes at a price. The inability to control some independent variables means that researchers are not able to demonstrate a direct cause-and-effect relationship between the independent variable and the dependent variable or outcomes. In other words, accommodating life's realities in the quasi-experimental design comes at the price of certainty.

Quasi-experimental intervention studies differ from experimental studies in another respect: They may not include control groups. In some quasi-experimental designs, a control group may be unnecessary if a researcher is interested only in the impact of an intervention on the study participants. In such cases, all participants are assigned to the same condition. However, without a control group, the researcher loses the ability to compare the outcomes of the intervention to another group. Absent this comparison, researchers cannot claim a cause-and-effect relationship, nor can they generalize their findings to a larger population.

Summary

Health psychologists may use a number of different research methods to explore the health status or changes in health outcomes of a specific study sample. These include qualitative studies such as case studies, focus groups, and interviews, as well as experimental studies that may rely on pre-posttest, pre-post-post-test, random clinical trials, or longitudinal or cross-sectional methodology. Health researchers can also use quasi-experimental designs that employ a modified version of the techniques used in experimental studies. The choice of research methods will be determined by the hypothesis or questions posed by the researcher and the type of data to be collected.

SECTION III. RESEARCH ETHICS AND POLICY

We began this chapter on research methods with a story describing the death of a research subject in a New York State Psychiatric Institute study on Parkinson's disease. The story illustrated two important points about conducting research. First, all studies using human subjects are governed by regulations that define ethical research practices. Second, study participants may experience real and severe consequences when researchers fail to follow the regulations.

To understand some of the problems posed by the Psychiatric Institute study and to prepare for our discussion on research ethics, we reviewed research concepts and methods in Sections I and II. We can now continue our examination of research ethics and researchers' responsibilities introduced in the opening story.

Reactions to the Word *Research*

What do you think when you hear the word *research?* For some people, the word brings to mind experimenters in white lab coats or research volunteers viewing images projected on screens. Perhaps your views on research were influenced by firsthand experiences, by books, or movies. For others, research is associated with outcomes such as advancements in science or new lifesaving discoveries. Still, others may view research as potentially harmful or abusive, involving the mistreatment of subjects or the use of people as human "guinea pigs."

Which view of research is most accurate? The history of research in the U.S. and other countries provides ample evidence that research has made significant contributions to society. Unfortunately, it is also true that a small number of studies have caused fatal injury or harm to participants. We begin this section by examining two studies, each of which caused harm to large numbers of participants in distinctly different ways. (And yes, this is part two of the history lesson on ethical issues in research methods). For some, this information will be new, and for others, it will be a review of stories you may have heard, perhaps incorrectly. Whatever the case, it is worthwhile to review these classic studies because they remind us of the need to carefully consider ethics whenever we decide to conduct research.

The famous *Tuskegee Syphilis Study*, conducted in the U.S. from 1932 through 1972, is an example of an egregious breach of research ethics that caused irreparable harm to the medical and mental health of the participants. To this day, some African Americans cite this study as a reason for their mistrust of research (Smirnoff et al., 2018).

By contrast, Philip Zimbardo's *Study of Interpersonal Dynamics* (sometimes referred to as the *Stanford prison experiment*) in social situations caused no physical harm to the participants but raised concerns about the potential of studies to cause psychological or emotional injury. During our discussion of the Tuskegee and Zimbardo studies, we will identify the historical events that led to the establishment of the codes of conduct for human research. These include the Nuremberg Code, the Declaration of Human Rights, and the Declaration of Helsinki. You will become familiar with the U.S. National Research Act of 1974, the Belmont Report, and the British Psychological Society's Code of Human Research Ethics (Oates et al., 2021). Finally, we will review three fundamental principles for the protection of human subjects.

The Tuskegee Syphilis Study

The Tuskegee Syphilis Study employed two unethical procedures: deception and disregard for the rights and welfare of human subjects in experiments. This longitudinal study was designed initially as a nine-month investigation to examine the course of syphilis and its impact on neurological functioning. Unfortunately, it evolved into a 40-year experiment following its "volunteers" to their deaths. The volunteers were not informed that the goal of the study was to demonstrate the neurological impact of syphilis on the brain. Nor did they know that the "demonstration" could be accomplished only by autopsies. To be clear, an autopsy is conducted on an individual after death. Thus, the volunteers in the Tuskegee study were unaware that they were expected to die to fulfill the goals of the study. The details of the deception by government agencies, educational institutions, medical care providers, researchers, local institutions, and individuals are provided in Box 2.4.

Box 2.4 Syphilis Victims in U.S. Study Went Untreated for 40 Years

The longest non-therapeutic experiment on human beings in medical history.

(Jones, 1981)

In the late 1920s, a group of researchers wanted to observe the effects of syphilis on different races. Some researchers theorized that untreated syphilis in its *latent*, or noncontagious, stage affects races differently. Some proposed that for blacks, syphilis affected the cardiovascular system, whereas others contended that syphilis in whites affected their neurological systems (Jones, 1981; Thomas & Quinn, 1991). Research published in Norway at about the same time demonstrated that untreated syphilis caused cardiovascular damage and not neurological damage in whites. This finding ran counter to popular theories in the U.S. at the time.

Concurrent with ongoing research on syphilis, the Rosenwald Fund designed a survey to measure the prevalence of syphilis among African Americans in five southern rural counties in the U.S. (Parran, 1937). The aim of this survey was to establish that clinics were needed in these areas to provide needed health care (Roy, 1996). The first stage of the survey revealed that approximately 40% of all groups tested in Macon County, Alabama, tested positive for syphilis. Consistent with the treatment goals, the Rosenwald Fund program also sought to make the standard treatment for syphilis available to African Americans in rural communities: injections of arsenical compounds and mercury or bismuth ointments that were applied to the skin (Tuskegee Syphilis Study Legacy Committee, 1996). The treatment program was to be a collaborative effort between the Rosenwald Fund and the U.S. Public Health Service (USPHS).

There is some disagreement over what happened next, but most historians contend that in the aftermath of the Great Depression (1929–1930) in the U.S., the Rosenwald Fund lost a significant part of its endowment and had to cut its funding for the project (Landau, 2010). Without the financial support of the Rosenwald Fund, the USPHS could not afford to conduct the proposed public health program. If, however, the program was redesigned as a scientific experiment, the U.S. government could fund the project. So, in 1932, the USPHS began a research study to document the long-term consequences of syphilis. The goal of the study, however, differed from the goal of the program proposed by the Rosenwald Fund. The USPHS study was not designed to provide medical testing and treatment to rural African Americans; rather, it proposed to study the effects of untreated syphilis, following the study subjects to the "endpoint" – in essence, to their death.

The USPHS service enlisted the help of many local and state agencies and individuals to find and recruit rural African American men in Macon County. Included among the organizations that assisted researchers were the Macon County Medical Society, the Tuskegee Institute, the Boards of Health in the state of Alabama and in Macon County, the Milbank Memorial Fund, as well as some leaders of local black churches, public schools, and plantation owners (Thomas & Quinn, 1991). Using trusted institutions and individuals as recruitment agents proved very successful for the USPHS study. In the end, 399 men were recruited with another 201 participants serving as the control group.

The study employed a number of unethical deceptions. The approximately 400 experimental and 200 control group participants were not told the true aim of the study. This was the first deception. In addition, they were not told that they tested positive for syphilis. Rather, they were told simply that they had "bad blood," a generic term common in the rural South to describe all forms of general ailments (Jones, 1981). Thus, the second deception was the inaccurate information given to the men about their health status. In fact, the men did not know that if untreated, their illnesses would result in death. With no access to other health care facilities, the men also had no ability to seek alternative care.

When penicillin became available as a more effective treatment for syphilis, the men were not given the new treatment. In fact, they were not advised that a new, more effective treatment for syphilis existed. Worse still, the USPHS took measures to ensure that the study participants would not be given penicillin. Ironically, during the course of the study, 50 study participants received letters from their local military draft boards. As part of their conscription for military service, they were required to take penicillin to treat their syphilis infections. Through an agreement between the USPHS and the U.S. draft board, these 50 men were exempted from treatment and from military service (Jones, 1981).

The study continued unimpeded until 1966 when Peter Buxtun, an investigator with the Public Health Service, raised moral and ethical concerns about the Tuskegee study. After several letters to Dr. Brown, the Director of Venereal Diseases at the time, the Centers for Disease Control and Prevention convened a panel in 1969 to review the study. The panel decided not to treat the Tuskegee Syphilis Study participants and to permit the Tuskegee study to continue (Thomas & Quinn, 1991). The Tuskegee study ended in 1972 only after Buxtun reported the study and his concerns to the Associated Press. It then appeared as the front-page story in the *Washington Star* on July 25, 1972. A second newspaper, the *New York Times*, followed with a full-page story the next day.

The final tragedy of this study involves more than deception and the deliberate withholding of lifesaving health care for study participants. The study may have caused physical harm to the participants' spouses and unborn children. Due to imprecise study protocol, it was impossible to ensure that all participants were diagnosed with latent syphilis – a less contagious stage of the disease. In essence, it is likely that many of the participants exposed and perhaps infected their spouses, their in utero children, or both to the disease (Hammonds, 1994).

In retrospect, we should ask the following questions about the Tuskegee study. How could this abuse happen, and who let it happen? Two factors contributed to this abuse: placing the quest for knowledge above the well-being of human subject participants and failing to regulate and monitor the conduct of research involving human subjects.

Who let this happen? Society and the community at large contributed to this outcome. The list of agencies and individuals who recruited people for the study demonstrates that such abuses require cooperation from many individuals. The responsibility was shared by individuals, communities, religious leaders, and government institutions. However, the greatest responsibility lies with those with full knowledge of the design and purpose of the study.

Dr. John Heller, the Director of Venereal Diseases at the U.S. Public Health Service from 1943 to 1948, rationalized the deception employed by members of the Tuskegee study research team by stating that "the [study participants'] status did not warrant ethical debate. *They were subjects, not patient[s], clinical material, not sick people*" (italics added; Jones, 1981). The Tuskegee study was terminated 40 years later in 1972, four years after the U.S. Civil Rights Act of 1968, when it was brought to the attention of the public through a newspaper article in the *Washington Star* and other publications, thereby provoking a public outcry (Jones, 1981; Thomas & Quinn, 1991).

The Tuskegee experiment was not the first use of human subjects as "clinical material, not . . . people." Medical records in the U.S. document smaller-scale yet no less disturbing abuses of individual rights in the name of research in the early to mid-1800s. For example, in Georgia in the early 1800s, a physician, Thomas Hamilton, conducted tests on African slaves in the U.S. to find a treatment for heatstroke (Boney, 1967). In one series of experiments, Hamilton placed a stool in a pit approximately three feet deep. He sat one of his slaves on this stool, naked, such that only his head was above ground. Hamilton then fed the slave different medications to test treatments for heatstroke (Boney, 1967).

During this same period, another physician, James Marion Sims, a pioneer in the field of gynecology, experimented on slaves by performing over 30 operations to develop a procedure for repairing vesicovaginal fistulas, an abnormal connection between a woman's vagina and the bladder. Each operation was done without the benefit of anesthesia, although anesthesia was widely available.

In retrospect, it seems obvious that the Tuskegee study and the lesser-known medical experiments placed scientific curiosity above the well-being of humans. They exposed all participants to serious risks, including death. If we are able to recognize the risks and danger to "study participants," you might ask why others failed to recognize the same. We will allow other authors to undertake a thorough analysis of that question! But interestingly, in 1946, midway through the Tuskegee experiment, abuse of human subjects in the name of science was brought to the attention of several national and international organizations.

The Nuremberg Code of 1947

Attention to the abuse of human subjects was prompted by discoveries at the end of World War II. Military personnel from the U.S. and Western European countries released survivors, largely Jews, from concentration camps run by the Third Reich, the ruling government in Germany at the time. The military, largely U.S. and Allied forces that liberated the camps, learned that many detainees of the camps were used as subjects in medical experiments in the name of science. The experiments included studies on procedures to change eye color by injecting chemicals into eye sockets, forced sterilization, and the effects of starvation on the lives of "volunteers," among others. When the experiments were revealed to the world, a U.S. military tribunal convened an international court known as the Nuremberg trials.

THE NUREMBERG TRIALS AND OUTCOMES One purpose of the Nuremberg trials was to hold the doctors and other persons responsible for conducting such research. One outcome of the Nuremberg trials was the *Nuremberg Code* of 1947, a list of ten conditions that regulated the use of human subjects in research (National Institute of Health [NIH], 2004; see Box 2.5). The Nuremberg Code was the first formal document defining the rules of conduct for research involving human subjects. Later, the Nuremberg Code was incorporated into the Declaration of Human Rights, a document developed and approved by the 51 original signers of the Charter of the United Nations. In 1964, the World Medical Society broadened the scope of the Nuremberg Code and the Declaration of Human Rights by adopting the *Declaration of Helsinki*: *Recommendations Guiding Medical Doctors in Biomedical Research Involving Human Subjects*. The documents have been revised several times, most recently in 2013 (World Medical Association, 2024).

Box 2.5 The Nuremberg Code of 1947

1. The voluntary consent of the human subject is absolutely essential. This means that the person involved should have legal capacity to give consent; should be so situated as to be able to exercise free power of choice, without the intervention of any element of force, fraud, deceit, duress, over-reaching, or other ulterior form of constraint or coercion; and should have sufficient knowledge and comprehension of the elements of the subject matter involved as to enable him to make an understanding and enlightened decision. This latter element requires that before the acceptance of an affirmative decision by the experimental subject there should be made known to him the nature, duration, and purpose of the experiment; the method and means by which it is to be conducted; all

inconveniences and hazards reasonable to be expected; and the effects upon his health or person which may possibly come from his participation in the experiment. The duty and responsibility for ascertaining the quality of the consent rests upon each individual who initiates, directs, or engages in the experiment. It is a personal duty and responsibility which may not be delegated to another with impunity.

2. The experiment should be such as to yield fruitful results for the good of society, unprocurable by other methods or means of study, and not random and unnecessary in nature.

3. The experiment should be so designed and based on the results of animal experimentation and a knowledge of the natural history of the disease or other problem under study that the anticipated results will justify the performance of the experiment.

4. The experiment should be so conducted as to avoid all unnecessary physical and mental suffering and injury.

5. No experiment should be conducted where there is an a priori reason to believe that death or disabling injury will occur; except, perhaps, in those experiments where the experimental physicians also serve as subjects.

6. The degree of risk to be taken should never exceed that determined by the humanitarian importance of the problem to be solved by the experiment.

7. Proper preparations should be made, and adequate facilities provided to protect the experimental subject against even remote possibilities of injury, disability, or death.

8. The experiment should be conducted only by scientifically qualified persons. The highest degree of skill and care should be required through all stages of the experiment of those who conduct or engage in the experiment.

9. During the course of the experiment the human subject should be at liberty to bring the experiment to an end if he has reached the physical or mental state where continuation of the experiment seems to him to be impossible.

10. During the course of the experiment the scientist in charge must be prepared to terminate the experiment at any stage, if he has probable cause to believe, in the exercise of the good faith, superior skill, and careful judgment required of him that a continuation of the experiment is likely to result in injury, disability, or death to the experimental subject.

Source: Retrieved from the U.S. Department of Health and Human Services, Office of Human Subjects Research, National Institute of Health (www.hhs.gov/ohrp/archive/nurcode.html).

In 1953, to monitor research in the U.S. involving human subjects, the U.S. National Institutes of Health (NIH) established an Institutional Review Board (IRB). The IRB is a system of national and local research review boards responsible for ensuring the protection of human subjects participating in research studies. The NIH defines research as "any systematic investigation designed to develop or contribute to generalizable knowledge", and "human subjects" are defined as living individuals from whom researchers propose to obtain information (data) through intervention with the person (National Institutes of Health, 2004).

The American Psychological Association (APA) joined the efforts to protect the rights of research volunteers by establishing codes of ethical standards for psychologists. The 1958 version of the APA standards for ethical behaviors for psychologists cautioned that conducting research with serious after-effects is possible only when the participant or someone authorized to speak on that person's behalf is fully informed (Committee on Ethical Standards of Psychologists, 1958). A revised code of conduct added that psychology researchers were required to show respect for the rights and dignity of individuals, concern for others' welfare, and social responsibility to human subjects in experiments (American Psychological Association, 1992). While the guidelines are not legally binding, they are enforceable by the APA and, if breached, can lead to loss of membership.

In spite of the guidelines, occasionally a study is conducted that does not adhere to the rules. The New York State Psychiatric Institute study on depression in Parkinson's disease is one example. Another is the Zimbardo Stanford prison experiment.

Study of Interpersonal Dynamics (Stanford Prison Experiment)

As early as 1964, over 51 countries, including the U.S., endorsed the code of conduct for use of human subjects in research. But in 1971, Philip Zimbardo designed a two-week study on interpersonal dynamics (Haney, Banks, & Zimbardo, 1973; Zimbardo, 1973) and sought to determine whether social contexts can influence, alter, shape, or transform human behavior (Haney & Zimbardo, 1998). Zimbardo intended to contribute to the then current research by examining the role of institutional environments on a person's behavior (see Box 2.6).

Box 2.6 The Social Power of Groups and Conformity: The Stanford Prison Experiment

Picture this scenario: A group of college students volunteer for a two-week research study exploring the effects of social contexts on human behaviors. The study takes place in a mock prison. Half of the students are randomly assigned to play the role of prison warden, and the other half are assigned the role of prisoner. The prisoners live in a mock prison for the full two weeks while the wardens work daily eight-hour shifts for the duration of the study. The "wardens" are permitted to make up their own rules for keeping order among the prisoners with one exception: Physical abuse is not permitted. Suddenly, after only six days, the investigator ends the study. What do you think caused its abrupt halt?

Perhaps the following background information will help answer the question. In 1971, Philip Zimbardo designed a study to determine whether social contexts can influence, shape, or transform human behavior. Specifically, Zimbardo questioned whether a "bad situation" can cause otherwise "good" people to act in ways inconsistent with their usual behavior. Zimbardo's Stanford prison experiment (SPE) was to test the research question. He converted the basement of Stanford's Psychology Department into a mock prison. He then recruited 24 male Stanford University students to participate in the study. All students were screened to ensure they were physically and psychologically healthy with no history of criminal behavior. Zimbardo wanted to ensure that all participants were, in fact, "good" people (Zimbardo, 2007). After the screening, the 24 participants were randomly assigned one of two roles, prison warden or prisoner. Zimbardo played the role of the prison supervisor.

To make the experiment as realistic as possible, Zimbardo arranged for the participants assigned to the prisoner group to be "arrested" by the Palo Alto police department and brought to the mock prison at Stanford at the beginning of the study. The "prisoners" were processed using some of the same procedures used in an actual prison. They were given identity numbers, stripped naked, and deloused (Zimbardo, 2007).

Unexpectedly, on the second day of the experiment, the prisoners staged an unplanned rebellion. The prison wardens, determined to end the rebellion, chose to deal harshly with the "dangerous prisoners." Within four days, prison wardens were observed becoming verbally and psychologically abusive toward the prisoners. For example, some wardens punished the prisoners by chaining their legs, repeatedly disrupting prisoners' sleep at night, and making prisoners engage in humiliating activities billed as "fun and games" (Zimbardo, 2007).

By the fifth day of the experiment, five of the student prisoners were allowed to end their participation because they suffered from extreme stress. In actuality, all prisoners had experienced psychological stress, trauma, and emotional breakdowns. The prisoners' changed emotional states were evident in their attitudes and demeanors. They became very compliant to the warden's hostile and abusive treatment.

Does this additional information provide clues that explain the abrupt termination of the study? There is one additional point. Zimbardo, the investigator and prison superintendent, initially did not realize the impact of the situation on the prisoners and the wardens. In fact, Zimbardo candidly confessed that he, along with visitors to the study while it was in progress, including colleagues, parents of the "imprisoned" college students, and a prison chaplain, did not question the impact of the study or the effect of the study on the student prisoners. So why did Zimbardo terminate the experiment?

Zimbardo credits a close friend who also visited the prison as the person who identified the study's dangers. After reviewing the friend's comments, Zimbardo realized that the mock prison environment had a profound effect on all participants, an impact far greater than either he or his colleagues imagined. In just six days, a mock prison environment converted the 24 Stanford students into either hostile and abusive wardens or submissive, compliant, and stressed prisoners. The impetus for the change was the prisoners' rebellion, an act perceived by the wardens as a threat to their authority. Their response was an excessive use of power to dominate and suppress the powerless – in this case, the prisoners.

Zimbardo's study found that a "bad" environment can have a profound impact on individuals. Even Zimbardo was affected. His inability to see the destructive effect of the mock prison setting on both groups of study participants was due, in part, to his role as the prison superintendent. The role conflicted with the investigator's responsibility to uphold the ethical standards of research.

The results of Zimbardo's study were indeed shocking. Yet the investigator's decision to end the study as well as his candid assessment of the dangers posed by his work serves as an example of the ethical standards of researchers. Zimbardo did not intend to cause psychological injury to his study participants. But when the injuries became apparent to him, he terminated the study. Today, Institutional Review Boards (IRBs) would not permit such a study. In the absence of IRBs, however, Zimbardo's actions are commendable.

Briefly, 24 male Stanford University students volunteered to participate in Zimbardo's experiment. They were randomly assigned to one of two roles: prison warden or prisoner. Prisoners were assigned to live in a mock prison for two weeks, while wardens worked eight-hour shifts "guarding" the prisoners for the duration of the study. The two-week study was terminated after only six days due to the prisoners' demonstrable and extreme psychological trauma and the increasingly hostile and abusive behavior of the wardens. Box 2.6 provides more detail.

Zimbardo answered his own research question in just six days. "Bad" social contexts or environments can alter the behavior of otherwise "good" people and, apparently, quicker than he thought. How is it possible that two questionable studies, one ongoing (Tuskegee) and another just beginning (Zimbardo), were conducted at the same time that the world was enacting regulations for the ethical conduct of research with human subjects? There are two possible explanations. First, the Zimbardo study was a social psychological study. Specifically, Zimbardo examined the effect of conformity expectations on people in institutional settings. The intent of the research and its design did not initially raise concerns about the potential harm to research participants, perhaps because there were few if any perceived risks of physical harm. In addition, some contend that Zimbardo's study was relevant to understanding human behavior given the events of World War II and the atrocities performed in the concentration camps. His study appeared to suggest that individuals may come to perform hostile or abusive behaviors when placed in a social context that permits or encourages such behaviors.

The rationale for continuing the Tuskegee study for decades after the adoption of the Nuremberg Code is less clear but may be linked to the U.S. regulations. Although the NIH established policies for the protection of human subjects in 1966, the policies were not binding. They were elevated to the status of regulations, an enforceable set of codes, only in 1974 – after the Tuskegee experiment and its abuses had been exposed nationally.

Following the public exposure of the Tuskegee experiment, the U.S. Senate Committee on Labor and Human Resources held hearings. One of the outcomes from these hearings included the "National Research Act of 1974 that required the (then) Health, Education, and Welfare Department to [formalize and regulate] its policy for the protection of human subjects to [establish] the National Commission for the Protection of Human Subjects of Biomedical and Behavioral Research."

The second outcome was the commission's final report: *The Belmont Report: Ethical Principles and Guidelines for the Protection of Human Subjects of Research*, published in 1979. The **Belmont Report** identified three fundamental, ethical principles for the protection of human subjects: *Respect for persons*, recognizing the dignity and autonomy of individuals and requiring special protection for people with diminished capacity; *beneficence,* requiring researchers to protect individuals further by maximizing the potential benefits and minimizing the potential harm or injury to them as research participants; and *justice,* requiring the fair and just treatment of participants, including the absence of bias in selection for or exclusion from research.

The new federal regulations, in addition to the Institutional Review Boards required at all major medical, academic, and other research centers, signaled the desire of the U.S. government and researchers to prevent the atrocities that occurred in Macon County, Alabama, as well as the debatable research ethics in Palo Alto, California, at Stanford University (see again Boxes 2.5 and 2.6).

To be clear, guidelines for human subjects research can be found in other countries as well. For example, the British Psychological Society's code of human subject research ethics prioritizes respect for the rights and dignity of the study participants (Oates et al., 2021). This includes: First, *respect* for the autonomy, privacy and dignity of individuals, groups and communities; second, *scientific integrity*, or a commitment to ensuring that their research is of a high scientific and scholarly standard, and to be accountable to this standard; and finally, *social responsibility,* aiming to generate knowledge that can contribute to the "common good" and supports and reflects respect for the dignity of individuals (Oates et al., 2021).

It is tempting to conclude here with the hope that no other abuses have been or will be committed post-Tuskegee or the Stanford prison experiment. Unfortunately, in 1993, then U.S. Energy Secretary Hazel O'Leary discovered, in the Energy Department archives, records of U.S. government experiments involving the use of radiation on U.S. residents from 1945 through the early 1980s (Tisdall, 1993). Ms. O'Leary noted that due to a "culture of deception" these activities remained hidden in files. The experiments included over 200 underground nuclear tests conducted in the U.S. between 1963 and 1990. Eighteen of these experiments occurred during the 1980s. While the records confirm the tests, no information is available at present that explains the reasons for the tests or the need for secrecy (Tisdall, 1993).

The main point here is that research abuses demonstrate the need to establish regulations and regulatory bodies that protect the health and well-being of study participants. Today, the vast majority of research studies are safe. Federal, state, and local regulations concerning the use of human subjects are effective in preventing research that may cause harm to study participants. It is true, however, that on rare occasions studies that are not in compliance with the regulations do take place. Yet, as we noted previously, many good and ethical studies are conducted and contribute to our understanding of health-enhancing and health-promoting behaviors. Therefore, at the conclusion of this chapter, we suggest ways to ensure that you can participate safely in research studies, should you desire to do so.

Research without Informed Consent

Does the title of this section seem confusing? We reviewed several extreme examples of abuses in research with human subjects, some of which pertained to the conduct of research on individuals without their informed consent. In fact, we just reviewed a number of regulations and codes that specified the need for informed consent. What is left to say?

The World Medical Association (WMA) in 1964 (revised as of 2013) stated that research is permissible on individuals from whom it is not possible to obtain consent *only if* the physical or mental condition that prevents research subjects from giving informed consent is a necessary characteristic of the research population (World Medical Association, 2013). In essence, the WMA states that, in limited instances, research on persons who are unconscious or have ***diminished mental capacity***, here meaning individuals who are unable to understand the research design and to give consent responsibly, is permissible if the persons' condition is due to their medical or mental illness and is a qualifying condition (eligibility criterion) for the study population. For example, when suffering a cardiac arrest – not a heart attack – a person instantly becomes unconscious. If researchers developed a drug to reverse the almost always fatal outcomes of cardiac arrests, they would not have an opportunity to obtain the consent of an unconscious cardiac arrest patient, someone who in this case is also a potential study participant, before testing the drug's effectiveness in reversing the fatal effects of a cardiac arrest. Emergency medical research on incapacitated persons is one example of a potentially lifesaving technique that must be tested on an eligible individual without his or her consent. To this end, the WMA developed broad guidelines for the conduct of this type of emergency medical or mental health research. Individual countries are expected to provide more specific regulations for the conduct of such research in their countries.

To that end, in 1996, the U.S. established new regulations that state that emergency medical research may be conducted without informed consent if all of the following conditions have been met: The patient is experiencing a life-threatening condition for which existing treatments are deemed either unsatisfactory or unproved; further evidence is needed to determine an experimental treatment's safety or efficacy; the participant is incapable of consent due to his or her medical condition; intervention is necessary before an authorized representative can be consulted; and researchers have observed a number of special protections including "community consultation" (Schmidt, Delorio, & McClure, 2006). Many of these conditions can be demonstrated easily. The condition of "community consultation," however, is more problematic because the definition of "community" and its role and authority in decision-making is a hotly debated proposition (Ragin et al., 2008).

Summary

National and international research studies have exposed a host of problems relating to the ethical conduct of research. Many of the problems have been addressed through the establishment of regulatory bodies, such as Institutional Review Boards, the National Commission for the Protection of Human Subjects of Biomedical and Behavioral Research, and the World Medical Association of the World Health Organization. Regulations including the Nuremberg Code, *The Belmont Report: Ethical Principles and Guidelines for the Protection of Human Subjects of Research*, The British Psychological Society's Code of Human Research Ethics, and U.S. federal regulations governing *research without informed consent* also were devised to guard against the abuse of human subjects. These governing bodies and regulations are effective but not fail proof, as we have seen. Therefore, the responsibility for the ethical conduct of research begins with the researcher.

Personal Postscript

RESEARCH STUDY NEEDS VOLUNTEERS: SHOULD YOU VOLUNTEER?

The next time you see a notice asking for volunteers for a study, you might hesitate. After reading this chapter and learning about the Tuskegee study, Zimbardo's social contexts and human behavior, the Johns Hopkins and the New York State Psychiatric Institute studies, not to mention the U.S. radiation experiments and other abuses, you might wonder whether it is safe to participate.

While there is some risk involved in all experiments, the vast majority of studies pose little physical or psychological risks to participants. This chapter highlighted four studies that entailed risk to the participants. But when considering the total number of studies conducted each year, it becomes clear that such risks are rare. Nevertheless, there are some precautions every potential study participant should take before agreeing to volunteer for any study.

First, be sure to read the informed consent form carefully. The consent form should explain in clear terms the activities required of each participant, as well as the risks and benefits of participating.

Second, be sure to ask questions if anything is unclear. The researcher is responsible for ensuring that all study participants understand the information presented in the consent form as well as the tasks to be performed.

Third, sign the consent form only if you understand the tasks involved and have had a chance to ask any questions you have about the study.

Fourth, insist on receiving a copy of the consent form. The experimenter should provide this automatically; but if the experimenter does not, remember to request a copy.

Fifth, study participants may discontinue their involvement *at any time* and *for any reason*. This too should be written in the consent form because it is a right of all study participants, regardless of the nature of the study.

Finally, if interested, request a copy of the results of the study when they are available. Researchers rarely share the raw data but can make available summaries of the main findings. Be patient, though. It may take several months or even years before results are ready and can be disseminated to the public.

Participating in a research study can be fun and informative, but do follow the steps outlined earlier for your protection.

If, on the other hand, you are the investigator and not the subject, be sure to follow these important steps as well as others as indicated by the OHRP and your local IRB. The safety of your participants could be in your hands.

Questions to Consider

1. Conducting research without informed consent is controversial in some research circles. What are the problems inherent in such an approach?
2. Why is "the absence of bias in selection for or exclusion from research studies" a problem even now when conducting research?
3. The rush to develop and distribute to the public a safe COVID-19 vaccine illustrated one of the difficulties scientists encounter when developing a potentially lifesaving vaccine using randomized clinically controlled study protocol. Explain the rationale for and against this research design when testing lifesaving medications.

True or False Questions

1. The Stanford Study of Interpersonal Dynamics was the last known example of a violation of ethical research standards in the U.S. True or False.
2. African American's mistrust of research is based on the effects of slavery in the U.S. True or False.
3. The five classic indicators of health are: incidence, prevalence, relative risk, distal, and mortality. True or False.
4. When comparing infant death across countries the preferred measure is raw data. True or False.
5. Interviews, when used in research studies, only yield qualitative data. True or False.

Important Terms

adverse event   29
atrial septal defect   39
baseline measure   49
Belmont Report   59
British Psychological Society's Code of Human Research Ethics   61
case study   41
cause-and-effect relationship   43

CHAPTER 3

Theories and Models of Health Behavior Change

Chapter Outline

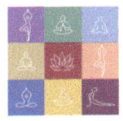

Source: 3xy/
Shutterstock.

Chapter Objectives

After studying this chapter, you will be able to:

1. Accurately define *expectancy value theory, social cognitive theory, the theory of planned behavior, health belief model,* and *the transtheoretical model of behavior change.*

2. Name and describe the key concepts of each theory and model.

3. Identify one contribution of each theory and model to understanding human health behavior.

4. Define social marketing.

5. Explain the four *P*s of marketing and their role in shaping behaviors.

6. Identify the five components of the social ecological model.

7. Describe the factors that limit access to health care.

8. Explain the effects of limited access to care on individual health outcomes.

9. Explain the goal of health policy initiatives for individual health behaviors.

DOI: 10.4324/9781003300670-3

OPENING STORY: EDDIE'S DILEMMA

Eddie is a 28-year-old single man who began smoking when he was 13 years old. He wanted to look mature like his older brother, who also began smoking as a teenager.

Eddie now smokes 20 to 30 cigarettes a day. He calls himself a "social smoker" because he smokes with his friends either after work or at social events. Recently he met Sarah, someone whose company he really enjoys. Sarah does not smoke. In fact, she detests the smell of cigarettes. After months of encouragement from Sarah, Eddie decided to stop smoking. On New Year's Day, Eddie threw away all the cigarette packs in his home and car.

For 11 days, Eddie managed without a cigarette. On the 12th day, he attended a birthday party for a friend. Many of his friends from work were at the party. When one friend offered Eddie a cigarette, Eddie accepted without hesitation and continued smoking ever since.

On occasion, Eddie tells himself he should stop smoking. Perhaps it is more accurate to say that Sarah tells him he should stop smoking. But he quickly dismisses the suggestion when he remembers his attempts to stop on New Year's Day. He remembers feeling fidgety and irritable on the fourth day without cigarettes. He dreads the thought of experiencing withdrawal symptoms once again, symptoms that were a sign that Eddie was physically addicted to cigarettes. In addition, he recalls the daily struggles to resist the temptation to smoke when his other friends who smoke were with him. He especially disliked their constant criticism of his efforts to quit.

Eddie's friends do not understand his desire to stop smoking and think that Sarah is being unreasonable when she makes Eddie choose between smoking and spending time with her. Unlike Sarah, they are not supportive of Eddie's efforts to change behaviors. Eddie commented recently to one friend that he feels like a yo-yo: Sarah pressures him to stop smoking while his other friends entice him to smoke.

Sarah understands his dilemma, but she is growing increasingly intolerant of Eddie's smoking habit. She never thought she would have a close relationship with a smoker and questions whether she can continue even now.

Now what? What if you were Eddie? What factors would support or undermine your efforts to quit smoking? ∎

The opening story identifies several social factors that influence Eddie's smoking behaviors. Without a doubt, friends, peer groups, and family all influence individual health behaviors (East, McNeill, Thrasher, & Hitchman, 2021; Elkington, Bauermeister, & Zimmerman, 2011; NHTSA, 2012a). But our behaviors are also shaped by other factors, including our attitudes, our knowledge of the health consequences of our behaviors, our environment, and our access to health care.

A number of theories and models in psychology explain human behavior. Some are designed specifically to identify factors that explain or predict health behaviors, whereas others are intended to explain general behaviors. In this chapter, we will examine five theories or models employed by health psychologists to explain a range of health behaviors: the expectancy value theory (EVT), the theory of planned behavior (TPB), the health belief model (HBM), social cognitive theory (SCT), and the transtheoretical model of behavior change (TTM). The EVT, the TPB, and the SCT were developed originally to explain general human behavior. They have been adapted for use in health psychology to explain healthy behaviors. Others, including the HBM and the TTM, were developed specifically as health behavior models. We will also examine a technique called social marketing which, although not a model, has been found to influence actions including health behaviors. Finally, consistent with the research in this field, we will explore blended models, a combination of several models designed to improve our ability to explain or predict health activities.

By the end of Section I, you will be able to describe five theories or models used frequently in health psychology to explain health behaviors. Section II introduces social marketing and its contribution to promoting behavior change. By the end of that section, you will be able to define and explain social marketing and its contribution to shaping an individual's or a group's health actions. You also will be able to describe blended models.

In Section III, we discuss a social ecological approach to health (See Chapter 1, An Interdisciplinary View of Health) by explaining the relative contributions of the individual, cultural or social networks, environment, health systems, and health policy on individual health outcomes. By the end of the section, you will be able to give examples of how each of these factors contributes to a person's health status. Finally, Section IV concludes the chapter with a discussion of the challenges to sustaining healthy behaviors.

While reading this chapter, you will want to remember one thing: The theories and models included were developed and tested primarily in developed countries. Their usefulness as global theories or as universal models of health behaviors is still being explored.

SECTION I. THEORIES AND MODELS OF HEALTH BEHAVIOR CHANGE

Expectancy Value Theory (EVT)

Fishbein's *expectancy value theory (EVT)* is one of three theories originally developed to explain human behavior. Health psychologists later adapted the EVT to explain health behaviors. The EVT states that two forces motivate behavior: the anticipated or expected outcome of the behavior and the value assigned to the outcome (Fishbein & Ajzen, 1975).

According to the EVT (see Table 3.1), every behavior has a consequence. Individuals anticipate these consequences and assign a positive or negative value to the outcome. The anticipated consequence of a behavior and the value assigned to it are based on an individual's past experiences with the behavior and its results. These experiences influence the decision to engage or not to engage in similar behaviors in the future (Borders, 2004; DelBocca, Darkes, Goldman, & Smith, 2002). In essence, the EVT describes a cognitive process whereby individuals assess their behaviors and evaluate the consequences based on the values they assign to the consequences.

We can examine the EVT using Eddie as a test case. In the opening story, Eddie is evaluating his smoking behavior and the consequence of smoking based on the value that he assigns to the consequence. Initially, Eddie enjoys smoking, especially "social smoking." Thus, he assigns a positive value to smoking. Based on this information, the EVT might predict that Eddie would continue smoking.

We see from the story, however, that Eddie's decision about smoking is not quite that simple. There are two additional factors that influence Eddie's smoking behavior: his peer groups and their views on smoking. Unfortunately, the EVT is designed to explain only one behavior. EVT can explain Eddie's smoking

TABLE 3.1 Theories and Models of Behavior Change

Author	Theory/Model	Defining Features	Limitations
Fishbein and Ajzen (1975)	Expectancy value theory (EVT)	Two forces motivate behavior: • Anticipated/expected outcome • Value assigned to outcome	Cannot explain effects of multiple factors on behavior
Bandura (1977)	Social cognitive theory	Individuals learn from cognitive assessment and consequences of behavior using four cues: • Direct experiences • Vicarious experiences • Persuasory learning • Inferred learning Self-efficacy is critical to learning	Reciprocal determinism (RD): • Behavior viewed in context of environmental factors, personal factors, and behaviors No way to test RD
Ajzen and Fishbein (1980)	Theory of reasoned action	Behaviors determined by intentions Intentions influenced by two factors: • Attitudes about behavior • Subjective norms	Cannot explain spontaneous, involuntary, habitual behaviors
Ajzen (1985)	Theory of planned behavior	Behaviors determined by intentions Intentions influenced by three factors: • Attitudes about behavior • Subjective norms • Perceived behavioral control	Self-efficacy (perceived behavioral control) strongest predictor of behaviors Does not explain spontaneous or habitual behaviors
Rosenstock, Strecher, and Becker (1988)	Health belief model	Motivational factors that influence health behaviors and health care seeking are: • Perceived severity • Perceived susceptibility • Perceived benefits • Perceived barriers Self-efficacy added as fifth factor	Self-efficacy accounts for many behavioral outcomes
Prochaska and DiClemente (1983)	Transtheoretical model of behavioral change	Change is a process that includes: • Precontemplation • Contemplation • Preparation for action • Action • Maintenance Recidivism explains setbacks	Fails to weigh effects of factors other than individual in process of change

behavior independent of group influences, but it cannot evaluate the effects of the second factor, peer groups, on the target behavior (Borders, 2004). As we indicated earlier, social influences affect behaviors, and these, too, must be considered.

Because the EVT cannot account for the effects of peer groups on Eddie's smoking behavior, it similarly cannot explain the impact of the negative or positive values of the group on Eddie's behaviors (Williams, Anderson, & Winett, 2005). For Eddie, there are negative outcomes associated with smoking and negative outcomes associated with not smoking. The outcomes are rooted in the values of each of the peer groups. For example, Sarah detests smoking. Therefore, one negative outcome associated with smoking is the loss of Sarah's company. On the other hand, Eddie's other friends enjoy smoking. Those friends represent a negative outcome associated with not smoking.

The EVT's inability to account for more than one factor that also influences behavior is a limitation of the theory. To address this limitation, Herrnstein (1970) and later Borders (2004) proposed adding the concept of matching law to EVT. The *matching law* states that decisions to engage in a specific behavior are influenced, in part, by reinforcements for the intended behavior as well as reinforcements for alternate behaviors (Herrnstein, 1961). If the reinforcement for an alternate behavior is greater than the reinforcement for the intended behavior, then the likelihood is greater that an individual will perform the alternate behavior.

How could EVT with matching law explain Eddie's behavior? Consider this: Eddie's intended behavior is smoking. One alternate behavior is spending time with Sarah. The reinforcement for spending time with Sarah is that Eddie enjoys her company. If Eddie determines that the reinforcement he feels from time with Sarah outweighs the reinforcement from smoking, then, according to the EVT with matching law, he will choose the alternate behavior, spending time with Sarah.

Research studies often test the explanatory power of theories. Their results are used either to support or to refute the theory in whole or in part. Research testing the EVT has produced findings that do both. For example, Finch and colleagues (2005) tested the EVT's ability to explain weight loss. They tested whether highly favorable outcome expectations would promote weight loss. Using a randomized clinical trial design (see Chapter 2, Research Methods) with 349 largely white (89.1%), female (86.7%) participants, Finch and colleagues (2005) found that positive expectations alone were not sufficient to predict weight loss. While Shang, Moss, and Chen's (2023) meta-analysis of 31 studies examining the EVT's ability to predict other health behaviors, such as physical activity, suggests support for the theory, other work suggests that the cost factor of behaviors, independent of expectancy and values, is critical when assessing this theory's relevance to students (Flake, Barron, Hulleman, McCoach, & Welsh, 2015).

Specific concepts introduced by the EVT theory have been incorporated into other models (Bandura, 1977; Fishbein & Ajzen, 1975). For example, *social learning theory* and the *theory of planned behavior* include values and expected outcomes as determinants of an individual's intention to engage in specific behaviors (Bandura, 1977; Fishbein & Ajzen, 1975). In essence, while there may remain some questions concerning whether EVT with matching law adequately explains behaviors, researchers generally accept that some concepts included in EVT are important determinants and should be integrated into other theories.

Social Cognitive Theory (SCT)

LEARNING PROCESSES Albert Bandura's *social cognitive theory (SCT)*, originally the *social learning theory*) proposes that cognitive processes are critical to the acquisition and regulation of behaviors (Bandura, 1977). Bandura contends that individuals learn from the consequences of their behaviors. He calls this concept *learned behavioral consequences*. Consequences are communicated through "response information" cues that are acquired in one of four ways. First, information can be acquired through *direct experiences*, that is, an individual engaging in a behavior that results in a specific behavioral outcome. For example, a person who touches a hot stove and withdraws their hand in pain will learn through direct experience that a hot stove causes pain. The experience of touching a hot stove resulted in a negative association. The behavior of touching the stove, together with the negative outcome conveys information to the person about the behavior. By linking behaviors with informational cues, Bandura links direct learning with our cognitive process. The pairing occurs as a conscious effort by the actor. It is not automatic.

Information also comes in the form of *vicarious experiences*. Here, Bandura suggests that learning can occur as a result of observing the outcomes of another individual. We will return to our example of touching a hot stove. In a vicarious experience, we may witness someone else touching a stove that we know to be hot. We may see the other person withdraw his or her hand quickly from the stove and cry out in pain. We learn through the other person's experience that the hot stove causes pain. There is no need to repeat the same act to determine the outcome. Like direct experiences, vicarious experiences also require cognition because the person observing the behavior deduces that similar behavioral outcomes would accrue to him or her if engaging in the same behavior.

Persuasory learning is the learning that occurs from the judgments expressed by others about specific behaviors. Persuasory learning requires no action on anyone's part. It is a wholly cognitive learning process. We may not ever witness the behavioral outcomes, yet we acknowledge and accept them as valid based on the credibility and/or authority of those rendering the judgment. For example, we may never experience, or see firsthand, lung cancer that resulted from long-term smoking behavior, but we credit the judgment of the experts who tell us that lung cancer is a possible outcome of smoking.

Finally, *inferred learning* is learning derived from a person's own knowledge. The application of logic or rules allows an individual to posit an outcome without having to engage in the act. As with persuasory learning, inferred learning requires no action. Rather, our cognitive process of deduction allows us to derive a set of probable behaviors and their corresponding outcomes based on our knowledge of both the behaviors and our application of rules.

SELF-EFFICACY Self-efficacy is a fifth and critical component of Bandura's theory. *Self-efficacy* is defined as a person's conviction that his or her actions will produce the expected outcomes. It is related to the concept of outcome expectancies. While the term *outcome expectancies* refers to our expectation of positive or negative results owing to our performance (Williams et al., 2005), self-efficacy characterizes our judgment about our ability to perform a specific task. According to Bandura, our strong belief in our ability to perform a behavior will increase the probability of performing the behavior. Conversely, serious doubts about the ability to perform a specific behavior will almost certainly result in the behavior not occurring. Bandura contends that efficacy expectations vary on three dimensions: magnitude, referring to the level of difficulty; generality, pertaining to the level of mastery needed to accomplish a specific task; and strength, here meaning strength of the expectation, which will be weak or strong (Bandura, 1977).

Does self-efficacy help explain Eddie's behaviors in the opening story? It may be difficult to determine based on the information presented. Initially, Eddie's self-efficacy about ending his smoking habit was high, as evidenced by the fact that he attempted to stop and successfully stopped smoking for 11 days. In the story, Eddie's reluctance to try to stop smoking for a second time is attributed to the negative sensations of nicotine withdrawal and the negative reinforcement of his close friends. It is also possible that Eddie now perceives the task as very difficult, a perception that may lower his overall self-efficacy to try again to quit. Eddie is aware that he failed to stop smoking once before and may believe that he lacks the level of mastery needed to accomplish his goal.

The self-efficacy concept in Bandura's SCT is compelling and appears to be an important factor in determining behaviors. It has been used in a number of studies that report strong correlations between self-efficacy and behavioral outcomes. For example, Shiaw-Ling, Charron-Prochownik, Sereika, Siminerio, and Yookyung (2006) tested three theories to determine which best predicted the reproductive health intentions of adolescent diabetic women. They found self-efficacy to be one of the best predictors of intention to use birth control. Alyahya, Al-Sheyab, Alqudah, Younis, and Khader (2021) found that targeting self-efficacy also increased study participants' beliefs about and initiation of physical activities among people with Type 2 diabetes.

RECIPROCAL DETERMINISM Overall, Bandura's theory offers an interesting approach to understanding human behaviors and specifically health behaviors. The principal problem with Bandura's SCT is the inability to test a concept he calls *reciprocal determinism*. Another key concept, reciprocal determinism, states that behavior must be viewed in the context of environmental events (*E*) and personal factors (*P*) that influence behaviors (*B;* Kohler, Grimley, & Reynolds, 1999). Bandura proposes that each of these variables interact significantly with the other two. Specifically, environmental events influence personal factors; likewise, personal factors can and do influence environmental events. Similarly, personal factors influence behaviors, and reciprocally, behaviors influence personal factors. Finally, behaviors influence environmental events and vice versa. Unfortunately, the simultaneous interaction of all three variables makes it almost impossible to isolate one of the variables, such as the environment, to test its effect on the other two.

In essence, the social cognitive theory of behavior is compelling conceptually but difficult to test. On the other hand, the concept of self-efficacy, which has been supported in subsequent research and included in many theories and models of health behaviors, can be tested. It appears to be central to behavioral outcomes.

Theory of Planned Behavior (TPB)

The *theory of planned behavior (TPB)* proposed by Ajzen (1985) builds on an earlier theory known as the *theory of reasoned action (TRA)* (Ajzen & Fishbein, 1980). We include a brief review of TRA because it is the foundation for TPB and because some studies continue to test the predictive validity of TRA.

THEORY OF REASONED ACTION Briefly, TRA states that an individual's behavior is determined by his or her intentions. Intentions, however, are influenced by two factors: attitudes about the behavior and subjective norms. The TRA does not suggest that attitudes influence subjective norms or vice versa. Rather, according to the model, attitudes and subjective norms appear to independently influence behavioral intentions, which then influence actual behaviors.

Take this as an example. Seeing a traffic light at an intersection change from green to yellow, a motorist must decide either to continue through the intersection or to slow to a stop, anticipating the red stoplight. If the motorist decides to continue without stopping at the light, then, according to TRA, that motorist's behavior is preceded by the intention to continue regardless of the changing signal. The intention is based on a belief about the likely outcome of the behavior (Madden, Ellen, & Ajzen, 1992). One likely outcome the motorist may anticipate is safe passage through the intersection.

The TRA also proposes that the behavior and the expected outcome are determined by two factors: the motorist's attitude about performing the action and the subjective norm associated with the behavior. A positive attitude about the behavior of continuing through the changing traffic light means that the motorist associates the decision to proceed with a positive outcome, such as saving time or safe passage through the light (Kohler et al., 1999). A negative attitude about proceeding might be based on an expectation of a negative outcome, such as getting a traffic ticket or having a traffic accident. Thus, a negative attitude would lead to a decision to stop at the light.

The second factor influencing both intentions and behaviors, according to TRA, is *subjective norms*. Here the authors are referring to the motorist's belief about what others would think about his or her behavior. The concern here is not what others, in general, think. What matters is the opinion of people who are important to the motorist. This might include family members, close friends, or perhaps her or his employer.

Do people really base their behaviors on the thoughts and beliefs of people close to them? Theories like TRA suggest that an individual's behavior may be shaped by the opinions of close friends or family members. But, at other times, individuals engage in behaviors that are inconsistent with the attitudes or values of their closest associates. For example, in many cases, illegal drug use or acts of theft are not supported or valued by an individual's friends. To account for behaviors that are at odds with the values and beliefs of one's social group, TRA proposes that we must consider a person's motivation to comply with the expectations of the social group. For example, if the motorist's friends think that refusing to stop when a traffic light changes to red is acceptable or even "cool," *and* if the motorist cares about the group's approval, it is likely that the motorist will adopt this behavior. If the motorist does not strongly seek the approval of the group or is not inclined to comply with the subjective norms of the group pertaining to driving through red lights, then the motorist will be less likely to adopt this behavior (Kohler et al., 1999).

SIMILARITIES BETWEEN EVT AND TRA We mentioned earlier that researchers have applied some of the concepts introduced by the expectancy value theory (EVT) to explain human behavior. A closer examination reveals similarities between the EVT and the TRA. The EVT identifies anticipated outcomes and values as determinants of human behaviors. The TRA identifies attitudes and subjective norms as the principal factors influencing behaviors. Yet attitudes and behaviors reflect values, and values are influenced, in part, by the subjective norms of an individual's peer groups.

It seems intuitive that attitudes about a behavior will affect the likelihood of performing the behavior. If we dislike a behavior, we may be less likely to repeat that act. Similarly, if our group's subjective norms are inconsistent with a specific action, we are less likely to perform that act. In many instances, a group's approval or disapproval of a person's behavior often influences that person's decisions.

Researchers continue to test the predictive validity of the TRA but, as was the case for the EVT, support for the TRA is mixed. In most instances, research supporting the TRA focuses on the ability of the theory to predict the intention to act but not the actual behavior (Poss, 2001). For example, Ross and colleagues (2007) tested the TRA's ability to explain African American men's intention to obtain information about prostate cancer. Their findings suggest that both attitudes and subjective norms were important predictors of the intention to seek information. They did not indicate whether the men actually obtained the information. Similarly, Dewi and Zein (2017) found that TRA predicted the intentions of women to do breast self-examinations. Specifically, this study suggests that women were more likely to perform breast self-examination if they believed that breast self-examination was instrumental in the early detection of breast cancer, and also believed this was a normative belief among their peer/family group. It did not indicate whether women actually performed the self-examination.

Other criticisms of the TRA include the association among subjective norms, behavioral intentions (Johnston, White, & Norman, 2004), and their effects on volitional acts, a subset of behaviors that are under a person's direct control. If, according to the TRA, intentions determine behaviors, then the theory cannot explain addictive, habitual, or involuntary behaviors. This is a major omission because addictive, habitual, and involuntary behaviors occur frequently in most humans. Think about this: Few people who engage in addictive behaviors do so to obtain the negative outcomes often associated with those behaviors. For example, smokers who are addicted to nicotine do not intend to put themselves at higher risk for lung or throat cancer. Nor do they intend to allocate ever-increasing amounts of their disposable income to sustain their habit.

Likewise, the TRA is unable to explain behaviors that are largely habitual, such as brushing one's teeth in the morning before leaving for work or school or other hygiene habits that are done without prior thought. Spontaneous behaviors also cannot be explained using this theory because intent assumes some level of thought and purposefulness, which is, by definition, the opposite of spontaneity.

THEORY OF PLANNED BEHAVIOR To address these omissions, Ajzen proposed the theory of planned behaviors (TPB). The TPB includes the concept of *perceived behavioral control* (Ajzen & Madden, 1986) to account for nonvolitional actions. The TPB suggests that peoples' belief that they possess the resources and the opportunities needed to perform a behavior is directly related to their perceived control over their behavior. The greater the perceived behavioral control, the greater the likelihood that the behavior will be performed. Note here that like the theory of reasoned action, which suggests that attitudes and subjective norms independently influence behavioral intentions, the TPB similarly suggests that attitudes, subjective norms, and now perceived behavioral control all independently influence behavioral intentions and ultimately influence one's actual behavior.

The concept of perceived behavioral control presented here is quite similar to Bandura's concept of self-efficacy, that is, the belief that one has the ability to achieve the intended behavior. Some research that tests the TPB suggests that the revised theory does indeed predict both intentions and adherence to new health behaviors. For example, in a study of adherence to treatment regiments for diabetes and hypertension among South Africans residing in a rural region called the Western Cape, the TPB variables of attitude, perceived behavior control, and subjective norms were the strongest predictors of behavioral outcomes (Kagee & van der Merwe, 2006). Similarly, TPB was strongly associated with self-management of rheumatoid arthritis (Strating, Schuur, & Suurmeijer, 2006) and regulation of sugar intake in Tanzania (Masalu & Astrom, 2003). More recently, the TPB was validated in a test of hand washing and limited social contacts during the first two months of the COVID-19 pandemic and lockdown in Belgium and France. In this study, Wollast, Schmitz, Bigot, and Luminet (2021) found that four factors influenced an increased likelihood of hand washing and limited social contact: positive attitudes, social norms, higher perceived control, and higher intentions (Wollast et al., 2021). What is important to note in all of these studies is the role of self-efficacy (perceived control) in explaining or predicting behaviors. In all four studies, self-efficacy was cited as a critical factor that increased the likelihood of performing the targeted behaviors. That, together with attitudes and subjective norms, boosts the predictive value of this model.

The theory of reasoned action and the theory of planned behavior identify two constructs – attitude and subjective norms – that contribute to explaining human behavior. The models also rely heavily on self-efficacy as a determinant of behavior. But to explain spontaneous, habitual, or unplanned behaviors, we must turn to other models and theories.

Health Belief Model (HBM)

A model designed to examine the motivational factors specifically associated with health behaviors is the *health belief model (HBM)*. Irwin Rosenstock introduced the health belief model in 1974 to understand why and under what conditions a person uses preventive health services. Examples of preventive health services include annual physical examinations, sometimes referred to as well-care medical visits, or annual dental examinations. Understanding the factors that motivate people to engage in behaviors that allow for early detection and diagnosis of diseases is the first step toward the goal of promoting and effecting changed health behaviors (Rosenstock, 2005). The health belief model seeks to explain the preventive health behaviors of persons who believe they are healthy and who attempt to maintain that state by preventing disease or by detecting and treating a disease in its earliest, asymptomatic stages (Rosenstock, 2005). The goal coincides with the public health goals of prevention, early detection, and disease control. As such, the HBM was also considered a useful tool in the field of public health.

The central concepts of HBM derive from work by Kurt Lewin (1935), a social psychologist. Drawing from Lewin's theory, the HBM attempts to explain and predict an individual's health behavior using the individual's own subjective frame of reference. For this reason, the HBM is considered a psychosocial model. The subjective focus of this theory is evident in the five key concepts used to explain health behaviors: perceived susceptibility, perceived severity, perceived benefits, perceived barriers, and cues to action. A sixth concept, Bandura's self-efficacy, was added to the model when it was determined to be a critical component of barriers to action (Bandura, 1977, 1982). Perceived susceptibility and perceived severity together contribute to the perceived threat of a disease, whereas perceived benefits and perceived barriers directly affect the likelihood that a person will take action against the disease.

PERCEIVED SUSCEPTIBILITY AND PERCEIVED SEVERITY *Perceived susceptibility* is the degree to which an individual feels at risk for catching a disease or illness. It is measured on a continuum. For example, a person may deny any possibility of contracting a disease. Conversely, a person may concede that contracting a disease is possible but highly unlikely. Finally, a person may concede a high probability of catching a disease and feel that they are in imminent danger (Rosenstock, 2005).

Consider for a moment the probability of farmers in Des Moines, Iowa, contracting the avian influenza A virus (avian flu). You will read about this in Chapter 4, Global, Communicable, and Chronic Disease. Briefly, the Avian flu was identified first in Hong Kong in 1997. It was the first known case of animal-to-human transmission of influenza A virus, spread from infected poultry. At its onset, the avian flu accounted for six deaths and 12 illnesses (Centers for Disease Control, 2006a). Initially, poultry farmers in Des Moines, Iowa, may not have perceived themselves as susceptible to the avian flu from Hong Kong, given the distance between Hong Kong and Des Moines. Reasonably, therefore, Des Moines farmers may have perceived their susceptibility to avian flu as low to nonexistent.

When avian flu was detected in poultry in China, Greece, Türkiye, and England, the Des Moines farmers may have reassessed their susceptibility to the virus. The spread of the virus to other countries, some a long distance from Hong Kong, changed the statistical probability of contracting the disease among people who raise or handle poultry. Des Moines farmers may have conceded the possibility of contracting the disease given its spread to other countries. Still, the farmers may have determined that their risk of catching the disease remained low because Iowa is an ocean away from all of the affected countries. But when avian flu was detected in the U.S. in 2009, the farmers probably perceived a marked increase in their susceptibility to the disease.

Perceived severity, or the perception of the seriousness of a disease, also varies by person; it is a subjective value. Perceived severity is shaped, in part, by two factors: a person's emotional response to the illness and the perceived impact of the disease on the person's life. For example, for some individuals, the possibility of suffering irreversible loss of sight in one eye due to glaucoma may be a frightening prospect. Yet the fact that the loss of sight is limited to one eye may be reassuring. For others, however, loss of sight, whether in one eye or two, could be emotionally devastating and could entail unwelcome changes in lifestyle or behaviors.

The perceived severity of a disease, however, refers to more than just the impact of the disease on the infected person. Severity could include the effect of the disease on people's daily functioning or on their responsibilities for their family. In some cases, the physical limitations caused by the disease may be less disruptive than the impact of the disease on the person's familial responsibilities. When combined, a perceived high susceptibility to and a perceived high severity of the disease should result in a strong perceived threat of the disease, perceptions that should lead to action.

PERCEIVED BENEFITS AND PERCEIVED BARRIERS The HBM proposes that individuals also calculate the *perceived benefits* and *perceived barriers* to health behaviors. Perceived benefits and perceived barriers help individuals transition from potential to actual behavior change. When calculating the perceived benefits of a healthy behavior, individuals consider the physical benefits of performing the behavior as well as the psychological benefits of preventing the onset of an illness or of controlling its effects. Here the influence of social psychology is evident again. The perception of benefits is highly subjective.

Consider the benefits of testing to determine whether one has been infected with the human immunodeficiency virus (HIV). We discuss HIV more fully in Chapter 5, Risky Health Behaviors, Part I. Briefly, HIV is a virus that attacks the body's immune system and for which there is currently no cure, only life-extending treatment. Prior to the introduction of antiretroviral drugs (ART) to treat HIV in the late 1990s, HIV was considered a fatal disease. For many individuals, knowing one's HIV status during the 1990s and 2000s may have provided a psychological benefit, especially if the individual did not have the disease. Knowledge may relieve worry.

However, some of the actions that people must take to obtain the benefit may present barriers. Consider this: In the early stages of this disease, health care workers in southern Africa thought that knowing one's HIV status would be seen as a benefit for villagers in rural areas. The increased incidences of HIV throughout southern Africa led many villagers in rural areas to be wary of the disease. Health workers surmised that an HIV test would provide reassuring information for those who tested negative and give those who tested positive an opportunity to obtain early counseling and treatment. Instead, researchers discovered that, for the villagers, testing triggered an unanticipated barrier: stigma (Pendry, 2001). In some villages, individuals who were tested for HIV were suspected of having the virus even before the results were known. Thus, villagers who were tested were ostracized by their community whether or not they tested positive for HIV. Some individuals were ostracized even by family members, who feared that the village would generalize their reactions to the entire family regardless of whether other family members also sought testing. In this case, the anticipated benefit of testing to determine one's HIV status was outweighed by the barrier of certain stigma for the individual and his or her family (Mills, 2006).

Similar barriers to testing during that time period have been reported in other countries. In studies among HIV-positive gay and bisexual men, heterosexual African men and women in England, as well as among HIV-positive women in the U.S., respondents also cited a fear of ostracism in their communities as a deterrent to HIV testing (Abel, 2007; Dodds, 2006). Thus, a community's social norms can create a psychological barrier that prevents some individuals from performing beneficial health behavior in order to prevent societal stigma.

It is important to note that, in some instances, society's stigma may be triggered by the behavior that led to the disease rather than the disease itself. For example, many societies discourage specific behaviors, including multiple sex partners, sex in exchange for money or goods, or illicit drug use. It just so happens that these are the same behaviors that increase the risk of contracting HIV. It is possible, then, that society's reaction is directed at the behaviors that cause HIV – behaviors that are inconsistent with society's values – rather than the disease itself.

Do the HBM concepts really explain our health behavior process? Can the HBM predict a person's likelihood of using preventive health services? The answer is an equivocal "sometimes." In a review of 29 studies testing the explanatory power of the HBM, Janz and Becker (1984) found strong evidence to support three of the four principal constructs of this model. Perceived barriers were found to be the strongest of the four constructs in explaining both preventive health behaviors and "sick role behaviors," that is, behaviors of people diagnosed with an illness and who are receiving medical treatment. Perceived susceptibility explained only preventive health behaviors, and perceived benefits explained only sick role behaviors. Perceived severity explained little in the way of behaviors (Janz & Becker, 1984). And, in an update, Carpenter (2010) conducted a meta-analysis of 18 studies which aimed to test the predictive abilities of the HBM. He found that only two of the five predictors – benefits and barriers – were consistently reported as the strongest predictors of health behaviors.

In sum, health benefits, real or perceived, may be negated by barriers. We define barriers as any impediment, real or perceived, that prevents an individual from performing activities that would be beneficial to their health. Barriers include tangible factors such as money, time, and effort, as well as psychological factors such as stigma or a loss of social standing among one's peer groups.

CUES TO ACTION The fifth variable in the HBM, ***cues to action***, prompts an individual to act when several conditions are met: The person perceives they are susceptible to a disease, the person views the disease as serious, or the person positively views the benefits to action and identifies few if any barriers to action.

There are several types of cues. A cue could be a tangible or visible factor such as a physiological reaction or symptom of illness. Psychological prompts such as concern on the part of the susceptible person or by family or friends also motivate action. Finally, environmental cues such as an advertisement or other stimuli external to the individual may also evoke action.

How important are cues to action? Some researchers suggest they are important predictors. For example, a study by Karimy and colleagues (2021) tested how well the HBM predicted COVID-19 preventive behaviors for 1,090 people in the Khuzestan Province in Iran. Their findings showed that four constructs – internal cues to action and external cues to action, in addition to perceived benefits and perceived barriers, best predicted such preventive behaviors, particularly for the female participants.

SELF-EFFICACY Perceived benefits, barriers, susceptibility, and severity provide the analytic framework for deciding on a healthy course of action. But health-enhancing behaviors assume that a person feels he or she can perform the behavior successfully. Hence, Bandura's self-efficacy was added to the HBM.

Additional studies provide support for the role of self-efficacy and perceived barriers in explaining health behaviors. For example, findings from longitudinal studies by Walter and colleagues (1992, 1993, 1994) suggest that self-efficacy is crucial for adolescents when attempting to adopt health-enhancing behaviors. Specifically, Walter and colleagues (1992, 1993) examined factors associated with AIDS risk behaviors among over 1,000 New York City high school students, grades 10 and 11, testing the role of perceived benefits, barriers, susceptibility, and severity of HIV and the role of self-efficacy in engaging in preventive HIV risk behaviors. In addition, the studies sought to measure the intention of students to use condoms when engaging in sexual intercourse. Condom use was considered a perceived benefit for HIV prevention because it reduces the risk of contracting the disease.

High school students in the studies were presented with an eight-week educational intervention program designed to impart knowledge, teach skills, and build confidence (self-efficacy) in negotiating safer sexual behaviors. Pre and posttests (see Chapter 2, Research Methods) measured the effectiveness of the intervention in reducing intentions to engage in risky sexual behaviors linked to HIV/AIDS. Walter and colleagues (1992, 1993) found that students readily accepted the benefits of condom use in reducing the risk of HIV. They even believed that the skills-building exercises that taught them to negotiate safer sexual behaviors (also a benefit) could be effective. However, the study revealed that students believed their self-efficacy in negotiating safer sex would be compromised severely if they consumed alcohol or used other substances before any attempt to negotiate such activities. Unfortunately, students also reported that the compromising agents (alcohol or drugs) are often consumed in venues like parties or other social events where they face a greater likelihood of engaging in unplanned sexual activities. In addition, students believed that other socioenvironmental factors, including perception of friends' behaviors and the student's personal values about the preventive behaviors, would mitigate their ability to practice safer sex. In essence,

Walter and colleagues (1992, 1993) demonstrated that self-efficacy is important for performing a behavior, but it can be undermined by substance use, by attitudes about the behaviors, and by the perceived subjective norms of the peer group. The latter two constructs are core to the theory of planned behavior.

The findings by Walter and colleagues (1992, 1993) were replicated by Naar-King, Wright, et. al. (2006) in their study of the relationship between substance use and the decreased use of condoms. They reaffirmed the role of self-efficacy in influencing behaviors associated with unprotected sexual behaviors.

Other studies that support the role of self-efficacy as a predictor of health behaviors include research on women's perceived severity, perceived susceptibility, or self-efficacy with respect to osteoporosis and colon and breast cancer (Dassow, 2005); women's intention to use hormone replacement therapy to control the physiological and emotional effects of menopause (McGinley, 2004); and women's and female student's dietary and nutritional behaviors (Schwarzer et al., 2007; Vahedian-Shahroodi et al., 2021).

The findings from recent studies that highlight the role of self-efficacy do not negate the importance of the four HBM concepts of perceived severity, perceived susceptibility, perceived benefits, and perceived barriers for explaining health behaviors. They do suggest, however, that self-efficacy is an essential component for action but one that is vulnerable to psychological and socioenvironmental factors.

TESTING THE HBM It seems only fitting that we use Eddie's case once again to test the HBM as a predictor of health-seeking behaviors. In the opening story, Eddie does not consider the health consequences of smoking. He does not consider his susceptibility to illnesses associated with smoking or the severity of such illnesses. Therefore, when applying the HBM to Eddie, we focus on the perceived benefits and perceived barriers of smoking cessation and on Eddie's self-efficacy. For Eddie, not smoking will result in both benefits and barriers. In the story, Eddie perceives that Sarah's support and friendship are the only benefits if he stops smoking. By comparison, the barriers to ending his smoking behaviors include the lost companionship and support of his other friends and the physical discomfort of withdrawal symptoms. At this point, it appears that the barriers outweigh the benefits.

Finally, Eddie's self-efficacy seems to be diminishing. His failed effort to stop smoking, in addition to the physical discomfort he experienced during that time, seems to suggest a waning belief in his ability to quit for a second time. If using the HBM to assess Eddie's behavior, we might conclude that Eddie will not stop smoking. However, this is an incomplete test because the health consequences of smoking are not included in this assessment.

Taking stock of the theories to date, we notice a pattern. Each theory identified factors that contribute to the likelihood of performing a healthy behavior. Notice also that the theories borrow or adapt concepts from other theories. This is a common practice. Rather than discard a theory entirely, researchers may borrow concepts from existing theories in an effort to build a stronger model to explain human behavior. Take, for example, research by Shmueli (2021) testing the combined role of the health belief model and the theory of planned behavior in predicting the likelihood of Israelis getting the COVID-19 vaccine. Results from this online survey with almost 400 participants showed that participants who perceived a benefit to getting the vaccine, perceived greater severity of contracting the virus, perceived more cues to action, expressed higher levels of self-efficacy, and perceived greater social norms were more willing to get the vaccine. Thus, in this example, the four constructs from the health belief model and one from the theory of planned behavior together best predict the likelihood of participants doing the target behavior.

As we continue with this chapter, you will see more examples of the practice of "borrowing" concepts to strengthen models.

Transtheoretical Model of Behavioral Change (TTM)

Prochaska and DiClemente's (1983) *transtheoretical model of behavioral change (TTM)* explains change as a process, not an event. This is an important distinction that differentiates the TTM from other models. The TTM asserts that change takes place over time. The developmental process of change described in the TTM leads us to classify this model as a stage model. Each stage of change is completed before moving to the next or more advanced level.

Prochaska and DiClemente (1983) contend that people must progress through five stages in order to obtain successful behavioral change: precontemplative, contemplative, preparation for action, action, and maintenance. Essential to this model is an accurate assessment of a person's readiness for change. According to TTM, a major reason that programs and individuals fail to attain their stated health behavior goals is that programs misjudge an individual's level of readiness for change. Recidivism, a sixth level, is included to reflect the process of failure to maintain the new behavior.

PRECONTEMPLATIVE STAGE The *precontemplative stage* is best characterized as the "not-ready-for-change" stage (see Figure 3.1). Individuals at the precontemplative stage are engaged in unhealthy or risky health behavior but are not thinking about changing their behaviors. For example, we may encounter numerous print advertisements or radio or television announcements about a health behavior that pertains to us. Our friends or family members may even talk with us about changing our behavior. For the most part, these messages will go "over our heads." We do not attend to or process the information. In fact, we may become defensive when hearing the message repeatedly.

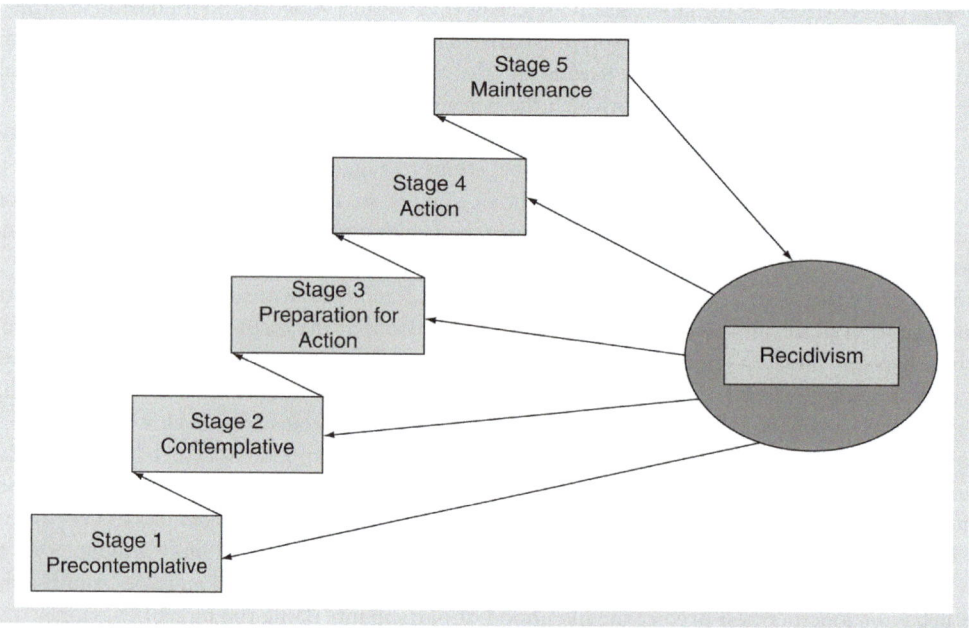

FIGURE 3.1 The diagram illustrates the five stages of the Transtheoretical Model. Each builds upon the preceeding stage like stair steps. Precontemplative (Stage 1) is the base, Contemplative (Stage 2) is the next step, followed by Preparation for Action (Stage 3), Action (Stage 4) and Maintenance (Stage 5). A person can move to Recidivism from Stage 5, but reenter the model at any point between Stages 1 thru 4.

Think about Eddie again. Before meeting Sarah, he was in the precontemplative stage of behavior change. He was not thinking about changing his smoking behavior. In fact, he enjoyed the behavior. He may have been aware of the dangers of smoking, as are some individuals in this stage. But if Eddie or others in the precontemplative stage are aware of the health consequences of their behaviors, the consequences have not prompted them to change their activities.

CONTEMPLATIVE STAGE The *contemplative stage*, the second stage in TTM, signals the beginning of the change process. In this stage, the person is thinking about change, although no action is involved. For example, people in this stage may begin to pay attention to commercials that address their behaviors. They also may listen more carefully to comments about their behavior by family members or friends. Finally, individuals in this stage may seek information about their health condition or behaviors.

Think about Eddie again. When he began listening to Sarah's comments about smoking, he was in the contemplative stage of TTM. He was receptive to her comments and considered her advice. But as is the case for many people in this stage, the disadvantages of not smoking were barriers to change. Eddie also contemplated the missed companionship and his friends' lack of support for his efforts to stop smoking. In essence, individuals in the contemplative stage weigh the benefits of the changed behavior against the barriers to change.

PREPARATION FOR ACTION After successfully transitioning through the contemplative stage, an individual will move to the third stage, *preparation for action*. The third stage signals a readiness to change behaviors. When preparing for action, an individual plans the activities needed to effect change. For Eddie, preparations included selecting the day he would stop smoking and deciding how to dispose of his supply of cigarettes in his home and car. Eddie chose to stop smoking on New Year's Day. He decided to put all packs of cigarettes in the garbage. In retrospect, we see that Eddie also should have developed a strategy for refusing cigarettes from friends and perhaps a plan to avoid his favorite smoking hangouts.

For other health behaviors, the preparation for action stage may involve more detailed plans. For example, if the planned behavior change involves a new diet, a person might specify the number of meals to be consumed each day. The person might plan the time of day each meal would be eaten as well as the types and quantity of foods to prepare. Finally, the person might plan either to prepare the meals at home or to purchase them, as many weight-loss programs sell prepared meals to participants as an essential part of their programs. Or, as we will see in Chapter 5, Risky Health Behaviors, Part II, a person may seek a prescription for a new medication shown to be effective in helping people lose weight.

ACTION The fourth stage is the *action stage*. This is, as the name suggests, the time to enact the plan and to perform the new health behavior. Prochaska and DiClemente (1983) note that stage four is a highly active stage because an individual must work diligently to adhere to the new behaviors. The action stage requires constant monitoring and attention to the new behavior. It also requires active resistance against old behaviors. The action stage usually lasts about six months before an individual transitions to the fifth stage, maintenance.

Eddie successfully entered the action stage. He even managed to stop smoking for 11 days. But he fell far short of the six months needed to solidify his new behavior. Eddie encountered difficulties when offered a cigarette by a friend. With no strategy for refusing cigarettes when offered, Eddie returned to his old behavior, apparently without much forethought.

MAINTENANCE Maintenance is the fifth stage. In theory, the *maintenance stage* requires far less active monitoring and attention to the new behavior than the action stage, in part because, by this time, an individual has adopted the new behavior. In practice, however, the maintenance stage is not static. In fact, many longitudinal studies of health behavior change report inconsistent adherence to the new behavior by their study participants after about six months, or the beginning of the maintenance stage (Swardh, Biguet, & Opava, 2008; Tsiros, Sinn, Coates, Howe, & Buckley, 2008; Wood & Neal, 2016). Alternatively, some also report that participants have regressed back to their old health behaviors. In the TTM, the regression to old behaviors is called recidivism.

RECIDIVISM *Recidivism*, according to Prochaska and DiClemente (1983), is part of the process of change, although it is not a formal stage. During recidivism, individuals may revert to the action stage to restart the new behavior and again try to adhere to the plan. They may return to the preparation for action stage and may temporarily cease the new behavior while they revise the plan for action or construct a new plan. Alternatively, individuals may revisit the contemplative stage, reconsidering the need for change but not acting on their thoughts. Finally, a person may return to the precontemplative stage. Frustrated or discouraged about the inability to sustain the new behavior, an individual may abandon all thoughts and efforts to change. On reflection, which of the five stages best characterizes Eddie's current level?

Prochaska and DiClemente's TTM proposes that people approach the process of change from different starting points. For example, one person may plan to lose weight by thinking about the amount or type of food he eats. Another person may begin with a detailed plan to eliminate the offending foods and substitute them with high-fiber, low-fat foods. Still another may forgo thorough preplanning and make decisions about her food consumption prior to each meal. The different approaches to change suggest that individuals have different levels of motivational readiness (Kohler et al., 1999). Prochaska and DiClemente contend that successful behavioral outcomes are more likely when people, and programs, carefully consider a person's level of readiness for change.

The novel aspect of TTM is that it accounts for individuals' successes, near successes, and failures when changing behaviors. Again, we turn to Eddie as an example. According to TTM, Eddie worked through the precontemplative, contemplative, preparation for action, and action stages. His 11-day adherence to his new behavior, however, means that he did not reach the maintenance stage before showing recidivism.

DECISIONAL BALANCE AND SITUATIONAL SELF-EFFICACY The concept of stages and processes of change are two of the four core constructs proposed in TTM. Prochaska and DiClemente include two others: *decisional balance* (pros and cons) and *situational self-efficacy*. These concepts may look familiar, because they appeared in earlier models. The theory of reasoned action (TRA) proposed pros and cons in decision-making using the concepts of behavioral outcomes and values. Rosenstock (2005) also introduced pros and cons into the health belief model (HBM) through perceived benefits and perceived barriers. According to the TTM, a person also calculates the pros and cons of engaging in a new behavior when undertaking a change process. This process begins in the contemplative stage and may continue through the preparation for action stage. Using the decisional balance, the TTM proposes that, like the HBM, when the benefits outweigh the cost, there is a good likelihood that a person will adopt and maintain the new behavior.

Many theories and models endorse the importance of self-efficacy, a person's belief that he or she can perform the intended behavior. So, too, does the TTM. In this model, situational self-efficacy influences the likelihood that an individual will be effective in planning and performing the new behavior. The study by

Naar-King, Wright et al. (2006) reported earlier in this chapter used the TTM to test students' likelihood of using condoms when engaging in sexual behaviors. Their findings revealed that self-efficacy mediated the relationship between stages of change and unprotected sexual behaviors. In essence, self-efficacy was the best predictor of use of condoms, not stages of change.

Other studies provide stronger support for the TTM as a predictor of health behaviors. The TTM has been used in health behavior programs to address issues of weight loss, physical activity, and nutrition (de Freitas et al., 2020). The TTM has also been used to establish a framework for weight management intervention programs, including managing healthy eating, exercise, and managing emotional distress (Johnson et al., 2008). More recently, the TTM was incorporated into a smoking cessation intervention program. Chang, Fu, Hsu, Okoli, and Guo (2024) found that using a TTM-based intervention program with 200 smokers improved participants' knowledge on smoking cessation, and also facilitated participant's progression through the stages of the model.

Although the TTM can be effective when used in health behavior programs, research studies stress the importance of self-efficacy in combination with the TTM when predicting health outcomes. Self-efficacy, in addition to attitude toward the behavior, subjective norms, barriers to action, and readiness for change, seems to be a strong predictor of behavior change.

SECTION II. SOCIAL MARKETING: A TECHNIQUE TO PROMOTE BEHAVIOR CHANGE

Many of the theories presented so far address motivation for change. The motivations were either internal or external, such as friends, family values, or societal expectations. Social marketing explores another type of external motivation for behavior change: the marketplace. *Social marketing* may seem like a strange topic to include in a health psychology textbook. The name suggests something more appropriate for business or advertising. Yet many would agree that commercial marketers are quite effective at influencing the behaviors of a target audience.

Social marketers aim to influence behaviors also, but they focus specifically on health behaviors. Thus, social marketing uses commercial marketing techniques to change behaviors for a social good. For this reason, it is appropriate to include social marketing in our discussion of theories and models that explain changes in health behaviors.

Consider this example of commercial marketing. Many people own cell phones, even young children. Think of a young child you know who has a cell phone, perhaps a close friend or family member. Why did the parents decide to purchase a phone for their child? Many times, parents cite a "need" to have a phone while at school. Notice we place the word *need* in quotations. Truthfully, for most children, a cell phone is not a needed item. By using marketing techniques, however, product manufacturers have convinced their target audience (parents) of just the opposite. In fact, today, many parents cannot think of a time when they thought that their children did not need a cell phone. Undoubtedly, cell phones facilitate immediate contact between individuals (they are convenient), but this hardly rises to the level of "need." Cell phone marketers have reshaped their audiences' perceptions such that many parents view the desire for quick and convenient communication as a "need." In this way, commercial marketers have changed both behaviors and attitudes about communication.

Similarly, social marketing aims to effect a change in attitudes and behaviors. In social marketing, however, the goal is to encourage an audience to adopt an intangible idea or a belief that will lead to behavior change. In almost all cases, the intended change will improve health outcomes. To effect change, social marketing uses commercial marketing principles to plan, execute, analyze, and evaluate a program "designed to influence the voluntary behavior of target audiences in order to improve their personal welfare and that of their society" (Andreasen, 1995). Thus, the goal of social marketing is to produce social change by causing outcomes that will benefit the individual and, by extension, society.

Social marketing programs have been used as a technique in a number of health promotion programs, including enhancing environmental preservation behaviors in Canada (McKenzie-Mohr, 2000); improving mother-to-child nutrition in Senegal (Aubel, Touré, & Diagne, 2004); encouraging condom use to promote safer sexual behavior in Myanmar, the Russian Federation, Bulgaria, Haiti, Cuba, Cameroon, Colombia, Türkiye, and the U.S. (Cohen, Farley, et al., 1999; UNAIDS, 2001); and reducing risky drug use, violence and risky sexual behaviors among an adolescent immigrant group (Edberg et al., 2022).

Social marketing campaigns are favored among some health researchers because they emphasize results. They have been effective in fostering sustained behavior change because they follow a pragmatic program plan. The plan includes careful selection of an activity to be promoted, careful identification of barriers to the activity, a strategy to overcome the barriers, a pilot test of the strategy, and an evaluation of the impact of the program once implemented (McKenzie-Mohr, 2000). Notice that, once again, the concepts of barriers to action and self-efficacy appear. Like other theories, social marketing borrows constructs from existing theories and integrates them with four marketing principles – *promotion*, *product*, *place*, and *price* – to produce change. The four principles are called, by some, the "four Ps."

The Four Ps

PROMOTION Effective promotion requires the selection of a target audience who is the intended recipient of the message. The process is referred to as *market segmentation*. Commercial marketing analysts know that a message designed to appeal to a broad audience may create awareness of the message but may not produce behavior change. Therefore, a successful message-promotion strategy must appeal to the specific demographics or behavioral characteristics of a target group in order to attract and retain their attention and to motivate them to initiate the intended behavior.

A classic study by Kelly and colleagues (1991) on HIV prevention with gay men is a good example of market segmentation. To promote the idea of safer sexual practices to reduce the transmission of HIV, Kelly and colleagues trained 39 men identified as the opinion leaders among gay men in two small, southern U.S. communities. The role of the trainees was to become behavior change endorsers to their social network. The leaders were chosen because they reflected the demographic mix of the target audience (gay men) and because they were identified by the target group as leaders within that network.

The leaders received training in the epidemiology of HIV, high-risk behaviors, protective behaviors that can reduce HIV transmission, and misconceptions about the risks. As part of the training, role-play activities taught leaders the elements of successful health promotion messages and encouraged them to practice effective delivery of such messages. Once trained, they were to engage their social network groups in discussions about HIV precautionary behaviors.

PRODUCT Unlike commercial marketers, social marketers do not have a tangible product to sell. They are not encouraging the purchase of a bar of soap or a new car. Rather, in social marketing, the product is the desired outcome. A desired outcome may be stopping a behavior like domestic violence (Ragin et al., 2000) or stopping littering in parks. At other times, social marketing may be used to modify behaviors such as dietary habits to improve nutrition (Dharod, Drewette-Card, & Crawford, 2011; Parker et al., 2011). To reinforce the behaviors, however, social marketers must associate an intangible concept with a tangible symbol that evokes the concept. The symbol serves as a reminder of the target behavior. Logos or slogans work well for this purpose.

Consider again Kelly and colleagues' (1991) study. The trained leaders needed a way to begin conversations with their social groups. Walking up to a group of acquaintances and saying, "I learned some interesting information about HIV prevention" would not necessarily catch the interest of a group intent on enjoying a night out in a club. Instead, Kelly designed a logo for HIV precaution in the shape of a traffic light. In the logo, a red light represented high-risk behaviors, yellow was linked to moderate-risk behaviors, and green indicated behaviors with a low risk of contracting HIV. The traffic light was fashioned into a lapel pin, and leaders were instructed to wear the lapel pins when going to their social clubs. In addition, posters with the logo were displayed prominently in the same clubs. As anticipated, the lapel pins and the posters prompted club patrons to ask about their meaning. The questions allowed the leaders to explain the analogy of the stoplight to the precautionary behaviors for HIV (Kelly et al., 1991). The traffic light lapel pin and posters were tangible symbols that were linked to the intangible product of safer sexual behaviors to reduce the risk of HIV infection.

PLACE Once motivated to adopt a new behavior, the target audience needs to know where to obtain the product, materials, or services to assist them in performing the new behavior. For example, condoms are the materials in Kelly and colleagues' (1991) study that enable the precautionary behavior of safer sex. The audience needs to know where to obtain the condoms. The place that distributes the product is called the ***distribution channel*** (see Figure 3.2). Place in social marketing is a location for gaining access to the tools needed to perform the new behavior.

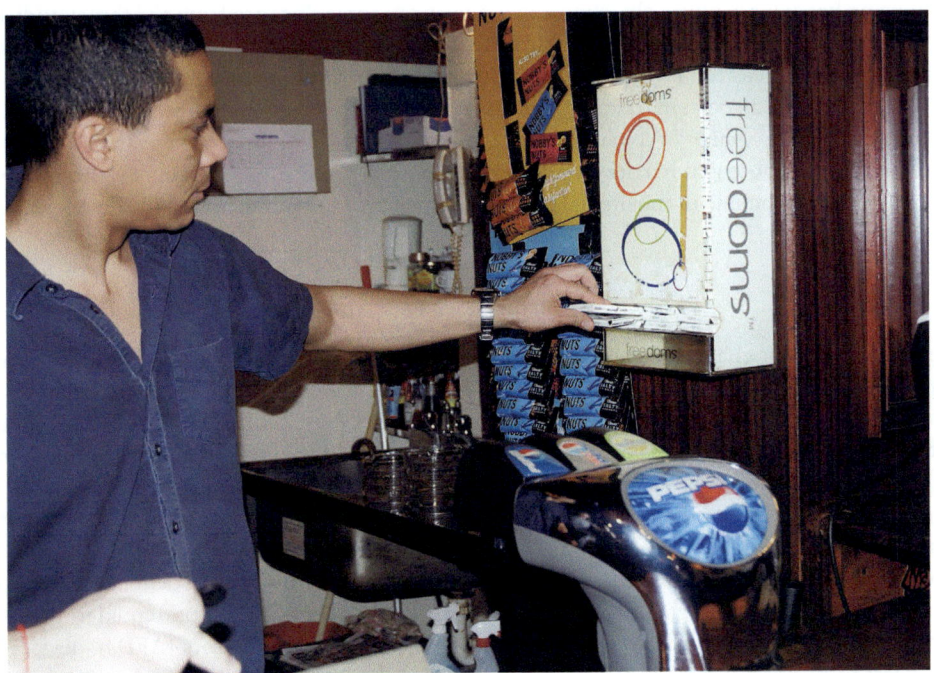

FIGURE 3.2 This photo shows a person taking a condom from a publicly accessible condom dispenser mounted on a wall in a publicly available space in a school.

Source: Alamy AF2W04.jpg

Earlier theories suggested that a good distribution channel is one that minimizes barriers to gaining access to the product. A place frequented by the target audience is an ideal distribution channel because it requires little time or effort and does not involve new behaviors. Although Kelly and colleagues' (1991) study did not specify a distribution channel, we can suggest possible places based on the study sample. Kelly and colleagues' study included white gay men who were, on average, 29.1 years of age, who resided in small towns in either Mississippi or Louisiana, and who frequented a specific nightclub in their respective towns. For this group, the researchers could have chosen a site in the nightclubs for distribution. Alternatively, they could have chosen a store or pharmacy in each town frequented by the targeted community.

PRICE Finally, social marketing, like the health belief model, includes a calculation of the price for adopting the new behavior. This includes the tangible costs associated with performing the new behavior such as monetary costs, time, or distance, as well as the intangible costs, which may include the emotional or social price of the new behavior. We saw in the health belief model that the price of adopting a new behavior, such as HIV testing, may be perceived as too great and may present barriers to action due, in part, to social stigma.

In Kelly and colleagues' (1991) study, selecting a pharmacy as a distribution channel could pose similar problems for the participants. Consider this: Purchasing condoms from a store close to one's home or place of work may expose the target audience member to comments or observations by other members of the community. The comments could evoke a social stigma. And, as we saw earlier with HIV testing in rural communities in southern Africa, the fear of stigma may present insurmountable barriers to performing health-enhancing behavior. Conversely, choosing a pharmacy some distance from the target audience's place of work or home may cost participants valuable time. Put another way, the distance to the distribution channel may be perceived as too far to make it an effective place to acquire the needed materials.

Thus, when designing a social marketing program, planners must anticipate the costs to participants and identify methods for overcoming or avoiding such barriers. Again, in Kelly and colleagues' (1991) study, one way of overcoming potential barriers to obtaining condoms from stores would have been to place condoms in a vending machine in the nightclubs. The audience could purchase the product without undue notice or comment.

Blended Models

Social marketing programs offer a technique for "selling" an audience on a need and a procedure for obtaining health behavior change. The theories and models discussed earlier in this chapter offer an explanation for why change may or may not occur. When blending a model or theory of behavior change together with the social marketing process, psychologists may be able to put forth a compelling combination of a theory and an implementation strategy that could lead to successful and long-term behavior change. The transtheoretical model of behavior change (TTM), when paired with social marketing techniques, is one example of a *blended model* that may guide a target audience through the change process.

This blend was tested in a retrospective analysis of a study of public access to defibrillators to prevent deaths due to cardiac arrests (Ragin et al., 2005a). The details of this study are presented in Box 3.1. The goal of the study was to test the effectiveness of automated external defibrillators (AEDs), devices used to return the heart to its normal rhythm after a cardiac arrest, when used by trained laypersons in selected communities. Specifically, the study tested whether laypersons in a community could be trained to provide immediate care to out-of-hospital cardiac arrest victims. Such assistance would shorten the medical response time to victims and improve their chances of survival.

Results of this study showed that a community layperson could be trained to use AEDs effectively. But the study also demonstrated that the response to cardiac arrest victims was best in settings in which the community already demonstrated a readiness for change (Ragin et al., 2005a). In other words, communities that were already in the preparation for action stage were most able to use and implement successfully the new behavioral response introduced by the social marketing techniques.

Box 3.1 Cardiac Defibrillators in the Community: A "Blended Model" Approach to Behavior Change

You may have seen automatic electronic defibrillators (AEDs) on television or in a movie. An AED is a small machine, about 11 inches by 13 inches, with two detachable paddles. It is used to provide emergency medical treatment when a person suffers a sudden cardiac arrest. In sudden cardiac arrest, a person experiences an abnormal heart rhythm that results in the failure of the heart to pump blood to other organs (Becker, 1996; Eisenberg, 1995). This type of heart failure always results in an immediate loss of consciousness.

When using an AED on a cardiac arrest victim, the technician places the detachable panels on the victim's bare chest. The defibrillator then sends an electric current to the victim's heart via the panels to jolt the heart back into a normal rhythm. This procedure buys valuable time until the person can receive professional medical care.

AEDs have been proven effective in reducing deaths due to sudden cardiac arrests when used by trained medical personnel or trained emergency responders. But the majority of cardiac arrests occur away from medical personnel, usually in private homes, parks, or other public places. And approximately 95% of all out-of-hospital cardiac arrests result in death. The problem is how to get immediate assistance to out-of-hospital cardiac arrest victims and how to train laypersons to provide that assistance using AEDs.

This was the goal of an international study of Public Access to Defibrillation (PAD): to determine whether community volunteers could be trained to respond to sudden cardiac arrest victims in their communities using AEDs. From a medical perspective, the key to providing a rapid response to sudden cardiac arrests victims is the number of AEDs available and the number of people trained to use them (Valenzuela et al., 2000). However, the community plays a crucial role in the implementation and outcome of the program.

Thus, from a social science perspective, the key to the PAD programs is not equipment or training but rather changing a community's behavior toward the health condition (Ragin et al., 2005a). In social marketing terms, therefore, the product was a new community response to cardiac arrest. So how do we change a community's health response?

The Public Access to Defibrillation (PAD) Trials Study investigators in New York City needed to design a process to inform and instruct the target community about the new medical emergency response system for cardiac arrests. The program they designed resembled a social marketing approach to behavior change, although it was not originally planned with social marketing concepts in mind. The NYC PAD Trials investigators recruited 59 residential buildings and two museums to participate in the study. From the 59 buildings, the investigators recruited 351 volunteers who agreed to be trained to use the AEDs and to respond to calls to assist cardiac arrest victims.

In addition, the investigators developed an eight-step implementation process to introduce the new emergency activation system at the participating sites. Essentially, the investigators needed to teach the community a new response to a medical emergency. Included in the eight-step process was a detailed information campaign. The researchers developed and disseminated brochures and posters designed to educate the community about the PAD Trials study and about cardiac arrests. The materials described the signs and symptoms of cardiac arrests, introduced the new emergency response system, alerted residents to the availability of trained volunteers on-site, and instructed residents on ways to contact the volunteers in their buildings in the event of a real or suspected cardiac arrest. Additional information was delivered to residents through on-site information sessions. The sessions provided residents with information about the product (their new response to arrests) and the materials (the new response system), promoted the system through written and oral communication methods, and explained how and where to activate the new system (place).

The good news is that residents were able to activate the emergency response system established by the PAD Trials investigators. The disappointing news is that the residents called the on-site trained volunteers for only 25% of the cardiac arrest incidences.

When reviewing these findings, the NYC PAD Trials investigators determined that limitations in their project design accounted for the low activation rate. First, the investigators noted that the informational materials were designed for the general PAD audience. While some of the written materials were available in Spanish, Chinese, and Russian in addition to English, investigators acknowledged that the content of the materials was the same in each language. They did not change the content to reflect the cultural or behavioral practices of the different linguistic or cultural groups. In other words, they did not use market segmentation to design their informational brochures. The "one-size-fits-all" message may have contributed to the low response rate by residents.

A second problem pertained to the residents' level of preparedness for change. In the PAD Trials study, some building sites activated the new medical response system, and others did not. Of the sites that activated, 70% already had a dedicated emergency response system specifically for medical emergencies prior to their participation in the PAD Trials Study. By comparison, of the nonactivated sites, fewer than half (43.5%) already had a dedicated medical emergency system. The investigators concluded that the sites with preexisting medical emergency response systems may have responded at a higher rate because they were at a higher level of preparedness for change. If, by using the transtheoretical model of behavioral change, investigators could have designed a special message and a special training and implementation procedure for the sites without the preexisting medical emergency systems, they might have found an increase in activations.

Finally, it is important to distinguish social marketing approaches from social advertising. Social marketing includes a message and a program. Social advertising includes a message but no program. Social marketing campaigns for condoms known as CONDOMIZE! and sponsored by UNAIDS throughout Africa, Asia, and Eastern Europe all include programs to distribute condoms and monitor their use (UNAIDS, 2012). Another example of social marketing programs are public service announcements for childhood immunizations in the U.S. that are supported by immunization centers to serve the demand for vaccinations created by the message. A limited ban on lobster traps, however, that requests that fishers voluntarily refrain from catching lobsters, is a social advertising campaign because it includes no programmatic support for the message.

While social marketing approaches can be successful in promoting health behavior change, they are somewhat less successful than commercial marketing campaigns for three reasons. First, commercial marketers can entice individuals by delivering immediate gratification. For example, immediately after parents buy a cell phone for their child, the child can show it to their friends, receive calls, make calls, and try the new features. Parents can also show it to other parents and receive validation for their decision, if that is a social norm of their peer group. But after beginning a new program of behavior change, such as a weight-loss program using social marketing techniques, a person must wait for the reinforcing positive outcomes of that change. Thus, they must delay gratification.

Second, the appeal of having a tangible object, and not a symbol, should not be underestimated. While a symbol or logo is a tangible reminder of the goal of the health program, the goal of the program is not the symbol. Finally, commercial marketers have the advantage of impulse. An attractive, well-promoted garment or piece of jewelry that can be acquired easily may lead to an impulsive purchase, one executed without planning or careful thought. But social marketers cannot rely on impulse. The process of behavior change, like weight loss, requires planning and sustained action over time. While some people may begin a behavior change process on an impulse, long-term maintenance or compliance with the new behavior requires sustained attention and effort. Such efforts are always subject to review and alteration and may be discontinued at any time.

SECTION III. THE ECOLOGICAL APPROACH TO HEALTH: FACTORS THAT INFLUENCE HEALTH BEHAVIORS

As much as we like to think of ourselves as independent-minded decision makers, the truth is that many of our behaviors are shaped by external factors or factors outside of our control. The previous sections explored the impact of some of these factors, including social groups, group norms, and commercial marketers. As mentioned at the beginning of this chapter, however, individual health behaviors are also shaped by other community, environmental, health systems, and health policy determinants.

Marks summarized this view when he noted that "historical, cultural and [economic] determinants of individual behavior are . . . robust and resistant to change" (Marks, 2002). This is not to suggest a pessimistic view of an individual's ability to choose or effect change. Rather, Marks's view is consistent with the social ecological health model: Individual health outcomes are influenced by factors that include but are not limited to the individual. In this section, we review factors that influence individual health outcomes, including the individual, cultural and social networks, the environment, health systems, and health policy.

Individual Factors

Earlier in the chapter, we explored the impact of social norms on an individual's behavioral intentions and decisions when reviewing theories and models used to explain health behavior change. What we did not emphasize is that some social norms are shaped by individual factors or characteristics that are either beyond our control or difficult to change. For example, each culture or group adopts a set of social norms associated with gender. As we will see shortly, gender is one of several individual-level variables that affect health but, for most of us, are largely outside of a person's control. Others include age, ethnic group, and culture (Valentine, Verdes-Tennant, & Bonsel, 2015). Gender norms are shaped by society and may vary by family, cultural heritage, and country of origin. There are, however, some similarities with respect to gender roles and health behaviors across cultures, as demonstrated by research.

GENDER AND HEALTH-SEEKING BEHAVIORS Health-seeking behaviors, defined here as actions taken to obtain guidance or assistance with health-related issues, have a direct impact on the quality of an individual's health status. Yet research shows that gender influences such behaviors. What is more, this appears to be a cross-cultural phenomenon. For example, VanDervanter and colleagues (2005) found that, among adolescents, boys were significantly less likely to use health care services than were girls, even when participating in intervention programs designed to increase preventive health care–seeking behaviors among adolescents.

In their study, VanDervanter and colleagues (2005) assigned adolescents to one of four groups. Half of the males were assigned to an all-male control group, while the other half were assigned to an intervention group for males that received guidance on seeking medical care. Similarly, half of the females in the study were assigned to an all-female control group, while the other half were placed in an intervention group for females only that was identical to the male intervention group. VanDervanter and colleagues found a significant increase in health care utilization for females who received the intervention when compared to females with no intervention. However, there was no difference in care-seeking behavior for males in the intervention versus the control group. The results also indicated that although males did not perceive specific barriers to gaining access to care, they did not perceive benefits to seeking care either (VanDervanter et al., 2005).

This finding is not unique to the U.S. South African researchers Otwombe and colleagues (2015) also report a significant gender difference in health care–seeking behaviors among adolescents (14- to 19-year-olds) in Soweto. Their survey of 830 adolescents found that females were significantly more likely to seek general health care services in addition to reproductive health care and counseling. In addition, research from Australia which examined the unmet mental health needs of adolescent and young adult males reported similar gender differences (Rice, Purcell, & McGorry, 2018). Specifically, these researchers note that as they approach adolescence, males tend to "disengage" from health care services. When they do seek health services, they then must contend with contravening societal norms and stigma (Rice et al., 2018).

Differences in health care–seeking behavior by gender occur in adults as well. Work by Gili, Roca, Ferrer, Obrador, and Cabeza (2006) on the cancer-screening behaviors of adult sons and daughters of people diagnosed with colorectal cancer illustrates this point. Research shows that the offspring of parents with a confirmed diagnosis of colorectal cancer are at the highest risk of contracting the same form of cancer. Despite this known risk, Gili and colleagues' study showed that male offspring were significantly less likely than females to seek a screening test to detect early stages of colorectal cancer.

Why does there appear to be a gender difference in health care–seeking behaviors? Hunt, Adamson, and Galdas (2010) suggest that men tend to dismiss their health needs, consistent with their concept of masculinity. Additional reasons men give for delaying health care include not recognizing the symptoms, a disinclination to express emotions or appear overly concerned about health, anxiety and fear about one's health, or gender role expectations and responsibilities, believing that a man would appear weak or nonmasculine if seeking medical care (Olanrewaju & Adeniyi, 2019; Yousaf, Grunfeld, & Hunter, 2013). In fact, the issue of gender socialization appears often in studies examining male health care–seeking behaviors. For many men, the social norm states that seeking health care is antithetical to masculine normative behaviors (Galdas, Cheater, & Marshall, 2005; Sobralske, 2006). Thus, some research suggests that there is nothing about gender per se that shapes health behaviors. Rather, the gender socialization process in many cultures subtly discourages health care–seeking behaviors among men.

One additional example of the gender difference in health-seeking behaviors is seen in research examining workplace absences. Even though statistics show that, in general, women tend to have longer life expectancies, studies suggest that women also report more frequent absences from work due to sickness than men (Antczak & Miszczyńska, 2021; Avdic & Johansson, 2013). Think about it: Greater longevity but more absences due to illnesses suggests that health care–seeking behaviors such as taking "sick days" to recuperate or to obtain medical care are more common and likely to be more socially accepted for women than men.

MULTIPLE INFLUENCES ON HEALTH CARE-SEEKING BEHAVIORS As we saw earlier, some studies report that gender is only one of several variables that influence health care–seeking behaviors. Consider culture (Galdas et al., 2005). In cultures that place a strong emphasis on masculine behavior or what is sometimes referred to as "machismo" (Davis & Liang, 2015; Hawkins et al., 2017), both culture and gender are thought to contribute to the lower rate of health-seeking behaviors among men.

KNOWLEDGE AND HEALTH-SEEKING BEHAVIORS Finally, researchers have shown that individuals' knowledge about risky or unhealthy behaviors also affects their health-seeking behaviors. Separate studies examining adolescents' and adults' knowledge of the risks associated with smoking and smoking behaviors support this fact. In a study examining adolescents' beliefs about smoking "light" cigarettes, Kropp and Halpern-Felsher (2004) found that adolescents believed they were at significantly lower risk for lung cancer, heart attacks, and deaths due to smoking-related diseases when smoking "light" versus regular cigarettes. In addition, adolescents thought it would be far easier to quit smoking when using "light" versus regular cigarettes (Kropp & Halpern-Felsher, 2004).

Adolescents who believe that "light" cigarettes lower the risks associated with smoking may also be less likely to seek help to stop smoking because they think their behavior puts them at less risk than other smokers. There is just one problem. "Light" cigarettes do not reduce the risk of smoking-related illnesses. Misinformation about the apparent advantages of "light" cigarettes is due, in part, to cigarette manufacturers' marketing campaigns that promote "light" cigarettes as a healthy alternative to regular cigarettes. Research refuting that claim is widely available (Dunlop & Romer, 2010; National Cancer Institute, 2010); however, adolescents are either unaware of this information or have not changed their views in spite of research results.

Some adult smokers also hold erroneous beliefs about smoking. Cummings and colleagues (2004) assessed adult smokers' beliefs about the health risks of smoking and the benefits of smoking filtered and low-tar cigarettes. Of the 1,046 adults surveyed, these researchers found that adult smokers who were the most misinformed about the risks of smoking were 45 years of age or older, smoked ultralight cigarettes, believed they would stop smoking before experiencing a serious health problem, never used medication to stop smoking, or were smokers with lower levels of education. Such misperceptions would make it unlikely that such individuals would seek assistance to stop smoking and would support the proposition that multiple factors affect health-seeking behaviors.

Current studies show that many adults still harbor these beliefs. A survey of over 1,700 adult smokers in the Republic of Korea reports that 25% of those surveyed believe that "light" cigarettes are less harmful than regular cigarettes and an additional 25% believe that such cigarettes contain less tar (Green et al., 2015). One more thing: Recent studies show that adults over 65 years of age in the U.S. believe that individuals cannot easily change their smoking behaviors. Interestingly, they are also less likely to have tried smoking cessation tools (Kulak & LaValley, 2018).

Clearly, individuals need accurate information about the health risks associated with their behaviors to adopt healthy actions. Yet, sound knowledge alone does not guarantee that individuals will adopt health-enhancing behaviors. Consider this: If individuals always did what was in their best health interest based on knowledge of the risks, their behaviors would be highly predictable and consistent. No doubt you can think of several people who are very knowledgeable about the health risks of, perhaps, smoking or consuming a high-fat diet but show no signs of changing their behaviors. In addition, cross-cultural research on views about smoking and the dangers of secondhand smoke in the U.S. and in Burkina Faso also shows that individuals often override their knowledge about risks in order to continue engaging in unhealthy behaviors (Halpern-Felsher, Biehl, Kropp, & Rubinstein, 2004; Ouedraogo, Ouedraogo, Ouoba, & Sawagodo, 2000).

At other times, individuals may have extensive and accurate knowledge about a health issue yet are still unable to change behaviors. For example, Lando and Labiner-Wolfe (2006) conducted a focus group to assess individuals' interest in having nutritional information posted on quick-service restaurant menus and billboards. They found that although focus group members indicated an interest in having the nutritional information displayed – a health-seeking behavior, of sorts – study participants indicated they would not consistently use the information when eating at the restaurants. The study suggests that knowledge does not always translate into behaviors and is not always sufficient to override intended behaviors.

Other studies suggest a complex relationship between nutrition information (including caloric information) and food choices. For example, Tandon and colleagues' (2010) study of fast-food selections that mothers make for themselves and for their children revealed that when mothers were provided with nutritional and caloric information about food items on a McDonald's menu, mothers ordered, on average, foods with 102 fewer calories for their children than did mothers without such information. Interestingly, there was no such difference when mothers ordered for themselves. The calorie content of foods ordered by mothers for themselves was similar regardless of whether mothers had the menu with the caloric information.

Another study found that calorie count information, while helpful, may not provide enough information to result in a reduced-calorie meal. Roberto, Larsen, Agnew, Baik, and Brownell (2010) examined the food-choice behaviors of study participants in a restaurant diner when assigned to one of three conditions: menu with no caloric information, menu with calorie labels only, or menu with caloric labels and with recommended daily calorie intake for the average adult (calorie plus). Their findings were both predictable and surprising. These researchers reported that study participants in both of the calorie-label conditions (calorie only and calorie plus) consumed on average 14% fewer calories than individuals in the no-caloric-information condition. In addition, participants in the calorie-plus condition consumed on average 250 fewer calories than participants in either of the other conditions. The surprising finding, however, was that individuals in the calorie label–only condition reported consuming more calories after the study dinner than did participants in the no-label or the calorie-plus conditions.

What do these findings suggest? First, as noted in other studies, information (knowledge) alone does not always result in changed behaviors. Tandon and colleagues (2010) demonstrated that a mother may apply the new knowledge when addressing the nutritional needs of her child but not when making food choices for herself. Similarly, Roberto and colleagues (2010) showed that, in some settings, limited knowledge (calorie label only) may result in short-term but not longer-term behavior change. In addition, Roberto and colleagues' study suggests that knowledge (information) may be maximally effective when placed in context. Calorie-count information together with the recommended average calorie intake for adults lead to changes in both short- and longer-term food choices for adults in the calorie-plus condition.

Finally, research shows that, in some instances, knowledge about a health issue may be secondary to practical social, socioeconomic, or cultural barriers. For example, in a classic study of knowledge, attitudes, and beliefs about sickle cell anemia in children in East Africa, researchers found that 75% of caregivers of children with sickle cell anemia knew that the disease was hereditary, and 55% knew the symptoms associated with the disease (Macharia, Shiroya, & Njeru, 1997). Researchers then examined five individual factors to determine which best predicted caregivers' health-seeking behaviors for their child: education, monthly income, occupation, religion, and family size. Only family size best predicted attitudes and behaviors. Why would family size affect the likelihood of seeking care for a child with sickle cell anemia? Simply put, a parent may be well educated about the illness but may encounter time, logistics, or even economic barriers when caring for the special needs of one of several children in the family.

Cultural and Social Networks

Studies of immigrant populations in the U.S., as well as studies of health-seeking behaviors in other countries, further demonstrate how culture may influence health care behaviors. We explore the role of culture and traditional medicines on health behaviors more fully in Chapter 6, Emotional Health and Well-Being. For the moment, however, it is important to note that in studies of barriers to health care access for those in the Latino and Native American communities, researchers have learned that convenience, affordability, cultural and linguistic preference, a preference for traditional medicine practices or holistic health, and use of *curanderos* (cultural healers; see Chapter 6, Emotional Health and Well-Being) all affect the likelihood that members of these communities would seek traditional health care (Cruz et al., 2022; Reese, Dang, & Liddell, 2024).

PEER GROUPS AND HEALTH-SEEKING BEHAVIORS The theories we reviewed earlier noted the effect of peer groups on individual health behaviors using the construct of subjective norms. There is an extensive body of literature on the impact of peer groups on adolescent health, and we examine some of that work in Chapter 5, Risky Health Behaviors, Part I. For the moment, we note that much of that work focuses on the effects of peer groups on encouraging or discouraging substance use, including the use of cigarettes, alcohol, and drugs, as well as risky sexual behavior (Balsa, Homer, French, & Norton, 2011; Park, Kim, & Kim, 2009; vanRyzin, Fosco, & Dishion, 2012). For example, studies testing the social cognitive theory (see pages 69) to explain smoking behavior among adolescents find that adolescents are influenced by models of smoking in their environments. And once again, Eddie's experience may be helpful in understanding this phenomenon. His role models for smoking were his older brother, who also began smoking as a teen, and his closest friends.

Interestingly, however, similar findings appear not to apply to African American adolescents. For example, a study of the smoking behaviors of white and African American adolescents revealed that having a close friend who smoked predicted initiation into cigarette smoking for white adolescents, but this finding was not true for African American adolescents (Hoffman, Sussman, Unger, & Valente, 2006). An interesting finding from a focus group of 99 African American teens and young adults (18–29 years of age) suggests that strong antismoking messages from mothers, respect for elders, and preference for marijuana accounted for the low levels of cigarette smoking as adolescents (Cheney & Mansker, 2014).

Other studies point to the effect of *acculturation*, the adoption of behaviors and values of a majority group, on health behavior. Studies examining the role of acculturation on health behaviors suggest that individuals who are influenced by the norms and behaviors of the dominant cultural group in their communities attempt to imitate the same health behaviors (Bethel & Schneker, 2005). Specifically, studies report a significant association between the degree of acculturation to Western culture and the use of substances including cigarettes, alcohol, and marijuana (Bell, Ragin, & Cohall, 1999; Trinidad, Unger,

Chih-Ping, & Anderson, 2005). In general, the research shows that the more an adolescent attempts to acculturate to the dominant culture – in this case, Western culture – the greater the likelihood of experimenting with substances including cigarettes, alcohol, and drugs. We note some exceptions to these general findings in Chapter 5, Risky Health Behaviors, Part I.

MEDIA AND HEALTH-SEEKING BEHAVIORS Earlier in this chapter, we discussed the impact of media and advertising on health behaviors. We made the point that mass-media advertisements can effectively shape behavior. In fact, they can shape both positive and negative health behaviors. An example of the role of the media in shaping positive health behaviors can be found in Ogata Jones, Denham, and Springston's (2006) study of breast cancer screening among younger versus older women. In a sample of 284 participants, these researchers found that older women responded more positively to mass-media appeals to obtain breast screening exams than younger women. The younger group responded best to personal communication.

Conversely, there are a host of examples of the media's role in encouraging negative health behaviors. The role of media in promoting cigarette smoking is well known (Braun, Mejia, Ling, & Perez-Stable, 2008). Perhaps less well known is the role of cigarette manufacturers in promoting tobacco use among the U.S. military (Haddock, Jahnke, Poston, & Williams, 2013; Pebley et al., 2023).

Joseph, Muggli, and Pearson (2005) documented a 10-year campaign by cigarette manufacturers to promote tobacco use among U.S. military personnel. According to this study, the military is an ideal target audience for cigarette manufacturers because of the volume of people, the availability of a target audience already preselected by socioeconomic class, the common culture of the military, and the promise of a carryover of the product (cigarettes) to the civilian market – in effect, free advertising to a secondary group. The example of marketing to the military is also an excellent illustration of the benefits of market segmentation when promoting a product. The military is one of the cigarette manufacturers' most loyal customers.

Physical Environment

We acknowledged that other people, values, cultures, and social norms are external factors that affect health. Another type of external factor is the environment, here meaning the physical environment. We can examine the relationship between individual health outcomes and the environment by examining the health consequences to individuals caused by environmental contaminants. Before proceeding, however, it is important to state that, in many instances, the environmental contaminants that adversely affect individual health are caused by human behaviors that change or alter the environment.

CLEAN AIR AND WATER ACTS For more than 45 years, the U.S. government has led or supported national and international efforts to become better stewards of the environment. Nationally, the U.S. has enacted federal regulations to protect two vital national resources, air and water. The Clean Air Act of 1970 established National Ambient Air Quality Standards (NAAQS) designed to protect both the environment and the health of the public (Environmental Protection Agency, 2007a). In 1977, the U.S. government followed with the Clean Water Act. The Clean Air Act and the Clean Water Act regulate the quantity, type, and frequency of pollutants that can be released by industry into the air and water, respectively. Both acts are administered by the U.S. Environmental Protection Agency (EPA). While the primary goal of these acts is to protect valuable environmental resources, they also ensure clean water and air for human consumption.

More importantly, on the international front, 194 countries plus the European Union have agreed to a legally binding treaty known as the Paris Agreement, which aims to mitigate climate change. In this agreement countries pledge to reduce their greenhouse gas emissions, something that in addition to mitigating the impact of climate change would also significantly improve air quality (United Nations, Climate Action, n.d.). Why? Because greenhouse gases are natural and artificial substances in the atmosphere that help warm the Earth's surface by trapping heat. Examples of greenhouse gases include water vapors, carbon dioxide, methane, and ozone that are emitted when we burn fossil fuels, such as coal, natural gas and coal (USEPA, n.d.). These substances contribute to air pollution. Therefore, global efforts to reduce such emissions would also reduce air pollution.

Clearly, greenhouse gas emissions negatively impact our health and our planet. When exposed to these gases in the long term, they can affect the respiratory system, causing bronchitis, exacerbating asthma, and also affecting the cardiovascular and central nervous systems (Naiyer & Abbas, 2022). If this claim seems a bit extreme, consider this: On some days you have probably heard weather forecasters warn people in specific geographic areas of poor air quality. On such days they advise people with respiratory illnesses and other vulnerable groups (usually older or younger individuals) to remain inside. If you wondered why these events happen, one explanation is the contributions of greenhouse gases to the air pollution index. In sum, then, the Paris Agreement, while aimed principally at reducing greenhouse gases and mitigating climate change, will also greatly benefit global health.

SUPERFUNDS *Superfund sites* are another example of the impact of environmental pollutants on human health. In 1980, the U.S. Congress created the Superfund, a program administered by the federal government to clean up its *hazardous waste sites*. The term *hazardous waste sites* refers to land and water sites that contain toxic chemicals or other substances that pose a current or future threat to human health or to the environment.

Superfund sites identify areas in which toxic waste products from various industries have been dumped onto land or into waterways. The toxic substances seep into the soil, the water, and often the underground water systems that supply drinking water to residents in nearby communities. As a result, the sites contain contaminants. The EPA estimates there are currently approximately 1,333 hazardous waste sites that have been prioritized for cleanup throughout the U.S. (U.S. Environmental Protection Agency, 2022).

The existence of contaminated environmental sites is distressing enough. The problem is compounded, however, by a host of health problems that have been linked to Superfund sites. In states such as New York, Massachusetts, New Jersey, California, and others, health problems have been associated with such sites including lung and breast cancer, leukemia, bloodborne illnesses, excessive bleeding, skin rashes, bronchitis and other respiratory diseases, and some unknown illnesses. Efforts to remove toxic substances from the land and water are underway and represent an important step in controlling the adverse health outcomes caused by contaminated environments.

Health Systems

We address health care systems and policy more thoroughly in Chapter 12, Health Care Systems and Health Policy: Effects on Health Outcomes. Briefly, we note that while there are a number of different health care systems in the world, the most common system appears to be universal health care systems where care is provided by the government or government-sponsored systems. The U.S., however, operates a very distinct system.

Access to health care in the U.S. has been a cause for debate for well over a century. Over the past 30 years, the debate has intensified again as economists and health policy experts determined that limited access to care is one of the factors contributing to the current crisis in the U.S. health care system. Access to care is defined as having the means to afford health care or having a person responsible for one's medical care needs. Before October 1, 2013, almost 50 million Americans were either uninsured or **underinsured**, meaning that their health care insurance did not adequately cover their medical needs (Institute of Medicine, 2000).

While there have been recent, significant, and positive changes to the U.S. health care system, Americans continue to face barriers to health care. First, the inability to pay for needed medical care at the time of service can cause individuals to postpone care for otherwise treatable illnesses, usually resulting in more serious health problems. For example, when uninsured or underinsured individuals postpone seeking care when first needed, these individuals are three times more likely to experience adverse health outcomes and more than four times more likely to experience **preventable hospitalizations**, meaning hospitalizations for conditions that could have been treated in a physician's office or in an outpatient visit.

A second problem with the system is access to a medical care provider. Individuals who do not have a primary care provider responsible for their care are also more likely to delay needed treatment. Without access to regular care, some individuals may seek medical treatment from emergency service centers such as hospital emergency departments (EDs), a more costly and less effective treatment, especially for ongoing health issues (see again Chapter 12, Health Care Systems and Health Policy).

Contrary to popular belief, in the U.S., the frequent users of emergency medical services for routine care issues are not individuals with limited or no access to care. Rather, they are those who are dissatisfied with their health care options. A nationwide study examining the reasons why patients sought care from hospital EDs illustrates this point. In their study of 28 hospital EDs nationwide, Ragin and colleagues (2005b) identified five main reasons why patients sought emergency medical treatment: a medical emergency (95.0%), preference for the ED (88.7%), convenience (86.5%), affordability (25.2%), and limitations of insurance (14.9%). Few people consider an ED a convenient source of care, and fewer still think of it as a place where they prefer to go for care. So, what do these results mean?

Ragin and colleagues (2005b) reported that for some individuals, the hospital – although not necessarily the ED – was their regular source of care. For others, however, the affirmative preference for hospital EDs may reflect their negative assessment of the quality of care available in other community health care settings. Thus, the 88.7% of persons who "preferred" the ED may suggest that the quality of care available in their community is inadequate, not that there is a dearth of service or that such services are inaccessible.

Ragin and colleagues (2005b) also found that 86.5% of people cited convenience as a reason for seeking emergency care. To understand that statistic, consider this: Many individuals with primary care physicians report waiting two to three weeks for an appointment for routine care. And, when needing emergency medical care, some individuals report waiting several hours or days because the primary care provider could not accommodate an emergency visit or because the office is closed. The restricted hours of service, even for emergencies, is considered inconvenient.

Such limitations are not the case in hospital EDs; hence, they are more convenient. In addition, at many primary care practices, appointments for nonemergency health care visits are available only during business hours, usually between 9:00 am and 5:00 pm on Mondays through Fridays. Individuals unable to take time from work or other family commitments to schedule medical visits during these times – hours that often conflict with an individual's work or school commitments – often postpone medical care.

Thus, when care is unavailable or inconvenient, people often choose one of two options: Find alternative sources of care, such as hospital EDs, or forgo care entirely. The first choice is expensive, and the second often leads to more serious health problems in the near future because of delayed care (see Chapter 12, Health Care Systems and Health Policy).

The Institute of Medicine's (2000) report on access to health care emphasizes additional factors such as socioeconomic status, ethnicity, and limitations of insurance as other likely barriers to care. Their study found that poor and minority groups in the U.S. are more likely to have limited access to adequate health care. As a result, these groups have poorer overall health outcomes than others in the U.S. (Bentacourt, 2006; Institute of Medicine, 2000).

We make one additional observation: Insured individuals may also face limitations of care. For example, many individuals opt to enlist in health insurance plans offered by health maintenance organizations (HMOs), a network of health care providers who have been preapproved to offer health care services to any patient who is a member of the organization. We review health care systems, including HMOs, more fully in Chapter 12, Health Care Systems and Health Policy. For now, however, we briefly note that even individuals who are members of HMOs encounter limitations of service.

HMOs define the type and frequency of service available as well as the providers authorized to render the services. These restrictions can and often do present conflicts for patients and care providers who may want or need care that is denied by the HMO. Individuals who can pay for the added care are not greatly affected by the regulated services. For others, however, such limitation means no treatment even though they are insured.

In sum, health care systems offer affordable options that improve access to care for many. However, here, too, in the U.S. the restrictions on the types of service and authorized providers will impact an individual's health outcomes.

Health Policy

Health systems regulate the type of services available to their members. Health policy, however, involves another form of regulation: government regulations intended to improve the overall health of a community, region, or nation. We review international health policies more fully in Chapter 5, Risky Health Behaviors, Part I. Here, however, we will briefly highlight smoking regulations and new restrictions on the types of foods available in school vending machines in some U.S. states – examples of two new health policies at the national and state levels designed to improve health outcomes.

SMOKING AND HEALTH POLICY In 1998, the U.S. federal government banned smoking on all domestic airline flights (GPO Access, 2008). Two years later, U.S. Federal Law 106–181, section 252.3, extended this ban to include international travel on U.S. carriers (Pan, Barbeau, Levenstein, & Balbach, 2005). The smoking ban on airplanes was one of the earliest in a series of smoking regulations designed to limit exposure to *secondhand smoke*. Since that time, broader smoking restrictions have been enacted in a total of 29 states, the District of Columbia, Puerto Rico, a number of territories, and the Navaho Nation (Campaign for Tobacco-Free Kids, 2024). Some states and cities also regulate or restrict smoking in restaurants, movie theaters, the workplace, and even in bars. This, too, is an example of health policy, but at the state or municipal level.

Health policies that restricted smoking venues were supported by health research that demonstrated the dangers of secondhand smoke to nonsmokers. *Secondhand smoke* is defined as the smoke from cigarettes, cigars, and pipes that is inhaled by people who themselves are nonsmokers. Health policy experts were able to demonstrate that environmental tobacco smoke is a carcinogen, an agent that causes cancer in humans (Environmental Health Information Services, 2000). In fact, tobacco smoke is so potent that the EPA cannot identify a safe level of exposure to secondhand cigarette smoke that would result in no harm to an individual (Environmental Health Information Services, 2000).

To put this in perspective, environmental tobacco smoke is the leading cause of preventable deaths, and the leading cause of deaths due to disease worldwide (WHO, 2022a). These data, combined with studies specifically linking secondhand smoke to deaths due to heart disease in women, and poorer health outcomes for those with asthma, have convinced policy makers that secondhand smoke is a health hazard to the public (Eisner et al., 2005; Kaur, Cohen, Dolor, Coffman, & Bastian, 2004). Such conclusions led to health policy aimed at improving the outcomes of a population, the primary goal of health policy initiatives.

Remember Sarah, Eddie's girlfriend in the opening story? She clearly dislikes smoking. Perhaps her dislike was based, in part, on her knowledge of the adverse consequences of secondhand smoke.

NUTRITION AND HEALTH POLICY New health policies were developed to reduce negative health outcomes among schoolchildren in New York City and other urban areas. Consider this: Michael Bloomberg, mayor of New York City from 2002 to 2013, banned soda, candy, and sugary snacks from vending machines in New York City schools, citing recent statistics on childhood obesity and juvenile diabetes (see Box 4.2, and Chapter 5, Risky Health Behaviors, Part II). The new health policy for the New York City public schools was intended to remove from schools all foods and beverages thought to contribute to the possible development of obesity or diabetes in children and adolescents.

In essence, the new policy seeks to adjust the dietary habits of children. The belief is that by shifting schoolchildren's snacking preferences from high-sugar, high-fat foods to those higher in fiber and lower in fats, schools may stem the increase in childhood obesity and Type 2 diabetes. The full impact of this intervention will not be known for several years.

Box 3.2 "Taking Candy from Children?"

Yes, it is true. In the summer of 2003, New York City's schools chancellor, Joel Klein, announced new restrictions on items sold in school vending machines and new standards for school lunches. The new regulations eliminated candy, soda, and juices containing less than 100% fruit from vending machines in schools (Goodnough, 2003). What is more, school lunch menus were revised significantly. More fresh or frozen vegetables and fruits were added to menus, and the number and quantity of high-fat foods were decreased. Items such as macaroni and cheese and potato salad were eliminated from lunch menus entirely. And students' favorites, chicken nuggets and cheese pizza, would be served in smaller portions.

The changes in school lunch menus and vending machine offerings were prompted by a study of obesity and diabetes conducted by New York City's Department of Health and Mental Hygiene and the Department of Education. City departments collected survey data on the height, weight, age, and gender of the city's elementary schoolchildren in kindergarten through fifth grade. The results of the survey, reported in 2003, revealed that 43% of the city's school-aged children in grades K–5 weighed more than the recommended weight for their height and age; 19% of children were considered overweight, and 24% were determined to be obese. This represents an increase of 4% in the number of obese school-aged children in New York City from 1996 to 2003 (Perez-Pena, 2003).

The obesity statistics are even more alarming when compared with national statistics for school-aged children. In that study, 34% of school-aged children nationwide were found to be overweight, of whom only 16% were determined to be obese (Wang & Beydoun, 2007).

New York City's decision is an example of a government health policy implemented to change the eating behaviors, and hopefully the health outcomes, of thousands of children. The goal of the policy is to reduce the amount of fatty foods consumed by children in school lunches and from vending machines. The unstated goal, however, may be far more significant. If New York City can succeed in influencing or changing the dietary preferences of elementary school-aged children through the new policies, it may be able to influence later eating behaviors. It is a step in the direction of controlling and possibly reducing childhood obesity or diabetes.

SECTION IV. CHALLENGES TO SUSTAINING HEALTH BEHAVIOR CHANGE

Looking back on this chapter, you may think it is a wonder that anyone manages to initiate or sustain health behavior change. In this chapter, we identified a host of individual, cultural, social network, environmental, health system, and health policy influences on health behaviors. These factors, singly or in combination, challenge our ability to adopt healthy behaviors. We may be aware of the obvious influences on our behaviors by family members and friends, but other factors, such as advertisements or environmental influences, may be more difficult to detect. In this section, we consider two additional challenges to maintaining healthy behaviors.

Short- versus Long-Term Adherence

The transtheoretical model of behavior change (TTM) identified short- and long-term behavior outcomes. Eddie's 11 days of abstinence from smoking is an example of a short-term outcome – very short term! Yet research shows that the average duration for new health regimens is about six months. During these six months, the individual performing the changed behavior may encounter a number of challenges. These include challenges to one's self-efficacy to maintain the changed behavior given temptations from the environment and emotional or psychological dependence on the old behaviors. In the opening story, Eddie encountered all of these challenges when trying to quit smoking. One or several of these factors may have resulted in Eddie's decision to return to smoking.

How could Eddie maximize the likelihood of sustained behavioral change? For some behaviors, efforts to change require a change in lifestyle. For Eddie, changing his group of friends, his preferred activities, and the emotional satisfaction he derived from smoking with his friends could make him more successful in his smoking cessation efforts, but radical changes in lifestyles often result in limited long-term success.

In addition, after several months of adherence to a new behavior, we may believe that the old behavior is no longer a risk or temptation. We may erroneously think that we have the situation under control. For example, how many times have you heard someone who has stopped smoking say, "I think one won't hurt me." The question is not whether one cigarette would "hurt" but whether that person can stop after just one. Individuals struggling with smoking cessation say that the notion that one can smoke just one cigarette is often incorrect. One cigarette is the prelude that leads them back to their original behavior. According to the TTM, recidivism back to the old behaviors is due to diminished adherence to the new health behaviors.

The Appeal of Unhealthy Behaviors

A second challenge individuals face when adopting new behaviors is the marketing savvy of producers of risky or less healthy products. In truth, advertising agencies are excellent psychologists. Through their careful research on targeted populations, they craft marketing messages that are very persuasive. For example, the concepts of product, promotion, price, and place all come together to determine that the best placement for the single bars of chocolate candy in a supermarket is at the checkout counter – the place where you wait rather impatiently before totaling and paying for your groceries. No doubt the time it takes to shop combined with the smell of the various foods in the store are guaranteed to stimulate the appetite. One chocolate bar, packaged attractively for just one person, would help pass the time while standing in line and would take care of the growl in the stomach at the same time. And although few people enter grocery stores to buy a single serving-size candy bar, the convenience of the individually sized candy in the checkout line satisfies a "need." It therefore provides immediate gratification for that unplanned "need."

Personal Postscript

BE ALERT, BE AWARE: INCREASE YOUR ABILITY TO IDENTIFY TARGETED ADVERTISEMENTS

Young women and teens were treated to an new ad for Camel cigarettes in the 1990s designed especially for them. At least that is what the manufacturers intended. The manufacturers of Camel cigarettes realized that few women smoked their brand. Thus, they developed a new ad campaign targeted to young women and teenage girls to increase their likelihood of buying and smoking Camel cigarettes.

How does this work? First, the ad depicts a box of Camel cigarettes in shades of pink and yellow. Pink is a color associated with females. The use of pink and other pastels is intended to appeal to a female aesthetic. Next, the company chose the tag line "light & luscious," again, words that resonate with a female audience more than a male audience. Finally, they call their new product "Camel No. 9." This name just might happen to make the target audience (females) think of perfumes with a similar name, like Chanel No. 5 or Chanel No. 19. The product name, the colors, and the tag line all are designed to attract the attention of females and to increase their interest in this new product.

Now imagine that one of your female relatives saw that advertisement. Would the ad attract her attention?

Questions to Consider

1. How might new school health policies that eliminate sugary drinks and candy from vending machines support the belief that subjective norms help shape behaviors?
2. Self-efficacy is a critical factor in many theories/models of health behavior change. But as Walter et al. (1992, 1993, 1994) show, it is subject to external influences. What strategies can health psychologists propose to help individuals develop sustainable self-efficacy that resists external influences when engaging in behavior change?

3. How do Superfund sites illustrate the complex relationship between people, the environment, and health outcomes?

True or False Questions

1. Social advertising programs include, as part of their design, a message and a program. True or False.
2. In the transtheoretical model of behavioral change, the action stage is where an individual begins planning to change their behavior. True or False.
3. Reciprocal determinism is the concept in the theory of planned behaviors that states that behavior must be viewed in the context of environmental events and personal factors. True or False.
4. One of the "Four Ps" of social marketing is purchasing power. True or False.
5. The Public Access to Defibrillation study tests whether the public could be trained to use an automatic electronic defibrillator on someone suffering a cardiac arrest. True or False.

Important Terms

acculturation   *91*
action stage   *79*
asymptomatic   *339*
blended models   *84*
contemplative stage   *79*
cues to action   *76*
decisional balance   *80*
direct experiences   *69*
distribution channel   *83*
expectancy value theory (EVT)   *67*
hazardous waste sites   *93*
health belief model (HBM)   *67*
inferred learning   *70*
learned behavioral consequence   *69*
maintenance stage   *80*
market segmentation   *82*
matching law   *69*
outcome expectancies   *70*
perceived barriers   *74*

Global, Communicable, and Chronic Disease

Chapter Outline

Opening Story: The Worst Pandemic in 100 Years

Section I. Global Health Problems

Section II. Chronic Diseases

Section III. Global Health Organizations

Section IV. Health Policy

Section V. The Economic Consequences of Poor Health

Personal Postscript

Questions to Consider

True or False Questions

Important Terms

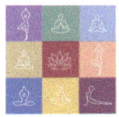

Source: 3xy/ Shutterstock.

Chapter Objectives

After studying this chapter, you will be able to:

1. Define epidemics, pandemics, and endemics.
2. Define communicable, recurring, and chronic diseases, and give three examples of each.
3. Compare the health consequences of communicable diseases in developed (high- and upper-middle-income) and developing (low-middle- and low-income) countries.
4. Compare the health consequences of chronic diseases in developed versus developing countries.
5. Examine the impact of vaccine hesitancy or vaccine resistance on health outcomes.
6. Explain the role of chronic diseases in assessing quality of life.
7. Identify and describe the mission of three international health organizations.
8. Explain how health policy contributes to individual health outcomes.
9. Explain the effects of individual health outcomes on the family, community, society, and country.

DOI: 10.4324/9781003300670-4

OPENING STORY: THE WORST PANDEMIC IN 100 YEARS

*December 12, 2019. A "cluster" of people in Wuhan, China, were diagnosed with "atypical" pneumonia like symptoms, in other words an infection caused by a bacteria other than those more commonly associated with pneumonia (CDC, 2023a; Icahn School of Medicine at Mount Sinai, 2023). Unfortunately, news of this new and deadly disease was not shared immediately. In fact, 19 days later, on December 31, 2019, the China office of the **World Health Organization (WHO)**, an international health organization that coordinates and at times implements global health policy (see Section III, Global Health Organizations, page 144), happened to find a statement about cases of "viral pneumonia" on the website of the Wuhan Municipal Health Commission. That same day, another division of the WHO discovered a similar media report about a number of cases of "pneumonia of unknown cause," also in Wuhan.*

What happened afterwards? There was a flurry of actions by the WHO and many countries as scientists hurriedly searched for more information about this new disease and its likely consequences.

The very next day, January 1, 2020, the WHO requested and received more information from China's National Health Commission and shared this information with all countries who were members of WHO's Event Information System. WHO then held multiple teleconferences to inform countries about the disease. They obtained and shared the genetic sequence of the virus with scientists and others worldwide (WHO, 2023c). But, while the WHO took steps to understand the etiology of this illness and its implications for the rest of the world, it was blamed for failing to require China to be fully transparent about the origins of this disease and its potential impact.

One week later on January 9, 2020, China preliminarily identified the new illness as a novel coronavirus (WHO, 2023d). Most experts believed that the likelihood of human-to-human transmission of the novel coronavirus was limited, a view that changed quickly when health care workers caring for patients with the coronavirus also became ill (WHO, 2023). On January 23, one month after the first cases of coronavirus appeared, 581 incidences of this illness were reported, the overwhelming majority (571) of which were in China.

*Meanwhile, the novel coronavirus was already spreading to other countries. Japan and the Republic of Korea each reported one case and Thailand reported four. More cases quickly followed. If the SARS-CoV-2 crisis were confined to Asia, it would have been labeled an **epidemic**, a disease that affects large numbers of a population within a geographic area. When the first case of coronavirus occurred in the U.S. on January 23, and more cases appeared in other countries in the Americas, the crisis was reclassified as a **pandemic**, a disease that is transmitted through large geographic regions of the world or worldwide (see Figure 4.1).* ∎

And the rest, as "they" say, is history. Many details about this deadly disease after January 2020 are known, except for its origins. Scientists and governments continue to debate this point.

One important final note. While scientists around the world worked feverishly to identify the ***genomic sequence*** of this new virus – here meaning determine the sequence or order of the letters that make up the virus's genetic material (Morgan, 2022) – the virus was changing, or ***mutating***, creating slightly different

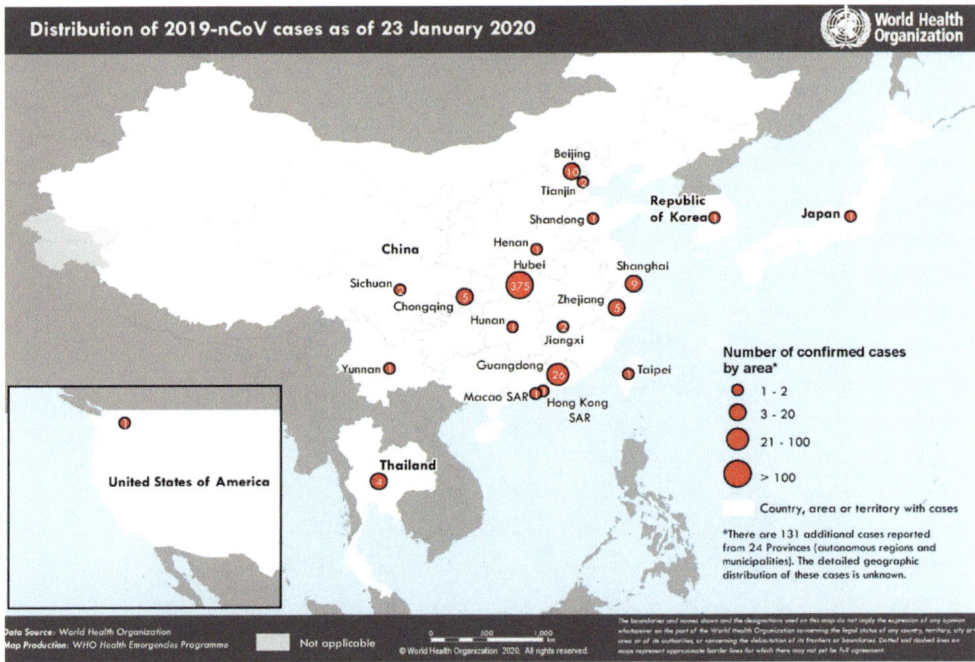

FIGURE 4.1 A map of COVID-19 cases as of January 23, 2020 shows the largest number in China's Hubei (375 cases), Guangdong (26 cases), and Beijing (10 cases) provinces. Other provinces in China, and other Asian countries (e.g., Japan, Republic of Korea, Thailand) reported between one and nine cases. The U.S. reported one case.

Source: World Health Organization (2023). Novel Coronavirus (2019-nCoV) Situation Report-3. Situation Report – 3 (who.int).

versions, or **variants**. These variants not only changed the "look" of the virus but also resulted in different symptoms. Thus, while some researchers were still studying the original virus and its properties, other scientists were working in real time to identify the various mutations. In southern Africa, the Botswana/Harvard AIDS Institute Partnership (BHP), led by Dr. Sikhulile Moyo (see Figure 4.2), the Lancet Laboratory in Pretoria, South Africa, and the Lancet Molecular Pathology Department in Johannesburg, South Africa, were the first to successfully sequence and identify one of the variants: Omicron (Feldscher, 2023; Lister & McKenzie, 2021).

As of the end of 2023, there is still no agreement on the likely origins of this disease, but scientists suggest two probable theories. Theory one states that the coronavirus escaped from a laboratory while scientists were researching coronaviruses. It is a fact that the Wuhan Institute of Virology in Wuhan, China, was engaged in research on coronaviruses. Supporters of the lab error theory suggest that the virus became airborne, leaked from the lab and infected the population (Stolenberg & Mueller, 2023). To be clear, lab accidents do happen. For example, the CDC in the U.S. revised its biosafety practices following laboratory accidents in 2014 involving anthrax and the avian bird flu (Stolenberg & Mueller, 2023). But there is inconclusive evidence to support claims that the coronavirus outbreak in Wuhan was the result of a research-related lab accident.

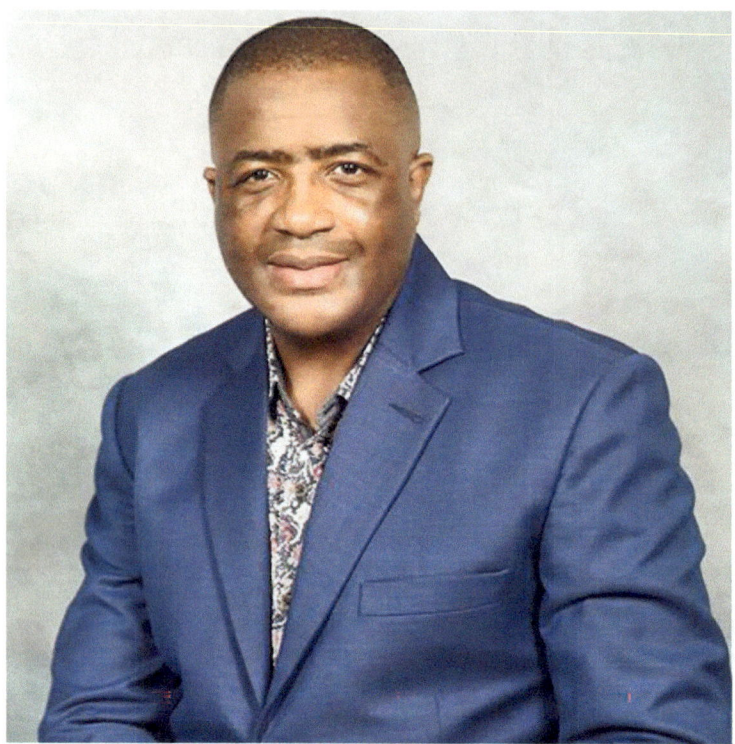

FIGURE 4.2 A photo of Dr. Sikhulile Moyo, leader of the South African team of researchers who were first to genetically sequence the Omicron variant of the Sars-CoV-2 virus in South Africa.

Source: Botswana Harvard Health Partnership (https://bhp.org.bw/dr-sikhulile-moyo).

A second theory is that the virus emanated from animals, a not uncommon occurrence. The transfer of diseases from animals to humans, a phenomenon known as ***zoonotic spillover***, has been documented in the past and continues even today. Such transmissions occur many ways, such as through air, food, or through direct or close contact with an animal's saliva, blood, or feces (Millbank & Vira, 2022). The *zoonotic spillover* theory has gained traction as a plausible explanation of the coronavirus crisis because one of the first cases of **SARS-CoV-2** appeared to have come from the Huanan Seafood Wholesale Market in Wuhan (Stolenberg & Mueller, 2023). Specifically, some scientists claim that in the early stages of the pandemic, the virus was contracted by people working in or shopping at the market (Stolenberg & Mueller, 2023). Other suggest that consuming the meat of wild animals can be another means by which the virus was transmitted to humans (Millbank & Vira, 2022).

We will not resolve the debate about the origins of the coronavirus here. But the likelihood of a *zoonotic spillover* is relevant to health psychologists. By explaining how some people catch viruses associated with animal populations (e.g., close contact with animals or consuming the meat of infected animals), health psychologists can identify behaviors that may increase the likelihood of contracting illnesses. Remember, one aim of health psychologists is to change behaviors that increase the risk of illnesses. And, just to be clear, SARS-CoV-2 is only one of many examples of possible animal-to-human transmission, even in recent times.

Does this claim seem unrealistic? Then consider the case of the avian bird flu in 2005 or the "swine flu" in 2009. In 2005, and again most recently in 2024, the world became aware of a health crisis involving a virus that was transmitted from birds to other animals and humans. Between 2005 and 2006, more than 200 people in 13 different countries contracted the highly pathogenic avian influenza (H5N1) strain of A influenza, abbreviated A/H5N1. At the time, many governments were unaware of the virus until incidences of the disease were reported among their populations. By the time international health organizations, such as the WHO, learned of the widespread impact of the avian flu, people in China and other countries in Southeast Asia, northeast Africa, the Middle East, and Europe were becoming ill. A delay in notifying health officials allowed the virus to spread among both the avian population and people in close contact with infected birds. Current data show that as of 2023, 878 cases of the 2006 A/H5N1 and 458 deaths were attributed to this virus (WHO, 2023e).

By comparison, Mexican authorities acted more quickly and with fuller disclosure when, in April 2009, incidences of a deadly "swine flu," known medically as Type A/H1N1 influenza, were discovered in the Mexican population. Within days of notifying WHO, 11 more countries reported incidences of the disease (see Box 4.1). Some, like the U.S., even reported deaths associated with the illness. The A/H1N1 flu was an international health crisis because people in many different, noncontiguous countries contracted the disease.

Box 4.1 Two 21st-Century Pandemics?

Did we really have two, 21st-century pandemics? The WHO, an international health group, seemed to think so.

A/H1N1 "Swine Flu"

We begin with the "swine flu." The origin of this disease and its progression is traced to Mexico. The first case is believed to have occurred as early as February 2009. By April 2009, authorities identified one source of the outbreak: a single case reported at a pig farm in La Gloria, Veracruz, Mexico, which eventually led to 444 confirmed cases in the same town of 2,600 inhabitants (World Health Organization, 2011a). While some officials in Mexico were challenging the assertion that these incidences of A/H1N1 were associated with pig farming, two children in southern California were diagnosed with the illness at the same time. It, too, was a variant of influenza that the Centers for Disease Control and Prevention said suggested a pig origin A/H1N1. Because of its prior association with pigs, the new disease was nicknamed the "swine flu."

Epidemiologists knew that the A/H1N1 Influenza was common among pigs. But now it appeared to be spreading to humans. A disease that at first was communicated only from animals to humans had changed its method of transmission. Health researchers observed that the disease could also be transmitted by humans to other humans, a process referred to as ***human-to-human transmission***. Contact with an infected animal was no longer necessary.

When WHO officials realized this new danger of A/H1N1, they became concerned. Like other influenzas that are passed from person to person, A/H1N1 was now capable of spreading quickly through a population. In fact, within weeks, more than eight countries reported actual or suspected cases of the flu. In response to the escalating threat, WHO issued a Phase 4 global threat warning to notify all countries of the potential of an imminent global health crisis. The threat level was elevated to Phase 6 by late June 2009 (see Figure 4.3).

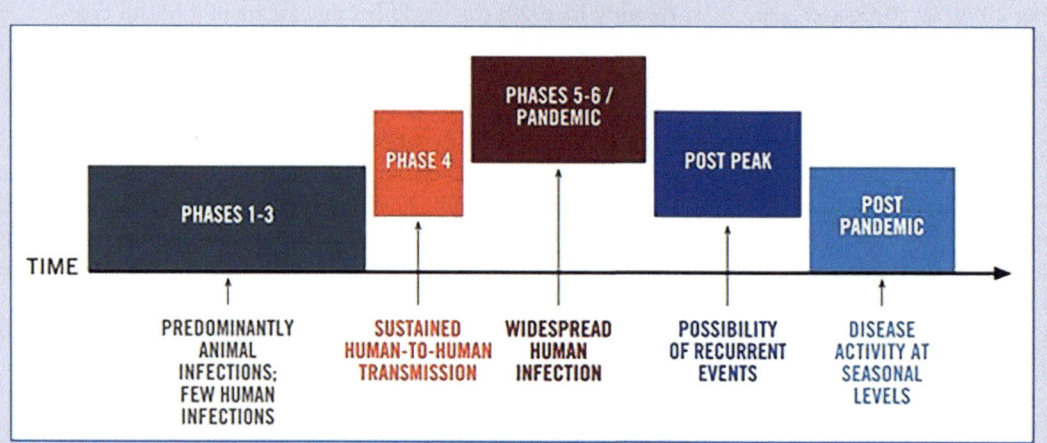

FIGURE 4.3 A bar graph shows WHO Pandemic Influenza Five Phases: Phase 1–3, Predominantly Animal Infections: Few Human Infections; Phase 4, Human-to-Human Transmission; Phases 5–6, Widespread Human Infections; Post Peak, Possibility of Recurrent Events; Post Pandemic, Disease Activity at Seasonal Levels. By June 2009, the WHO elevated the global threat level of the A/H1N1 virus to phase 5–6/pandemic levels.

Source: World Health Organization (2009c). Pandemic Influenza Preparedness and Response: A WHO Guidance Document Retrieved on December 8, 2023, from GIP CORE A4 INGILIZCE.fh11 (who.int).

The story worsened with each passing day. As of June 9, 2009, 73 countries were reporting a total of more than 26,563 confirmed cases of A/H1N1 virus and 115 deaths (World Health Organization, 2011a). The U.S. accounted for 8,975 of the cases but only 15 of the deaths. By comparison, only 5,029 of the global cases of A/H1N1 were officially reported in Mexico, the site of origin of the disease (World Health Organization, 2010a). Yet Mexico was responsible for more than 97 deaths. The statistics made some wonder about the actual number of cases of A/H1N1 in Mexico. With more A/H1N1 cases resulting in death, some researchers suggested that the over 5,000 cases of A/H1N1 in Mexico underreported the total number of cases.

On the other hand, the difference in infections and deaths between the U.S. and Mexico caused by the flu led to other possible explanations. For example, some epidemiologist speculated that people in the U.S. and other countries had contracted a less severe strain of the flu than individuals in Mexico. Others suggested that better access to medical care in the U.S. and other countries may have reduced both the intensity and duration of illness.

Equally uncertain are the final effects of the flu. A/H1N1 is a new variant of Type A influenza. The latest update on A/H1N1 shows that approximately 115 countries reported at least one incidence of this flu, resulting in more than 81,000 cases globally and approximately 18,631 laboratory confirmed deaths (Simonsen et al., 2013; World Health Organization, 2023m). Given the initial spread of this illness, it may not be surprising to learn that the U.S. and Mexico reported the highest numbers of cases (33,985 and 8,279 respectively; World Health Organization 2023m). Even now, the virus continues to circulate seasonally throughout the world, changing its designation from a *pandemic* to an **endemic** disease – here meaning a regularly occurring disease.

SARS-CoV-2, Also Known as Coronavirus Disease (COVID-19)

The A/H1N1 pandemic pales in comparison to SARS-CoV-2 also known as COVID-19. The A/H1N1 pandemic resulted in an estimated 18,631 laboratory confirmed deaths in the first year. We are, as of this writing, in the third year of the COVID-19 pandemic with an estimated 6,897,025 deaths globally (see Table 4.1; World Health Organization, 2023b). You do the math.

TABLE 4.1 Confirmed Cases and Deaths due to COVID-19 as of April 13, 2023

WHO Regions	Confirmed Cases 4/13/2023	Confirmed Deaths 4/13/2023	Proportion of Deaths to Cases
Europe	275,220,560	2,212,212	0.80%
Western Pacific	202,153,158	409,585	0.20%
American	191,814,966	2,945,187	1.50%
Southeast Asia	60,867,951	804,273	1.30%
Eastern Mediterranean	23,324,249	305,417	1.30%
Africa	9,519,504	175,388	1.80%
Global	762,791,152	6,897,025	0.90%

Source: World Health Organization (2023e). Weekly epidemiological update on COVID-19–13 April 2023 (who.int).

As noted in the opening story, in January 2020, the WHO identified only one case of a novel coronavirus in the Americas and 571 in China. And, because this virus appeared to cause respiratory infections ranging from mild to severe, the WHO originally called this disease novel coronavirus–infected pneumonia (Hafeez, Ahmad, Ali Siddqui, Ahmad, & Mishra, 2020). The name was later shortened to coronavirus disease 19, or COVID-19. Just over three years later – April 13, 2023 – the number of confirmed COVID-19 cases had risen to 191,814,966 in the Americas and 60,867,951 confirmed cases in Southeast Asia (World Health Organization, 2023b), with more in other parts of the world. It is fair to say that the COVID-19 disease erupted worldwide over these three years.

Researchers have identified a genetic link between this new virus and two earlier versions of coronavirus, both of which are attributed to *zoonotic spillover*. The first, SARS-CoV, originated in bats, and was first reported in humans in Guangdong, China, in November 2002. The second, Middle East respiratory syndrome (MERS), occurred in 2012. It is a virus also linked to bats but is transmitted to humans via the camel. It was first reported in Jeddah, Saudi Arabia. SARS-CoV-2 shares approximately 96% of its structure with another virus found in horseshoe bats (World Health Organization, 2021). Collectively, the total number of mortalities for SARS-CoV and MERS was less than 1,600 (Ganesh et al., 2021). Clearly, SARS-CoV-2, especially the early variants of the virus, accounted for far more deaths.

Why so many deaths? Unlike the A/H1N1 pandemic, but similar to SARS-CoV and MERS, the usual transmission route for SARS-CoV-2 is through respiratory droplets released when people cough or sneeze (Hafeez et al., 2020). These airborne particles can easily infect others particularly in crowded areas. And while all three – SARS-CoV, MERS, and SARS-CoV-2 – could result in pneumonia or severe respiratory distress, among other symptoms, SARS-CoV-2, particularly the earlier variants of this virus, disproportionately affected older persons and people with preexisting health conditions, such as cancer, kidney, liver or lung diseases, diabetes, heart diseases, or immune compromising conditions (CDC, 2023b). For such individuals, SARS-CoV-2 was a serious illness at best, and at worse, fatal.

The novel coronavirus (SARS-CoV-2), the avian bird flu, and the A/H1N1 flu are examples of viruses linked to zoonotic spillover. In addition, these viruses are all pandemics which have traveled across borders and infected large populations in many countries. Consequently, they present global health problems and challenges for health professionals, including health psychologists. Interestingly, such global health problems also give health psychologists an opportunity to study the effects of different health determinants on outcomes, such as individual and cultural behaviors; physical, social, and cultural environments; health policy; and health systems.

In this chapter, we explore the impact of each of these determinants on global and communicable illnesses and their impacts on the health status of people in countries around the world. We pay particular attention to differences in the health outcomes of people in economically prosperous nations, referred to by the World Bank as high- and upper-middle-income countries, versus those in less economically advantaged nations, including low- and lower-middle-income countries (see Chapter 2, Research Methods). Because the World Bank sometimes refers to both the low- and lower-middle-income countries as *developing economies*, we will continue to use the term *developing* when referring to these countries, and refer to upper-middle and high-income countries as *developed economies.*

In earlier versions of this textbook, we began Section I with a brief review of seven of the best-known communicable diseases past and present and explained their effects on communities. As of this edition, we have experienced several more global viruses and now include them in our review of pandemics. After a brief review of the selected pandemics, we continue with a discussion of childhood viral illnesses and the disparities in health outcomes for children who contract childhood infectious diseases in developed versus developing countries. We conclude Section I with an explanation of the role of childhood immunizations – an effective tool for improving health status, specifically mortality and morbidity rates, among children worldwide.

In Section II we explore *chronic diseases*, illnesses that result in lingering health problems and may limit an individual's daily functioning. In this section, we examine two chronic illnesses: diabetes and chronic respiratory illnesses. (Other chronic illnesses, including heart disease, cancer, and arthritis, are explored in greater detail in Chapters 9 through 11). Again, taking a global health approach, we explore the impact of chronic illnesses on populations in developed versus developing countries to illustrate the role of socioeconomic status and access to health care (a health systems determinant) on health outcomes.

In Section III, we introduce three international health organizations that provide health care and health policy assistance to countries unable to provide such services themselves. We explore the international organizations' roles in addressing the specific health promotion and health maintenance needs of the region.

Section IV compares the health policies of two countries in their efforts to contain the spread of a deadly disease. In both examples, the countries adopt policies that help protect the well-being of the community while restricting individual rights. By the end of Sections I through IV, you will be able to distinguish between chronic and communicable diseases and describe the global consequences of each, explain how individual behaviors, demographic factors (such as socioeconomic status), access to health care, and health policy influence health outcomes, and finally compare the health of people living in developed versus developing countries.

Finally, in Section V, we look at the economic consequences of poor health. In this section, we examine how one individual's health status can adversely affect his or her immediate family in addition to the well-being of the community, society, and nation.

SECTION I. GLOBAL HEALTH PROBLEMS

Communicable Diseases: Human-to-Human Transmission

EPIDEMICS AND PANDEMICS History shows us that for centuries, communicable diseases have caused severe illness and death throughout the world. Table 4.2 identifies 12 major global diseases over more than 3,000 years (between 1350 BCE and the present) based on historical records. While in some cases these diseases were the result of *zoonotic spillover*, it is the human-to-human transmission that results in the epidemics and pandemics that can lead to human deaths.

TABLE 4.2 Selection of Major Global Pandemics

Years	Name	Location	Cause	Duration	Outcome
1350 BCE to 1980 CE	Smallpox	North and West Africa, East and South Asia, Europe, the Ottoman Empire, the "New World" (U.S.)	Zoonotic spillover, trade	3,000 years	Hundreds of millions (exact figures unavailable)
1347–1350	Black Death	Europe, Asia, Middle East	Movement of military and trade	3 years	Total death toll >137 million
1580	Influenza: First documented influenza pandemic	Origin: Asia Spread: Africa, Europe, the Americas		6 months	>8,000 deaths in Rome Some Spanish cities decimated
1781–1782	Influenza pandemic	Origin: China Spread: Russia west to Europe and North America		8 months	Very high infection rates: St. Petersburg, Russia, >30,000 ill per day Rome, > 50% of population ill Britain, rampant illnesses in 1782
1790	Influenza pandemic	Origin: Russia Spread: Europe and the entire "known" world		3 years	High death rates Distinct "waves" of the pandemic Deaths highest in subsequent waves
1816 to present	Cholera	India, Russia, Europe, North America, South Asia, Africa	Trade and commerce	Endemic	Death toll >1 million
1830–1833	Influenza pandemic	Origin: China Spread to Philippines, India, Russia, North America		3 years	Moderate death rate, but estimated 20%–25% of world population became ill
1918–1920	Influenza pandemic "Spanish Flu" "Mother of all influenza pandemics"	U.S. military bases Spread to France, England, Spain, Germany, Russia, North Africa, India, China, New Zealand, and the Philippines	Movement of military during World War I	3 years	Estimated 40–50 million deaths (1.5–2 million in Africa; 7 million in India; 25% of population in Samoa and Alaska) Infection rate >50% of world population People aged 20–40 most affected

(Continued)

TABLE 4.2 (Continued)

Years	Name	Location	Cause	Duration	Outcome
1957–1958	Influenza pandemic	Origin: China Spread: Hong Kong, Singapore, Taiwan, Japan, India, Australia, North and South America, South Africa	Travelers over land routes from Russia to Scandinavia and through a large international conference in Iowa (U.S.)	2 years	1 million dead 40%–50% of world population ill Disproportionately affected very young and very old
1980 to present	HIV/AIDS	U.S., Africa, Asia, Europe	Risky, unprotected sexual behavior	Ongoing	Estimated deaths: 40.1 million Estimated HIV positive: 84.2 million
2009–2010	Influenza A/H1N1 pandemic	North and South America, Europe, Middle East, Asia	Zoonotic spillover from pigs Transition to human-to-human transmission	1.5 years	Estimated deaths: 151,700 to 575,400 in first year
2020 to present	SARS-CoV-2 pandemic	Origin: China Spread: Neighboring Asian countries, Western Europe, Australia, U.S., South America, Africa	Unclear: Either Zoonotic spillover or lab leak	3+ years	Deaths: 6.9 million confirmed; 14.83 million excess deaths

Sources: Beveridge (1991); Crosby (1989); Nickol and Kindrachuk (2019); UNAIDS (2023); Walters (1978).

As we noted in the opening story, diseases that affect large numbers of a population within a geographic area are called epidemics, from the Greek words *epi* meaning "upon" and *demos* meaning "people." In comparison, diseases that spread through large geographic regions of the world or occur worldwide are pandemics. Again, the origin of this word is Greek, derived from the words *pan* meaning "all" and *demos* meaning "people." All diseases listed in Table 4.2 were considered pandemics because of their impact on multiple populations and millions of people across many global regions. We will quickly review a few of the pandemics here.

Smallpox Table 4.2 lists *smallpox* as the earliest documented communicable disease (see also Box 4.4). A highly contagious disease, smallpox caused hundreds of millions of deaths over its more than 3,000-year history (WHO, 2023f). The telltale symptoms – fluid-filled pustules or lesions on the body, plus high fevers and vomiting – could be severe, lasting about two weeks. For many, it was a fatal illness. Fortunately, this deadly pandemic has been largely eradicated since 1980.

Athenian Plague Another deadly pandemic was the *Athenian plague*. This disease inflicted a number of symptoms on its victims in Greece in 430 BCE, including fever; inflammation of the eyes, tongue, or throat; gastrointestinal symptoms, such as diarrhea or vomiting; and rashes covering the entire body. The victims usually died within seven or eight days of contracting the disease. Historians have been unable to estimate accurately the number of deaths attributed to the Athenian plague, but some contend that the plague resulted in death to thousands in the city of Athens.

To this day, archeologists and epidemiologists dispute the actual name of this disease. Some liken it to *glanders*, another fatal disease caused by zoonotic spillover, which was eradicated in the early part of the 20th century, while others claimed it was more similar to the Ebola virus (Eby & Evjen, 1962; Holden, 1996).

Ebola Does the name "Ebola" sound familiar? You might recall news reports about the Ebola outbreak that garnered worldwide attention between 2014 and 2016 and claimed the lives of over 11,000 people, principally in three countries in West Africa: Guinea, Liberia, and Sierra Leone (Barbiero, 2020). This fatal disease that spreads quickly between people is not a new disease. Ebola is a *hemorrhagic fever*, belonging to a family of viruses that first appeared in Europe as early as the 14th century (Mangat & Louie, 2023). It is related to the *Marburg hemorrhagic fever* that reappeared in Germany in 1967 (El Sayed et al., 2016). In Africa, the disease first appeared in the Democratic Republic of Congo (DRC) in 1976, near the Ebola River, hence its name (Farmer, 2020).

VIDEO #2/60

Chapter 4: Global, Communicable, and Chronic Disease

- *Ebola virus*
- *Website: www.youtube.com/watch?v=sZD5e2BfHiE*
- *The Medical University of South Carolina is publicly accessible as it provides free medical-based information and resources to the public. (https://muschealth.org/)*

If you are familiar with the 1995 American film *Outbreak*, starring Dustin Hoffman, Rene Russo, Morgan Freeman, and others, you may think that hemorrhagic viruses look and progress like the fictional "Motaba" ebolavirus depicted in the movie. Not so. Remember, that was a fictional presentation of a hemorrhagic virus. Less than 10% of the West African patients with Ebola had bleeding disorders (Farmer, 2020; WHO Ebola Response Team, 2016). Nevertheless, Liberia and Sierra Leone suffered the highest mortalities with 4,810 and 3,956 deaths, respectively (see Figure 4.4). In total, this dangerous disease resulted in an average mortality rate of 50%. The Ebola virus in the DRC was the deadliest variant, with a reported mortality rate of 90%.

Black Death Perhaps a more infamous pandemic was the plague of 1346, often referred to as *Black Death*, which decimated villages throughout Europe, Asia, and the Middle East from 1346 to 1353 CE. An estimated 25 million people died during the first two years of the plague. Unfortunately, there were seven reoccurrences of the Black Death, the last of which appeared in the 18th century. Together, the eight episodes of this plague were responsible for the deaths of over 137 million people.

"Spanish Flu" Finally, we cannot forget the ill-named "Spanish Flu" pandemic of 1918. We say "ill-named" because this virus actually appears to have originated in the U.S. This 1918 pandemic viral strain has been credited with contributing to every global, seasonal flu epidemic since, including the major flu pandemics of 1957, 1968, and, of course, the 2009 A/H1N1 pandemic (Nickol & Kindrachuk, 2019). Consequently, the 1918 virus strain has earned the title "The Mother of All Influenza Pandemics" (Taubenberger & Morens, 2006; see Box 4.2).

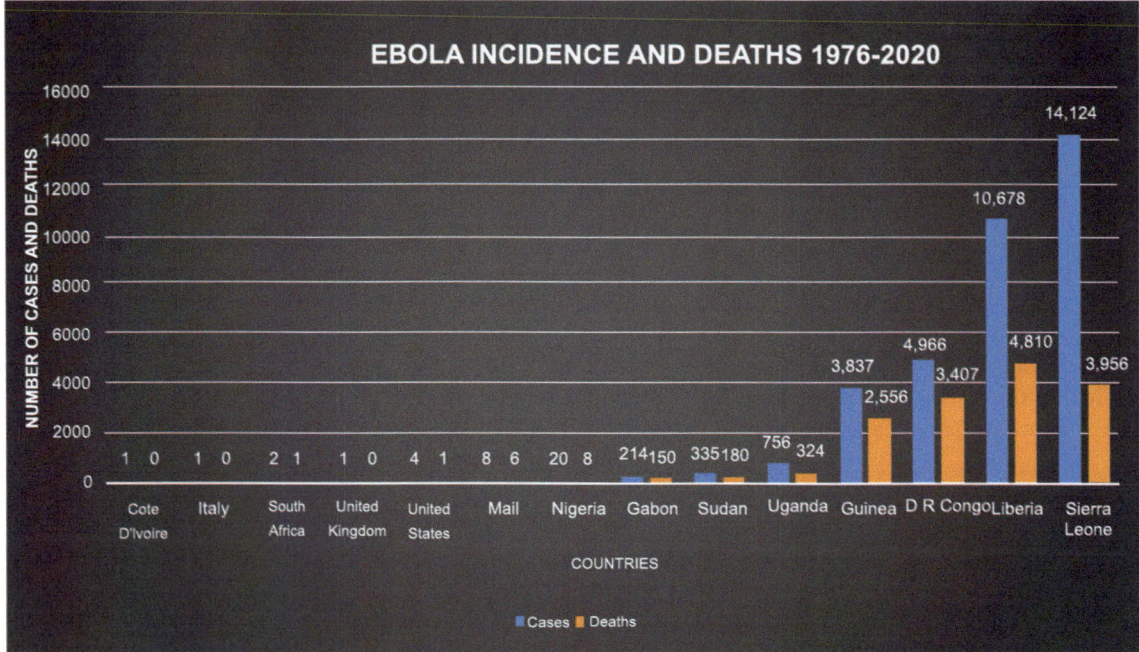

FIGURE 4.4 A bar graph shows the Ebola incidences and deaths between 1976 and 2020 in 14 countries. Largest number of incidences and deaths were reported in 7 countries: Sierra Leone (14,124 incidences, 3,956 deaths), Liberia (10,678 incidences, 4,810 deaths), DRC (4,966 incidences, 3,407 deaths), Guinea (3837 incidences, 2556 deaths) Uganda (756 incidences, 324 deaths), Sudan (335 incidences,180 deaths), and Gabon (214 incidences, 150 deaths). Seven other countries (Nigeria, Mali, U.S., U.K., South Africa, Italy & Cote D'Ivorie) each reported fewer than 20 incidences and fewer than 10 deaths.

Sources: CDC (2019), 2014–2016 Ebola Outbreak in West Africa, 2014–2016 Ebola Outbreak in West Africa | History | Ebola (Ebola Virus Disease) | CDC; CDC (2023) Ebola Disease Distribution Map: Cases of Ebola Disease in Africa Since 1976, www.cdc.gov/vhf/ebola/history/distribution-map.html

Box 4.2 The 1918 "Spanish Flu"

For some, the COVID-19 pandemic is reminiscent of the 1918 Spanish Flu pandemic. Like COVID-19, the origins of the 1918 pandemic were unclear in the beginning. Although its name implies that it originated in Spain, that is incorrect. The actual source of the "Spanish Flu" now appears to be the U.S. One of the first cases reported was at Fort Riley, a U.S. military base in Kansas (Fujimura, 2003). As Fujimura notes, this highly contagious disease spread quickly at Fort Riley and became a global pandemic in four months. One important contributor to its spread was World War I. The transcontinental and transnational movement of large numbers of military personnel from the U.S. and other countries enabled the virus to spread globally.

As we explain in the opening story, communicable diseases can be epidemics or pandemics. Influenza epidemics have and continue to occur annually whereas influenza pandemics happen sporadically (Nickol & Kindrachuk, 2019). We do note some similarities between the influenza pandemic of 1918 and COVID-19.

One similarity between the 1918 and the COVID-19 pandemics is that both the 1918 and the COVID-19 pandemics had multiple "waves": three for the 1918 pandemic and, so far, three for COVID-19. Unlike COVID-19, however, the second wave of the 1918 pandemic was the deadliest (Nickol & Kindrachuk, 2019). For COVID-19, the first wave accounted for more deaths.

The second similarity is the symptoms and the course of the illness. The 1918 pandemic presented with, among other things, shivering, high fever, weakness, loss of appetite, and cough (Radusin, 2012). People who contracted COVID-19 reported some of these same symptoms, but also included – at least initially – a loss of taste, muscle or body aches, and mild or severe respiratory distress (CDC, 2022b). Finally, in some instances, people who caught the 1918 flu virus and those who contracted COVID-19 seemed to "rebound" to better health, only to quickly return to a critical state that often resulted in death (Radusin, 2012).

In spite of these similarities, there is at least one major difference. Typically, most fatal influenzas affect people younger than five years of age and those over 65 years of age (Nickol & Kindrachuk, 2019). COVID-19 disproportionately affected the older population and those with preexisting health conditions. With the 1918 pandemic, however, the older population was not adversely affected. More than 95% of all fatalities attributed to the 1918 pandemic occurred among people younger than 65 years of age. In fact, those between the ages of 20–40 accounted for approximately 50% of all fatalities (Krammer et al., 2018). Why the difference? Some contend that 20- to 40-year-olds lacked a preexisting immunity from prior exposures to the influenza A virus. It is also possible that the high contagion rate in the U.S. military and the unsanitary conditions at the bases and battlefronts also contributed to a higher infection and death rate among the military and younger population.

The bottom line: Both the 1918 and COVID-19 pandemics were devastating, global pandemics. There were no vaccines to arrest the spread of the 1918 pandemic. In fact, scientists only successfully isolated the first human influenza virus in 1933. Similarly, initially, there were no effective vaccines against the SARS-CoV-2. One lesson we learned from the 1918 pandemic and subsequent infections is the need to quickly develop a vaccine that could arrest the spread of the virus, or at least lessen its symptoms and fatal outcomes.

There is one more important note, especially for health psychologists. Slowing the spread of a pandemic is not relegated just to pharmacological treatments. Teaching people how to protect themselves from the SARS-CoV-2 virus while waiting for the pharmaceutical treatment to "catch up" is important. This approach to health preventing behaviors is sometimes called **non-pharmaceutical intervention**, or **NPI**. Health psychologists can make significant contributions to NPIs by developing effective health messaging, intervention techniques, and strategies targeted to specific groups to encourage the use of NPIs until more effective treatment is available. Techniques such as mask-wearing, social distancing, frequent and repeated testing, and, if necessary, isolation, if messaged well could be immensely helpful in slowing the rate of transmission for the next pandemic.

Taken together, the last five major pandemics – the influenza pandemic of 1918, the human immunodeficiency virus (HIV), A/H1N1 influenza, the influenza of 1957–1958, and SARS-CoV-2 – account for more than 97 million deaths worldwide. The newest addition to the list of deadly pandemics, SARS-CoV-2 is, as of this writing, still impairing the health and well-being of millions of people. We reviewed the SARS-CoV-2 pandemic and its impact in Box 4.1 (see page 105). But one fact bears repeating here: if indeed SARS-CoV-2 is the result of *zoologic spillover*, as was the case with the A/H1N1 and MERS viruses, health researchers and environmentalists may need to reassess health protocol and human behaviors to help minimize the transmission of future animal-to-human viruses.

In summary, the viruses that caused the pandemics listed in Table 4.2 became major global health crises when they became capable of human-to-human transmission. In some instances, as with the pandemic of 1918, military troop movements during World War I facilitated transmission of the virus to countries around the globe. In other examples, as in the A/H1N1 and SARS-CoV-2 viruses, commerce and travel facilitated the rapid spread of the disease. All are effective methods for spreading diseases between people and over great geographic distances.

TUBERCULOSIS (TB) Tuberculosis fits the definition of a communicable disease because it can be transmitted from one living organism to another. Briefly, **tuberculosis (TB)** is caused by the *Mycobacterium tuberculosis* germ, sometimes called **bacilli**, that can spread when *TB* germs are propelled from a contagious person's cough, sneeze, talk, or spit, sending it airborne to other persons sharing the same airspace (Centers for Disease Control, 2007b; World Health Organization, 2007b).

Researchers have shown that a person with an **active case of TB**, here meaning someone who is untreated or ineffectively treated, can infect, on average, one person per month. At that rate, a contagious individual can infect 10 to 12 persons per year. Once infected, a person may become sick with active TB bacteria within a year (World Health Organization, 2007b). By comparison, a person with a **latent case of TB** will test positive for the bacteria but will not show signs of illness, will not be sick, and cannot communicate the disease to others.

TB is not a new illness. In fact, archeologists found evidence of tubercular decay in the spines of Egyptian mummies as early as 5,000 BCE (Donoghue et al., 2009; Nunn, 1996). It was a common ailment also in ancient Greece in 570 BCE (Daniel, 2006).

More recently, health records indicate that the U.S. and Europe experienced major TB epidemics in the 18th and 19th centuries. We describe the history and treatment of TB in the U.S. in Section IV of this chapter. For the moment, however, we call attention to current trends in global versus U.S. TB rates that, once again, illustrate the importance of a global perspective on health. First, the good news. The WHO's data on worldwide TB rates shows a 25% reduction in TB rates for the WHO European Region between 2015 and 2020 (WHO, 2023g; see Figure 4.5). Similarly, the WHO Africa Region, specifically countries in southern Africa, reported a 4%–10% decrease in TB rates for the same time period. Of the 30 "high TB burden" countries identified by WHO, six have successfully reached the WHO's annual 4%–5% targeted decline in TB rates each year: Ethiopia, Kenya, Myanmar, Namibia, South Africa, and the United Republic of Tanzania (WHO, 2023g).

All of this is good news. Now, the not-so-good news. Health experts feared that the SARS-CoV-2 virus would result in a worldwide acceleration of TB cases in many countries in 2022 and 2023. Unfortunately, they were right. For example, in Brazil, the rates of TB had begun to increase slowly between 2016 and 2020, and the pandemic is credited with a continued increase in cases there. In other countries, it appears that the disruptions to health care caused by the SARS-CoV-2 pandemic resulted in delayed testing

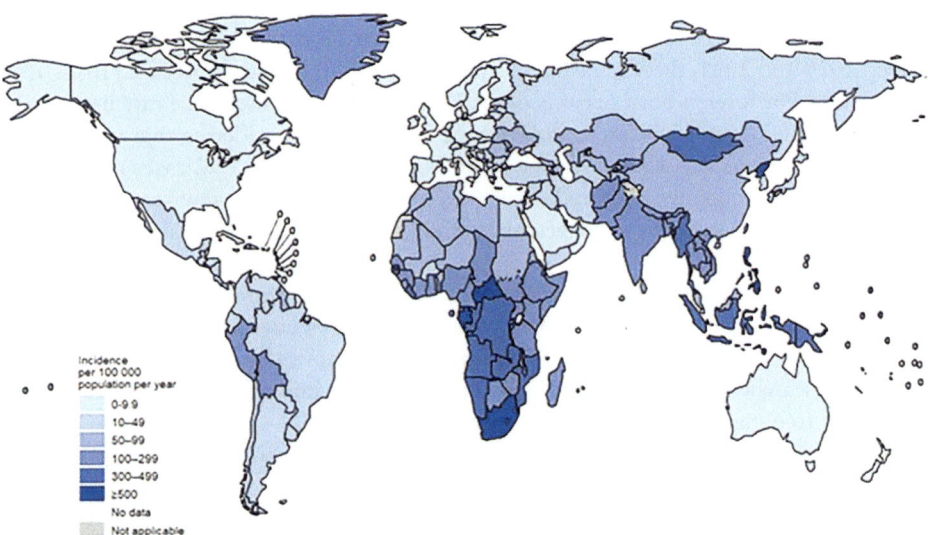

FIGURE 4.5 A map of global tuberculosis incidence rates shows the highest rates are in sub-Saharan Africa, south and southeast Asia, north central Asia and Greenland.

Source: WHO (2023g).

and notification of positive TB test results to people in countries within the WHO's Southeast Asia and Western Pacific Regions. These regions, which include the countries of Bangladesh, Democratic People's Republic of Korea, and Indonesia, among others, accounted for more than 86% of the global reductions in TB *notifications* (WHO, 2023g). In total, the WHO now estimates that 4.1 million people who have tuberculosis are either undiagnosed or unreported to health agencies. In 2019, that figure was only 2.9 million (Kirby, 2021).

The TB data for the U.S. show a similarly disturbing pattern. Again, the good news first. The TB rates in the U.S. are still low relative to some other countries. The not-so-good news is that these rates are increasing slightly. In fact, the 2022 TB rates in the U.S. increased for a second year in a row (CDC, 2023g; CNN, 2023), due principally to two factors: a slower reduction in the rate of TB cases and an increase in the actual rate.

Let's unpack that beginning with the slower reduction in TB cases per year. Prior to the pandemic, the CDC reported that the average decline in TB rates in the U.S. for 1993 through 2002 was 6.6% per year. In other words, there were 6.6% fewer TB cases each year in the U.S. between 1993 and 2002. From 2003 through 2006, however, there were only 3.1% fewer cases of TB per year, and the rate of decline from 2013 to 2014 was only 2.2%, the slowest decline in more than 10 years (CDC, 2015b). The slower reduction means more cases of TB in the U.S. from 2003 through 2014.

The second reason for the increase in TB cases is the increase in actual cases. With the onset of the COVID-19 pandemic, the U.S. and other developed countries saw an increase in TB cases, from 2.4 cases per 100,000 in 2021 to 2.5 per 100,000 in 2022. This may seem like a small difference, but remember, the total population of the U.S. is almost 340 million. You do the math.

In the U.S., one possible reason for the slower decline and subsequent increase of TB rates was linked to immigration. Foreign-born U.S. residents have higher rates of TB than do U.S.-born residents (CNN, 2023). Between 2020 and 2021, the TB incidence rates for U.S. born persons increased from 0.71 to 0.79 per 100,000 persons. For foreign-born persons in the U.S., however, the incidence rate increased from 11.7 to 12.2 per 100,000 (Filardo, Feng, Pratt, Price, & Self, 2022). Considering that in 2014 the TB rate for foreign-born U.S. persons was 15.4 cases per 100,000, this new rate of 12.2 cases per 100,000 is an improvement. Nevertheless, an upward trend (from 11.7 to 12.2) in the past few years is a trend in the wrong direction. Thus, the data seem to suggest that immigration plays a role in slowing the decline of TB rates in the U.S.

At this point you may be wondering why global and U.S. TB rates are relevant to health psychologists. Simply put, these statistics are relevant to health psychologists who study the health status of communities, especially if their work involves immigrant communities. For example, these statistics suggest that community-based researchers and health providers who work with immigrant communities should include measures of TB risk to obtain a complete community health profile.

Equally as important, health psychologists who design or contribute to intervention programs to reduce TB rates in the U.S. could use these statistics to identify groups of people at greatest risk for contracting TB. They could design intervention, prevention, and treatment programs tailored specifically to the higher-risk groups to maximize the likelihood of successful health outcomes. The statistics suggest that one high-risk group is select immigrant populations.

CHILDHOOD VIRAL DISEASES Measles, mumps, rubella, chickenpox, diphtheria, whooping cough, and polio: Do these diseases sound familiar to you? Most children in developed countries like the U.S. are medically protected from such *childhood viral diseases*. In fact, few would recognize names like whooping cough or mumps, and fewer still would come in contact with such diseases. For millions of other children, however, the same diseases often lead to serious illness or death. In this section, we examine three childhood diseases that continue to pose health problems for the global community: measles, chickenpox, and polio (see Box 4.3). We examine childhood viral diseases as part of our study of health psychology because the diseases have one thing in common: They are *all* preventable. Preventable illnesses are of special interest to health psychologists because they suggest an opportunity to improve health outcomes through changes in individual or community behaviors, or through improving access to health care. And, as we saw in Chapter 3, Theories and Models of Health Behavior Change, one goal of health psychologists is to motivate individuals to adopt behaviors that will improve their health status.

Box 4.3 Do These Viral Infections Sound Familiar?

How many childhood illnesses have you had? What about your friends? Chances are, not many. In many developed countries, incidences of measles, polio, and now even chickenpox are very low. Childhood immunization programs in many developed countries have made such diseases a rare occurrence. For that reason, we present a brief summary of three diseases that are uncommon in most developed countries but still occur at alarmingly high rates in developing countries.

Measles

Measles is a viral infection seen most commonly in children. Early symptoms usually include a cough, fever, runny nose, red and watery eyes, and small white spots inside the cheeks. The most prominent symptom is a rash that appears first on the face and neck, eventually spreading to other parts of the body. The symptoms last approximately 10 to 12 days (WHO, 2023h).

The illness itself is not as dangerous as the likely complications. Pneumonia, severe diarrhea leading to dehydration, or encephalitis (a dangerous inflammation of the brain) are the more serious complications and can lead to death (WHO, 2006b). Measles is especially fatal for children five years of age or younger who are malnourished, have weakened immune systems, or have vitamin A deficiencies.

Chickenpox

More uncomfortable to children than dangerous, chickenpox is characterized by an itchy rash that often turns into a blistering pox and, when ruptured, secretes a small quantity of pus. Children who catch chickenpox often complain of fever in addition to the uncomfortable itchy sensation from the blisters.

Less common are complications that arise from chickenpox, including encephalitis, pneumonia, or secondary bacterial infections (Varela et al., 2019). Overall, in 2014 the WHO reported approximately 4.2 million cases of serious complications among adults and children, associated with the varicella virus that causes chickenpox. That resulted in approximately 4,200 deaths (World Health Organization, 2014).

Prior to 1995, the U.S. reported approximately 4,000 cases of chickenpox per year, mainly among children. In those years, parents sometimes purposely exposed their non-infected children to others with active cases of chickenpox so that non-infected children would catch the disease which, for children, is essentially harmless. However, for adults who were never exposed to chickenpox, the disease is not as benign. Approximately 10% of adults in the U.S. are susceptible to chickenpox and can suffer complications that can include respiratory diseases such as pneumonia.

Polio

Like chickenpox and measles, polio is a viral disease. Unlike the other two, however, polio can be a crippling disease. The effects of the disease can vary from a mild, flu-like infection, including fever, nausea, and fatigue, to partial or total paralysis of the arms or legs.

When thinking of adult polio cases, many recall Franklin D. Roosevelt, the 32nd president of the U.S. President Roosevelt contracted polio in 1921 at the age of 39. His case demonstrates that adults afflicted with polio experience more severe symptoms, such as paralysis, than do children.

Thanks to the effectiveness of a vaccine discovered by Jonas Salk and eventually administered worldwide, polio is considered largely a disease of the past, at least in the U.S.

Measles, Chickenpox, and Polio *Measles* is a viral infection most commonly found in children. It can result in respiratory illness and even death. For that reason, it is the most serious of the preventable childhood infections (WHO, 2023h).

Until very recently, this illness was more prevalent in developing countries, due to weak health infrastructures in which children who were merely exposed to the measles virus were likely to contract the disease (WHO, 2023h). In many cases, the disease resulted in fatalities. In 2005, over 216,000 people in Africa – mostly children – and Southeast Asia died of measles. The high mortality rate associated with measles in developing countries is one of the reasons its prevention is considered the highest medical priority for children. What is more, WHO statistics showed that, in emergency settings, such as natural disasters or refugee camps, 25% of all child deaths are attributed to measles (WHO, 2006b).

But, here, too, there is good news and not-so-good news. As before, good news first. In 2018, the number of total deaths due to measles dropped to approximately 140,000. The reason? Vaccines. We will explore the role of vaccines in reducing transmissible illnesses and decreasing deaths in the following section. For the moment, it is only important to note that the measles vaccine is credited with a 73% drop in measles deaths between 2000 and 2018 (WHO, 2023h).

VIDEO #3/60

Chapter 4: Global, Communicable, and Chronic Disease

- *Measles: 5 Things You Need to Know About Measles in 30 Seconds (YouTube.com)*
- *Website: https://www.youtube.com/watch?v=0vySz5-fJlc*
- **The NFID is publicly accessible. The NFID is a nonprofit organization and provides valuable resources to the public and other organizations for free. National Foundation for Infectious Diseases-Healthier Lives for All through Effective Prevention and Treatment (nfid.org)**

VIDEO #4/60

Chapter 4: Global, Communicable, and Chronic Disease

- *Chickenpox: A Family's Story (60 second video PSA)-YouTube*
- *Website: https://www.youtube.com/watch?v=2LsJdS46Bw8*
- **All videos that are publicly posted on YouTube are publicly accessible to the public. PKIDsOrg is an educational YouTube channel that informs its audience about different medical conditions.**

Now, the not-so-good news. Recently, the U.S. and Europe have seen an uptick in measles. In 2019, the U.S. reported over 1,200 cases of measles, a record high for a country that classified measles as virtually eliminated in 2000 (Patel et al., 2019). In Europe, reported measles cases increased from more than 5,000 in 2015 to over 82,000 in 2018, just three short years later (WHO, 2023i).

What is the reason for this increase? Researchers and health officials cite many possible reasons, one of which is the increase in the number of unvaccinated children. While some children may be unvaccinated because they come from countries where vaccinations were not available, a more pressing problem in other countries is vaccine hesitancy, a health behavior. We will explore vaccine hesitancy in greater detail in the following section. For now, just remember that one cause for an unexpected rise in measles cases is due to this health behavior, specifically the health beliefs and behaviors of parents. Here, again, health psychologists can and should be involved in listening to, understanding, and addressing the beliefs and health behaviors that have contributed to the increased rates of measles among children.

Chickenpox, or the *varicella-zoster virus*, as it is known in the medical community, is a highly transmissible disease, although transmission is less efficient in tropical climates (New Zealand Government, Ministry of Health, 2022). It is an uncomfortable but rarely serious illness when contracted during childhood. Before 1995, approximately 90% of U.S. children experienced and successfully overcame chickenpox by age 10. As with many other childhood diseases, a person who has the disease becomes immune for life. Thus, by age 10, over 90% of children in the U.S. were effectively immune from contracting chickenpox a second time. But, as noted in Box 4.3, adults who contract the illness may face more serious health complications and a higher risk of death.

Finally, *poliomyelitis*, referred to commonly as *polio*, is a highly contagious viral disease that damages cells in the spinal cord and specifically attacks the muscle-controlling nerves (Wilson, 2005). Polio only results in flu-like symptoms for over 90% of people who contract the illness. For approximately 2%, however, the disease causes more severe health issues such as partial or full paralysis of the arms or legs.

During the first half of the 1900s, the U.S. experienced many waves of polio, often referred to as polio epidemics. The most serious epidemic occurred in 1916, followed by a succession of epidemics occurring from 1930 through 1960. The number of people affected by polio during that time exceeded 400,000 (Wilson, 2005).

VACCINES The statistics on measles, chickenpox, and polio may seem unreal. After all, when was the last time you heard of someone dying of measles? In fact, when was the last time you remember hearing that someone even contracted measles? The extremely low rate of measles – even with this recent uptick in cases – and other childhood communicable diseases in developed countries is no accident. Incidences of childhood viral illnesses are infrequent in many regions of the world primarily because many children with access to health care receive vaccines that *immunize* them against the diseases.

VIDEO #5/60

Chapter 4: Global, Communicable, and Chronic Disease
- **Vaccine: The Importance of Vaccines in 60 Seconds**
- *Website: https://www.youtube.com/watch?v=-UJ_LBVS8qU*
- *The Alliance of Aging Research is publicly accessible because it provides health-based information to the public for free (www.agingresearch.org/advocacy/vaccines/)*

Vaccines are medicines that contain a small amount of the virus (dead or live) from the disease in question (see Box 4.4). Introducing a controlled amount of a virus to the body encourages the body's immune system to build *antibodies*. We explore the body's immune system more fully in Chapter 8, Psychoneuroimmunology. Briefly, antibodies are proteins that identify and destroy bacteria and viruses that are foreign to the body. The immune system then retains some antibodies to recognize and destroy the virus if an individual becomes exposed to it at a later time. Teaching the body to recognize and destroy a controlled amount of the virus enables the body to protect or immunize the vaccinated individual from severe versions of the disease or from future occurrences.

Box 4.4 Vaccination: In Brief

The history of vaccines is quite fascinating. Historians credit a process called variolation, a forerunner to the current-day vaccines. This process actually began in China, India, and countries in Africa in response to smallpox, a nearly 3,000-year-old global pandemic. As noted previously, smallpox is a highly contagious disease that caused millions of death over its more than 3,000-year history, but fortunately has been eradicated since 1980 (World Health Organization, 2023f).

The first documented cases of the smallpox virus were found in 1350 BCE in Egyptian mummies (World Health Organization, 2023n). Subsequently, smallpox has been documented across the world in China, Greece, Arabia, and in various regions in Africa. Documents also show that in China, Arabia, and North Africa, **variolation** was introduced (as early as 200 BCE in some areas) to reduce the severity of the disease and reduce the incidences of death. Variolation involved extracting some of the liquid contained in a smallpox nodule and injecting or rubbing the liquid into a scratch or incision of the person being inoculated. When successful, this process effectively protected a person from severe cases of smallpox which could lead to death (Behbehani, 1983; Ranscombe, 2022).

Variolation techniques varied across countries and cultures. And, while it was effective in many instances, it was not risk-free. Variolated people who received too much of the smallpox liquid could develop full-fledged smallpox or risk transmitting it to others. Additionally, this process risked transmission of other illnesses from the infected person, albeit a rare occurrence (Behbehani, 1983).

Written records show that variolation was practiced in the 14th century in China, in the early 17th century in Türkiye, and in the 18th century in India, although some historians believe the practice was in effect long before then (Behbehani, 1983; Boylston, 2012). Somewhat later, in the early 18th century, the practice was hotly debated in Europe, England, and the British colonies of the New World, now called the U.S. In the new colonies, an African slave who was called Onesimus, told his slave master of this practice that was unknown in the U.S. colonies but common among the Garamante people from the Fezzan region of present-day Libya (Behbehani, 1983). Other African slaves also confirmed that variolation was a common practice on the continent. At about the same time, Lady Mary Wortley Montagu of the U.K. learned of this practice in the Ottoman Empire while living in Türkiye with her husband, an ambassador to Türkiye. Controversy over the safety and efficacy of variolation delayed its adoption in England until later in the 18th century. Finally, in 1796, scientist Edward Jenner developed a safer method of protecting people from smallpox by using cowpox, a viral source that proved to be less dangerous (Stewart & Delvin, 2006). Whether using variolation or Jenner's new vaccine, these techniques largely protected people either from contracting or spreading dangerous diseases.

Effectiveness of Vaccines How effective are vaccines in preventing the spread of childhood viral illnesses? Consider this: In 1973, Dr. Michiaki Takahashi developed the chickenpox vaccine in Japan by producing a live but weakened strain of the varicella zoster virus (Ozaki & Asano, 2016). The vaccine was certified by the WHO in 1984 as the most effective chickenpox vaccine (Cosdon, 2022). Six years after it was licensed for use in Japan, the Japanese government conducted safety and efficacy assessments and found that clinical symptoms of the varicella-zoster (chickenpox) virus were reported in only 6.9% of children (Asano, 1996). Worldwide, studies have shown that two doses of this vaccine provide 100% effectiveness against all forms of the varicella-zoster virus (Varela et al., 2019).

In 1995, the U.S. added the chickenpox vaccine to its arsenal of childhood vaccines. Today, two administrations of the varicella-zoster virus vaccine protect 95% of children from the disease (Chaves et al., 2007; Tugwell et al., 2004). Put another way, before Dr. Takahashi's discovery, more than 4 million people in the U.S. contracted chickenpox each year. Currently, the U.S. experiences fewer than 150,000 cases of chickenpox each year, and less than 30 deaths annually due to this disease (CDC, 2022c). In addition, vaccinating children to protect them from chickenpox reduces the exposure risks for unvaccinated adults, who are more likely to develop serious and sometimes fatal complications when contracting chickenpox.

The success of vaccine programs in many countries, including Australia, India, Italy, Japan, New Zealand, Singapore, South Africa, and the U.S. is due in part to public health regulations that strongly recommend that, by age six, children should have received all vaccines for measles, mumps, rubella, chickenpox, diphtheria, whooping cough, polio, and other infectious diseases usually contracted in childhood (University of Oxford, 2022). Is it a coincidence that public health officials chose to mandate immunization of children by age six? Not at all. In many countries, children are required to attend school by age six or earlier. Thus, millions of children spend five days a week acquiring knowledge and sharing germs in a common space. Unvaccinated children in such an environment could easily spark a mini-epidemic of childhood illnesses. To protect the health and well-being of all children, their families, and the community, most health policies require that children be immunized before starting school.

To summarize, a goal of health officials across the globe is to reduce the incidences of childhood diseases and to minimize the chance of children experiencing illness or death associated with serious, but preventable, diseases such as measles. Consequently, for countries with established immunization programs, measles and other serious childhood diseases are rare occurrences.

Vaccines have proved effective not only in preventing children from becoming seriously ill or disabled but also in protecting the health and well-being of a community. Yet, as we see from the changes in polio statistics worldwide (see Box 4.5 and Figure 4.6), not all children are vaccinated.

Box 4.5 Vaccines to Prevent Contagion

We can understand the beneficial impact of vaccines by examining an incident in 2003 when polio vaccines were suspended in Nigeria. Until 2003, polio was thought to be under control in all regions of the world. However, a new outbreak of polio was reported in seven west and central African countries: Burkina Faso, Cameroon, the Central African Republic, Chad, Ghana, Nigeria, and Togo. The source of the outbreak appeared to be Nigeria, where the government suspended its polio immunization campaign in the northern part of the country (see Figure 4.6). The reason for the suspension is unclear. What is clear is that the change in Nigeria's national immunization policy appears to be the principal cause of the resurgence of polio that affected seven countries in Africa. Nigeria's changed health policy is a good example of the effect that health policy may have on individual health outcomes.

Now, fast forward to 2022 and a new global outbreak of polio. This time it affected three high-income countries in different regions of the globe: England, Israel, and the U.S. The WHO Global Polio Laboratory in London, England, detected the **Sabin-like type 2 poliovirus**, one of three types of wild polio virus, in sewage samples taken in London. (Not to distract, but scientists have found that a reliable way to test for the presence of some communicable diseases is by sampling and testing waste or sewage water in selected geographic areas!) In 2016, sewage samples of the Sabin-like type 2 poliovirus were found also in Hyderabad and Ahmedabad, India, after the country changed the type of polio vaccine it had used in the past (Bahl et al., 2017). Sound familiar?

The polio outbreak in 2022 may be attributable to several factors. Some countries, for example Brazil, the Dominican Republic, Haiti, and Peru, experienced declines in polio vaccination rates during the COVID-19 pandemic (Torkington, 2022). This phenomenon was reported in other regions of the globe and has resulted in a spike in polio cases worldwide.

In other instances, unvaccinated persons traveling to areas where the population has not achieved what is called **herd immunity**, or the minimum number of people in a community who have immunity to a disease due to either vaccination or prior contact with the disease and have developed protective antibodies to protect against the illness (Mayo Clinic, 2022), can spark an outbreak. In the U.S., the majority of the new cases of polio occurred in New York State, specifically in Rockland, Sullivan, and Orange Counties. The polio vaccination rates in these three counties were 60%, 62%, and 59%, respectively (Torkington, 2022). Herd immunity for polio requires a vaccination rate of at least 80%. You do the math.

The proven effectiveness of vaccines is one reason why international aid organizations such as the WHO and the United Nations Children's Fund (UNICEF) have placed a high priority on global immunization programs for children. An equally compelling reason to prioritize immunizations is the minimal cost. In 2021, there were approximately 128,000 deaths due to measles, affecting principally unvaccinated or vaccinated children less than five years of age (World Health Organization, 2023h). For less than $1.00 per child, international aid agencies could vaccinate all children five years of age or younger to control and eventually to eradicate childhood infectious diseases (World Health Organization, 2023h). The cost for such a program in 2021 would have been approximately $128,000 – a minor sum for most developed countries.

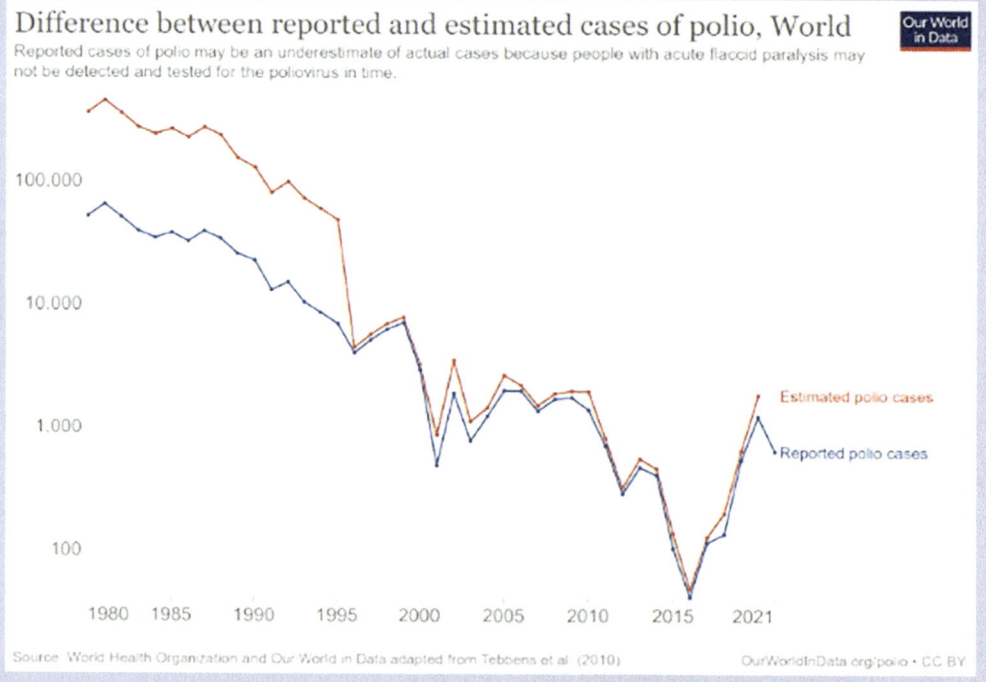

FIGURE 4.6 A line graph shows in 2021, there were just under 1,000 reported polio cases and just over 1,000 estimated cases, significantly more than the less than 100 reported or estimated cases in 2015. In 1980, there were approximately 90,000 reported cases and 140,000 estimated cases. Reported and estimated polio cases worldwide have increased since 2016, reversing a steady decline since 1990.

What would prevent someone from vaccinating a child to protect against a serious or potentially fatal disease? Health psychologists ask this question often to understand the factors that influence an individual's decision to obtain health-enhancing or health-sustaining treatments.

Vaccine Hesitancy/Vaccine Refusals In the case of childhood illnesses, we note that cultural or religious beliefs (individual, family, and cultural factors), fear of the consequences of vaccines (individual factors), the cost of vaccines (affordability, a demographic factor), access to health care (health systems factor), and vaccine programs (a health policy factor) all determine the likelihood that a child or an adult may forgo vaccinations. We explored the factors that influence health-enhancing behaviors from a health psychology perspective in Chapter 3, Theories and Models of Health Behavior Change. However, in light of reported increases in vaccine hesitancy and vaccine refusals for childhood immunizations, and the response to the COVID-19 vaccine in some countries, this issue deserves attention in several places, including here.

It is important to mention, first, that with respect to childhood illnesses (e.g., measles, mumps, chickenpox, rubella), *vaccine hesitancy*, here meaning parents rejecting or delaying specific vaccines beyond the schedule recommended by health care professionals, and *vaccine refusals*, or parents opting out of vaccines altogether, is not new (Reich, 2021). We will encounter this issue again in Chapter 11, Cancer, when discussing the human papillomavirus (HPV) vaccine for pre-teens. Here, we address, briefly, issues related to parental hesitancy or refusal to immunize their children against childhood illnesses and more recently the resistance to the new COVID-19 vaccine.

It should come as no surprise that parents would be wary of newly developed vaccines. The safety and efficacy of such treatments are not fully known, and few parents wish to have their children serve as experimental "guinea pigs" or learn of adverse effects of the vaccines well after the fact. Indeed, according to Kajetanowicz and Kajetanowicz (2016), parents' decision not to vaccinate their children is due mainly to their desire to protect them. Yet, in spite of a long record of safety and efficacy for the measles, mumps, chickenpox, rubella and polio vaccines, researchers and health care providers are at a loss to explain why, in the last 20 years (2001–2020), there has been a 10% decrease in the number of American parents who agree to vaccinate their children (Reinhart, 2020).

Box 4.6a Vaccine Hesitancy and Refusal: A Challenge for Health Psychologists

There are many reasons for vaccine hesitancy or vaccine refusal. In some instances, new risk factors created by a vaccine shakes public confidence in both the new and existing vaccine regimens resulting in a loss of public confidence in both. Such was the case in the Philippines when the newly introduced dengue vaccine was found to increase risks to people not exposed to the illness (Larson, Hartigan-go, & de Figueiredo, 2019). In other cases, erroneous information and false media reports can undermine vaccine confidence and uptake. This was the case in Japan when uptake of the human papillomavirus (HPV) vaccine, a vaccine to protect individuals from the virus that can cause cancer in a number of places in the body, including the cervix or vagina in females, and the penis in males (see Chapter 11, Cancer), plummeted from 70% to less than 1% in three years. The reason? Erroneous reports of adverse health effects linked to the HPV virus were picked up and spread through the media (Simms, Hanley, Smith, Keane, & Canfell, 2020).

Research in the U.S. suggests that the cultural context of parents and families can also explain vaccine hesitance or vaccine refusal. Parents of children in a private, Waldorf Steiner school, who themselves were highly educated and knowledgeable about vaccines, rejected them because they viewed them as unnecessary, developmentally inappropriate, toxic, and a source of profit for the pharmaceuticals (Sobo, 2015).

Perhaps, contrary to expectations, access to facts and more information about vaccines do not necessarily change opinions or intentions to vaccinate, especially among parents. In a 2014 study to identify effective messaging techniques that encourage parents to vaccinate their children, Nyhan, Reifler, Richey, and Freed (2014) randomly assigned parents 18 years of age or older who have children 17 years of age or younger, into one of four messaging treatment conditions. In Condition One, parents received information from the CDC explaining the lack of evidence that the measles, mumps, and rubella (MMR) vaccine caused autism. In Condition Two, the message provided information about the dangers of the diseases caused by MMR which could be prevented by the MMR vaccine. Condition Three shared visual images of children who had contracted the exact diseases that could be prevented by the MMR vaccine. Finally, Condition Four shared a dramatic but true narrative from the CDC about a child who almost died from measles (Nyhan et al., 2014). The results were not what the experimenters expected. None of the four conditions increased parent's intentions to vaccinate their child. In fact, in some cases they *decreased* parent's intention to vaccinate!

For health psychologists this is very disturbing news. But it also offers an opportunity to learn and to explore, develop, and promote effective messaging to change perceptions and influence the health behaviors of parents to increase intentions to vaccinate their children.

One study offers health psychologists a possible approach. Work by van der Linden, Clarke, and Mailbach (2015) suggests that presenting what they call "consensus information" helps to increase public support for vaccines. In this study, parents were also randomly assigned to one of four treatment conditions. The first was a descriptive norm condition where participants were shown a pie chart indicating that "90% of medical scientists agree that vaccines are safe." The second, a prescriptive condition, showed participants a pie chart revealing that "90% of medical scientists agree that all parents should be required to vaccinate their children." The third condition provided participants with both pie charts, and the final condition was the control group who received no information. Following these conditions, study participants answered eight questions (in addition to demographic questions) to ascertain their views on vaccination, including, for example, "I believe that vaccines are a safe and reliable way to avoid the spread of otherwise preventable diseases," and "More people ought to vaccinate themselves and their children." Van der Linden and colleagues (2015) found that the consensus messaging significantly reduced vaccine concerns and significantly increased consensus about vaccine safety.

Is this result surprising? Perhaps not, considering the information presented earlier about cultural context. If parents and others believe that vaccines are safe, their viewpoints are reinforced, and they receive support from others whose views they trust (see Chapter 3, Theories and Models of Health Behavior Change), these affirmations help to solidify their views. Thus, a lesson for health psychologists: one way to challenge opposing viewpoints on vaccine safety and effectiveness might be consensus messaging.

Global patterns in vaccine hesitancy and confidence in vaccines show similar results. An extensive study of vaccine confidence in 149 countries, conducted between 2015 and 2019, shows regional disparities in the belief of the importance, safety, and efficacy of vaccines. Briefly, de Figueiredo, Simas, Karafillakis, Paterson, and Larson's (2020) survey, which included over 284,000 individuals, measured an individual's perception of vaccine safety ("I think vaccines are safe"), importance ("I think vaccines are important for children to have"), and effectiveness ("I think vaccines are effective"). Study participants with children were also asked whether they vaccinated at least one of their children according to routine immunization schedules (de Figueiredo et al., 2020).

The researchers report that confidence in the importance, safety, and effectiveness of vaccines fell in six countries from 2015 to 2019, including Afghanistan, Indonesia, Pakistan, the Philippines, and South Korea (de Figueiredo et al., 2020). What is more, in three of these countries (Afghanistan, Indonesia, and Pakistan), along with Azerbaijan, Nigeria, and Serbia, there was a marked increase in the number of people who disagreed with the statement, "I think vaccines are safe." Only some European Union countries, specifically France, Italy, Finland, and Ireland reported increased confidence in the vaccines (de Figueiredo et al., 2020).

Other researchers such as Arce et al. (2021) report findings from 15 countries where parents express a belief that childhood vaccines are largely effective (67%–99%), safe (48%–97%) and important for children (80%–99%). And, in contrast to de Figueiredo et al. (2020), Arce et al. (2021) suggest that acceptance is generally higher in low- to middle-income countries. These and other studies, such as those noted in Box 4.6a, help explain why this issue is of particular interest to health psychologist and identify a role for them in changing health outcomes.

So much for childhood immunizations, what about the COVID-19 vaccine? Box 4.6b provides some of the background and current thinking about opposition to the COVID-19 vaccine. It is important to state again, however, that new vaccines, particularly ones that introduce a technique perceived by the public to be new or novel, will raise concerns. What the public did not know at the time the COVID-19 vaccine was first made available was that scientist had been working on and experimenting with the *messenger RNA (mRNA)* technology used in the COVID-19 vaccine for over 60 years (Martinon et al., 1993). Thus, while this technique is new to the public, scientist were much more optimistic of its likely success and minimal risks because of their 60 years of experience. Still, one of the challenges encountered by scientists and health psychologists when introducing and promoting the COVID-19 vaccine was its perceived newness.

Box 4.6b The SARS-CoV-2 (COVID-19) Vaccine

It is no exaggeration to say that the SARS-CoV-2 virus was causing fear and pandemonium worldwide.

In approximately one month, COVID-19 spread to over 581 people in four countries. It then accelerated to spread at alarming rates across Africa, Asia, Europe, and North and South America. Between March 2020 and October 2021, COVID-19 was the third leading cause of death in the U.S., after heart disease and cancer. (National Institutes of Health, 2022). Msemburi and colleagues (2023) and the World Health Organization (2023c) estimated that the true death toll of COVID-19 – including excess deaths directly related to COVID-19 in addition to the indirect impact due to, for example, a disruption of essential health care – was 14.83 million people worldwide.

Scientists in every country and at the WHO knew that the only way to truly combat this disease was to develop a vaccine that would at least minimize the harm to individuals who contracted the disease – here meaning lessen the likelihood of hospitalization and/or death – and hopefully prevent others from contracting it altogether.

While it is true that a number of vaccines were being developed concurrently to combat the virus, including vaccines that employed existing technology of inactivated viruses or live, attenuated viruses used to successfully develop vaccines against the childhood illnesses discussed previously (see, for example, Seo & Jang, 2020; Xia et al., 2021), what the public did not know at the time was that scientists had been studying a "new" approach, **mRNA** vaccines, for well over 60 years before COVID-19 became a global threat (see for example, Martinon et al., 1993).

mRNA is a genetic molecule that helps cells make proteins (Kolata & Mueller, 2022). Scientists first experimented with *mRNA*'s ability to command cells to make small viruses that would strengthen the body's immune system (Kolata & Mueller, 2022). Soon thereafter, biotechnology companies in Canada that were engaged in research on **gene therapy** – here referring to the process of repairing genes to treat diseases – were also experimenting with ways to protect fragile genetic molecules, such as *mRNA*, so that they could successfully embed these into the human body. These efforts, together with a third leg of research on genetic molecule, initially focused on producing a vaccine to prevent HIV/AIDS, led researchers to explore the "spikes" on the HIV virus and later to focus on the "spikes" of the coronavirus (Kolata & Mueller, 2022). When scientists successfully identified and mapped the coronavirus spikes, they were then able to encode that information into *mRNA* molecules and embed this molecule into the coronavirus vaccine. Thus, while this vaccine technique was new to the public, the over 60-year history, discovery, and development of *mRNA* technology was anything but new. For this reason, scientists were more confident in its potential success – at least in experimental settings.

The public, however, was another matter. Saad Omer, director of the Yale Institute of Global Health, notes that just "educating" the public about the virus and the vaccine is not helpful. In fact, he notes that that can be viewed as patronizing (Tavernise, 2021). Rather, Omer notes that to many "vaccine skeptics," scientists and policy officials were less credible (Tavernise, 2021). Research conducted in Australia (Rossen, Hurlstone, Dunlop, & Lawrence, 2019) and work by Hornsey, Harris, and Fielding (2018) confirm these findings, showing that participants with anti-vaccination attitudes had a low tolerance for any impingement on their freedom and held highly individualistic and/or hierarchical world views. It was also the case, Hornsey et al. found, that those with anti-vaccination attitudes were more likely to hate needles and to espouse conspiratorial ideas. In essence, it is about "gut beliefs."

Are health psychologists equipped to work with these gut beliefs to hopefully change health behaviors? Maybe. But current research suggests that health psychologists should work first to understand that they will encounter beliefs that are rooted in more than just misinformation. Health psychologist must be prepared to hear and respond to strong individualistic beliefs. They must give people convincing reasons to change their behavior without forgoing their independence and their freedom. For example, Hornsey and colleagues (2018) suggest helping people who have strong beliefs in independence and who abhor things that impinge on their freedoms to see that an anti-vax movement is a high-pressure, high-conformist approach that is contrary to their strong beliefs in independence and freedom.

It is a tall task, but it is not impossible.

Recurring Diseases

A second type of communicable disease is recurring diseases such as cholera, malaria, and dracunculiasis, sometimes called Guinea worm (see Box 4.7). These diseases present special challenges to the global health community because they are transmitted to humans from insects or bacteria that breed in unsanitary environmental conditions. In other words, for many recurrent diseases, environmental conditions are a predisposing factor (see Chapter 2, Research Methods) that contributes to the disease.

Box 4.7 *Dracunculiasis medinensis* (Guinea Worm)

Not all **parasites** are as easy to detect and treat as the cestode, or tapeworm (See Parasites, pg. 130). For example, some developing countries continue to combat an extremely painful and debilitating parasite known as **Dracunculus medinensis**, or **Guinea worm**. Like the cestode, Guinea worm disease is contracted when a person consumes a contaminated substance. Because the Guinea worm lives in contaminated water, a person can contract this parasite when drinking water that contains **copepods**, or small crustaceans that contain the larvae of the Guinea worm (Centers for Disease Control, 2004a). If consumed, the copepods die, but the larvae continue to live. The larvae will grow in the host (in this case, a person) for approximately 12 months until it becomes an adult worm.

After maturing, the female worms leave the host site, here meaning the human body. But the process by which the worm leaves the body is the painful and debilitating part of the disease (The Carter Center, 2023). To leave a host's body, the female worm forms a blister on the skin of the host, usually on the lower leg or foot. The worm ruptures the blister when it exits, causing an open wound in the skin. The rupture causes a burning pain so intense that most infected persons try to relieve the discomfort by placing the blistering part of the body in water. While the water certainly relieves the discomfort for a moment, it also puts the worm once again in water, the preferred environment to exit the body and to infect others. To speed the process, some individuals help the worm exit by pulling it as it exists in water. Now in the water, the female worm, once again, deposits a fresh supply of larvae. The cycle then begins again for another individual.

The entire process of extracting the worm is slow and painful. And for the majority (58%), the process of extracting the worm is so debilitating that they are unable to walk for a month afterwards.

There is good news, however. Guinea worm disease is rarely life-threatening. Most people are able to resume normal functioning after recuperating from the process. In addition, through concerted efforts by international aid organizations, Guinea worm disease has been reduced by 99.7%. In 1986, global estimates of Guinea worm disease totaled 3.5 million cases. As of 2005, fewer than 11,000 cases of the disease were reported worldwide (Hopkins, 2006). But even more exciting, in 2022 only 13 – that's right, THIRTEEN – cases of Guinea worm disease were reported worldwide! (The Carter Center, 2023). This outcome is so phenomenal that it bears repeating. In 30 years, the number of cases of Guinea worm has dropped to 13 total cases in 2022 from 3.5 million in in 1986. It is now one of two diseases targeted for full eradication by international health organizations.

How will the organizations eradicate the remaining cases? Remember that the disease is contracted through contaminated water. By providing clean, safe drinking water to the approximately 20 countries in Africa and Asia where the disease is most prevalent, eradication of the Guinea worm may be achievable in the very near future.

CHOLERA Like measles, very few people contract *cholera* in developed countries. The low rates of cholera in developed countries are attributable, in part, to local and national health policies that protect important infrastructure. Recall that in Chapter 1, An Interdisciplinary View of Health, we noted the important role of health policy in ensuring access to safe, clean water for the majority of the population.

VIDEO #6/60

Chapter 4: Global, Communicable, and Chronic Disease
- *Cholera: Why areThere So Many Cholera Outbreaks in 2022?*
- *Website: https://www.youtube.com/watch?v=mbflhWyHvqw*
- *Doctors Without Borders is publicly accessible since it provides medical-based information to the public at no cost (www.doctorswithoutborders.org/)*

Vibrio cholerae bacteria cause the intestinal infection that we call cholera. The bacteria are usually found in contaminated food or water or in human fecal matter. An individual who eats contaminated food, drinks contaminated water, or is in contact with human fecal matter infected with the bacteria can contract cholera (World Health Organization, 2008c). Approximately 80% of the time, cholera causes mild or moderate symptoms that usually include diarrhea and stomach cramping. In 10%–20% of the cases, however, diarrhea can be so sudden and severe that it causes severe dehydration, kidney failure, or death.

Cholera is closely linked to poor environmental management and unsafe water conditions. Countries with limited water treatment facilities, such as areas within Mexico, the Dominican Republic, Costa Rica, and Thailand, encounter frequent problems with water contaminants. In some instances, travelers to these and other countries are warned not to drink the water. In other instances, these factors, in addition to climate change (see Chapter 3, Theories and Models of Health Behavior Change), create conditions ripe for cholera. Climate change is credited with erratic and violent weather conditions, including excessive rainfalls, that flood communities and overwhelm or damage existing water or sewage infrastructure. Extreme weather conditions in addition to weak infrastructure have been credited for more than 4,000 deaths in the past two years in southern Africa and for a dramatic increase in cholera cases (Eligon & Moyo, 2024).

Even developed countries, however, may experience a disruption of water sanitation systems that jeopardize the water supply. Hurricane Katrina (see Box 4.8) damaged water treatment systems and prompted concern by health officials about a potential outbreak of cholera in the U.S.

In essence, cholera is a preventable disease but, like vaccinations for childhood viral illnesses, it is best addressed through health policy interventions. And, as we indicated previously, local, regional, or national governments are best equipped to develop the health policies that provide the environmental and safety systems needed to ensure safe water supplies.

Box 4.8 In the Wake of Hurricane Katrina

Hurricane Katrina, the Category 5 hurricane that severely flooded and damaged New Orleans and the Gulf Coast of Mississippi, is a well-known example of a natural disaster that created the perfect conditions for a cholera outbreak.

Katrina destroyed the water levees that protect New Orleans from the Gulf of Mexico and Lake Pontchartrain. Massive amounts of water flooded into the city when the levees failed, disrupting the city's infrastructure, causing major damage to sewer systems, and contaminating water supplies as well as other systems. Raw sewage and other waste products flowed into the waters that flooded streets and neighborhoods, especially in the Lower Ninth Ward and Chantilly, two neighborhoods in New Orleans.

Once the storm ended, many health workers braced for an outbreak of cholera. Why? The scarcity of clean drinking water and the contaminated water in streets and homes meant that people were exposed daily to microorganisms (see Chapter 1, An Interdisciplinary View of Health) that increased their risk of infections. Fortunately, no major outbreaks of cholera were diagnosed. There were, however, over 140 cases of diarrhea and more than 289 cases of other infectious diseases reported in the first days after the storm (Centers for Disease Control, 2005a). The point is that even in developed countries, like the U.S., cholera outbreaks are high-risk events that can occur in times of natural disasters like Hurricane Katrina. The U.S. was very fortunate this time that no such outbreak occurred.

MALARIA Mosquitoes! For many people the word *mosquito* conjures annoying images of insects that leave irritating welts after biting and an itchy sensation that can take days to subside. For others, the word *mosquito* is linked to insect sprays or other repellents that help avoid irritating sensations. Hot, humid weather and large bodies of stagnant water offer an ideal breeding ground for mosquitoes. And in countries with extensive hot or humid seasons as well as large bodies of stagnant water and large populations of mosquitoes, these insects can be more than just annoying: They can mean death if they carry the *malaria* virus.

VIDEO #7/60

Chapter 4: Global, Communicable, and Chronic Disease
- *Malaria: Malaria 3D Animation Shows How the Infection Spreads in the Body*
- *Website: https://www.youtube.com/watch?v=reKlLpbTHFs*

How does a mosquito become a carrier of the virus? The process begins with a parasite called *Plasmodium*. The *Plasmodium* parasite infects humans, but then it is transmitted from person to person with the aid of the female **Anopheles** *mosquito* (World Health Organization, 2007a). When the *Anopheles* mosquito bites an infected person, it injects a small amount of fluid that causes the skin irritation associated with mosquito bites. It then withdraws a small amount of blood from the infected person. The *Anopheles* mosquito then moves on to its next victim. When biting the next victim, some of the blood from the first person is injected into the newly bitten person along with the mosquito's fluid. In this way, the mosquito transmits malaria from one person to another.

Over 90% of the deaths from malaria occur in sub-Saharan Africa, where children disproportionately are the victims. Although hot, humid, tropical climates are the preferred breeding grounds for mosquitoes, in truth any area with favorable breeding conditions for mosquitoes is a potential malaria region. For this reason, high rates of malaria infections have been reported in Southeast Asia as well as in Central America and northern South America.

Like cholera, malaria is preventable. Anti-malarial medications widely available in the U.S. in addition to precautions such as mosquito repellents, protective clothing, and protective bed nets sprayed with repellent help to reduce the risk of contracting malaria (see Box 4.9). These treatments, in addition to two new vaccines just approved to treat symptomatic malaria, give new hope that malaria rates will decrease in the near future. While some note that these vaccines are only moderately effective, it is a start and a much-needed contribution to the toolbox for combatting malaria (MedicalNewsToday, 2024).

Box 4.9 Combatting Malaria

In 1998, a Roll Back Malaria campaign supported by WHO proposed and implemented three strategies to combat and control the spread of malaria: drug treatments, repellent-treated mosquito nets, and education. The drug treatment approach was aided by the discovery of the drug *artemisinin*. Artemisinin is an ancient Chinese herbal therapy that has been found to be effective against a number of types of malaria organisms (Miller & Su, 2011). When combined with a second antimalarial medicine, artemisinin is far more effective in controlling the illness than previous drug treatments. Currently, over 40 countries have changed their health policies and adopted the new combination drug treatment regimen (World Health Organization, 2005b).

The second strategy, sleeping under mosquito nets treated with insect repellent, effectively reduces the number of mosquito bites and therefore the number of persons infected with malaria. Because mosquitoes are most active from dusk to dawn, individuals are at increased risk of being bitten at night and while sleeping. The simple solution of sleeping under treated nets further reduces mosquitos' access to unsuspecting sleeping victims (Malaria No More, 2010).

The third strategy introduced by Roll Back Malaria is a global education campaign. The aim of the third strategy is to teach mothers, shopkeepers, and other village residents in malaria-infested areas to recognize the symptoms of malaria and to treat malaria with the artemisinin-based combination therapy (ACT; World Health Organization, 2005b).

Does this work? Yes, in many instances. Recently, Belize, a country southeast of Mexico, has eliminated malaria by using a combination of insecticide-treated nets, intensive malaria surveillance, and training for health care workers to recognize and treat malaria cases. These techniques helped Belize to reduce the number of malaria cases from 10,000 in 1994 to 0 – yes, zero – in 2019! (World Health Organization, 2023o).

There is one more bit of exciting news about combatting malaria. As of 2023, the WHO has approved two new vaccines to protect against malaria in children: RTS,S/AS01 in 2022 and R21/Matrix M. These vaccines, together with other malaria prevention efforts lead experts to have high hopes for a significant reduction in incidences of malaria (World Health Organization, 2023p). Like cholera and measles, malaria is treatable, but only with concerted national and, in some cases, international efforts.

PARASITES The U.S. Food and Drug Administration (FDA) frequently warns us of the danger of eating raw or undercooked beef or pork. These warnings are really meant to protect us from consuming meat products that are contaminated with the *Cestode parasite*, commonly known as *tapeworm*.

The Cestode parasite lives in the intestines of animals such as cattle or pigs. People can be infected with the parasite if the meat they consume from such animals is not cooked long enough or at a high enough temperature to kill the organism. Infected beef may contain the parasite *Taenia saginata*, whereas the parasite found in contaminated pork is called *Taenia solium*. When consumed, either parasite is capable of causing diarrhea, abdominal pain, and weight loss. In severe cases, the parasite can cause brain damage when left untreated. It is important to point out that the *T. solium* parasites found in pigs are not related to the agents that cause the A/H1N1 disease.

SECTION II. CHRONIC DISEASES

Until recently, health researchers believed that communicable diseases, like TB, cholera, and malaria, were the principal health problems for developing countries. On the other hand, *chronic diseases*, here defined as long-term (three to six months or longer), complex illnesses that can be controlled but not cured, were thought to be the main health concerns for developed countries like the U.S. (O'Halloran, Miller, & Britt, 2004). Because of such views, chronic diseases were given the nicknames "*diseases of affluence*" and the "*Western diseases*" (Ezzati, Vander-Hoorn, & Lowes, 2005). We now know that chronic and communicable diseases are widely prevalent in all countries. As we will see, the high rates of cardiovascular disease (a chronic disease) in developing countries and the prevalence of HIV, TB, and COVID-19 (communicable diseases) in developed countries demonstrate that diseases do not discriminate based on a country's economic status.

VIDEO #8/60

Chapter 4: Global, Communicable, and Chronic Disease

- **Chronic Diseases**
- *Website: https://www.youtube.com/watch?v=IP92d0Rf-UY*
- *Columbia University Medical Center is publicly accessible since it provides medical-based information to the public at no cost (www.publichealth.columbia.edu/)*

Chronic diseases include illnesses such as arthritis, asthma, cancer, chronic heart disease, chronic renal disease, chronic respiratory diseases, depression, diabetes, osteoporosis, stroke, and others (see, for example, Table 4.3). The symptoms associated with chronic diseases vary according to the illness. Yet one thing is common across all illnesses; the symptoms may occur intermittently, or they may be continuous and worsen over time.

Earlier in the chapter, we introduced childhood and other infectious diseases that afflict millions of people each year. Some of these diseases can be fatal. But it may surprise you to know that the leading causes of death *worldwide* are chronic diseases, not infectious diseases. This is true for both developed as well as developing countries. Statistics from WHO underscore this fact.

Statistics for the year 2019, shown in Table 4.3, show the ten leading causes of death worldwide for each of the four countries' income levels. These data show that of these causes of death, the majority are due to chronic illnesses. For example, among low-income countries, the chronic illnesses listed accounted for 409.5 deaths per 100,000, or approximately 42.4% of deaths. For low-middle income countries, approximately 76.2% of deaths are attributed to these same illnesses, while for upper-middle and high-income countries, the figures are 96.1% and 100%, respectively. Clearly, chronic illnesses are a critical health issue for all countries, regardless of income.

TABLE 4.3 Estimated Ten Leading Causes of Deaths by Country's Income Levels 2019

Rank	Low Income	Deaths per 100,000	Low-Middle Income	Deaths per 100,000	Upper-Middle Income	Deaths per 100,000	High Income	Deaths per 100,000
1	Neonatal conditions	77.6	Ischemic heart disease	106.3	Ischemic heart disease	126.7	Ischemic heart disease	141.3
2	Lower respiratory infections	62.3	Stroke	59.5	Stroke	114.9	Alzheimer disease and other dementias	66.5
3	**Ischemic heart disease**	56.8	Neonatal conditions	43.7	COPD	46.1	Stroke	64.6
4	Stroke	50.0	Chronic obstructive pulmonary disease (COPD)	42.6	Trachea, bronchus, lung cancers	33.6	Trachea, bronchus, lung cancers	47.7
5	Diarrheal disease	39.3	Lower respiratory infections	38.5	Lower respiratory infections	21.9	COPD	45.0
6	Malaria	28.5	Diarrheal disease	37.9	**Diabetes mellitus**	20.8	Lower respiratory infections	34.2
7	Road injury	28.3	Tuberculosis	28.7	Hypertensive heart disease	18.1	Colon and rectum cancers	27.1
8	Tuberculosis	25.5	Cirrhosis of the liver	21.1	Alzheimer disease and other dementias	18.0	Kidney disease	22.0
9	**HIV/AIDS**	24.1	**Diabetes mellitus**	20.5	Stomach cancer	17.9	Hypertensive heart disease	18.0
10	**Cirrhosis of the liver**	17.1	Road injury	17.3	Road injury	16.8	**Diabetes mellitus**	16.5
	Total per 100,000	409.5	Total per 100,000	416.1	Total per 100,000	434.8	Total per 100,000	482.9
	% deaths due to chronic diseases	42.4%	% deaths due to chronic diseases	76.2%	% deaths due to chronic diseases	96.1%	% deaths due to chronic diseases	100 %

Note: Of the ten leading causes of death, chronic illnesses (in bold type) account for almost half of the deaths in low-income countries and virtually all deaths in high-income countries.

Source: World Health Organization (2023r).

When examining Table 4.3 closely, it is evident that some chronic illnesses, such as tuberculosis, cirrhosis of the liver, and lower respiratory illnesses result in higher mortality rates in low- and lower-middle income countries than in developed nations. The economic disparities between nations means that populations in low- and lower-income countries are contracting and dying from illnesses that are highly treatable in higher-income countries. This economic disparity between nations led health psychologists and other researchers to propose that one probable explanation for the discrepancy in health outcomes between the higher-income or developed countries and the lower-income or developing countries is the lack of access to health care. Research shows that people with infrequent or irregular medical care have a higher mortality rate associated with chronic illnesses than people with a regular source of care or medical treatment. And, just to be clear, one reason for the lack of access is the low gross national income (GNI) *per capita* of individuals in developing nations. Thus, higher death rates due to certain chronic and communicable illnesses in developing countries could be caused, in part, by an individual's inability to afford health care or by a nation's inability to provide medical care to its neediest citizens – health systems and health policy determinants.

It is important to note, however, that lack of access to medical care is a problem in developed countries as well. In such instances, however, it is usually low-income or poor individuals who experience such outcomes.

CAUSES OF CHRONIC DISEASES Researchers almost unanimously agree that there are three principal causes of chronic illnesses: unhealthy diets, physical inactivity, and tobacco use (Jayedi, Soltani, Abdolshahi, & Shab-Bidar, 2020; Strong, Mathers, Leeder, & Beaglehole, 2005). In other words, the main determinants of chronic illnesses are the choices people make about their diets, their activities, and their habits. We add to these principal determents two *confounding factors*, here meaning variables that do not cause but may exacerbate the problem: socioeconomic class (specifically income) and race/ethnicity. In this section, we explain the causes and the confounding factors for chronic illness by examining two prevalent chronic diseases in the U.S.: diabetes mellitus and chronic respiratory diseases. We will explore other chronic illnesses, specifically cardiovascular diseases, arthritis, and cancer, in greater depth in Chapters 9 through 11.

DIABETES MELLITUS *Diabetes mellitus* is a chronic disease that occurs when the pancreas, an organ below the stomach, does not produce enough *insulin*, here meaning a hormone that controls the blood sugar levels in the body, or when the body cannot use the insulin it produces. When either of these occurs, it results in too much blood sugar in the bloodstream – an event that over time can cause damage to the heart, kidneys, or the eyes (CDC, 2023d).

There are two principal causes of diabetes. *Type 1 diabetes* is usually genetic in origin and is caused by the body's failure to produce insulin. There are no good estimates of the prevalence or incidences of Type 1 diabetes globally, but in the U.S., 5%–15% of Americans have Type 1 diabetes (Mayo Clinic, 2023a; Mobasseri et al., 2020).

The second type of diabetes, formerly called *adult-onset diabetes*, is now referred to simply as *Type 2 diabetes*. This is the most common form of diabetes both in the U.S. and worldwide. According to the International Diabetes Federation, in 2019, approximately 463 million adults globally were diagnosed with Type 1 or Type 2 diabetes resulting in a prevalence rate of 9.3% (Saeedi et al., 2019). This represents more than double the prevalence rate of 1980, which stood at 4.7% (Jung et al., 2021). Unsurprisingly, the prevalence rates for diabetes are higher in high-income (10.4%) than low-income countries (4.0%; Saeedi et al., 2019). But the important point here is that globally, approximately 90% of all incidences of diabetes are classified as Type 2.

VIDEO #9/60

Chapter 4: Global, Communicable, and Chronic Disease

- **Type 1 Diabetes: Conditions Associated with Diabetes – Scientific Animations**
- *Website: https://www.youtube.com/watch?v=XW7_V8ykoAI*
- **SAWBO creates educational animations on topics such as agriculture, health, and women's empowerment. Their videos are freely available for educational purposes.**

VIDEO #10/60

Chapter 4: Global, Communicable, and Chronic Disease

- **Type 2 Diabetes: Conditions Associated with Diabetes – Scientific Animations**
- *Website: https://www.youtube.com/watch?v=ZsTSoLhl3Y4*
- **SAWBO creates educational animations on topics such as agriculture, health, and women's empowerment. Their videos are freely available for educational purposes.**

Type 2 diabetes is caused by insulin resistance or the inability of the body to use insulin properly. Individuals with Type 2 diabetes could have a family history of diabetes that would predispose them to a greater likelihood of the disease (see Chapter 2, Research Methods). However, researchers have determined that the largest single contributor to its onset is unhealthy diets. In addition to poor dietary habits, however, Type 2 diabetes rates are escalating because of the increasingly *sedentary lifestyles* of people, especially in Western industrialized countries.

VIDEO #11/60

Chapter 4: Global, Communicable, and Chronic Disease

- **Insulin: Do You Have Diabetes? (60 Seconds Health Check)**
- *Website: https://www.youtube.com/watch?v=YUMp-Pm0eYi*
- **Yes, i-medics is publicly accessible. It is a platform where creators earn support for producing their content which informs the audience about medical education.**

VIDEO #12/60

Chapter 4: Global, Communicable, and Chronic Disease

- **Sedentary lifestyles: Combatting a Sedentary Lifestyle**
- *Website: https://www.youtube.com/watch?v=d4g7bPS_8pk*
- *Penn State Health is publicly accessible since it provides medical-based information to the public at no cost (www.pennstatehealth.org/)*

Researchers generally agree that we can reduce the incidences of chronic health problems, like diabetes, through relatively small changes in lifestyles and health behaviors. Specifically, reducing the consumption of foods with high concentrations of saturated fats and salt, increasing consumption of fresh fruits and vegetables, and increasing physical activity would help prevent many types of chronic illnesses (World Health Organization, 2005c).

Consider nutritional habits first. The nutritional habits of Western cultures, such as the U.S., are often referred to as Western diets. They have an abundance of highly processed foods and foods with high-fat and high-calorie but low fiber content. Unsure about this claim? Try this exercise. Next time you have lunch at a fast-food establishment or other restaurant with friends, count the number of high-fat, high-calorie items on the menu. To help you in this process, be sure to include the following: pizza, hamburgers, cheeseburgers, French fries, onion rings, cheesesteak sandwiches, and nachos with cheese. And don't forget the drinks. Sodas or other sugary drinks, including Starbuck's Frappuccino blended coffees, count also! When consumed in excess, such foods contribute to the increasing obesity rates in the U.S., a precipitating factor for diabetes mellitus and other chronic health issues. Thus, these highly processed, high-fat items are excellent examples of foods to limit or avoid to reduce the likelihood of developing chronic health problems later in life (Scott, 2007; World Health Organization, 2005c).

When should health psychologists begin advocating for healthy diets? We now know that it is never too soon to address dietary habits. Consider this: In 2003, the American Academy of Pediatricians, a professional organization for medical doctors in the U.S. who treat children from infancy to age 18, acknowledged the link between obesity and diabetes. Later that same year, the Academy asked pediatricians to include screenings for obesity as part of their annual or biannual checkups for patients. The aim was to monitor and address the increasing rates of obesity in American children (Wartik, 2003; and see Figure 4.7a-b). Their fear: If left unchecked, obese children will be more likely to develop diabetes as adolescents, a previously uncommon phenomenon.

In their 2030 edition of clinical practice guidelines, the Academy cited new data that show an increase in obesity as children age into adolescents (Hampl et al., 2023; see Figure 4.7a-b). These guidelines acknowledge the myriad of sociodemographic, environmental, and genetic factors that contribute to childhood obesity. In addition, they specifically note the role that many different providers and entities can play in the evaluation and treatment for obesity, including, but not limited to physicians, nutritionists, nurses, psychologists – and here we specify health psychologists – social workers, families and others (Hampl et al., 2023).

Diabetes and Lifestyle Choices Earlier we mentioned the contribution of sedentary lifestyles to diabetes. What does that mean? Television viewing and leisure use of computers and smartphones are examples of sedentary behaviors. When done in moderation, they are relaxing activities that may be part of a balanced regimen of active and passive behaviors. However, researchers are finding that the amount of time children and adolescents engage in such sedentary activities is increasing over time (Mahumud et al., 2021; Nelson, Newmark-Strainer, Hannan, Sirard, & Story, 2006).

Earlier studies, for example, a longitudinal study of adolescents' activities between 1999 and 2004, found that girls and boys show a decrease in physical exercise and an increase in leisure computer use that begins in early adolescence and continues well into the late adolescent years (Nelson et al., 2006). More recently, Mahumud and colleagues (2021) show that sedentary behaviors and low levels of physical activity, in addition to unhealthy diets, are even affecting children in low-middle income countries. Their sample of over 282,000 children, ages 11–17 years, found that sedentary behaviors were contributing to a global problem of overweight and obesity among children in both low-middle and high-income countries.

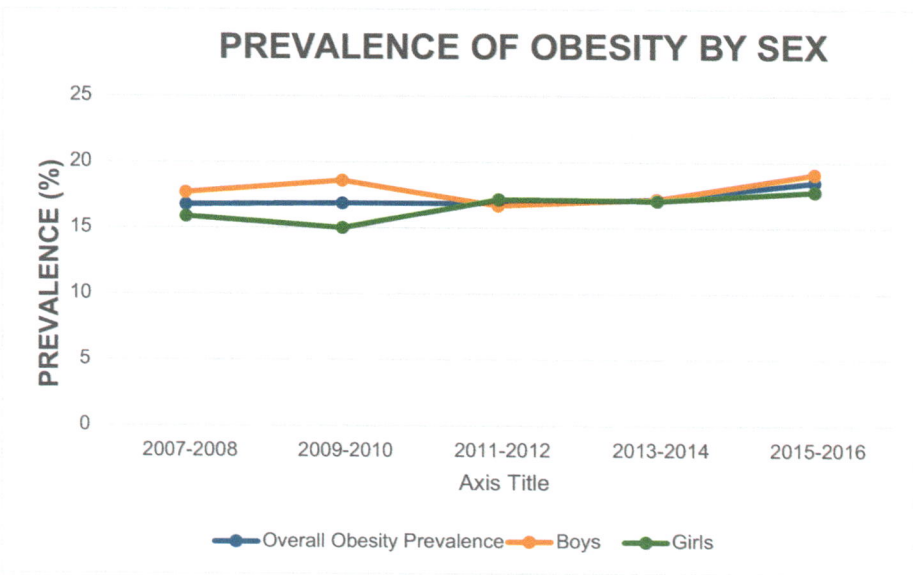

FIGURE 4.7a A line graph shows the prevalence of obesity by sex from 2007 thru 2016. Boys were slightly more likely to be obese than girls in 2009–2010 (18% vs. 15% respectively), a difference that narrowed in 2016 (approximately 18.5% for boys vs. 17% for girls).

Source: Hales, Fryar, Carroll, Freedman, and Ogden (2018).

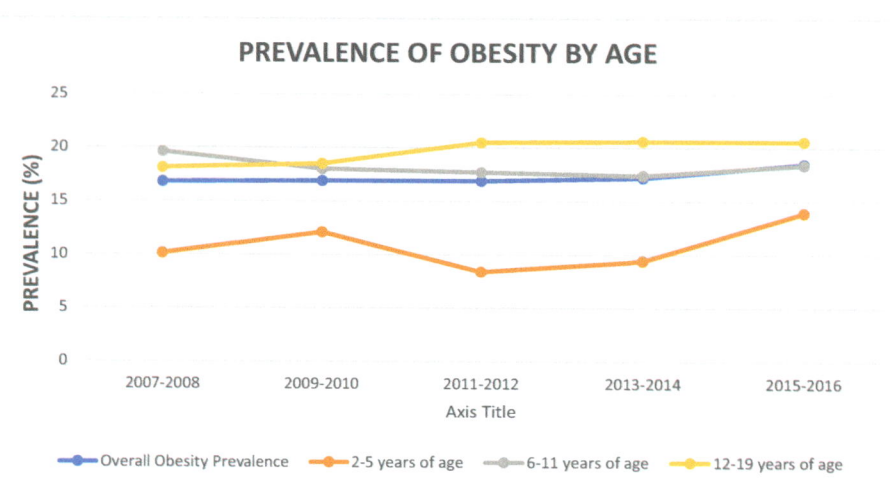

FIGURE 4.7b A line graph compares the prevalance of obesity by three age groups between 2007–2016: 2–5 years, 6–11 years and 12–19 years. An increase in obesity for children 2–5 years (10% in 2007 vs. 14% in 2016), a slight decrease for children 6–11 years (20% in 2007 vs. 18% in 2016) and an increase for children 12–19 years (18% in 2007 vs. 20.5% in 2016) was reported.

Source: Hales, Fryar, Carroll, Freedman, and Ogden (2018).

Diabetes Diagnosis Diabetes can go undetected and undiagnosed for considerable periods of time. In fact, globally 50% of people are not aware that they have diabetes (Saeedi et al., 2019). How is this possible? Symptoms of diabetes can be nonspecific and easily overlooked. For example, a frequent need to urinate or an extreme thirst may not be associated at first with diabetes. In addition, some symptoms are nonspecific. Unusual weight loss, increased fatigue, and irritability may signal the onset of diabetes. Yet, they could also be warning signs of some forms of cancer (Mayo Clinic, 2023a).

The most reliable method for detecting diabetes is through a blood test. But consider this: Unless a person has a reason to suspect that they are experiencing early warning signs of diabetes, he or she may either overlook the symptoms or fail to mention them to their physician. Lack of awareness of the symptoms of diabetes or a lack of access to health care for testing can delay diagnosis and treatment. Delays in treatment, or nontreatment of diabetes, can lead to health complications including blindness, amputation of extremities (arms or legs), or kidney failure, which can also lead to death.

We stated earlier that Type 2 diabetes is preventable. Therefore, we might be tempted to assume that anyone who contracts the disease has only themself to blame. Although such a conclusion may be accurate when individuals have access to nutritious foods, balanced diets, health care, and safe environments that allow for physical activity, it is less accurate when explaining the incidences of diabetes among individuals in developing countries with limited resources and fewer opportunities to obtain care, or for those in developed countries with no or limited access to healthy food alternatives or safe spaces for recreational activities. For diabetes, therefore, national or regional health policies are needed that ensure access to healthy options and offer preventive or early detection options that can reduce the onset or adverse consequences of diabetes. Here again, health policy can play a crucial role in an individual's health outcome.

CHRONIC RESPIRATORY DISEASES *Chronic respiratory diseases* are a class of chronic illnesses that affect the airways and damage lung function over time. Examples of chronic respiratory diseases include asthma, chronic obstructive pulmonary disease (COPD), respiratory allergies, and occupational lung diseases such as mesothelioma (see Table 4.4).

Like other chronic diseases, the cause of chronic respiratory disease can be both biological and environmental. For example, a biological cause of *asthma*, a partial obstruction of the airways that can cause wheezing or impair breathing, may be a family history of asthma that predisposes an individual

TABLE 4.4 Common Chronic Respiratory Diseases

Disease	Defined
Asthma	Partial obstruction of the airwaves (lungs) that causes episodic attacks of wheezing and difficulty breathing. Attacks can be triggered by allergies to pollen, mites, house dust, or other agents.
Chronic obstructive pulmonary disease (COPD)	Damage to the airway (lungs) caused by irritants such as tobacco smoke, pollution, chemical fumes, or dust. COPD causes coughing, mucus, sneezing, shortness of breath, chest tightness, and other symptoms.
Respiratory allergies	A physical response or hypersensitivity to foods, plants, animal hair, or other elements based on a misdirection of the body's immune system.
Mesothelioma	A form of cancer of the lungs that develops in the lining of the chest cavity, caused principally from inhaling asbestos fibers that cause irritation and damage to the lungs.

Source: Centers for Disease Control, 2004f.

to experiencing asthma-like symptoms or to having the illness (see Table 4.4). On the other hand, environmental triggers such as cigarette smoke and animal fur may cause an irritation of the airways that also results in asthma. Cigarette smoke is the most significant contributor to respiratory ailments, specifically asthma (Strzelak, Ratajczak, Adamiec, & Feleszko, 2018). This is true for individuals who smoke, as well as for individuals exposed to secondhand smoke on a regular basis (Stämpfli & Anderson, 2009).

VIDEO #13/60

Chapter 4: Global, Communicable, and Chronic Disease

- **Asthma: Asthma Attack**
- *Website: https://www.youtube.com/watch?v=svbSVnyISlc*
- *First Aid for Life is publicly accessible because it provides health-based information to the public for free (https://firstaidforlife.org.uk/)*

VIDEO #14/60

Chapter 4: Global, Communicable, and Chronic Disease

- **Secondhand Smoke: Secondhand Smoke PSA**
- *Secondhand Smoke PSA (YouTube.com)*
- *Website: https://www.youtube.com/watch?v=f_Auh61aN9Y*
- **The ADHD website is publicly accessible and serves as a valuable resource. Arizona Department of Health Services (azdhs.gov)**

COPD and Access to Care Obtaining an accurate estimate of the incidences of asthma or other chronic illnesses is difficult. Take, for example, *chronic obstructive pulmonary disease (COPD)*. Underdiagnosis of COPD is common due both to the difficulty of diagnosing the disease and to a lack of access to regular medical care. Herrera et al. (2016) illustrate this problem. In their study, which tested over 1,500 persons for COPD in four Latin American countries – Argentina, Columbia, Venezuela and Uruguay – 77% of study participants were underdiagnosed. Those in the underdiagnosed category were likely to be black, have a body mass index of more than 30, have a milder form of airway obstruction, and have no signs of wheezing or related hospitalizations.

Falagas, Vardakas, and Paschalis (2007) and Scott (2007) note that, in addition to difficulty in diagnosing, testing for COPD is infrequent. In developing countries, less than half (44.6%) of the people suspected of having COPD receive a pulmonary function test, a basic test that measures how well the lungs take in and expel air. Of those, fewer than 24% received an official diagnosis confirming COPD. But consider this: For individuals in developing countries, making repeat visits to doctors, being tested, and receiving the results of tests is a costly and time-consuming process that many cannot afford, especially when testing for a long-term and debilitating, but not necessarily fatal, disease.

In case this sounds a little shortsighted, consider another example. In developed countries, it is not uncommon for an individual to postpone seeking treatment for what appears to be a minor cough. You may know of someone who feels this way. A person with a minor cough may postpone seeking medical care even when the cough worsens and causes a heavy feeling in the chest. That person's rationale for not seeking treatment may be that the cough is not serious, they can still perform daily tasks, or the person cannot afford the time off from work or school to seek treatment. The cost factors that an individual considers when determining whether to seek treatment may be similar regardless of whether the individual lives in a developed or a developing country. Alarm bells should be sounding about now, as these are the issues that health psychologists can and are equipped to address.

Researchers who examine the morbidity and mortality statistics for chronic respiratory diseases find the data sobering. The research group GBD Chronic Respiratory Disease Collaborators (2020) placed the number of deaths due to chronic respiratory disease in 2017 at just less than 4 million worldwide. East Asia and South Asia reported the highest rates of chronic respiratory disease deaths, largely due to higher levels of air pollution and smoking (Institute for Health Metrics and Evaluation, 2023). More specifically, chronic obstructive pulmonary disease (COPD), which accounted for approximately 3.3 million deaths, was the primary cause of deaths globally (GBD Chronic Respiratory Disease Collaborators (2019). In the U.S. alone, approximately 148,000 Americans died of complications associated with COPD in 2020 (American Lung Association, n.d.), with the highest death rates reported among white males (43.6 per 100,000) and white females (37.9 per 100,000).

The long-term nature of most chronic illnesses leads many to view chronic diseases as less threatening to one's health than infectious diseases. But remember, as these statistics show, and as we noted at the beginning of the section on chronic diseases, more deaths are attributed to chronic illnesses worldwide than to infectious diseases, a fact that should encourage us to reconsider the impact of chronic diseases on individual or community health outcomes.

SOCIOECONOMIC CLASS, RACE/ETHNICITY, AND CHRONIC DISEASES Socioeconomic class and race/ethnicity are two confounding factors that contribute to chronic illnesses. Yet many researchers contend that socioeconomic class and race/ethnicity are indirect contributors to chronic illnesses because they entail lifestyle choices and access to care.

Research conducted by the WHO and the Institute of Medicine (IOM), a U.S.-based institution that examines health care systems and access to care, demonstrates the effects of race/ethnicity and socioeconomic factors on health care outcomes, as shown in two classic studies in Box 4.10. Briefly, the findings suggest that individuals in the lower socioeconomic groups (people who, by income levels, would be considered poor or lower-middle income), are less able to obtain quality health care when needed than are individuals in the middle and upper-middle socioeconomic groups (Institute of Medicine, 2002b). This is true whether comparing people in high-income countries, such as the U.S., or comparing across countries of different income categories (Emadi, Delavari, & Bayati, 2021).

Equally alarming, however, is that even when there is no disparity in socioeconomic status, researchers found inequities in health care based on ethnicity and race (Kelley, Moy, Stryer, Burstin, & Clancy, 2005; Mahajan et al., 2021). As Mahajan and colleagues (2021) report, differences in health status, access to care, or access to affordable care as a function of socioeconomic status has persisted for over 20 years in the U.S. (1999–2018). Earlier studies by Kelley and colleagues (2005) found largely similar results.

Box 4.10 Health Care Disparities in the U.S.

Do individuals experience differences in health care treatment in the U.S. based on their socioeconomic status or race/ethnicity? Some researchers think so.

Sonel and colleagues (2005) designed a study to examine this question for patients with coronary or heart-related illnesses. A total of 400 hospitals participated in a program called CRUSADE (Can Rapid Risk Stratification of Unstable Angina Patients Suppress Adverse Outcomes with Early Implementation of ACC/AHA Guidelines?). Hospitals in the CRUSADE study agreed to provide data for Sonel and colleagues (2005) to determine whether there were differences in medical care for heart patients of different ethnic/racial or socioeconomic classes. Specifically, Sonel and colleagues reviewed the medical records of over 43,000 patients, of whom approximately 84% were white and 13% were African American, to determine whether African Americans and whites received different types of treatment for largely similar heart-related illnesses when seeking care in hospitals.

Their results revealed significant treatment differences between the two groups. In general, Sonel and colleagues (2005) found that African American patients were more likely to be in poorer health and to have less access to health care. Demographically, African Americans were more likely to be younger than the white patients and to be female. Healthwise, African Americans were more likely to have a diagnosis of hypertension (high blood pressure), to have a confirmed diagnosis of diabetes, and to have a history of smoking and of heart disease. With respect to access to health care, African American patients were less likely to have health insurance through either a health maintenance organization (HMO) or other private insurance. That means they were more likely to be self-insured or have no insurance and less likely to have a cardiologist as their primary care physician at the hospital.

Sonel and colleagues' (2005) study demonstrates clear differences between African Americans and whites with regard to health status and access to health care. But do the differences extend to the types and quality of health treatment? The answer to that question also appears to be yes. When examining the type of treatment given to the two groups, Sonel and colleagues found that while African Americans were as likely as whites to receive the standard treatment, such as aspirin, for acute coronary (heart) problems, they were 20%–40% less likely to be given the newer, more resource-intensive treatments.

Why is there such a difference? One study alone cannot address that question. However, an earlier study suggests that ethnicity plays a role. Whittle, Conigliaro, Good, and Lofgren (1993) examined the rates of four types of cardiovascular procedures on African American and white patients in a Veterans Administration (VA) Hospital. By choosing a VA hospital, the researchers controlled for the possible confounding effect of income or insurance on access to resource-intensive treatments. Remember, U.S. veterans' health care is funded by the government. Yet here, too, the researchers found that African American patients were 1.38 to 2.2 times *less* likely to receive the more invasive surgical procedures for their cardiovascular illness than were whites. Now, with income and insurance not a factor, the only remaining factor appears to be ethnicity.

Studies like these have prompted the Institute of Medicine, a U.S. research and policy organization, to caution and advise U.S. health care providers about the continuing problems of disparities in health care in the U.S. due to race/ethnicity and socioeconomic class.

There is, however, a twist. In the aforementioned studies, socioeconomic class and race are often correlated and their findings suggest that both factors are positively associated with poorer health and higher mortality rates. Now examine an innovative study by Gong, Phillips, Hudson, Curti, and Phillips (2019). This U.S. based study examined the overall well-being and mortality outcomes in rural versus urban communities in all 50 U.S. states. Specifically, they examined the health outcomes of people within and across states by comparing five variables: rural versus urban residence, well-being (measured using the Wellbeing Index; see Box 4.11), primary care physician supply, the percentage of uninsured residents, and the percentage of racial/ethnic groups in the communities (Gong et al., 2019). Their findings revealed that, unsurprising to many in the U.S., rural areas reported higher mortality rates. What might be surprising, however, is that three factors best predicted this higher rural mortality rate: socioeconomic deprivation, physician shortage, and lack of access to health care (Gong et al., 2019). What is missing here? Race! Two of the three factors that best predicted higher mortality rates in rural areas measure lack of health care, not race/ethnicity.

Box 4.11 World Health Organization (WHO)-5 Wellbeing Index

The WHO-5 Questionnaire

Instructions:
Please indicate for each of the five statements which is closest to how you have been feeling over the past 2 weeks.

Over the Past 2 Weeks . . .	All of the Time	Most of the Time	More Than Half the Time	Less than Half the Time	Some of the Time	At No Time
I have felt cheerful and in good spirits	5	4	3	2	1	0
I have felt calm and relaxed.	5	4	3	2	1	0
I have felt active and vigorous	5	4	3	2	1	0
I woke up feeling fresh and rested.	5	4	3	2	1	0
My daily life has been filled with things that interest me.	5	4	3	2	1	0

Scoring principle: The raw score ranging from 0 to 25 is multiplied by 4 to give the final score from 0 representing the worst imaginable well-being to 100 representing the best imaginable well-being.

Source: https://ogg.osu.edu/media/documents/MB%20Stream/who5.pdf

---

What might be even more surprising is that this study also revealed a negative association between the percentage of Hispanics and mortality rates, which, according to Gong and colleagues (2019), exhibits what has been called the "Hispanic Paradox." In essence, Hispanics have been found to have better health outcomes than non-Hispanic whites, even though, on average, Hispanics have a lower socioeconomic status than whites. The final surprise from this study is Gong and colleagues' explanation for the higher mortality rates among African Americans in southern states, a cause they attribute more to the socioeconomic status of African Americans than to their race.

So, what does all this mean? It means that while in many places in the U.S. socioeconomic status and race are highly correlated, it is imperative that when attempting to address chronic health issues, we disaggregate race and socioeconomic status to offer a more sophisticated analysis and targeted treatment.

Measures of Life Expectancy, Quality of Life, and Chronic Illnesses

We mentioned in Chapter 2, Research Methods, that mortality rates are a gross measure of the health of a nation. In general, countries and communities with higher life expectancies are believed to have a healthier population because longevity is an indication of healthier living conditions. Now, however, we can use more precise measures to assess the overall health of a population by estimating the effect of chronic illnesses on overall well-being.

The *Disability Adjusted Life Expectancy (DALE)* measures a population's health status adjusted for *quality of life*. Here, *quality of life* is defined as the number of years of good, full functioning ability (see Box 4.12 and Table 4.5). It is important to point out that the DALE estimates the number of years of healthy, unimpaired functioning, not life expectancy. As such, some health researchers question its usefulness as a measure of the health status of a population because it measures healthy function and not mortality. For some illnesses, however, health impairments are morbidity factors (see Chapter 2, Research Methods) that contribute to mortality. Hence the DALE may measure an individual's *overall life expectancy*.

Box 4.12 Calculating Disability Adjusted Life Expectancy (DALE)

To calculate the adjusted life expectancy using the Disability Adjusted Life Expectancy (DALE), we determine first the number of years the person is expected to live under completely healthy conditions, that is, without impairment. Life expectancy data, sorted by country and gender (published by the World Bank; see Table 4.5, provide the vital statistics needed for the first part of the calculation.

TABLE 4.5 Life Expectancies by Birth Year: Top 40 Countries by Descending Overall Longevity

COUNTRY	Life Expectancy in Years (2021)
Hong Kong (People's Republic of China)	85
Japan	84
Sweden	84
Switzerland	84
Italy	83
Singapore	83
Spain	83
Australia	83
Canada	83
Israel	83
Luxembourg	83
Malta	83
Norway	83
Belgium	82
Finland	82
France	82
Ireland	82
New Zealand	82

(Continued)

TABLE 4.5 (Continued)

COUNTRY	Life Expectancy in Years (2021)
Austria	81
Channel Islands	81
Denmark	81
Germany	81
Netherlands	81
Portugal	81
Slovenia	81
Cyprus	81
Greece	80
U.S. Virgin Islands	80
Puerto Rico	80
Chile	79
Costa Rica	77
U.S.	76
Cuba	74

Source: World Bank (2023). Life expectancy at birth (in years). Accessed at: https://data.worldbank.org/indicator/SP.DYN.LE00.IN

Using Table 4.5, we can take, as an example, an individual from New Zealand. The overall life expectancy in New Zealand is 82 years. Using the information in Table 4.5 and the DALE, we can calculate the adjusted life expectancy of an individual in New Zealand if we know that person's current health status, that is, his or her current illnesses. For this exercise, assume that a Kiwi man (Kiwis is how New Zealanders refer to themselves) contracted cancer at age 60. We compute the number of years of expected ill health (that is, less than fully functional health) based on his current health status and the severity of any current illness. For cancer, some would estimate a loss of approximately five years due to ill health while undergoing treatment. We subtract five years from the overall life expectancy for a Kiwi man (82 years) according to Table 4.5 to obtain an adjusted life expectancy of 77 years.

Country	Overall Life Expectancy	Years Expected Ill Health	Adjusted Life Expectancy
Kiwi	82 yrs	5 yrs	77 yrs.

In addition to estimating an individual's number of years of fully functioning health, the DALE also measures a population's likely productivity based on the health of its population. Using the DALE, WHO estimates that developed countries lose about 9% of their population's productivity to disability, whereas less developed countries lose approximately 14%. In essence, the DALE serves as a measure of overall well-being that also helps to predict a country's likely economic health based on its most valuable resource: the health of its workforce.

To review, chronic illnesses are the leading causes of deaths worldwide. For this reason alone, health care providers and health psychologists should include healthy lifestyles and their impact on chronic illnesses as an important determinant of an individual's health status. Surprisingly, many do not. In Part III of this book, we devote three chapters, Chapters 9 through 11, to three of the leading chronic illnesses in the U.S. in an effort to refocus needed attention on the impact of chronic illnesses on overall well-being.

SECTION III. GLOBAL HEALTH ORGANIZATIONS

We indicated that a country's health needs are usually addressed by local or national health care systems or policy organizations within countries. In some countries, however, local or national governments do not have the personnel, financial, or material resources to meet even the most basic health care needs of their populations or to establish policies to do the same. In such cases, *global health organizations* help bridge the gap between needed and available resources. We examine the contributions of such organizations in this section because health care systems and health policy are two important determinants of individual health outcomes.

Although there are a host of organizations that provide health care services globally, in this section, we focus on three of the best known organizations that provide health services and assistance to the international community: the World Health Organization (WHO), the Federation of Red Cross and Red Crescent Societies (IFRC), and Médecins Sans Frontières (MSF, also known as Doctors Without Borders).

World Health Organization (WHO)

Throughout the chapter, we have presented facts and statistics on global health issues published by the WHO. It should come as no surprise, therefore, that WHO is considered one of the leading international health policy organizations. WHO is a specialized agency created by the United Nations in 1948 to help people live healthy, productive lives and to address the social, economic and political determinants of health (WHO, 2023j). As of 2023, the organization consists of 194 member states (countries). Led by a director general, the WHO oversees the work of over 8,000 doctors, public health experts, epidemiologists, scientists, and managers with the aim of coordinating health responses to emergencies such as the COVID-19 crisis, promoting overall well-being across the globe, helping prevent disease, and expanding health care to all (WHO, 2023k).

In 2015, the UN, the WHO's parent organization, developed 17 Sustainable Development Goals aimed at improving the lives of people everywhere. The vast majority of these goals impact health in one way or another, however eight goals directly impact and contribute to health: SDG 2 (Zero Hunger), 3 (Good Health and Well-Being), 6 (Clean Water and Sanitation), 10 (Reduced Inequalities), 13 (Climate Action), 14 (Life Below Water), 15 (Life on Land), and 16 (Peace, Justice and Strong Institutions). You may have noticed that the goals are similar to some of the objectives espoused by health psychologists. Thus, another reason for us to examine WHO's work is because they share some common goals with health psychologists.

WHO promotes its health goals using a three-step process. It assesses the health needs of a population, develops policy initiatives, and, to a limited extent, implements policies in targeted regions of the world. One example of WHO's needs assessment work is shown in a publication titled *Preventing Chronic Diseases: A Vital Investment* (World Health Organization, 2005c), considered the most authoritative source of information on chronic illnesses worldwide. *Preventing Chronic Diseases* has led some health providers to reclassify chronic illnesses as an important, perhaps even critical, unmet need in all countries. More recently, WHO has partnered with two private agencies, Bloomberg Philanthropies and Vital Statistics, to launch Partnership for Healthy Cities, a network of 73 cities worldwide committed to enhance health by preventing chronic (now called noncommunicable) diseases and preventing injuries (Partnership for Healthy Cities, 2023).

Second, WHO formulates and adopts policy initiatives aimed at eliminating specific health problems. This is a critical role because, as we have indicated, some countries do not have the resources to develop and adopt health policy initiatives themselves. For example, according to the WHO, people with untreated mental health conditions are more likely to encounter other communicable and noncommunicable physical health conditions (WHO, 2019). What is more, pandemics, like COVID-19, contribute to mental health crises that, according to the WHO, lead to a 25% increase worldwide in depression and anxiety (WHO, 2023l).

To respond to the health needs of people with mental illnesses, WHO developed programs to assist countries in adopting mental health legislation for their citizens. In its most recent report, the WHO advocates for the integration of mental health services into primary health care, and the development and strengthening of mental health services that are community-based – a departure from the psychiatric care model in place in many developed countries that may be unaffordable in many developing countries (WHO, 2023l).

The organization plans for and implements policy changes at the national, subnational (regional), and individual level. Consider this: In response to the recurrent problem of malnutrition, WHO developed a high-protein food that, when given to children suffering from disease, or the impact of war or displacement, decreases mortality rates due to malnutrition.

Finally, WHO examines the *macroeconomic impact of ill health* on individual nations and on the world. What does this mean? We explored this briefly when explaining the uses of the DALE in assessing worker productivity. There are several ways to calculate the effect of an individual's ill health. For much of this chapter, we have focused on the impact of illness or disease on either the individual, their family, or the immediate community. However, another reason that countries establish national health policies is to help sustain the economic health of the country. Countries realize that highly contagious or chronic diseases can reduce the number of able-bodied workers. A reduction in the workforce reduces the quantity of products produced, and a reduction in the quantity of products will reduce the country's ability to export goods for sale to sustain its own citizens. For example, HATI International, a health care information technology firm based in Malaysia, notes that a 10% improvement in life expectancy at birth, could translate to a 0.3–0.4% increase in the economic growth of a country (Das, 2019). And remember, life expectancy is directly impacted by a person's quality of health and the availability of health care in a country.

How does one person's illness affect a country's productivity? In truth, one physically impaired or sick person would have little if any impact on a country's economy. A number of people suffering from the same or related illnesses, however, would affect productivity. Here is an example. New research suggests that investing $1.50 per person per year, between 2015 and 2030, in 20 low- and lower-middle income countries with the highest deaths due to cardiovascular diseases would save 15 million lives and result in 8 million fewer cases of ischemic heart disease and 13 million fewer incidences of strokes in these 20 countries (Bertram et al., 2018). In other words, for a minor investment, millions of people could realize improved longevity and improved health status that could contribute to the economic health of their respective countries. WHO recognizes that individual health affects more than just the individual. It has the potential to affect the economic health of a country as well.

The Federation of Red Cross and Red Crescent Societies

The *Federation of Red Cross and Red Crescent Societies* was established as an international committee to provide relief to wounded soldiers. The founders believed that any organization that provides medical care to soldiers wounded on the battlefield should be a neutral entity in war and therefore free from attacks by either side.

The Federation began as a collection of smaller, unaffiliated organizations. In 1919, the smaller organizations banded together to form an international organization known then as the League of Red

Cross Societies. The Federation – renamed in 1991 – currently consists of over 180 societies and is currently the world's largest humanitarian organization (IFRC, 2023).

The Federation's mission is to provide assistance to individuals irrespective of nationality, race, religious beliefs, class, or political opinion, and to improve the lives of people by mobilizing the power of humanity. The federation focuses on four key areas: promoting humanitarian principles and values, disaster response, disaster preparedness, and health care in communities. However, it is probably best known for its work in the area of disaster relief.

Remember our discussion earlier in the chapter about Hurricane Katrina? (see Box 4.8). To use the Federation's familiar tag line, "The Red Cross was there." It provided temporary shelter, meals, and general assistance to the thousands of people displaced by Hurricane Katrina. Their goal was to provide for individuals' basic needs, including food, shelter, and emergency health care. But this is just one example. Over the decades the Federation has provided invaluable relief assistance to hundreds of thousands of people injured and displaced. Some of these examples include assistance after a tsunami destroyed parts of Indonesia and southern Thailand in December 2004 that resulted in approximately 110,000 deaths and left hundreds of thousands of others homeless; assistance after the Nepalese earthquake in Karnali, in October 2023; vital support and assistance for victims of the September 2023 earthquake in Morocco; and assisting Asia Pacific countries experiencing floods and tropical cyclones resulting from significant climate change.

Thus, in contrast with WHO, the Federation focuses on providing emergency medical and humanitarian aid to people as a result of a natural or a human-made disaster. It does not address policy issues.

Médecins Sans Frontières (Doctors without Borders)

Médecins Sans Frontières (MSF) shares some of the goals of the Federation of Red Cross and Red Crescent Societies. Like the Federation, MSF is an international humanitarian organization that provides emergency aid to persons in need. Specifically, however, MSF responds to the medical care needs of people affected by armed conflict (wars), epidemics, and natural or human-made disasters and to persons who have no access to health care. It was founded in 1971 by French doctors as a non-governmental organization to provide emergency medical assistance to people in need and to document the plight of the people it served. Currently, MSF is based in 19 countries and has provided aid and assistance to over 70 countries.

MSF is known throughout the world for its work in establishing emergency feeding stations in famine-stricken areas such as East Africa. For example, MSF has been at the forefront of the effort to use ready-to-use therapeutic food (RUTF), including peanut butter paste, to combat malnutrition, an effort also spearheaded by WHO (Medicines Sans Frontières, 2017). Equally as important, MSF is a vital lifeline for refugees in countries adversely affected by war or civil conflicts.

In addition to therapeutic feeding stations for displaced persons, MSF provides medical care. While this work often falls under the category of immediate care, MSF also trains health care providers in each region or country in order to support existing medical care and to improve the overall quality of care. In this way, MSF endeavors to help develop the in-country personnel resources needed to provide long-term and sustained medical care once they depart. In essence, MSF contributes to both immediate and long-term health care systems.

WHO, the Federation of Red Cross and Red Crescent Societies, and Médecins Sans Frontières supply some of the basic health and humanitarian services that are unavailable or unaffordable in developing and some developed countries. In essence, they provide the basic health systems infrastructure unavailable in some regions of the world.

National Policy: Global Implications

At first glance, this section may seem redundant. After all, we have discussed national health policy throughout the chapter. For example, we explained the benefits of immunization policies on families and communities and examined the effect that termination of such policies has on the health of an entire nation or region.

But national policies can have a negative effect as well. For example, in some instances national policies prioritize the health of the community over the rights of the individual. The isolation and containment policies that limited the spread of TB in the 19th and 20th centuries in the U.S. and the containment policies adopted by some countries during the COVID-19 pandemic serve as good examples.

Isolation and Containment for TB, HIV/AIDS, and COVID-19

Let's take TB first. In the late 19th and early 20th centuries, local and federal agencies in the U.S. identified TB as a contagious disease that posed a public health threat to the population (Snider, 1997). To prevent the risk of infection of whole communities, several states constructed *sanatoriums*, lodge-like facilities to isolate and treat TB patients. The primary goal of the treatment centers was to contain the spread of the highly contagious TB disease by preventing individuals with the disease from interacting with noninfected persons. A second goal was to treat TB patients before returning them to their communities. Local and state governments could and often did force TB patients to reside in a sanatorium, sometimes for as long as a year, before returning them to their homes. In essence, local and national health policy prioritized the public health and welfare of the population by treating and forcefully isolating (if necessary) individuals with TB, sometimes against their will.

The first sanatorium of record in the U.S. was opened in 1885 in Lake Saranac, New York (Davis, 1996). Later, other states constructed similar treatment sanatoriums. By the 1950s, over 800 sanatoriums were operating in the U.S., serving over 70,000 patients (Davis, 1996; Snider, 1997). The screening and isolation of TB patients, in addition to a rise in the socioeconomic conditions of the U.S. population, jointly helped reduce the prevalence of TB (Binkin et al., 1999).

Cuba used a similar containment strategy for HIV in 1986. When HIV was first detected in Cuba, the Ministry of Health isolated individuals who tested positive for the virus in order to treat them and their sexual partners. The aggressive policy of isolation, containment, and treatment of HIV-positive individuals helped reduce the HIV prevalence rate in Cuba to 0.1% by 2001 (AMFAR, 2006). Compared with a global HIV rate of 1.0%, Cuba's prevalence rate for HIV was, essentially, negligible.

Containment and isolation policies always raise concerns about the rights of the individual. But when COVID-19 hit in 2020, countries worldwide undertook several different strategies to contain this new, highly contagious, and deadly disease. What worked best? We still do not have an answer to that question. What is clear, however, is that there is no one-size-fits-all strategy. China, for example, implemented perhaps the most extensive containment strategies, limiting the movement of individuals through lockdowns, school and business closures, isolation and self-isolation, face masks, and other strategies (Jiao et al., 2022). The first full lockdown in Hubei province in 2020 did not eradicate the virus, however. A second lockdown followed in Jilin province (Clennett & Yiu, 2022).

Other countries faced similar dilemmas and reoccurrences of the virus using somewhat less extreme lockdowns. For example, by March of 2022, stay-at-home restrictions for people who tested positive for COVID (except those hospitalized) were in place in a number of countries including Canada, France, India,

Libya, Pakistan, Portugal, Spain, the U.S., and a host of others (Mathieu et al., 2020). One year later, while the U.S. relaxed restrictions to "recommended," many countries in South America, including Argentina, Brazil, Chile, and Venezuela, as well as most of Western Europe, and almost 20 countries in Africa, including Algeria, Angola, Libya, South Africa, Zimbabwe, and others, had imposed required at-home restrictions (Mathieu et al., 2020). While such lockdowns and forced isolation did not eradicate COVID-19, it did the next best thing: it slowed the spread of the disease.

In spite of the benefits of public health policies that protect the community, we cannot deny that such policies carry a cost for the individual. For the U.S. TB patients in the 19th and 20th centuries, HIV-positive individuals in Cuba, and people around the world during COVID-19, the individual may not be free to determine whether or how to address his or her health issue.

SECTION V. THE ECONOMIC CONSEQUENCES OF POOR HEALTH

Who Is Affected?

When thinking about health and illness, we often focus on the sufferer, the person afflicted with the illness. That is a sensible place to start. But consider for a moment an individual's health from another perspective. Suppose a 40-year-old man is the major wage earner for his family, which includes a wife and three children. His work in a textile factory, together with his spouse's income as an assistant in a local bakery, provides them with enough money to buy a small but adequate house for themselves and their children and to pay for daily necessities. This income does not allow enough, however, to afford health insurance in a country without universal health care.

Suddenly, the man suffers a stroke. After several weeks of medical care and daily exercise, he is able to move about without assistance, but he cannot return to his old job. His job required manual labor: lifting and transporting heavy containers. Unable to do the same job and unable to find a less physically demanding job, he is now unemployed.

The man's wife takes a second job to make up for the lost earnings, but her two jobs still pay considerably less than her husband's old job at the factory. What is more, due to working two jobs the woman finds that she is often exhausted and more prone to catching colds and other minor viral infections.

Seeing the desperate economic condition of the family, the oldest son decides to leave school in the 10th grade to find work and help the family. Because he is a talented student, the family hoped the son would study engineering at a university near them. With a degree in engineering, the son could have helped support his family. Perhaps he can return to school in the future. For now, however, he is needed at home to provide additional economic support for his family.

This is a sad but all-too-common story in many parts of the world. One person's illness can have a domino effect on the health and well-being of an entire family. It is easy to see the physical costs of the illness on the man and on the economic stability of the family. Less easy to see is the effect his illness has on his emotional state as he sees his wife and son work harder to compensate for his limitations or the emotional and health strains experienced by other family members.

One clear impact of the changed financial circumstances on the wife is her need to work two jobs. The additional responsibility is clearly more demanding physically. But there are emotional health costs as well. With less time at home, she has less time to devote to her role as the primary caregiver of the younger children. The story could go on. We could look at each of the younger children to assess the impact of the changed circumstances on their physical and emotional health, but the likely effect is clear. One person's illness can affect an entire family. The family's well-being is jeopardized by this economic downturn, and as a result the family can easily slip into poverty and poor family health.

Individual Health and Community Outcomes

The family certainly suffers from ill health and loss of productivity of one of its members – but so does the community. We noted previously that communities, and in some cases whole countries, can be adversely affected when large numbers of their working-age population are compromised by ill health. To illustrate this point, we consider the case of workers in Lesotho, a landlocked country in southern Africa. Lesotho, a country the size of the state of Maryland, has little industry to employ its people or to help them earn an income. As a result, many travel into South Africa, an hour's journey by local transport, to find jobs as domestic workers, day laborers, or other similar jobs.

Lesotho's HIV/AIDS prevalence rate was 40% for much of the 2000s, meaning that 4 in 10 adults were infected with the disease. In some cases, whole communities had been affected, leaving children and grandparents as the principal wage earners. In essence, in Lesotho, almost half of a generation of adults – 20 to 40 years of age – were becoming ill and dying at an alarming rate. Their illnesses devastated not only the family but the community and the country as well. The young adults would have assumed roles in their communities as employed laborers but also as local organizers for social events, such as fundraisers to raise money for irrigation ditches, or as coaches of local football teams. But, as a result of HIV, these same adults were either unable to work or volunteer due to their illnesses. As a result, businesses fail or relocate to countries with a larger supply of workers, and community life becomes a shadow of its former self.

The loss of Lesotho's workforce can be measured in the country's economic profile. The loss to Lesotho's families and to their community is much harder to quantify.

Summary

Many would agree that access to health care should be the right of all individuals. Yet we have been reading about many instances in which, unfortunately, this is not the case. In both developed and developing countries, large segments of societies are unable to obtain health care due to a host of individual, community, systems, and policy factors. The lack of access to health care leads to poorer outcomes and more costly procedures.

It may not be immediately obvious how a health policy positively impacts an individual's health. In fact, most often the impact may be indirect. Yet health policies that ensure access to clean water and air and safe neighborhoods or that provide direct medical care benefit each individual in society.

Personal Postscript

DO GLOBAL HEALTH POLICIES AFFECT YOU?

Simply stated, yes! We may not be aware of the ways in which global health policies affect us given the vast and well-established health care systems and infrastructure in developed countries like the U.S., but they do.

First, most developed countries are members of the WHO. U.S. representatives to WHO help shape the policy decisions and plan the health activities and projects to be undertaken throughout the world. The effects of these policies are more evident in less developed countries, but even developed countries must continue to strive toward the 17 Sustainable Development Goals, particularly those that directly or indirectly impact health.

In addition, organizations like the Federation of Red Cross and Red Crescent and Médecins Sans Frontières send their aid workers to assist in disasters and to provide needed medical care in all countries, even in developed countries. The Red Cross and Médecins Sans Frontières were two of the many aid organizations that provided valuable assistance to many countries around the world. Assistance also pours in from other countries around the world, in part because these nations see it as their responsibility to help provide for the health and well-being of their global neighbors especially in times of crises, regardless of their nationality.

Remember also that diseases and illnesses can cross borders. Throughout history, we have seen the effects of epidemics and pandemics that, by definition, do not respect borders. More recently, we have experienced the effects of SARS-CoV-2, Ebola, the avian flu, and the A/H1N1 (swine) influenza, which have caused illness and death to thousands globally. Therefore, another reason to be mindful of global health policy is to safeguard and protect your own health as well as that of others.

Questions to Consider

1. Many countries do not have the resources to develop and implement policies to improve the psychological health of their citizens. How might the WHO assist such countries?
2. What environmental and health policy factors help explain the disappointingly low life-expectancy ranking of the U.S. or other developed nations?
3. Vaccine skeptics and vaccine refusers have grown in number over the past decade. What are the potential national and global implications of such a movement? What role can health psychologists play in addressing the concerns of parents while also helping to protect communities from preventable illnesses?

True or False Questions

1. Measles has been fully eradicated in developed nations. True or False.
2. Dr. Takahashi of Japan developed the most effective vaccine against polio. True or False.
3. Dr. Moyo's team of researchers in South Africa contributed to the effective sequencing of the Omicron coronavirus variant. True or False.
4. Médecins Sans Frontières (MSF) assists in health policy development and implementation across the world. True or False.
5. The new vaccines against malaria are almost 90% effective in preventing the disease. True or False.

Important Terms

Risky Health Behaviors: Part I

Chapter Outline

Opening Story: 70-Year-Old Lungs in a Teenage Wrestler: Is Vaping the Cause?

Section I. Substance Use and Abuse: Cigarettes and E-Cigarettes

Section II. Alcohol Use and Abuse

Section III. Risky Sexual Behaviors

Personal Postscript

Questions to Consider

True or False Questions

Important Terms

Chapter Objectives

After studying Part I of this chapter, you will be able to:

1. Identify and define risky health behaviors.
2. Describe the health consequences of cigarette smoking and vaping.
3. Identify and describe the health consequences of alcohol abuse.
4. Identify and describe the health consequences of illegal and prescription drugs.
5. Identify and describe factors that influence substance use.
6. Discuss the relationship between the brain's reward circuitry and substance abuse.
7. Discuss the pros and cons of three treatment options for substance abuse disorders.
8. Identify the factors that influence risky sexual health behaviors.
9. Explain the HIV infection and transmission process.

DOI: 10.4324/9781003300670-5

OPENING STORY: 70-YEAR-OLD LUNGS IN A TEENAGE WRESTLER: IS VAPING THE CAUSE?

Adam Hergenreder, an 18-year-old varsity wrestler, thought he was going to die! He was short of breath and breathing heavily, especially for someone his age. He was experiencing uncontrollable shivers and then started vomiting nonstop (Howard & Nedelman, 2019). It continued for three days.

*After trying an anti-nausea medication and seeing several doctors, one medical provider asked Adam whether he had been "JUUL-ing," here meaning using an e-cigarette or other vaping device (Clearing House for Military Family Readiness, 2023), or using **tetrahydrocannabinol** or **THC**, a psychoactive component of marijuana. Adam admitted he was doing both.*

*Adam said he first "started vaping just to fit in, because everyone else was doing it" (Howard & Nedelman, 2019). The **vape pods** – interchangeable cartridges that contain a liquid consisting of nicotine and more than 2,000 other chemicals, came in many flavors. Adam preferred the mango flavor made by the company JUUL. But JUUL also made other flavors, for example bubble gum, fruit flavors, mint, and popcorn, many of which appeal to a younger audience.*

Adam remembers that he liked the vape pods because they "didn't taste like cigarettes . . . [they] tasted good" (Howard & Nedelman, 2019) – most likely the aim of the manufacturers. He also remembered that vaping "gave him a little high," probably due to nicotine (Howard & Nedelman, 2019). According to his father, Adam smoked a pod and a half every other day. And, since one pod contains approximately the same amount of nicotine as an entire pack of cigarettes, Adam was inhaling a lot of nicotine! As for THC, Adam claims he got that from "a friend" or dealer.

*Only after doctors x-rayed Adam's lungs did the medical providers learn the full extent of the damage due to vaping. The X-rays showed severe lung disease. Yet, Adam was lucky. He could have suffered a collapsed lung, a condition known as **pneumothorax**, which can be a life-threatening event (Mayo Clinic, 2023b).*

By the time his story was published in 2019, Adam was recovering slowly. He continues to experience shortness of breath, for example when walking up stairs or doing other normal activities. Yet, he wants his story told so that other teens can be forewarned. Adam does not want others to go through a similar experience. ■

Let's call this opening story "The Dangers of Smoking 2.0." After reading about Eddie and his struggles to quit smoking, the dangers of cigarettes, and health policies designed to reduce smoking and related health effects in Chapter 3, Theories and Models of Health Behavior Change, it is disappointing to learn that a new smoking product has been introduced to the public which may reverse some of the progress against unhealthy behaviors over the past decades. But more on that in a moment.

Just to be clear, the full health effects of vaping are not yet known because it is a new product. However, from what we know so far, there is reason to be concerned. In 2019, the CDC noticed a sharp rise in the number of teenage hospitalizations associated with vaping (Yale Medicine, 2024). By 2020, the CDC recorded over 2,800 vaping-related hospitalizations and 68 deaths (Yale Medicine, 2024). Common vaping-related symptoms, including shortness of breath, cough, and chest pain, mirrored some of Adam's complaints. This vaping-related health condition was even given its own medical diagnosis and name: *"e-cigarette, or vaping product use associated lung injury,"* or *EVALI*.

VIDEO #15/60

Chapter 5: Risky Health Behaviors, Part I

- *Vaping: Reshaping the FDA's Regulations (In 60 Seconds)*
- *Website: https://www.youtube.com/watch?v=dD-fB3XjWfo*
- *American Enterprise Institute is a publicly accessible platform as it provides public policy research to the public for free (www.aei.org)*

We will address the specific arguments for (yes, there are some arguments for) and against vaping in Section I. For now, we will just point out that, again, while the product is essentially new and the research is "catching up," researchers have positively linked ***vitamin E acetate*** – a chemical frequently found in some vaping products that contain *THC* – to *EVALI* (Howard & Nedelman, 2019; Yale Medicine, 2024). Briefly, *vitamin E* acetate is safe when consumed in food or used on the skin. Its effects when inhaled, however, are not well understood and are a source of concern (WHO, 2021a). In fact, in a study conducted by Blount and colleagues (2020), researchers found that of their 150 study participants, all 51 patients diagnosed with *EVALI* also tested positive for *vitamin E acetate*. By comparison, *none* of the 99 healthy patients in the study tested positive for that substance.

Before we move on to explore the potential impacts of risky health behaviors, like vaping, there are three important points to remember. First, a number of risky health behaviors that begin during adolescence continue into adulthood. For this reason, much of the research on risky behaviors focuses on adolescents (Brender & Collins, 1998; Kulbok & Cox, 2002). Therefore, in this chapter we focus on studies that examine adolescent health risks in order to explore the origins, causes, and possible implications of such behaviors for adolescents as well as adults.

Second, the concepts of risk and risky behaviors need clarification. The World Health Organization (2002b) defines ***risk*** as the probability of an adverse outcome or the occurrence of an event that raises that probability. Likewise, we define a ***risky behavior*** as an action that increases the probability of an adverse outcome. Note, however, that the presence of a risk factor or risky behavior does not always lead to an adverse health outcome.

Finally, many studies tend to group together individuals who engage in a risky behavior once (or episodically) with repeat or frequent risk takers. That is to say, they divide adolescents into two groups: individuals who never engaged in a risky behavior versus those who ever engaged in such behaviors, even if only once (Kulbok & Cox, 2002). The never-versus-ever dichotomy seems a bit extreme. It does not distinguish between experimental risk-taking among adolescents that occurs infrequently and may not continue, versus behavior that continues over time or is habitual (He, Kramer, Houser, Chomitz, & Hacker, 2004). Clearly, the probability of an adverse event resulting from a risky behavior will be greater among frequent rather than infrequent risk takers. Therefore, whenever possible we will choose studies that examine risky health behaviors that adolescents engage in repeatedly and over time.

With those caveats in mind, in this chapter we focus on risky behaviors that have, unfortunately, increased over the past decade. First, we address substance use/abuse and the impact of culture, age, and gender on cigarette and e-cigarette use in Section I. In Section II we examine the effects of the same factors on alcohol use/abuse, and in Section III we examine the increased use of prescription and illicit drugs, specifically cannabis, prescription medications, and fentanyl. Finally, Section IV is dedicated to risky sexual behaviors, sexually transmitted diseases (specifically HIV), and teen pregnancy.

SECTION I. SUBSTANCE USE AND ABUSE: CIGARETTES AND E-CIGARETTES

In the current section, we examine the effects of substance use on health outcomes. We lead with this topic in this edition of our textbook because, unfortunately, statistics now show that the rates of substance use, here meaning cigarettes, vape products, alcohol, and drugs, are increasing. This activity is widely reported in the U.S., as well as other countries and regions of the world.

We first look briefly at the data on cigarette smoking and its impact on health. We also briefly explore how the marketing techniques used to promote these products lead to early onset of smoking by adolescents in some countries. We then explore the development of vape products and their adverse impacts on health.

Cigarettes

Why is smoking tobacco a problem? Consider this: Globally, smoking results in approximately 8.7 million deaths annually. It is and remains the leading preventable cause of death and the leading cause of death due to disease globally (WHO, 2022a). In fact, smoking causes more deaths than alcohol, homicides, illicit drugs, suicides, and traffic accidents combined (see Table 5.I.1). Thus, according to the WHO, smoking is "one of the biggest public health threats the world has ever faced" (WHO, 2022a). The only surprising thing about this assessment is that it was issued in the midst of the global COVID-19 pandemic!

VIDEO #16/60

Chapter 5: Risky Health Behaviors, Part I

·   **Substance Use and Abuse: Cigarettes: Influence of Culture, Age and Gender**

·   *7 Reasons to Be Smoke-Free*

·   *Website: https://www.youtube.com/watch?v=hCC1dgmwO_4*

·   *Nemours KidsHealth is a publicly accessible as it provides information regarding various health topics to the public for free (https://kidshealth.org/)*

·   *https://kidshealth.org/*

TABLE 5.I.1 Global Cause of Death Due to Substance Use

Cause of Death	Global Deaths
Alcohol	3,000,000[1]
Homicides	458,000[2]
Illicit Drug Use	494,492[3]
Smoking/Tobacco	8,710,000[3]
Suicides	703,000[4]
Traffic Accidents	1,190.000[5]

Globally, smoking and tobacco kill more people than alcohol, homicides, illicit drug use, suicides and traffic accidents combined.

Sources: [1]WHO Alcohol Fact Sheet; [2]United Nations Office on Drugs & Crime (2023). Global Study on Homicide/Vienna, Austria; [3]Our World in Data (2019). Deaths Attributed to Tobacco, Alcohol & Drugs. Deaths attributed to tobacco, alcohol and drugs, World, 2019 (ourworldindata.org); [4]International Association for Suicide Prevention (2022). Global Suicide Statistics. Global Suicide Statistics – IASP; 5World Health Organization (2023). Road traffic injuries. Road traffic injuries (who.int).

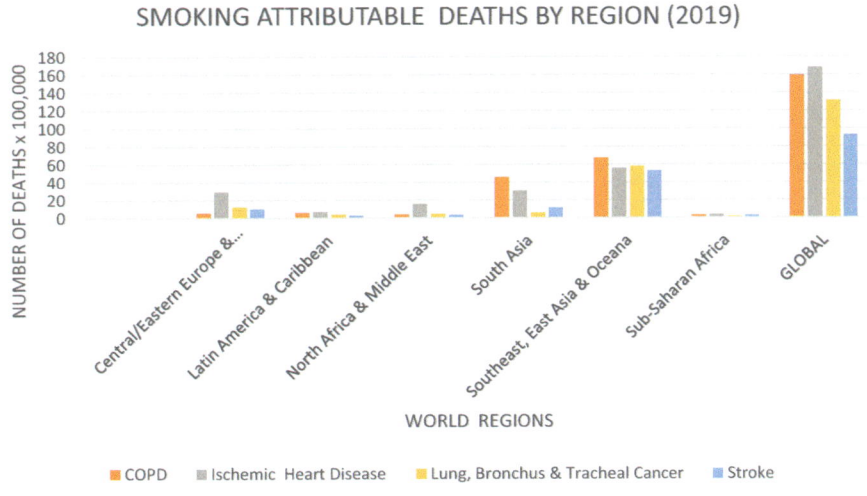

FIGURE 5.I.1 The comparative bar chart shows the smoking-attributable death rates for six WHO global regions: Central, Eastern Europe & Asia; Latin America and the Caribbean; North Africa & the Middle East; South Asia; Southeast, East Asia & Oceana; and Sub-Saharan Africa. Overall, Ischematic heart disease is the leading cause of smoking-attributable death rates for the world.

Source: Supplement to: GBD 2019 Tobacco Collaborators. (2021) Spatial, temporal, and demographic patterns in prevalence of smoking tobacco use and attributable disease burden in 204 countries and territories, 1990–2019: a systematic analysis from the Global Burden of Disease Study 2019. *Lancet* http://dx.doi.org/10.1016/S0140-6736(21)01169-7

Sound incredible? Just take a look at the data on smoking-related illnesses in Figure 5.I.1 that lead to death. This figure shows the number of deaths (per 100,000 persons) due to four of the most common, smoking-related causes of death in six regions of the world: chronic obstructive pulmonary disease (COPD), ischemic heart disease, lung/bronchus/tracheal cancer, and stroke. The region that includes countries in Southeast Asia, East Asia, and Oceania report the highest number of deaths due to these four conditions: COPD (672,000), ischemic heart disease (558,000), lung/bronchus/tracheal cancer (581,000) and stroke (530,000; GBD, 2023 Tobacco Collaborators, 2021). By comparison, the region that includes sub-Saharan Africa reports the lowest number of deaths for these diseases (COPD, 29,000; ischemic heart disease, 37,400; lung/bronchus/tracheal cancer, 16,500; and stroke, 27,800; GBD, 2023; Tobacco Collaborators, 2021).

Would it seem logical to assume that smoking-related deaths would be greatest in regions with the highest rates of smoking? Indeed! And there are statistics to support that assumption. Table 5.I.2 shows the 25 countries with the highest rates of age-standardized tobacco smoking in 2019, here meaning smoking rates (not number of smokers). In this comparison, using age-standardized data allows us to compare countries with different age distributions, since the age distribution of each country will, in part, impact smoking prevalence rates (Mathieu, 2023). Of the 25 countries with the highest rates, 18 are found in the Central and South Pacific and in Europe (World Health Organization, 2022a). Six island nations in the Central or South Pacific Ocean report some of the largest age-standardized prevalence rates of smoking. In fact, the rates in three countries – Nauru, Kiribati, and Papua New Guinea – are higher than those reported in Europe. However, approximately half of the 25 countries with the highest smoking prevalence rates are located in Europe, with the greatest rates reported in countries in Eastern Europe (see again Table 5.I.2).

TABLE 5.1.2 Age-Standardized Rates of Current Tobacco Smoking by Country (2019): Top 25 Countries

Country	Tobacco Smoking Rate (%) Both Sexes	Geographic Region
Nauru	44.7	South Pacific Ocean
Kiribati	41.7	Central Pacific Ocean
Serbia	40.1	Europe
Papua New Guinea	39.9	South Pacific Ocean
Bulgaria	39.4	Europe
Solomon Islands	37.8	South Pacific Ocean
Croatia	36.7	Europe
Tuvalu	36.0	West/Central Pacific Ocean
Bosnia/Herzegovina	35.5	Europe
Cyprus	35.5	Mediterranean
Latvia	35.2	Europe
Jordan	34.6	Middle East
Greece	34.5	Europe
Lebanon	33.9	Middle East
France	33.6	Europe
Timor-Leste	32.5	South East Asia
Indonesia	32.3	South East Asia
Hungary	32.2	Europe
Montenegro	31.8	Europe
Georgia	31.7	Europe
Slovakia	31.5	Europe
Tonga	31.1	South Pacific Ocean
Czechia	30.9	Europe
Türkiye	30.9	Europe/Asia

The good news, however, is that with very few exceptions, the overall rate of tobacco smoking is slowly declining for almost all countries worldwide, including these 25. It would be wonderful to assume that this decline is due to the great work of health professionals in changing smoking behaviors. While they do deserve credit, we will see shortly that the decline in cigarette smoking is also due, in part, to the rollout of a new smoking product. More on that in a moment.

Even though the prevalence rates of smoking in the U.S. are considerably less than in the Central/South Pacific or in Europe, the U.S. is facing its own set of challenges. Each day, more than 1,600 teens in the U.S. smoke their first cigarette. Is it any wonder, therefore, that more than 90% of U.S. adult smokers report that they began smoking before age 18 (CDC, 2023e)? Clearly, smoking is a critical health problem. But what leads teens to begin smoking, often at such early ages? And why do they continue?

There is no shortage of theories in psychology to explain why adolescents experiment with cigarettes and other substances or why they continue. In this section, we examine some of the social and intrapersonal factors that influence substance use. We then examine five groups of theories that offer explanations about early and habitual adolescent substance use.

SOCIAL NORMS AND ENVIRONMENTAL FACTORS In Chapter 3, Theories and Models of Health Behavior Change, we noted that product manufacturers skillfully promote and sell their merchandise to their intended audiences. The R.J. Reynolds company pioneered the first marketing campaign for mass-produced cigarettes in the U.S. in 1923. Its product, Camel cigarettes, was the first mass-marketed, nationally advertised cigarette brand in the U.S. (Wipfli & Samit, 2016).

Mass marketing and promotional materials that advertise a product are not inherently a problem. However, when cigarette manufactures use these strategies to promote smoking, they disproportionately attract the attention of younger smokers, leading to an early onset of smoking. In fact, advertisements that promote smoking as a *socially normative behavior* – here meaning a behavior widely accepted by society – have positively disposed younger age groups, specifically children and adolescents, to smoking (Hansen, Hanewinkel, & Morgenstern, 2020; Papaleontiou, Agaku, & Filippidis, 2020). If such a claim seems unlikely, consider this: Cartoon characters, smoking logos, and items with cigarette logos embossed on them are particularly popular with younger audiences. It is not uncommon to find cigarette manufacturers placing their logos on jackets, cigarette lighters, water bottles, coolers, and even, in past years, on candy cigarettes. Although the ads and products may be intended for adults, children and teens also find them quite appealing (Sargent et al., 1997). In addition, as Wipfli and Samit (2016) note, the tobacco industry is expert in their use of highly prized social attributes, such as freedom, rebellion, stress relief, weight loss, sex appeal, and even health and fitness, to sell their products. Linking smoking to these socially desirable attributes, in attractive and persuasive advertisements, or to desired objects, makes it doubly challenging for health professionals, and health psychologists in particular, to advocate against the use of these products. What is more, this "psychological warfare" has been reignited with the newest smoking product: e-cigarettes and vape products. As promised, more on that in just a moment.

But first, we take a moment to delve into the Joe Camel mass-marketing campaign pioneered by R. J. Reynolds, in part because it was extremely successful – scarily so, and also because it is an excellent example of an environmental factor that contributed to the early onset of smoking.

Cigarette ads were banned from television, radio, and print media in the U.S. after 2009 (Public Law Health Center, 2009). Before then, such ads were ubiquitous. Camel cigarette ads are but one example. These ads featured Joe Camel, a caricatured depiction of a camel used to advertise Camel cigarettes in the 1970s and 1980s. Joe Camel's 1950s attire – complete with a leather jacket, jeans, sunglasses, and a Harley-Davidson motorcycle – captivated young audiences. In fact, even children readily identified this cartoon figure. In a classic study by Fischer, Schwartz, Richards, Goldstein, and Rojas (1991), approximately 30% of three-year-olds were able to match the Joe Camel cartoon figure correctly with the cigarette, and more than 91% of six-year-olds were able to correctly pair the image of Joe with the product. Surprisingly, children were more successful at identifying Joe Camel than they were in correctly identifying Mickey Mouse, a Walt Disney cartoon character designed especially for children.

Similarly, when comparing adolescents' and adults' ability to recognize and identify the Camel advertisements, adolescents in grades 9 through 12 were significantly better at the task than adults. Not surprisingly, adolescents also found the ads to be more appealing than did adults (DiFranza et al., 1991). In fact, the Camel campaign with Joe Camel was so successful that Camel product manufacturers saw a 31% increase in their share of the illegal children's cigarette market (DiFranza et al., 1991).

Thus, returning to our question of what explains the early onset of smoking by adolescents, one possible explanation is the direct and indirect marketing of these products to young audiences. Just to be clear, we label marketing and advertisement campaigns an environmental factor that can influence health behaviors. Here we see that the well-recognized cartoon figures and the much-sought-after products emblazoned with cigarette logos show that the marketing strategy appears to have been effective (Klein & St Clair, 2000; Klein, Thomas, & Sutter, 2007).

SOCIAL ROLE MODELS If children and adolescents find cartoon cigarette advertisements attractive and appealing, would they also be attracted to models, such as actors, who smoke in movies? Research suggested that smoking on the silver screen has a ***direct*** and an ***indirect effect*** on adolescent smoking (Alzahrani, 2020). By indirect effect, we mean smoking behavior that is influenced or mediated by a secondary factor. The secondary or ***mediating factor*** can be peers, family members, or, as mentioned previously, actors in movies.

Let's look at smoking by movie actors. Research in six European countries and the U.S. suggests that teen smoking rates increase when the on-screen smoking is done by actors in movies, and, in the case of the U.S. study, by an adolescent's favorite movie star (Mejia et al., 2017; Morgenstern et al., 2013). In a seminal 2004 study of the impact of on-screen smoking on adolescents, Distefan, Pierce, and Gilpin (2004) found that, among adolescent girls who never smoked, the on-screen smoking behavior of their favorite actor strongly predicted smoking initiation. Nonsmoking boys were not as affected by the actions of their favorite on-screen actors, suggesting a gender effect of smoking models on later smoking behaviors.

In sum, there is ample research that shows that cigarette-product manufacturers have successfully attracted the attention of a young audience. Effective marketing may have encouraged children and adolescents to view smoking as a desirable or even an expected behavior, linked to socially desirable attributes. In addition, the studies suggest that adolescent smoking behavior may be encouraged by exposure to individuals who model smoking behaviors. Movie actors who smoke on-screen constitute one example of a model as do close friends who smoke.

CULTURE AND GENDER Adolescents also credit their family members and friends as smoking models. In fact, studies suggest that adolescents often initiate their peers into smoking, including friends, siblings, or other similarly aged relatives. Notably, however, few follow when their peers decide to stop smoking (Haas & Schaefer, 2014; Hall & Valente, 2007). Remember Eddie from the opening story in Chapter 3, Theories and Models of Health Behavior Change? His brother and his close friends helped to create a smoking culture that he found very appealing and difficult to avoid. And consistent with research findings, Eddie's friends did not follow his lead when he attempted to stop smoking.

There is one important caveat to add when examining the role of peers in adolescent smoking behaviors. A meta-analysis of 17 studies showed that it is not peers in general, but rather close friends, siblings, and parents, who significantly influence an adolescent's smoking onset (East et al., 2021). Looking again at Eddie, we see that his experience is consistent with this more limited explanation. It was Eddie's brother and his closest friends who initiated and sustained his smoking activities. This is an important distinction, especially for health psychologists who design and implement smoking cessation or smoking abstinence programs for adolescents. If, indeed, it is mainly close friends, parents, and siblings who influence adolescent smoking initiation, then health psychologists should focus on these three subgroups when developing smoking intervention programs.

Similarly, cultural practices also influence smoking patterns. Looking again at Table 5.I.2, we may wonder whether the high prevalence rates of smoking in Central and South Pacific countries, or in Eastern Europe, is because smoking is a common or perhaps even a socially accepted behavior.

Recall that there is some good news to add to this issue: recent data show a global decline in smoking. Overall, smoking prevalence has declined by 27.2% for men and 37.9% for women (Dai, Gakidou, & Lopez, 2022). While smoking prevalence appears to remain high in low- and middle-income countries in Asia and the Pacific Islands, in other countries, for example Brazil, smoking prevalence has reportedly decreased by almost 70% (Dai et al., 2022).

Consider, also, data on smokers in the U.S. and the U.K. In the U.K., smoking rates declined from a high of more than 45% of adults in 1974 to approximately 14.7% in 2020 (Foundation for a Smoke-Free World, 2022). In 1965, 42% of adults in the U.S. (18 years of age or older) smoked. Presently, just over 11% of adults in the U.S. are smokers, representing almost a two-thirds decline in smoking (CDC, 2023e; National Center for Health Statistics, 2006).

Similar declines have been reported also for adolescent smoking rates in the U.S. The National Youth Tobacco Survey, a voluntary, school-based, cross-sectional study, measured current use (within the past 30-days) of tobacco products among middle and high school students in the U.S. This survey revealed statistically significant declines in cigarette smoking among the sampled populations. Only 4.6% of the high school students sampled reporting smoking cigarettes, and only 1.6% of middle school students reported using cigarettes within the past 30 days (Gentzke et al., 2020). This compares with approximately 10.5% of adolescents who reported ever smoking daily in 2012 (Centers for Disease Control, 2012a). We do note that these statistics include any adolescent who ever smoked cigarettes in the past 30 days, not our preferred measure.

To what do we attribute the significant decline in smoking rates in the U.S. and other upper-middle and high-income countries? One possibility is that the extensive health promotion and smoking cessation campaigns in these countries, especially those conducted over the past 30 years in the U.S., have changed the culture of smoking. Now, in many places in the U.S., cigarette smoking is the exception rather than the norm.

In spite of these recent declines in U.S. smoking rates, researchers have noticed striking differences in smoking rates for adolescents by ethnicity. When comparing students across ethnicities, white high school students who are regular smokers – that is, individuals who smoked at least once in the 30 days prior to the survey – or who ever used cigarettes outnumbered Hispanic, black, or other smokers (Gentzke et al., 2020; see Figure 5.I.2). The same is not true for middle school students, however. Here, Hispanic students are more likely to report ever using or using cigarettes in the last 30 days (see again Figure 5.I.2).

Some researchers contend that ethnic differences in smoking may also reflect an *acculturation* process, here meaning the effort to change attitudes, values, or behaviors to adopt those of a dominant ethnic group (Burnam, Telles, Karno, & Hough, 1987). While acculturation may explain the smoking behaviors of some groups, it is not universal. For example, Ra and colleagues (2020) found that education levels impact smoking behaviors among some Asian immigrants. In their study, U.S.-born Asian women with some college education or less, as well as immigrant Asian men of similar education levels, were more likely to be smokers. Interestingly, East African immigrants to the U.S. who felt marginalized, here meaning felt a lack of attachment to both their host country and their home country, were four times more likely to smoke than acculturated individuals from the same region (Nakajima et al., 2023). So, what does this mean? Simply that level or degree of acculturation may explain some patterns of smoking among some immigrants or members of an immigrant community, but not all.

COUNTERING THE GLOBAL SMOKING "EPIDEMIC" Smoking and its impact on health is considered a global problem. To that end, WHO proposed the WHO Framework Convention on Tobacco Control (WHO, 2003). You will remember from Chapter 4, Global, Communicable, and Chronic Disease, that one of the aims of the WHO is to propose and develop policy guidelines and initiatives that address global health issues.

Joining with the Bloomberg Foundation, the two organizations proposed a new paradigm for tobacco control known as *MPOWER* (see Table 5.I.3). This tobacco control strategy suggests specific actions

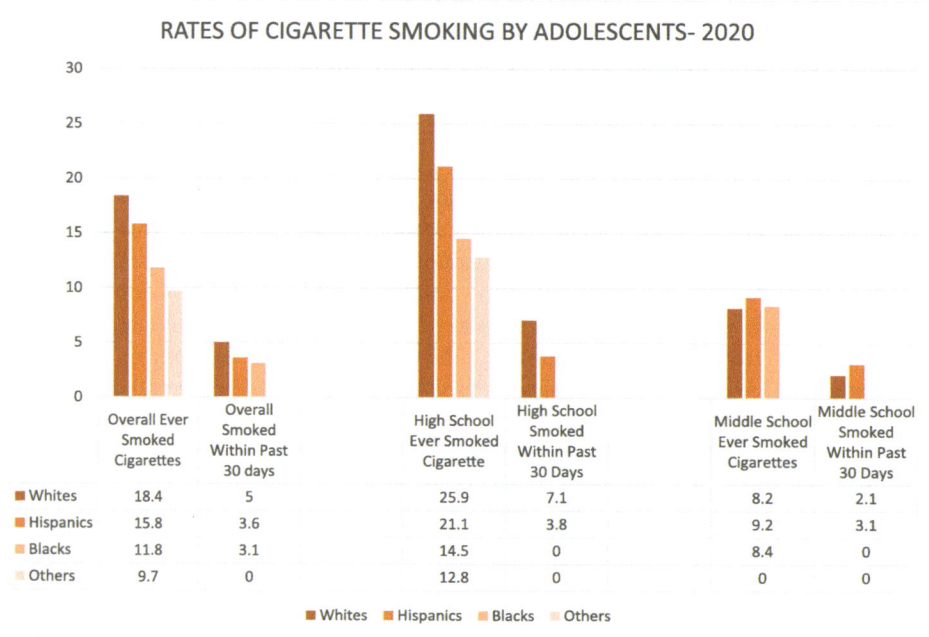

FIGURE 5.1.2 The comparative bar chart shows the rate of cigarette smoking by four adolescent ethnic groups: white, Black, Hispanic and the general category "Other." Overall, white adolescents report higher rates of ever smoked cigarettes (18.4 per 100,000) and smoked within the past 30 days (5 per 100,000). Specifically in high school, whites report higher rates than other ethnic groups for ever smoked (25.9 per 100,000) and smoked within the last 30 days (7.1 per 100,000). Hispanic and African American students report the highest rates of cigarette smoking in middle school.

Source: Adapted from Gentzke et al. (2020).

TABLE 5.1.3 MPOWER: Global Tobacco Control Strategy

M	Monitor tobacco use and prevention policies
P	Protect people from tobacco use
O	Offer help to quit tobacco use
W	Warn about dangers of tobacco
E	Enforce bans on tobacco advertising, promotion, and sponsorship
R	Raise taxes on tobacco

Source: World Health Organization (2021a).

countries can adopt to both educate and protect the public from the dangers of smoking, and to counter the messages from cigarette manufacturers that present smoking as socially desirable attributes. It is likely that the MPOWER health policy initiative would benefit health psychologists who are involved in designing and evaluating smoking reduction programs, especially among adolescents.

E-Cigarettes/Vaping

Just when the health professions, health psychologists, and global policy experts think they have made real progress in reducing unhealthy behaviors, like cigarette smoking, product developers introduce a newer, more attractive, and more enticing product.

Meet the latest clever devices: *e-cigarettes and vaping devices*. Just to be clear, these devices are not entirely new. Herbert Gilbert obtained a patent in the U.S. in 1963 for his invention, a "smokeless, non-tobacco cigarette" that would replace the then current version of cigarettes with a more "harmless" method of smoking (National Center for Chronic Disease Prevention and Health Promotion, 2016). This "harmless" smoking device could be marketed as a healthier option in part because it could reasonably claim to reduce non-smoker's exposure to secondhand smoke.

There is no doubt that e-cigarettes and many vaping devices reduce exposure to secondhand smoke. This is one of the positive aspects of e-cigarettes and vaping devices that we alluded to in the beginning of this chapter. But, some manufacturers claim a second benefit of these products: they help people to quit smoking. This second claim has not been validated and has been questioned by many researchers. Thus, the claim that e-cigarettes and vaping devices are "harmless" may be true for the nonsmoker while its benefits to the smoker are in question.

What we do know is that e-cigarette/vaping products have been updated and redesigned, and with each new update, prospective users seem keen to try the latest invention – similar to the desire to get the latest cell phone! The first generation of smokeless device (see right side of Figure 5.I.3) could only be used once, was not refillable or rechargeable, and was designed to look like the old-fashioned cigarette (CDC, n.d.-a). The second-generation e-cigarette, however, made significant "improvements," moving away from the old-fashioned cigarette look-alike to more mechanical-looking devices, nicknamed "vape pens," "dab pens" (CDC, n.d.-a), "rechargeable e-cigarette," or "vaping device." The key to these newer models was that they were reusable. A smokable liquid that comes in a pre-filled cartridge can be purchased and inserted, or users can refill the devices with their preferred agent, such as nicotine, cannabis, flavored liquids, or other substances. Remember Adam from the opening story? He regularly refilled his cartridge with THC and other flavored liquids.

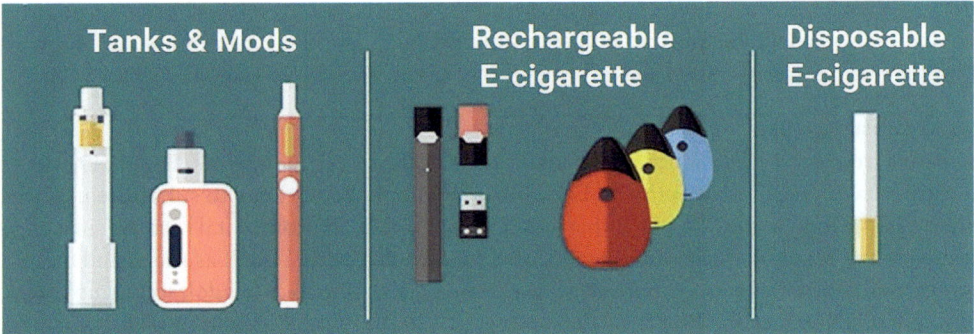

FIGURE 5.I.3 Three "generations" of vape devices are presented in this photo. First generation devices are disposable and look like cigarettes (right side of photo). Second generation products look like USB and/or elongated flash drive and are rechargable. Next generation devices are pear-like in shape and brightly colored, in this case red (middle panel). They are rechargeable and refilable. Newer products resemble pens and rectangular shaped boxes with a mouthpiece, also in bright colors.

Source: CDC (2023). E-Cigarettes quick facts. Accessed online at E-cigarettes Quick Facts | Healthy Schools | CDC. Retrieved on May 20, 2023.

An important part of this second-generation device is the **battery**, a rechargeable lithium ion battery that is designed to heat the **atomizer**, a coil that converts the e-liquid in the cartridge into aerosol (or airborne) droplets. These devices allow the battery to heat the atomizer up to 400°F.

The third- and fourth-generation devices are also designed to be used multiple times and to be modifiable, here meaning users can customize the substances that they put into the device. Additionally, users can change other elements of the pods, including the voltage, coils, and wicks. Finally, and perhaps to maximize consumer interest, some of these devices come in many different shapes, from USB-looking devices to rectangular shapes that resemble the old-fashioned cigarette lighters. It goes without saying that the colors vary widely also (see Figure 5.I.3; CDC, n.d.-a).

Yet, the question remains, are these e-cigarettes and vaping devices "harmless"? The opening story with Adam should make us wary of such claims. With over 2,000 reports of adverse health effects on teens and 68 deaths linked to vaping just in the U.S., Adam's story and that of Simah Herman – another teenage daily vaper who was put on a ventilator and then into a medically induced coma after she was unable to breathe unassisted for two days (ABC News, 2019) – should make us wonder. Similar to Adam, Simah did not think of herself as a smoker.

Given these data points, health psychologists now have a stronger position from which to argue that e-cigarettes and vaping products have potentially very dangerous health consequences. To assist them, health psychologists can follow the lead of the WHO, which again has promoted policies to regulate **electronic nicotine delivery systems (ENDS)**. Under their policy initiative, 32 countries have banned the sale of ENDS (18 middle-income countries and nine high-income countries), 30 countries have banned the use of ENDS in all indoor spaces, eight countries now require the use of large public warnings on all ENDS packaging, and 22 countries ban the advertising, promotion, and sponsorship of ENDS devices, e-liquids, or both (World Health Organization, 2021a). When compared to the over 50-year effort to reign in the tobacco industry and limit children's and teens' smoking, this effort by the international community to limit the reach and adverse health effects of e-cigarettes and vaping products in less than one decade is momentous. Health psychologists would be well advised to become very familiar with this internationally sponsored effort and include it in their program design.

To summarize, the effective promotion of cigarettes and e-cigarette/vape products, appealing to popular social attributes, social norms, culture, and gender, and the influence of close friends, family, and role models are social and environmental factors that influence smoking initiation and general smoking behaviors. One way to test the relative importance of these factors is by examining theories that assess their roles.

Theories of Substance Use

As noted earlier, research on substance use behavior tends to focus on adolescents. Examining the early onset of such behaviors helps to identify and assess the factors that contribute to substance use behaviors in the short and the long terms. We noted that studies suggest that environmental factors (such as product advertisements, and movie and television images of actors who smoke), as well as social and cultural factors (such as attitudes and behaviors of family and close friends), all contribute to adolescent smoking patterns (Alzahrani, 2020; Hansen et al., 2020; Papaleontiou et al., 2020; Wipfli & Samit, 2016). But can we say that these factors *cause* adolescents to initiate smoking behavior?

There is no shortage of theories that attempt to explain the cause-and-effect relationship of individual, environmental, social, and cultural factors on smoking among adolescents; there are far too many to review in this chapter. Fortunately, seminal work by Petraitis, Flay, and Miller (1995) offer an easy and succinct summary of the theories using five categories: cognitive-affective theories, social learning theories, conventional commitment theories, personality trait theories, and integration theories.

COGNITIVE-AFFECTIVE THEORIES According to Petraitis et al. (1995), one group of theories that can be used to explain substance use is best described as *cognitive-affective theories*. These theories propose that three factors influence adolescents' likely substance use: their positive attitudes about substance use, the endorsement of substance use by others, and an individual's decision that the benefits of substance use outweigh the costs. And, as you may have suspected, Azjen's theory of reasoned action and theory of planned behavior (1985), which considers attitudes toward intended behavior and social norms, are included in this first group of theories. Rosenstock's classic health belief model (2005; see Chapter 3, Theories and Models of Health Behavior Change), which weighs perceived benefits, barriers, susceptibility, and severity, also falls into this category.

How might these theories explain an adolescent's decision to smoke? Consider Eddie, the main character in the opening story from Chapter 3. Eddie was struggling to decide whether the benefits of smoking with his close friends outweighed the cost of losing his girlfriend, Sarah. Azjen might suggest that when making his decision, Eddie considered his own attitude about smoking, his close friends' attitudes and the benefits of sharing this activity with them.

SOCIAL LEARNING THEORIES *Social learning theories*, including Bandura's seminal social cognitive theory (1986) and Akers's social learning theory (1996), constitute the second category. Here substance use is explained as a behavior rooted in the attitudes and beliefs of the adolescent's role models, close friends, and parents (Petraitis et al., 1995). Social learning theories contend that, by observing the context in which role models use, for example, cigarettes, and the consequences of their use, adolescents form attitudes about smoking and the perceived likely consequences of their decision to smoke. Again, consider Eddie. His decision could be explained in terms of these social learning paradigms.

CONVENTIONAL COMMITMENT THEORIES Third are the *conventional commitment theories*, which view adolescents' level of attachment to conventional social institutions, such as the family, schools, religious institutions, or other structured systems, as buffers against substance use. In this case, *buffers* are the factors that protect an adolescent from initiating substance use behaviors. Conventional commitment theorists claim that weak bonds to structured systems will lead to a lack of commitment to the social norms of the institutions that help guide behavior. These weak bonds lead to a greater likelihood of involvement with other adolescents with similar weak ties, which can lead to "deviant" behaviors (Jessor, Donovan, & Costa, 1991; Kandel, Smicha-Fagan, & Davies, 1986).

What is meant by deviant behaviors in this instance? Consider this example: Members of one family neither smoke nor drink alcohol. The youngest child in the family has a weak attachment to the family and associates with other adolescents who similarly have weak familial attachments. At one point, the group of adolescents begins to smoke and drink alcohol. The resulting substance use behaviors of the adolescents are inconsistent with – deviant from – the behaviors of the family. It is important to point out that, according to conventional commitment theorists, the adolescent's behavior is not brought about by a desire to rebel but rather by an absence of close personal ties to the institution – in this case, the family.

Could these theories also explain Eddie's decision? Perhaps, but we do not have enough information about Eddie's familial or social institutional attachments to draw a conclusion.

PERSONALITY TRAIT THEORIES The fourth category is *personality trait theories*. According to these theories, the individual characteristics of the adolescents and their social settings may influence the timing and occurrence of substance use. Thus, generalized stress and generalized low self-esteem (Kaplan, Martin, & Robbins, 1984; Kumpfer & Turner, 1990–1991) may explain more about the likelihood of substance use than conventional commitment or social normative beliefs. Trait theorists hold that an individual's method of coping with highly stressful environments, rather than that person's commitment to institutions, the behavior of his or her role models, or his or her own views of the behavior, may shape the decision to smoke.

Here, too, we have insufficient information to determine whether these theories could apply to Eddie.

INTEGRATION THEORIES Finally, the fifth category consists of *integration theories*, which include elements of each of the four categories mentioned previously. Included in this group is the problem-behavior theory (Jessor et al., 1991), which examines early substance use behavior in the context of other problem behaviors that may occur. Jessor and colleagues suggest that adolescents who exhibit one problem behavior, such as substance use, are prone to engage in other problem behaviors also. Therefore, according to problem behavior theory, early substance use is just one of a number of risky behaviors that must be studied in context. Other theories included in this category are the peer cluster theory (Oetting & Beauvis, 1987; Petraitis, Flay, & Miller, 1995), which focuses on the role of peers in influencing substance use, and the model of vulnerability (Sher, 1991), which suggests a genetic or biological determinant of substance use.

Which cluster of theories best predicts early cigarette use? There is no definitive answer. What is clear, however, is that individual (age, ethnicity, and gender), social (close friend's influence and cultural norms as seen through family), societal/environmental (media), and biological factors all contribute. In addition, given the differences in smoking behaviors by demographic groups, one single theory may not apply to all. Instead, different theories or even blended theories (see Chapter 3, Theories and Models of Behavior Change) may be needed to explain the substance use behaviors of different populations.

SECTION II. ALCOHOL USE AND ABUSE

Cigarettes, e-cigarettes, and vape products are legal substances that can cause serious health consequences. Another potentially problematic substance is alcohol. In 15 countries, including the Oceania nations of Kiribati, Nauru, and the Solomon Islands, as well as the U.S., just to name a few, only adults 21 years of age or older are legally allowed to purchase and consume alcohol. However, for many other countries the legal age to drink alcohol is lower. For example, 20-year-olds can consume legally in Japan. In approximately 160 other countries people under 20 years of age can legally drink, and many countries have no age limit.

Is alcohol really a problem? Well, some studies suggest that moderate consumption of alcohol can be beneficial to one's health. For example, some types of red wine contain *plant phenolics* or chemical compounds that serve as *antioxidants* that protect against some forms of cardiovascular diseases, Type 2 diabetes, and cancer, and also improve systolic blood pressure, the pressure in the arteries when the heart beats (see Table 5.I.4 and Chapter 9, Cardiovascular Disease; Hrelia et al., 2023; Weaver, Rendeiro, Gettrick, Philip, & Lucas, 2021). If alcohol is legal and can have health-enhancing consequences, why, then, do we include alcohol in the chapter on risky health behaviors?

Alcohol itself is not the problem. It is the way we use alcohol – specifically, the excessive consumption or the abuse of alcohol – that makes it risky. Studies show that excessive alcohol consumption and the use of alcohol by adolescents 20 years of age or younger has been linked to a number of illnesses and death (Lees, Meredith, Kirkland, Bryant, & Squeglia, 2020; Merlin, Jager, & Schulenberger, 2008). Therefore, in this chapter, we focus on the misuse of alcohol and its impact on individual and community health outcomes.

TABLE 5.I.4 Substance Use: Perceived Benefits and Short- and Long-Term Health Consequences

Substance	Method of Use	Perceived Benefits	Short- and Long-Term Health Consequences
Cigarettes	Smoked (oral)	Suppresses appetite	Cancer of lungs and esophagus Emphysema Other respiratory problems Yellowed/stained teeth
Alcohol	Drink (oral)	Mild euphoria Reduces anxiety Induces relaxation Some types protect against cardiovascular disease, cancer	Impaired judgment Impaired coordination Cirrhosis of liver Gastrointestinal problems Heart disease or stroke Cancer of mouth, throat, liver, prostate Fetal alcohol syndrome (infants)
Marijuana	Smoke (oral)	Euphoria Giddiness Sedation Tranquility	Impaired coordination Impaired vision Increased anxiety Interference with short-term memory
Cocaine/crack	Sniff (nasal) or smoke (oral)	Prolonged stimulation Euphoria	Increased temperature, heart rate, blood pressure Irregular heart rhythms Excessive nose bleeds Gastrointestinal problems
Heroin	Inject	Short-term euphoria Long-term drowsiness, relaxed state	Severely impaired coordination Impaired mental functioning Collapsed veins Liver disease Depressed respiratory system

Excessive Alcohol Consumption

Researchers suggest that *excessive alcohol consumption* results in more than 3 million deaths worldwide, accounting for 5.3% of all deaths (World Health Organization, 2018a; see again Table 5.I.1). And while almost half (44.5%) of the world's population aged 15 years or older has never drank alcohol, almost the same proportion (43%) describe themselves as current drinkers (World Health Organization, 2018a). Global statistics also show that high alcohol consumption, here meaning consumption by more than 50% of the population, is concentrated in only three WHO regions: the European Region, with 59.9% of the population listed as current consumers; the Americas Region, with 54.1% as current consumers; and the Western Pacific Region, with 53.8% of the population as current consumers (see Figure 5.I.4).

In the U.S., an estimated 78.5% of the population 12 years of age or older (approximately 221.3 million people) report consuming alcohol at some point in their life in 2021. That statistic alone says little about the potential adverse effects of alcohol. So, consider this: In the U.S., alcohol accounted for more than 140,000 deaths a year, on average, between 2015 and 2019 (National Institute on Alcohol Abuse and Alcoholism, 2023). Men account for approximately 70% of these deaths – just over 97,000.

To understand what constitutes excessive consumption, however, we must first define non-excessive or "standard" consumption. According to the U.S. Department of Agriculture, a standard drink of alcohol is defined as one that contains approximately 14 grams of pure alcohol. That could take the form of 12

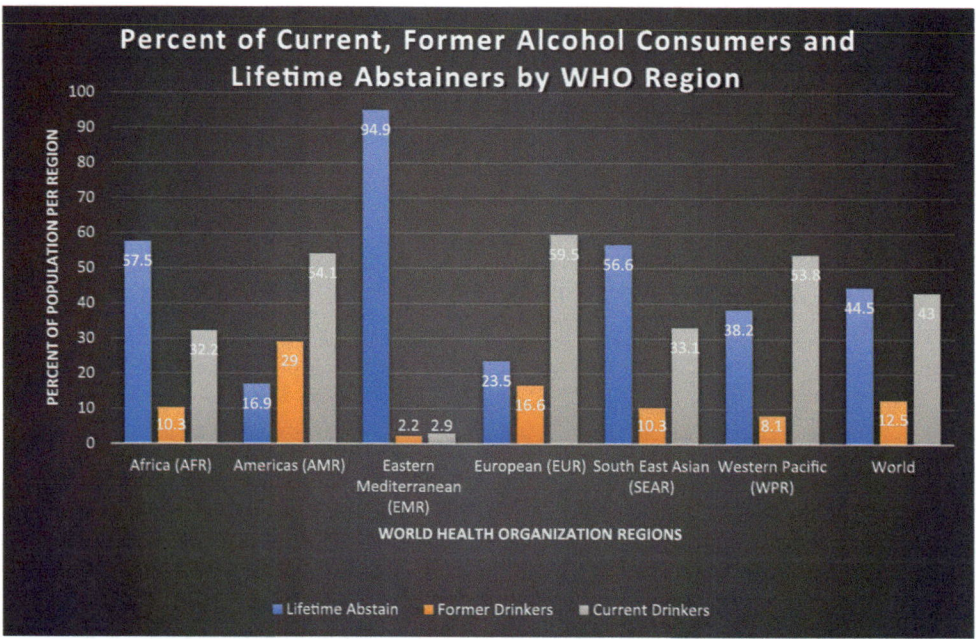

FIGURE 5.I.4 A comparative bar chart shows the percent of current and former alcohol consumers and lifetime abstainers in six WHO regions: Africa, the Americas, Eastern Mediterranean, Europe, Southeast Asia, and Western Pacific. The Eastern Mediterranean region reports the highest percent of abstainers (94.9%) followed by Africa (57.5%) and Southeast Asia (56.5%). Most current alcohol consumers are in Europe (59.5%), followed by Americas (54.1%) and Western Pacific (53.8%). Most former drinkers are in Americas (29%), followed by Europe (16.6%) and Africa & South East Asia 10.3% each.

Source: Adapted from World Health Organization (2018a).

TABLE 5.I.5 Defining Alcohol Consumption

Category	Women	Men
Moderate drinking	One or fewer drinks per day	Two or fewer drinks per day
Heavy drinking	One or more drinks per day	Two or more drinks per day
Binge drinking	Four or more drinks within two hours	Five or more drinks within two hours

Source: Based on U.S. Department of Agriculture (2020).

ounces of beer, 5 ounces of wine, or 1.2 ounces of a distilled 80-proof liquor such as rum, bourbon, or vodka (U.S. Department of Agriculture, 2020).

To define excessive consumption, health researchers calculate the number of alcoholic drinks consumed in a single setting as well as the average number of drinks consumed on a daily basis (see Table 5.I.5). Excessive alcohol consumption may also be characterized as heavy drinking or binge drinking. In general, *heavy drinking* is defined as consuming one or more drinks per day for women and two or more drinks per day for men (Centers for Disease Control, 2012b), whereas researchers consider four or more drinks in a setting (or within two hours) for women, and five or more drinks in the same time frame for men to be the definition of *binge drinking* (U.S. Department of Agriculture, 2020; see again Table 5.I.5).

VIDEO #17/60

Chapter 5: Risky Health Behaviors, Part I

· **Binge Drinking: What is Binge Drinking?**

· *Website: https://www.youtube.com/watch?v=vT55ShgKr6g*

· **The National Institute of Alcohol Abuse and Alcoholism is publicly accessible as it's a federal website that provides resources and information relating to alcohol abuse (niaaa.nih.gov)**

Excessive drinking, including heavy and binge drinking, poses serious health risks to the consumer and to others. In the U.S., of the 60% of adults who report consuming alcohol within the past 30 days, 18% report engaging in binge drinking (U.S. Department of Agriculture, 2020). For the consumer, excessive consumption has been linked to gastrointestinal problems, heart disease, strokes, and cancer of the mouth, throat, liver, and prostate (Centers for Disease Control, 2008e). It is responsible for serious liver diseases, including inflammation and scarring of the liver, known as *cirrhosis*, a disease that prevents the liver from properly carrying out its main function, removing waste products from the body. Cirrhosis can lead to liver failure, a fatal outcome (Centers for Disease Control, 2008e). Finally, excessive alcohol consumption also contributes to neurological and psychiatric problems and a greater likelihood of involvement in other risky behaviors such as risky sexual behaviors. But this just describes the risks to the excessive drinker.

Alcohol abuse can also affect family members, friends, and communities. In 2021 alcohol was implicated in 31% of all deaths due to traffic accidents in the U.S., totaling 13,384 people (National Highway Traffic Safety Administration, 2021a). Excessive drinking also exposes family members to increased risk of violence, including domestic violence. The link between alcohol abuse and aggression, established in the research literature, describes this association as enormous, causal, and unequivocal, including in incidences of intimate partner violence and child maltreatment (Cafferky et al., 2018; Centers for Disease Control, 2022d; Leonard & Quigley, 2017; Tomlinson, Brown, & Hoaken, 2016).

Finally, alcohol abuse by pregnant mothers can cause *fetal alcohol syndrome*, a condition that causes physical and mental abnormalities in the developing fetus. For example, it may result in abnormal facial features, growth deficiencies, and problems with the central nervous system. Children born with fetal alcohol syndrome carry these problems throughout life.

VIDEO #18/60

Chapter 5: Risky Health Behaviors, Part I

· **Fetal Alcohol Syndrome: A Pregnant Woman Never Drinks Alone**

· *Website: https://www.youtube.com/watch?v=cd6EUazxOVc*

· *The North Carolina Department of Health and Human Services is publicly accessible as they are a state department (www.ncdhhs.gov/)*

In sum, excessive alcohol use can cause a host of health problems for the consumer, the family, and the community. What is more, statistics on the rate of alcohol consumption, and the demographics of those who consume the greatest quantities, show that we have reason to be concerned about alcohol abuse in many countries.

ALCOHOL CONSUMPTION AND GENDER Early studies in the U.S., such as work by Moore and colleagues (2005), suggested that higher alcohol consumption was associated with specific demographic and behavioral characteristics, including being a white male, being married, having higher educational attainment and higher income, and being a smoker. Yet, current research by Kang, Min, and Min (2020), Keyes, Grant, and Hasin (2008), and Moinuddin and colleagues (2016) suggests that these demographic and behavioral characters may not describe current consumption patterns in many cultures. Instead, these studies and others suggest a rise in alcohol consumption by females and older adults, a new phenomenon that is occurring in many different cultures. We cite three of the studies here to illustrate this point.

The first study is by researchers in Norway. Stelander and colleagues (2021) measured changes in the prevalence of alcohol consumption in four groups of adults – alcohol abstainers, frequent consumers (more than 2–3 drinks per week), at-risk consumers (more than three drinks or 36 grams), or "heavy episodic" drinkers (more than six drinks or 72 grams) – over 22 years (between 1994–1995 and 2015–2016) – using a modified version of the Alcohol Use Disorders Identification Test–Consumption (AUDIT-C) scale. Almost 21,000 people 60 years of age or older participated in this study. Stelander and colleagues identified several significant outcomes. First, their results revealed that fewer men and women, in two age groups (60–69 years and 70+ years), reported abstaining from alcohol in 2015–2016 than in 1994–1995 (see Figure 5.I.5a-b).

In addition, the prevalence of frequent consumption of alcohol (two to three drinks per week) increased significantly between 1994–1995 and 2015–2016 for both men and women and for both age groups. Similarly, increases in the prevalence of at-risk consumption (more than three drinks per setting) was reported for all groups, with the exception of women 70 years or older (see again Figure 5.I.5b).

A second study by Keyes and colleagues (2008) also found a pattern of higher alcohol consumption among women. Their study examined rates of alcohol use, binge drinking, and alcohol dependency in four groups of adults in the U.S.: those born between 1913 and 1932, between 1933 and 1949, between 1950

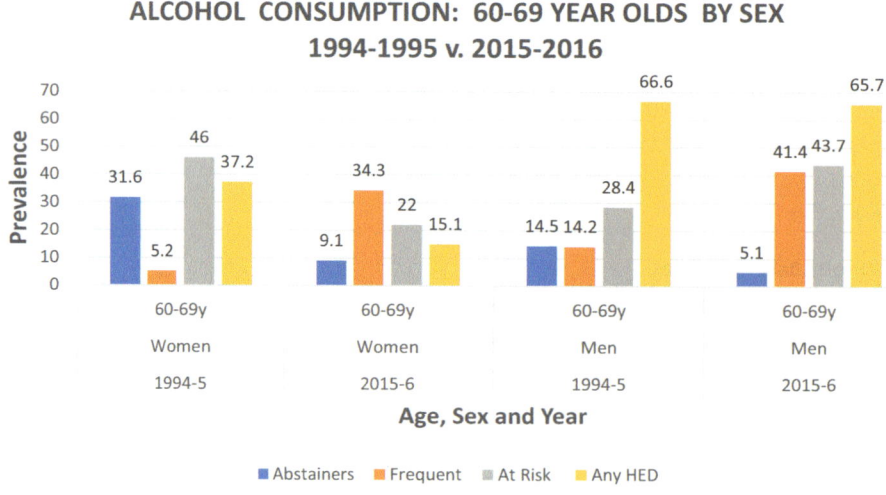

FIGURE 5.I.5a A bar chart compares alcohol consumption for two groups of men and women, 60–69 year old, at two points in time: 1994–1995 and 2015–2016. Over time, there was a decrease in women self-described as abstainers (31.6% vs. 9.1%) and an increase in women as frequent drinkers (5.2% vs. 34.3%). Men also reported fewer abstainers (14.5% vs. 5.1), more frequent drinkers (14.2% vs. 41.4%), and more at risk drinkers (28.4% vs. 43.7%).

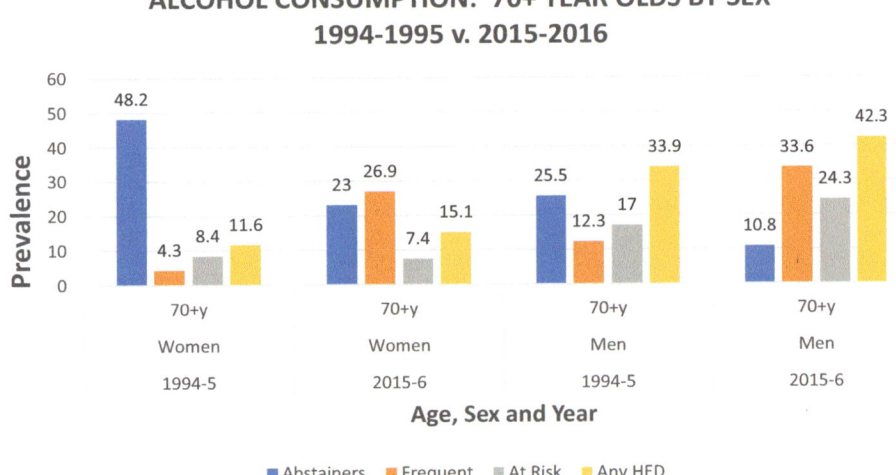

ALCOHOL CONSUMPTION: 70+ YEAR OLDS BY SEX
1994-1995 v. 2015-2016

FIGURE 5.I.5b A bar chart compares alcohol consumption for two groups of men and women, 70+ year old, at two points in time: 1994–1995 and 2015–2016. Over time, fewer women abstained from alcohol (48.2% vs. 23%) and more reported being frequent drinkers (4.3% vs. 23.9%). Men reported fewer abstainers (25.5% vs. 10.8%), more frequent drinkers (12.3% vs. 33.6%), more at risk drinkers (17% vs. 24.3%), and more involved in heavy episode drinking (33.9% vs. 42.3%).

Source: Adapted from Stelander et al. (2021).

and 1967, and between 1968 and 1984. Of the over 42,000 interviews collected, Keyes and colleagues discovered that among older adults, or those in the 1913–1932 and 1933–1949 birth years, males were still more likely than women to report excessive alcohol use, binge drinking, and alcohol dependency. However, the younger adult cohorts – those born between 1950 and 1967 and between 1968 and 1984 – reported a much smaller difference in excessive alcohol use by gender. In other words, younger women were more heavily represented among the excessive alcohol group than were older women. Interestingly, these findings are consistent with reports of heavy and binge drinking on college campuses by both men and women. Current reports from the National Center for Health Statistics (2022) also report an increase in consumption of alcohol between 2002 and 2019 for people 26 years of age and older, men and women, and white and black respondents (see Table 5.I.6).

Finally, in the Republic of Korea, Kang and colleagues' (2020) study of drinking patterns between 2007 and 2016 showed a similar narrowing of gender differences in drinking behaviors. Their retrospective analysis of data collected on over 73,000 South Koreans who participated in the Korean National Health and Nutrition Examination Survey found a significant decrease in the prevalence of heavy and binge drinking between 2007 and 2016 for boys (67.5% vs. 63.9%) and men (63.4% vs. 60.9%), but no significant difference for girls (50.2% vs. 50.4%) or women (30.6% vs. 32.0%) for the same period (Kang et al., 2020). Stated another way, while the prevalence of binge and heavy drinking decreased among boys and men over these nine years, there was no decrease among girls or women. Women and girls also began drinking, on average, six months earlier between 2007 and 2016, a change that was also reported as significant. There was no significant decrease in drinking age for boys or men.

TABLE 5.I.6 Use and Excessive Use of Alcohol, and Marijuana by Age, Gender, and Race: U.S. 2002–2019

Categories	Alcohol % Users by Year		Binge Drinking % Users by Year		Marijuana % Users by Year	
	2002	2019	2002	2019	2002	2019
AGE						
12–13 years old	4.3	1.7	–	0.5	1.4	1.0
14–17 years old	49.2	26.6	–	14.0	23.3	21.1
18–25 years old	60.5	54.3	–	34.3	17.3	23.0
26–34 years old	61.4	64.3	–	57.4	7.7	19.0
35+ years	52.1	52.8	–	21.5	3.1	8.2
SEX						
Male	57.4	54.3	31.2	27.8	8.1	13.9
Female	44.9	47.5	–	20.8	4.4	9.2
RACE						
White	55.0	56.1	–	25.0	6.5	12.0
Black	39.9	42.8	–	22.7	7.4	13.7
American Indian and Alaskan Native	44.7	32.1	–	20.9	6.7	12.0
Native Hawaiian and Other Pacific Islanders	–	41.5	–	23.8	4.4	10.6
Asians	37.1	37.6	–	13.4	1.8	4.4
Hispanics	42.8	42.7	–	24.2	4.3	9.5
Two or More Races	49.9	49.5	–	25.8	9.0	19.7

Source: National Center for Health Statistics (2022).

What conclusions might we draw from these data across three countries and continents? They indicate that alcohol consumption patterns are changing. As Moinuddin and colleagues (2016) remind us, alcohol consumption patterns do still differ by culture, socioeconomic status, and education, but the changes in consumption patterns for girls/women and older adults in high- and upper-middle income countries appear to follow a common pattern.

Theories of Alcohol Use

The five clusters of theories introduced in the previous section to explore early cigarette use can also be used to explain early and sustained use of all substances, including alcohol. We will not repeat the theories here. We will note, however, two interesting points. First, like the research on cigarettes, research on alcohol also suggests that many factors contribute to excessive alcohol consumption. Studies suggest that close friends (Andrews, Tildesley, Hops, & Li, 2002; Cavanagh, 2007: social learning theorists and integrationists) and stress (Harrell & Karim, 2008; Jukkala, Makinen, Kislitsyna, Ferlander, & Vagero, 2008: personality trait theorists) positively influence alcohol consumption, whereas social institutions (Delucchi et al., 2008; Wallace et al., 2007: conventional commitment theorists) have the opposite effect.

More recently, studies suggest that health policy can also influence drinking behaviors. For example, Harvard researchers Nelson, Naomi, Brewer, and Wechsler (2005) examined the effect of state health policies on binge drinking on college campuses in the U.S. Nelson and colleagues found that colleges located in states with more stringent restrictions on alcohol consumption reported the lowest level of adult binge drinking in general and lower binge drinking rates on college campuses. The finding seems to suggest that health policy at the state level can moderate drinking behaviors of college students as well as adults (Nelson et al., 2005).

Nelson and colleagues' findings are supported by several current studies. In a 2015 study by Xuan and colleagues, researchers developed an Alcohol Policy Scale to measure the strength of state-level alcohol policies in all 50 U.S. states and the District of Columbia. Their results showed that stronger state-level alcohol policies help reduce the likelihood of youth drinking and binge drinking. Similar outcomes were reported by Paschall, Grube, and Kypri in their 2009 study of the effects of alcohol control policies on adolescent alcohol consumption in 26 countries, including the U.S.

There are, of course, other possible explanations for alcohol consumption. For example, Kandel's *gateway theory* of substance use suggests that substance use develops progressively. She contends that adolescent substance use begins with substances that are legal for adults (Kandel, Yamaguchi, & Chen, 1992). This progressive model proposes that when adolescents first experiment with substances they begin with legally obtainable substances, here meaning cigarettes or alcohol. If continuing, adolescents will then progress to marijuana (cannabis) followed by other more potent illicit drugs. Even with alcohol, Kandel and her colleagues claim that adolescents almost always begin with beer or wine, the drinks with the lowest alcohol content per ounce, before trying other stronger substances. For this reason, Kandel has labeled cigarettes and alcohol the "gateway drugs" because, according to her theory, cigarettes and alcohol "open the gate" for experimentation or regular use of other drugs.

Kandel's theory was supported by longitudinal data from studies in the U.S. and Israel (Kandel et al., 1986; Nkansah-Amankra & Minelli, 2016; Yu & Williford, 1992). Recent studies, however, suggest that the gateway theory may not explain patterns and progression of substance use equally well for some populations. That is to say, some researchers suggest that there may be a progression from one drug to the next but not as predicted by the gateway theory. For example, a multinational study by Degenhardt and colleagues (2010) examined the drug use patterns and histories of adults in 17 countries: seven developing countries (Colombia, Lebanon, Mexico, Nigeria, People's Republic of China, South Africa, Ukraine) and 10 developed countries (Belgium, France, Germany, Italy, Israel, Japan, the Netherlands, New Zealand, Spain, and the U.S.). Their results revealed significant differences in the pattern and order of substance use across countries. Specifically, cannabis use was less strongly associated with higher-level illicit drugs, like cocaine, in the Netherlands than it was in Spain or Belgium. Additionally, Degenhardt and colleagues found that adult substance users in Japan and Nigeria were least likely to follow the gateway sequence of drug use. In sum, these studies suggests that other factors, such as age of onset of drug use, the availability of specific substances, frequency of use, or personality factors were better predictors of which substances were used first.

One final note. Studies examining risk-taking or other behavioral factors suggest that attention-deficit/hyperactivity disorder may also affect substance use (Treur et al., 2021; Zulauf, Sprich, Safren, & Wilens, 2014). Unfortunately, we do not have the space to fully address that here.

Legal, Illegal, and Prescription Drugs

An entire chapter could be devoted to a discussion of the use of *illicit* – that is, illegal – drugs; recently legalized drugs in some countries, such as cannabis; and their health consequences. In fact, it could require a separate book! But we limit our discussion here to three substances which, because of changes in laws or ever-increasing rates of abuse, have particular salience for many countries: marijuana (cannabis), prescription drugs, and fentanyl.

MARIJUANA Known by many names, including pot, weed, grass, ganja, and cannabis, among others, *marijuana* is the most commonly abused illicit drug worldwide (World Health Organization, 2024a). Marijuana is a mixture of the flowers, stems, seeds, and leaves of the hemp plant, smoked as a cigarette or cigar or used in a pipe.

We refer to this substance as illicit because in much of the world, this substance is illegal or highly regulated by law. As of 2023, 20 of 195 countries worldwide permitted the use of marijuana, although some place strict limits on the quantity and type of use (e.g., medicinal versus recreational). Uruguay was the first country to legalize marijuana in 2013, whereas in Canada, marijuana was legal for medicinal purposes in 2001 and legalized for recreational purposes in 2018 (Conde Nast, 2022). Worldwide, approximately 147 million people (2.5% of the world population) use cannabis in some form (World Health Organization, 2024a).

As of April 2023 in the U.S., marijuana is fully legal in 24 states and the District of Columbia, fully illegal in three states, and legal in limited circumstances (e.g., medicinal) in 38 states and the District of Columbia (Gorelick, 2023). The move to legalization in the U.S. was driven, in part, by a growing body of research suggesting that medical marijuana may be an effective pain medication for people with chronic illnesses, such as cancer, or for whom other forms of pain medication has failed to provide relief (Thaler, Gupta, & Cohen, 2011; Uritsky, McPherson, & Prudel, 2011; Mercurio, Aston, Claborn, Waye, & Rosen, 2019). The reasons for the legal changes that allow for recreational marijuana use go beyond the scope of this book. But, it is the case that this movement towards legalization has overshadowed marijuana's more common use and its adverse consequence when abused. Additionally, it is thought to be responsible for the increase prevalence in cannabis consumption. An estimated 17% of the U.S. population (56 million people) consumed cannabis in 2020 (Conway, 2023). Interesting, the country reporting the highest prevalence of cannabis use in the same year was Israel (27%; Conway, 2023).

Individuals who use marijuana recreationally report a variety of sensations when smoking the drug, depending on the person and the setting. The most common short-term sensation is one of euphoria and giddiness. Such reactions are commonly associated with drugs known as *stimulants*, or drugs that excite the nervous system. With marijuana, however, the excitation is often followed by feelings of sedation and tranquility, sensations often associated with drugs known as *depressants*, or agents that relax and quiet the nervous system. Other more specific short-term effects of marijuana include dizziness or trouble with coordination and with basic motor movements (NIDA, 2002).

What causes the alternate feelings of euphoria and sedation? Marijuana, like other drugs, interacts with the brain's communication system by tapping into the brain's neural activity and interfering with the way the brain sends, receives, and processes information through the nerve cells called *neurons*. We explain the body's communication system in Chapter 6, Emotional Health and Well-Being. Briefly, to send messages between cells, the body relies on *neurotransmitters*, or chemical substances manufactured in our bodies. Marijuana contains a chemical structure that is similar to some of our body's natural neurotransmitters. Because of this similarity, marijuana is able to mimic *dopamine*, one of the body's neurotransmitters that regulates, among other things, our sensation of pleasure (NIDA, 2006a). Specifically, marijuana floods the body with dopamine. The buildup of dopamine in the system intensifies and prolongs feelings of euphoria. Because the euphoria associated with marijuana is a pleasurable sensation, or as some call it, a "high," many users experience an intense desire to repeat the experience (NIDA, 2019).

The research on the long-term consequences of marijuana is incomplete. Earlier studies reported that regular users of marijuana may experience a variety of permanent health problems, including damage to the brain's short-term memory capabilities, increased risk of heart attack due to elevated blood pressure, cardiovascular disease, a weakened immune system, pulmonary disease, sexual dysfunction, and an increased risk of cancer (Friedman, Newton, & Klein, 2003; Gorelick, 2023; Roberts, 2019). A longitudinal study of the effects of cannabis use on adolescents also found that cannabis users performed worse on cognitive tests including tests of memory and attention (Jacobus et al., 2015). And even the American Heart Association warned that, based on studies with animals and observational studies with humans, cannabis can lead to cognitive abnormalities and other impairments (Testai et al., 2022).

VIDEO #19/60

Chapter 5: Risky Health Behaviors, Part I
- **Substance Use and Abuse: Influence of Culture, Age and Gender**
- *Website: https://www.youtube.com/watch?v=nhBIXw0LVvw*
- *Chico Unified School District is publicly accessible as they provide information regarding various topics aimed at the youth without cost to the public (https://www.chicousd.org/)*

Other researchers contradict some of these findings, especially the position that cannabis use causes a decrease in cognitive ability, or mental health problems. Rather, Schaefer and colleague's longitudinal study of 3,000 adolescent twins, whom they followed into their adult lives, found that cannabis use presented no adverse physical or mental health outcomes. It was, however, associated with poorer educational and occupation outcomes and lower incomes (Schaefer et al., 2021). It is unclear whether these lower socioeconomic outcomes are due to the cannabis or to behaviors associated with its use.

Another area that is hotly debated is whether marijuana is linked to cancer. In earlier editions of this text, we noted that marijuana contains between 50% and 70% more *carcinogens*, or substances that are known to cause cancer, than cigarettes (Hoffman et al., 1975; National Institute on Drug Abuse [NIDA], 2002). These facts are not disputed. Further, experts contend that the increased carcinogens, in addition to marijuana smokers' tendency to inhale more deeply and retain the smoke in their lungs longer than cigarette smokers, makes them more susceptible to cancers when smoking this substance than cigarette smokers (Hancox et al., 2010). Notwithstanding these findings, researchers have been unable to demonstrate conclusively a link between smoking marijuana and lung cancer (NIDA, 2002).

What is not disputed, however, is that in surveys conducted in several Midwestern states in the U.S., marijuana-related emergency department visits increased in Colorado by 54% and marijuana-related hospitalizations increased 101% after it was legalized in that state (Sabet, 2021). Similarly, increases in emergency department visits and hospitalizations were reported in three additional Midwestern states after legalization: Iowa, Missouri, and North Dakota (Midwest HIDTA, 2021).

It is important to restate that much more research is needed to understand the advantages and disadvantages of cannabis use. There is, however, one point of general agreement among researchers: cannabis is neither the cure-all for all ailments nor the horrible drug it was believed to be several decades ago.

PRESCRIPTION MEDICATIONS For some time, research on drug use focused almost exclusively on illicit drugs. Illegal drugs are often associated with crime, and the crime statistics they generate allow researchers to track, report, and measure illegal drug use behaviors. Abusers of prescription drugs, however, are less likely to generate crime statistics and therefore are less visible to researchers.

The term *prescription drugs* refers specifically to medication prescribed by a doctor to treat a person's specific medical condition. The drug is intended for use solely by the individual to whom it is prescribed. Prescription drugs are used illegally if they are used for nonmedical purposes or by people other than the person for whom the drug was prescribed.

There are three types of commonly abused prescription medications. *Opioids*, or drugs that treat pain, are one type. Such medicines include morphine- and codeine-based treatments. A second type, depressants, are used to relax or calm the central nervous system. They include barbiturates and benzodiazepines such as Valium or Xanax. Finally, stimulants are used to increase attention and enhance energy.

VIDEO #20/60

Chapter 5: Risky Health Behaviors, Part I

· **Opioids: Opioid Side Effects in 60 Seconds**

· *Website: https://www.youtube.com/watch?v=4vt5BR4hqxl*

· **The YouTube channel "Anaesthesia" is an educational YouTube video that makes educational videos for medical school students.**

VIDEO #21/60

Chapter 5: Risky Health Behaviors, Part I

· **Depressants:** *What Are Depressants? We Answer Your Common Questions about Depressants – Anaheim Lighthouse*

· *Website: https://anaheimlighthouse.com/blog/what-are-depressants-we-answer-your-common-questions-about-depressants/*

· **The Anaheim Lighthouse is publicly accessible.**

Precise statistics on the number of people abusing prescription drugs are difficult to obtain for two reasons. First, prescription drugs are obtained from licensed medical professionals. Doctors may not be aware that their prescriptions are being used for purposes other than those intended. Individuals who are misusing prescription medicines have no incentive to reveal their true intent to their doctor and would jeopardize their ability to obtain drugs in the future if they admitted to abusing their prescribed medication. Second, doctors who prescribe medicines for nonmedical purposes risk punishment and possible loss of their medical license. Because it is neither in the abusers' nor the doctors' interest to admit to misusing prescription drugs, statistics on prescription drug abuse capture only those individuals who encounter medical or legal problems as a result of their actions. But, recent studies report that more than 11.5 million Americans reported misusing prescription opioids in the previous year (CDC, 2017).

Additional data on patterns of misuse of prescription drugs are discernable through data on drug overdoses and drug-related deaths. Manchikanti and colleagues (2022) have identified four distinct waves of illicit drug overdoses and deaths in the U.S. from the 1990s to 2020. Specifically, they note that the increase in opioid prescriptions and later the easy availability of heroin contributed to the first two waves of overdoses and deaths from 1999–2013. A third wave of drug overdoses and deaths was attributed to the rise in the easy availability of synthetic opioids, such as fentanyl. The fourth wave appears to be attributed to a combination of factors, including revised guidelines from the CDC limiting prescription opioid distribution, the COVID-19 pandemic, the decrease in intervention options, and the increased availability of fentanyl (see Figure 5.I.6).

In 2000, the CDC reported a death rate of 3 deaths per 100,000 persons due to opioids in the U.S. But this rate grew to 21.4 per 100,000 persons in 2020 – an increase of 18.4 per 100,000 (CDC, 2022i; see Figure 5.I.6). Deaths due to *synthetic opioid analgesics*, here meaning synthetic drugs such as fentanyl or tramadol, but not methadone, yielded similar increases in death rates: 0.3 deaths per 100,000 persons in 2000 rising to 17.8 per 100,000 in 2020 (CDC, 2022i).

What is more, statistics also show that deaths due to drug overdoses are disproportionately affecting populations that were underrepresented in the past. Now, females, persons between 25 and 44 and those 55 years and older, non-Hispanic whites, and non-Hispanic blacks are increasingly represented in these opioid-related death rates in the U.S. (Rudd, Aleshire, Zibbel, & Gladden, 2016).

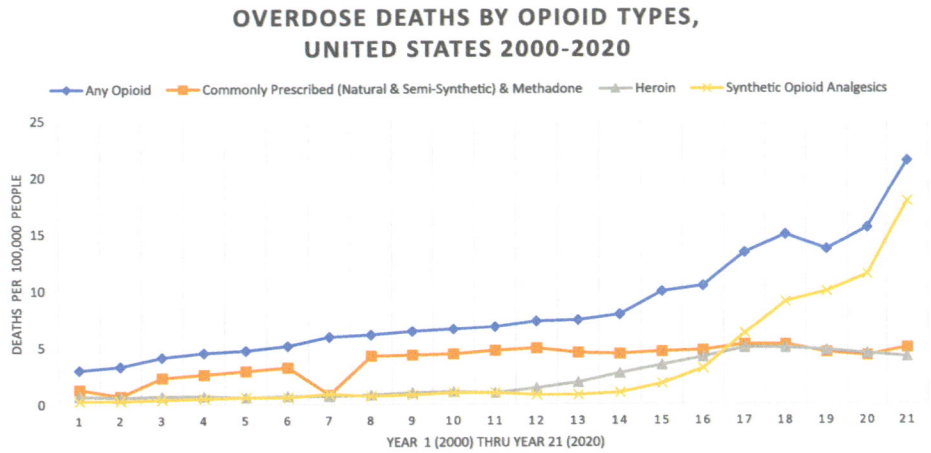

FIGURE 5.I.6 The line graph shows that death rates in the U.S. due to any opioid in 2000, including commonly prescribed opioids, heroin, & synthetic opioids, ranged from one to four persons per 100,000. In 2021, death rates from commonly prescribed opioids and heroin was four per 100,000, but deaths from synthetic opioids rose to 18 per 100,000, and approximately 22 per 100,000 for any opioid.

Source: CDC (2022i). Drug Overdose. Accessed online at www.cdc.gov/drugoverdose/data/od-death-data.html. Retrieved on May 30, 2023.

We noted previously that some people obtain their opioids from doctors. One cause of the increase in opioid-related drug overdose is the increase in prescribed pain medication. Simply put, when medical providers readily prescribe pain medication to their patients, patients may become dependent on these painkillers, fueling a demand for more. In Chapter 10, Chronic Pain Management and Arthritis, we discuss the heightened attention to pain and pain management by health providers. Briefly, we note that more than 45% of patients 65 years of age or older report frequent complaints of lower back pain (National Center for Health Statistics, 2021). And what medication is most often prescribed for such ailments? You guessed it: opioid pain medication. Undoubtedly, this has contributed to the overuse and in some cases overdose of opioids.

To be clear, the increased demand for painkillers is also caused by people seeking the drugs for non-medical reasons. Globally, more than 62 million people or 1.2% of the world's population uses opioids recreationally – here meaning for nonmedical use (UNODC, 2021). Currently, the continent of North America has the highest percentage of recreational opioid users per population, with 3.6% of users overall. Of growing concern, however, is the projected increase of opioid users in Africa and Asia. Researchers estimate the continent of Africa will see a 40% increase in opioid users by 2030 (UNODC, 2021).

In earlier editions of this text, we stated that the prescription pain abusers may turn to heroin (Rudd et al., 2016), a cheaper and thus more affordable form of pain relief. In fact in 2016, 75% of new heroin users claimed to have abused prescription pain medication before using heroin, and subsequent research illustrated this point with a marked increase in the overdose deaths due to heroin between 2010 and 2016 (see Figure 5.I.6). Now, however, fentanyl and other synthetic drugs have eclipsed heroin as a leading cause of overdose deaths, especially in the U.S.

VIDEO #22/60

Chapter 5: Risky Health Behaviors, Part I
· **Prescription Drug Abuse: Prescription Drug Abuse (60 Seconds of Health PSA)**
· **Website: https://www.youtube.com/watch?v=B63lJqJ0Oic**
· *Purdue University Extension is a publicly accessible platform as it provides research-based information and programs to the public for free. https://www.extension.purdue.edu/*

FENTANYL *Fentanyl* is a synthetic, here meaning a human-made drug produced in a laboratory setting either legally or illegally. It contains the same painkilling ingredients as natural opioids like codeine or morphine, with one exception: it is 50–100 times more powerful than these natural substances (NIDA, 2021).

When produced and used legally, fentanyl and related synthetic opioids are used to treat severe pain experienced by patients after surgery or for persons with chronic pain for which other opioids are no longer effective. When used illegally, however, this potent drug is often mixed with other substances such as heroin or methamphetamine. Unfortunately, the buyer of the illegal fentanyl is often unaware that the drug has been "cut" with other substances. This mixing, combined with the high potency of fentanyl, contributes to likely drug overdoses.

Like other opioids, fentanyl can initially produce feelings of euphoria, drowsiness, and nausea (NIDA, 2021). However, when used in excess it can slow or impair breathing and lead to unconsciousness and coma. If unaddressed, it can be life-threatening.

In sum, all three substances described earlier – marijuana, prescription painkillers, and fentanyl – when used in medically prescribed ways have some medicinal benefits. All three substances, however, can and have been linked to health risks and even death due to risky behaviors while under the influence of these drugs.

Alcohol/Drug Therapy

Undoubtedly, the overdose and death statistics for substance abuse reported in this section presents a discouraging picture, especially for health providers. The increase in alcohol consumption globally, and the increased use of cannabis, opioids, and fentanyl, seem to suggest that substance use is out of control. But, there is actually some good news, mainly in the treatment options for people with substance abuse disorders. Three treatment options are particularly noteworthy: glucagon-like-peptide-1, contingency management (nudge therapy to some), and pharmacological therapy.

GLUCAGON-LIKE-PEPTIDE-1 Perhaps the newest medication that may help to reduce alcohol use disorder is *glucagon-like-peptide-1 (GLP-1)*. This new drug was developed and intended for use for people with diabetes (see Chapter 4, Global, Communicable, and Chronic Disease) but was later discovered to be highly successful in helping people lose weight. We explore GLP-1s more fully in Chapter 5, Risky Health Behaviors, Part II, but briefly, this drug works to suppress the appetite and to reduce cravings by acting on the brain's pleasure pathways (Ouyang, 2023). Recently, researchers discovered that GLP-1s are also effective in reducing the desire for alcohol and some drugs. Researchers are still studying the exact mechanism by which this drug reduces the desire for these substances, but this is what is known to date. GLP-1 is produced in the brainstem, and GLP-1 receptors in the brainstem are thought to affect the brain's reward circuitry and addiction (Klausen, Thomsen, Wortwein, & Fink-Jensen, 2021; Vallöf, Kalafateli, & Jerlhag, 2020). Current studies suggest that taking additional GLP-1 helps reduce or eliminate the rewarding effects of alcohol when tested in animals. What is more, in their review of 17 studies examining the effects of added GLP-1s on alcohol, nicotine, amphetamine, and cocaine use disorders, Brunchmann and colleagues (2019) found GLP1s to be an effective treatment for the "behavioral effects" of these substances. If these findings are supported by additional studies, then GLP-1s may become a vital, new treatment for alcohol and drug use disorder.

CONTINGENCY MANAGEMENT This is both an old and a new strategy to effect behavior change or behavior modification. Some see this as an extension of B. F. Skinner's operant conditioning (McPherson, Parent, Miguel, McDonell, & Roll, 2022; you may remember this conditioning paradigm from your introductory psychology classes). In this paradigm, behavior is shaped and maintained through the consequences that follow. Using this logic and Skinner's operant conditioning techniques, studies have found that three components of this behavior modification technique are essential to maximize outcomes: frequent reinforcement (at least twice weekly); immediate reinforcement (the shorter the delay between the behavior and the reinforcer, the better); and the magnitude (here meaning the degree or amount of the reinforcer; McPherson et al., 2022). While a higher magnitude of reinforcement might increase the likelihood of behavioral change, the reinforcement cannot be so high as to result in a reversion back to the original behavior when the reinforcer is no longer present.

Consider this example: If trying to reduce the frequency of binge drinking on a college campus, a researcher (or health psychologist) might recruit volunteers who agree to be monitored for two to three months. The researchers select a reinforcer, for example a $15.00 gift certificate to the Panera Bread eatery on campus, a favorite hangout for students, to help shape student's behaviors. The health psychologists would then frequent the bars or restaurants that students prefer, to monitor the drinking behaviors of students. To reinforce the behaviors of students who refrain from binge drinking, the health psychologist would give the $15.00 gift certificate to student who refrained from binge drinking as they leave the bar or restaurant. The reinforcement is limited to two times a week.

For some, contingency management is similar to **nudge theory**. Essentially, nudge theory proposes that presenting people with choices of behaviors that do not restrict their behaviors in any way, or impact their incentives economically (Thaler & Sunstein, 2009), can be a motivator for people to choose behaviors that are more beneficial and yield the desired outcome. In essence, providing an incentive to choose a positive health behavior may motivate someone to unconsciously shape their preference for the desired behavior – say, perhaps, refraining from cocaine. Here, too, a gift certificate can be used to reinforce the behavior. If nudging a person to refrain from cocaine use, the gift certificate can be given to a person who produces a negative urine sample.

At this point, you may be thinking, "Of course people will change behaviors if they are paid!" But this is where the magnitude of reward or reward incentives become important. When selecting the reward, it is important to choose things that do not economically impact the recipient. In essence, the goal is to motivate a person (that is, to "nudge" them) to *choose* the preferred behavior, using the reward as an incentive, not a payment. Thus, choosing the target behavior (refraining from binge drinking or from cocaine use) becomes the goal for the person. The reward is just a form of encouragement to continue the behavior.

PHARMACOLOGICAL THERAPY For some people diagnosed with *alcohol use disorder (AUD)*, due, in part, to heavy alcohol use, there are medications approved for treatment. For example, the use of *naltrexone* or *acamprosate*, both approved by the U.S. Food and Drug Administration (FDA), results in a 5% lower risk of consuming alcohol and a 10% lower risk of binge drinking (Kranzler & Soyka, 2018). Pharmacological therapy is not new, but it is primarily used for people who have severe cases of AUD. Just to be clear, more than 29 million people 12 years of age or older were identified as having AUD in the U.S.

in 2022. This represents 10.5% of the population of those 12 years of age or older in the U.S. (National Institute on Alcohol Abuse and Alcoholism, n.d.).

For other substances, however, the pharmacological treatment options are more limited. For example, there are no FDA-approved pharmacological therapies for cocaine use disorder. However, there are some studies that suggest using a *dopamine agonist* helps address some substance use disorders. We explain more about dopamine in Chapter 5, Risky Health Behaviors, Part II, but briefly, dopamine is a chemical found in the brain that plays an important role in our experiencing and interpreting reward and pleasure (Cleveland Clinic, 2024b). A *dopamine agonist* is a drug that activates the dopamine receptors in the brain. Adding a dopamine agonist satisfies the reward and pleasure "craving" and is less addictive than the illicit drugs that perform the same role.

When using a dopamine agonist, researchers suggest that the key is choosing a medicine that triggers the same receptor as the drug, in this case cocaine (Kampman, 2019). When stimulated in this way, the pharmacological medicine will reproduce the effects of the drug in a less "abusable" form (Kampman, 2019). There is one drawback with cocaine, however: cocaine impacts multiple receptors in the brain. Therefore, pharmacological therapy for cocaine use disorder requires medications that target more than one receptor in the brain (Kampman, 2019).

In sum, yes, cigarettes, e-cigarettes, alcohol, cannabis, and illegal drugs can present unique problems of substance abuse and substance use disorders. And while there are treatments – both old and new – that have been identified for these disorders, there is no single best practice for reducing or eliminating substance use disorders. We have an arsenal of approaches and medications. But, effective treatment of these conditions will require not just medical intervention. In most cases, treatment for substance use disorders also entails psychological counseling and other programmatic interventions. Here, health psychologists can play a critical role in identifying intervention approaches that may be used in combination with pharmacological treatments.

SECTION III. RISKY SEXUAL BEHAVIORS

Is there a link between substance use or abuse and risky sexual behaviors? Absolutely! For several decades researchers have reported that alcohol and drug abuse lowers inhibitions against engaging in risky sexual behaviors (recall the Walter et al., 1992, 1993 studies on HIV prevention in Chapter 3, Theories and Models of Health Behavior Change). In fact, many researchers who examine the risky health behaviors of adolescents and young adults explore the correlations between substance use and sexual behavior. Therefore, it seems appropriate to follow our discussion of substance use with a discussion on risky sexual behaviors.

Defining Risk

Early in the chapter, we distinguished between risk and risky health behaviors. We further refine the definitions here for application to sexual behaviors. The term risky sexual behaviors describes a category of actions that increase an individual's likelihood of adverse consequences such as acquiring *sexually transmitted diseases (STDs)* – infectious diseases spread by sexual acts, usually through intercourse or through oral sex (see Table 5.I.7). Having sexual intercourse with multiple sex partners or not using a condom when having sex are two behaviors that increase the risk of adverse events.

Before proceeding, we need to make one observation. Sexual activity is a normal part of adolescent development and of adult behavior. As we explained in the section on alcohol, it is not the behaviors per se

TABLE 5.I.7 Summary of Selected Transmitted Diseases

Disease	Cause	Symptoms	Untreated Outcomes
Chlamydia	Bacteria *Chlamydia trachomatis*	Asymptomatic in women	Damage to women's reproductive organs
Herpes	Herpes simplex virus	Pain, itching in genitals Fever, headache Blisters, ulcers on genitals	Recurring bouts of blistering
Genital warts	Human papillomavirus (HPV)	Warts	Complication for pregnancy
Gonorrhea	Gonococcus bacterium	Painful urination Discharge from penis or vagina Discomfort in lower abdomen *or* asymptomatic	Sterility Infection of joints, skin, bone
Trichomoniasis	*Trichomonas vaginalis* parasite	Asymptomatic in 70% of persons infected Symptoms for remaining 30% can include itching, burning and irritation of genitals and discomfort when urinating	None, just discomfort
Syphilis HIV/AIDS	*Treponema pallidum* bacterium Human immunodeficiency virus	Canker sore on genitals, mouth, or rectum Fever, headache, loss of appetite Swollen glands Skin rash HIV: Early stages: No noticeable symptoms or flulike symptoms AIDS: Weight loss, cough, fevers, fatigue, diarrhea, low CD4 cell count	Paralysis Senility, insanity Opportunistic infections Death

Source: Based on Kunz (1982).

that increase the risk of adverse consequences. Rather, our focus here is on the risky sexual activities that can cause negative outcomes for at least one of the participants. Specifically, we focus on early initiation of sexual behaviors, engaging in sex without protection against diseases, multiple sexual partners, and combining substance use and sexual behavior.

Early Initiation Behaviors

In the section on theories of substance use, we noted that several integration theorists suggested that problem behavior, including early onset of sexual activity, may be an indicator of other problems in an adolescent's life. Specifically, problem-behavior theorists such as Jessor, Donovan, and Costa (1991) believe that early initiation of sexual behaviors may be a symptom of emotional, psychological, or social problems for teens (Chan et al., 2015; Gambadauro et al., 2018; Patton et al., 2016). Some studies have found that sexual intercourse in early adolescence is associated with poor family relationships and/or a lack of close relationships with friends or teachers (Makenzius & Larsson, 2013; Price & Hyde, 2011), a perspective shared also by conventional commitment theorists.

Other studies take a somewhat different view, endorsing a social ecological model to explain the onset of sexual activity in adolescents (Elkington et al., 2011; Zimmerman, Darnell, Rhew, Lee, & Kaysen, 2015). In these and related studies, researchers conclude that the sexual norms of adolescents' peers greatly influence the onset and risk-taking nature of their sexual activities. Specifically, adolescents who view their peers – and here we specify close peers/friends – as more approving of sexual activity and more sexually active will themselves engage in more sexual activity. And, teens who believe that their close friends engage in more risk-taking sexual behaviors will do likewise (van de Bongard, Reitz, Sandfort & Deković (2015).

Early engagement in sexual activities also increases teens' health risks by decreasing the probability that they will be well informed about protective behaviors that could minimize the spread of diseases to themselves or their partner. For example, research shows that African American adolescents engage in sexual behavior earlier than many other ethnic groups in the U.S. In one study on adolescents' and young adults' patterns of sexual behaviors, 55.6% of African American females and 61.8% of African American males between the ages of 14 and 19 reported ever having sex (Liu et al., 2015; see Figure 5.I.7). This number is higher than the average for all groups of the same age (49.2% females and 45.3% males) and higher than that for either whites or Mexican Americans, the other two ethnic groups sampled.

In spite of these data suggesting earlier sexual initiation behavior, Lindberg and Kantor (2022) found that African American and Hispanic males were less likely to receive formal sex education instruction before their first sexual experience. Specifically missing was information on birth control, where and how to obtain birth control, and sexually transmitted diseases including human immunodeficiency virus

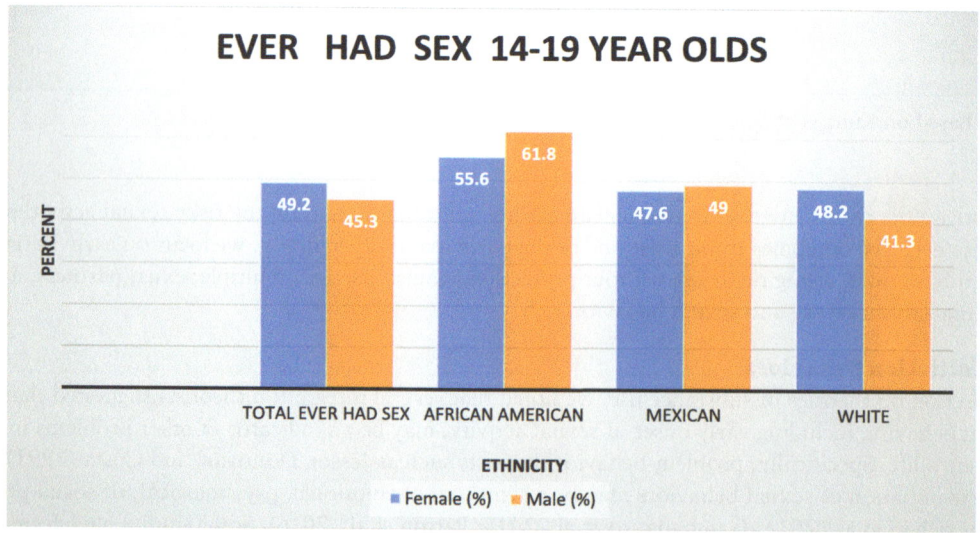

FIGURE 5.I.7 The comparative bar chart for 14–19 year olds who ever had sex shows that, overall, 49.2% of females and 45.3% of males reported having sex. African American females (55.6%) and males (61.8%) reported highest rates, followed by Mexican females (47.9%) and males (49%), and white females (48.2) and males (41.3%).

Source: Liu et al. (2015).

(HIV). Specifically, their data show that while 67% of white adolescents received instruction on methods of birth control, only 51% and 58% of African American or Hispanic males, respectively, received the same information. Additionally, 46% of white and Hispanic males received information on where to obtain birth control, but only 39% of African American males received similar information (Lindberg & Kantor, 2022).

The results for females were less dramatically different. While white, African American, and Hispanic females were almost equally likely to obtain information on where to obtain birth control (47%, 48%, and 49% respectively), African American females were significantly less likely to hear information on methods of birth control (58%) versus their white (63%) or Hispanic (68%) counterparts (Lindberg & Kantor, 2022). Thus, African American adolescents, specifically African American males who engage in early sexual behaviors, are likely to be the least informed about safer sexual practices, placing them at greater risk of negative outcomes, including unplanned pregnancies and, by extension, sexually transmitted diseases.

It should come as no surprise, therefore that studies also report that African American females have significantly higher levels of STD infections, specifically chlamydia, than other ethnic groups (Corcoran et al., 2021). The study by Corcoran and colleagues suggests that, for African Americans, early initiation of sex, combined with poorer access to health education and health care, increases the probability of adverse consequences.

VIDEO #23/60

Chapter 5: Risky Health Behaviors, Part I
- *Teenage Pregnancies: Teenage Pregnancy – What You Need to Know*
- *Website: https://www.youtube.com/watch?v=yYoyBdtGwx4*
- *Rehealthify is a public accessible platform that provides health-related information through online videos posted to Youtube (https://www.youtube.com/@rehealthify243)*

So, what can health psychologists do to address this issue? As researchers Astle and colleagues (2021) note, sex education, especially in the U.S., needs an update. When Astle and colleagues asked college-aged students for suggestions for improving the sex education they received – yielding something that would be both more useful and encourage safer sexual practices – these students suggested a plethora of ideas, including: lose the scare tactics about sex; provide basic information about sex, including relevant medical information; information about sexually transmitted diseases and safer sexual practices they can readily adopt; and offer a more holistic discussion about sex, including the social and emotional aspects of these behaviors (Astle et al., 2021). Health psychologists are well suited to respond to a need for an updated sex education program, or "Sex Education 2.0." Developing new health education programs and materials that encourage a wholesome discussion of the social and emotional aspects of sexual relationships, as well as implementing and assessing the effectiveness of such programs, are a core component of health psychologists' skill sets.

Human Immunodeficiency Virus (HIV)

With the preceding discussion in mind, we examine how all of us, including health psychologists, were less effective in mounting helpful programs when addressing the HIV pandemic.

By way of background, in the 1980s and early 1990s, HIV was more than an unfortunate, life-threatening disease. It was a stigma. One reason for the stigma was the lack of information about the disease and the populations most at risk. In an effort to quickly inform the public about the disease and to contain its spread, scientists released preliminary information and updates about the virus. Some of the information was found later to be inaccurate. For example, based on preliminary information, people who were diagnosed with HIV were assumed, often incorrectly, to be homosexuals, intravenous drug users, or Haitians. The assumption that HIV affected only these three groups obscured the fact that women, children, adolescents, sports celebrities – in other words, anyone – could contract HIV (see Boxes 5.I.1 and 5.I.2).

Box 5.I.1 Ryan White: An Agent of Change

Events of the 1990s shocked many sports fans. Basketball fans were stunned when the legendary Earvin "Magic" Johnson of the Los Angeles Lakers announced on November 7, 1991, that he had the human immunodeficiency virus (HIV), the virus that causes acquired immunodeficiency syndrome (AIDS). Tennis fans felt a loss when they learned that Arthur Ashe, the first African American man to win Wimbledon and the U.S. and Australian Opens, died of complications related to HIV/AIDS in 1993. And aquatic sports fans absorbed the announcement in 1994 by Greg Louganis, the winner of four Olympic gold medals, that he, too, had HIV. By comparison, few people heard about Ryan White, an adolescent who contracted the disease several years earlier (see Figure 5.I.8).

Ryan was not a famous athlete. But like Magic Johnson, Arthur Ashe, and Greg Louganis, his life was irrevocably changed by HIV/AIDS. Ryan was born with hemophilia, a rare bleeding disease that prevents blood from clotting normally. For hemophiliacs, ordinary scrapes, cuts, and nicks turn into potentially life-threatening scenarios due to excessive blood loss or damage to their internal organs (National Heart, Lung, and Blood Institute, 2007). To help control the bleeding, hemophiliacs are treated with blood products. Ryan was receiving treatment for his hemophilia when he was diagnosed with HIV in 1984. He was apparently given a blood product that was contaminated with the virus. Ryan was only 13 years old.

In 1984, HIV/AIDS was a rare and relatively unknown disease. At the time, the virus was associated with three groups: homosexual men, intravenous drug users, and Haitians, groups often stigmatized by society. Lack of knowledge about the disease and erroneous assumptions about individuals who were HIV positive caused many to fear or reject anyone with the virus. Ryan's neighbors in Kokomo, Indiana, were no exception. Reacting to Ryan's diagnosis of HIV, the school board in Kokomo banned Ryan from attending school based on the fear that he would expose other children to HIV/AIDS (U.S. Congress AIDS PAC, 2007). Ryan and his mother successfully sued the Kokomo school board. He won the right to return to school, but the family chose to move to Cicero, Indiana, instead; stigma and isolation by the Kokomo community created an unwelcoming environment for the White family.

Ryan died of AIDS in 1990. That same year, the U.S. Congress passed the Ryan White Comprehensive AIDS Resource Emergency (RARE) Act (Public Law 101–381), an act that provides $1.5 billion per year for health care and resources for people with HIV/AIDS (U.S. Congress AIDS PAC, 2007).

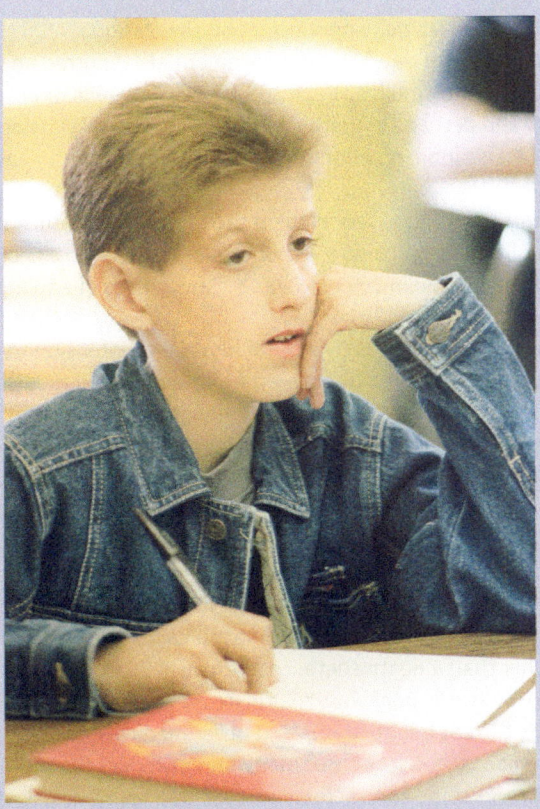

FIGURE 5.I.8 Headshot photo of Ryan White at about 13 years of age.

Source: Bettmann via Getty Images.

Box 5.I.2 Even Magic Johnson Has It, and He Looks Good

The Los Angeles Lakers' legendary star player, Earvin "Magic" Johnson, has everything: five National Basketball Association (NBA) championships, three Most Valuable Player awards, three NBA Finals Most Valuable Player awards, a winning personality, and a "magic" smile. What more could he ask for?

Actually, the question is what Magic did not ask for. In November 1991, Magic stunned the world when he announced that he was HIV positive. It seemed as if the world stopped and listened. "Sometimes you're a little naïve," he said, "and . . . think it could never happen to you. You only thought it could happen to . . . other people. . . . And it has happened but I'm going to deal with it" (American Rhetoric, 2001, p. 1).

That same November day, after Magic's announcement, the National AIDS Hotline received 40,000 calls, up from its usual 3,800 calls per day. The announcement also spurred an immediate increase in anonymous HIV testing (Gellert, Weismuller, Higgins, & Maxwell, 1992). Other researchers suggest that it created awareness of HIV and perhaps empathy toward people with HIV (Noormohamed, Ferguson, Baghaie, & Cohen, 1994). If Magic Johnson intended to get people's attention about HIV, he succeeded – at least for the moment.

Today, more than 30 years later, Magic seems to be the picture of health. A little heavier than he was in his days as a Los Angeles Laker, Magic is now a business entrepreneur; the principal donor to the Magic Johnson Foundation, which he created in 1991 to increase awareness of and attention to HIV/AIDS; and a spokesperson for World AIDS Day.

Magic is still strong and active, largely as a result of his careful attention to his health and excellent medical care. At that time, researchers had discovered a combination of medications, sometimes called a "drug cocktail," that, when taken in combination, not only prolongs the life of people with HIV but also improves their overall quality of life. Fortunately for Magic, the cocktail therapy is working well. Today, newer medications reduce the detectable levels of HIV in a person that prevents them from infecting others with the illness.

Ironically, Magic's success, and the discovery of new, more effective medications that prevent the spread of HIV, appear to undermine the message. Current research suggests many men believe that HIV is not such a problem after all. Among males who engage in risky sexual behaviors, researchers note that many are less fearful of HIV now than before. Some males believe that the newer medications make HIV a treatable disease rather than a death sentence. With such attitudes, some men may be inclined to continue engaging in the risky sexual behaviors that increase their susceptibility to HIV.

Without a doubt, Magic's current health status and other medical developments have improved our understanding and treatment of the disease. But many may still miss the more important message, specifically from Magic's case. First, he contracted a disease as a result of risky sexual behaviors. Health prevention messages were not effective in changing his behavior to reduce that risk. Second, Magic has access to unrestricted and excellent-quality health care that provides life-prolonging and health-enhancing HIV medicines. The same may not be true for the average male. Consider this: Research in health psychology shows that lack of access to quality health care is one cause of poor health outcomes (Clauss-Ehler, 2003; Coursen, 2009). It is unlikely that the average male (or female) will have the same access to health care Magic received, either as a current or former member of the Lakers basketball team.

In addition, HIV caused adverse emotional and psychological health outcomes for individuals with the disease and others in their social networks. Thus, absent a cure or treatment, one role for health psychologists in the early stages of the pandemic was to address the emotional and psychological health of infected individuals and their support groups.

By the early 1990s, scientists discovered that HIV was not associated with high-risk groups; rather, it was associated with specific high-risk behaviors. Scientists learned that HIV was transmitted by direct contact with blood or other body fluids that were contaminated with the virus (see Box 5.I.3). But the public – here meaning the nonscientific community – seemed to hold fast to earlier information that associated HIV with specific groups, illustrating how difficult it is to correct inaccurate information once it has been made public.

Box 5.I.3 What Is HIV?

HIV is a unique virus because it targets and attacks our immune system.

What makes HIV so distinctive? Simply stated, it is a retrovirus.

Many viruses we encounter are DNA viruses. DNA is deoxyribonucleic acid, the heredity material present in humans and other organisms. DNA is often called the "human blueprint" because it contains the information needed to construct the cells that make up our system.

DNA is housed in the cell nucleus, the control center for the activities of the cell, and consists of hundreds of strands packed with information. A DNA virus, however, contains only one strand of DNA. When a DNA virus enters the body, it copies its genetic code onto a viral RNA (ribonucleic acid), the agent that helps the virus reproduce. Thus, most DNA viruses are easily identifiable by the viral RNA code they display to the immune system.

HIV, however, is a retrovirus. Retroviruses store their genetic information in RNA. Put another way, the genetic material for HIV is RNA. Unlike a DNA virus that converts into a viral RNA that is easily recognized as a foreign element, the HIV virus does the opposite. The virus converts its genetic RNA into viral DNA. After recoding as viral DNA, HIV inserts itself into the cell nucleus and copies its genetic material onto the host cell's DNA, firmly imbedding itself into the cell (Goldsby, Kindt, Osborn, & Kuby, 2003). Once embedded, the HIV virus has a host that will help it reproduce when the time is right.

Compounding the problem, the HIV virus lies dormant for 8 to 10 years unless detected by medical tests. This means that it does not replicate immediately. Think of it this way: The HIV virus is like a fox, and the body's healthy cells can be compared to sheep. When an HIV fox enters a body full of healthy sheep cells, it attacks one of the sheep. It slowly destroys the sheep and then uses the sheep's wool to disguise itself as just another sheep. The disguised HIV fox is not recognized by the body as a foreign element. Slowly, HIV fox begins to multiply and invade other sheep.

HIV and the process by which it invades, converts, and destroys healthy human cells presented researchers with a unique challenge: how to identify, isolate, and destroy HIV (viral DNA) without killing other human cells necessary for survival. The challenge is one reason why scientists have been unable to effectively isolate and kill the HIV virus.

The revelation in the early 1990s that three sports celebrities had HIV – Magic Johnson, former star basketball player for the Los Angeles Lakers; Arthur Ashe, tennis pro and winner of 51 tennis tournaments including Wimbledon; and Greg Louganis, star athlete and winner of several Olympic gold medals for diving – in addition to more information about the virus, helped change the public's perception of the disease (see again Box 5.I.1). Slowly, many in the public began to accept that HIV was associated with risky behaviors that exposed individuals to contaminated human body fluids.

Increasingly, the public became aware that women, too, were being diagnosed with HIV. This revelation, together with celebrities contracting the illness, helped the public understand that HIV is a disease that can affect anyone regardless of gender, ethnicity, socioeconomic status, or profession. We now know that our behaviors, not who we are, influence our risk of contracting HIV. Thus, it is appropriately included in this chapter on risky health behaviors.

Unlike other contagious diseases such as measles, there is no vaccine to protect individuals from HIV. For quite a while the only proven method for controlling the spread of the disease was through behavior change: specifically, avoiding risky behaviors that may expose individuals to the virus. Fortunately, the discovery of antiretroviral drugs, a combination of drugs that together slow the rate at which HIV multiplies in the body (HealthwiseStaff, 2022), has dramatically slowed the spread of this disease, allowing the infected individual to remain healthy longer.

HIV ORIGINS, TRANSMISSIONS, AND HUMAN BEHAVIOR Many scientists contend that HIV is linked to a species of chimpanzees known as *Pan troglodytes*, found in West Africa (Gao et al., 1999). In other words, scientists suggest that the virus was probably transmitted through zoonotic spillover (see Chapter 4, Global, Communicable, and Chronic Disease). Humans may have contracted the virus as a result of a bite from a chimpanzee, from eating undercooked chimpanzee meat, or from contact with chimpanzees' virus-infected blood. When living in chimpanzees, the virus was a simian immunodeficiency virus (SIV) that is not fatal to that species. The infected primates show no signs of illness or dysfunction from the virus. Thus, although SIV is harmless in one species, it can be fatal in another.

Research by Faria and colleagues (2014) further explains how this disease made its way from areas populated with chimpanzees to the Western Hemisphere. They traced the transmission of the SIV from chimpanzees to human and then mapped its movement in the 1920s as it traveled with its new human host in much the same way that viruses have traveled for centuries. Remember that in Chapter 4, Global, Communicable, and Chronic Disease, we noted that whether through trade, travel, wars, or other methods, people from one region of the world brought their goods and diseases to another part of the globe. This was the case with HIV. Faria and colleagues traced the route of the virus along railways and water ways through the Democratic Republic of Congo (DRC) to the capital, Kinshasa (Faria et al., 2014). It appears that the virus then infected Haitian professionals who were in Kinshasa. When the Haitians returned to Haiti, the virus transmission changed from animal-to-human to human-to-human. This change led to the rapid spread of HIV to others in Haiti.

HUMAN-TO-HUMAN TRANSMISSION Researchers discovered the human-to-human transmission of HIV through case-study analysis (see Chapter 2, Research Methods) of people with HIV, such as Magic Johnson, Greg Louganis, and Arthur Ashe. We now know that many activities that result in an exchange of fluids from an HIV-positive person or that expose uninfected individuals to contaminated fluids could result in infection.

Medical studies have further determined that HIV is transmitted primarily through three routes: sexual intercourse, parenteral (bloodborne) transmission, or perinatal (mother-to-child) transmission (MTCT; see Box 5.I.4). Today, sexual transmission accounts for the majority of HIV cases.

Box 5.I.4 Three Primary Transmission Routes of HIV

By now most people know that HIV cannot be transmitted through kissing. Saliva is a very poor – indeed ineffective – conduit of the virus. But few may realize that HIV can be contracted through a few other ways. First, to be clear, HIV is carried in semen, vaginal fluids, and blood. Thus the virus can be contracted through heterosexual and homosexual intercourse. Case-study analyses of individuals who tested positive for HIV, such as Magic Johnson and Greg Louganis, helped establish the link between sexual behaviors and HIV infection. Although earlier studies on HIV emphasized the susceptibility of homosexual men to HIV infection, Magic Johnson's announcement offered a clear and compelling message to the public: Heterosexual men and women were also at risk for contracting HIV (see Box 5/I.2).

A second method of HIV transmission is parenteral, transmission, including blood transfusions, similar to the type received by Ryan White and Arthur Ashe, and infections from unsanitary needles such as those used by intravenous drug users. Accidental needle sticks, common occurrences among health care workers (Greenblatt & Hessol, 2001), also can result in transmission of HIV if the needle had been used on a patient who was HIV positive.

The third method of infection, perinatal, or mother-to-child, transmission (MTCT), occurs when an HIV-positive mother transmits the virus to her child during childbirth. Early in the HIV disease history, approximately one-third to one-half (35%–50%) of children born to HIV-positive mothers were thought to have been infected during delivery, a time in which the infant is exposed to a mother's infected blood and other body fluids as it journeys through the birth canal (UNICEF, 2002a, 2002b). In 1991, the U.S. reported that approximately 1,700 infants were infected with HIV at birth; this number declined to 73 infants by 2017 (McKenna & Hu, 2007; Vijayan, Naeem, & Veesenmeyer, 2021). Similar declines have been reported in other countries. For example, South Africa reported a 97% decrease in HIV infections in the over 300,000 infants exposed to HIV at birth (Slogrove et al., 2017).

The declines are largely attributed to antiretroviral postexposure prophylaxis – a drug that is given to HIV-positive mothers within six hours after birth. This has been shown to reduce the transmission rate of HIV from mother to child in 95% of cases (Vijayan et al., 2021). As of 2021, global estimates suggest that 82% of women with, or who have been exposed to, HIV receive this prophylaxis. Without such treatment, the risk of transmission of HIV from mother to child can be high. Consider this: Globally, in 2021, 160,000 children were positive for HIV. Of this number, 48% had mothers who had not been treated with the antiretroviral therapy, and another 22% had mothers who had discontinued treatment (Ruel et al., 2023).

Challenges to Health-Protecting Behaviors

KNOWLEDGE Using the HIV pandemic, we can examine health-protecting sexual behaviors. As we noted, one of the ways HIV is communicated is through unprotected sexual intercourse. And while sex is a natural human behavior, the consequences for engaging in this behavior in a risky manner, here meaning without the knowledge and tools to protect oneself from illnesses and diseases, may have more consequences.

We noted earlier that in many instances, adolescents who are sexually active at earlier ages may be less well-informed than those who wait, but this is not always accurate. Two studies help illustrate the point. A study conducted in Taiwan measured the sexual knowledge, sexual attitudes, and safe-sex behaviors of 823 fifth-year, junior college students of medicine, nursing, and/or management in Central Taiwan. Lou and Chen (2009) found that student's sexual knowledge had no effect on safe – or we should say, safer – sexual behavior. Their findings may seem surprising but they actually fit the old adage "knowledge does not equal behavior." This further underscores the point that adolescents may need help in applying their knowledge.

A related study among 156 second-year medical students and 63 second-year nursing students in France assessed their knowledge of sexually transmitted diseases, STI prevention, and sexual behaviors. Note that as part of their training, these students were required to contribute to the health education of middle and high school students, among others. The study by Raia-Barjat and colleagues (2020) found that while the majority of these medical and nursing students (83.3%) could correctly identify how HIV is transmitted, 13% believed that HIV was also transmitted by kissing (see again Box 5.I.4). Only 35% of these medical and nursing students were aware of the beneficial effects of antiretroviral drugs on life expectancy. And while almost all knew that condoms were effective as a barrier method to protect against HIV transmission, less than half knew that pre-exposure or post-exposure prophylaxis were available and effective (Raia-Barjat et al., 2020). Remember, these students were responsible for imparting essential sexual health information to others.

The main point of these studies is that knowledge does not always change behaviors. Indeed, if this were true, none of us would engage in unhealthy activities because we would automatically adopt the health-protective behaviors consistent with our knowledge. Clearly, this is not the case. In language more consistent with social marketing, our messaging must change if we are to be more effective in changing behaviors.

SUBSTANCE USE AND SEXUAL BEHAVIOR Studies suggest that both adolescents and adults indicate that substance use will undermine even the most confident individual's ability to negotiate safer sexual behavior. A classic intervention study by Walter and colleagues, mentioned earlier, designed to teach adolescents in grades 10 through 12 strategies to negotiate safer sexual behaviors revealed that adolescents felt unable to use the strategies learned in the eight-week intervention sessions if they drank alcohol or used drugs immediately before a sexual encounter (Walter et al., 1992, 1993), a finding that has been supported in more recent studies (Hunt, Sanders, Petersen, & Bogren, 2021). The main point here is that alcohol and drug use may compromise judgment and decision-making skills even when a person has demonstrated an ability to exercise sound judgment when impaired. Impaired judgment puts the individual at higher risk for adverse health outcomes.

TEENAGE PREGNANCIES It is probably true that, in a few cases, female teenagers intended to become pregnant as a result of sexual behaviors. In most instances, however, a teenage pregnancy is a surprising and unexpected outcome. Therefore, teenage births qualify as an adverse outcome.

Global data on children born to adolescents has shown a steady decrease in the number births to girls 15–19 years of age. This is true for all global regions. In 2000, four global regions reported the highest birth rates to girls ages 15–19: Western and Central Africa (134 per 100,000), Sub-Saharan Africa (129 per 100,000), Eastern and Southern Africa (123 per 100,000), and South Asia (103 per 100,000; UNICEF, 2024; see Table 5.I.8). But, in 2022, each of these four regions reported substantially lower birth rates. In fact, only Western and Central Africa reported birth rates to 15- to 19-year-old girls that exceeded 100 per 100,000. What is more, the birth rates in South Asia for this population fell significantly, resulting in only 28 births per 100,000 (UNICEF, 2024; see again Table 5.I.8). Decreases in births to 15- to 19-year-olds were also reported in other regions of the world. For example Europe reported a 50% decrease in births to this age cohort between 2000 and 2022 (25 per 100,00 vs. 13 per 100,000, respectively) and a two-thirds decrease in North America (44 births per 100,000 in 2000 vs. 14 per 100,000 in 2022; UNICEF, 2024).

This data on the decrease in teen births is very good news. As we mentioned, in most cases, teen births are unplanned and can present economic, psychological, and emotional challenges for the mother. It is, perhaps, one bit of good news in this chapter's discussion of adverse outcomes from risky health behaviors.

TABLE 5.1.8 Estimated Birth Rates by Global Regions: 15- to 19-Year-Olds

REGION	2000	2022
WORLD	65	42
Western Europe	14	8
Europe and Central Asia	25	13
North America	44	14
East Asia and Pacific	22	20
Eastern Europe and Central Asia	34	19
South Asia	103	28
Middle East and North Africa	44	34
Latin America and the Caribbean	84	52
Eastern and Southern Africa	123	94
Sub-Saharan Africa	129	99
Western and Central Africa	134	105

Western and Central Africa, Sub-Saharan Africa, and Eastern and Southern Africa top the list in 2000 and 2022 for the largest number of births per 100,000 for girls 15–19 years of age.

Source: UNICEF: Early Child bearing (2024). Accessed online at: https://data.unicef.org/topic/child-health/adolescent-health/

Summary

We highlighted here two specific risky behaviors that are sometimes related: substance use/abuse, including cigarettes, e-cigarettes, alcohol, cannabis and illicit drugs, and high-risk sexual behaviors. We noted that whereas use/abuse of cigarettes, alcohol, and drugs is on the increase worldwide, presenting new challenges to all health professionals, high-risk sexual behaviors appear to be declining. Adolescents report fewer sexual partners and fewer teen pregnancies over the past 20+ years. We also note that new treatment options that appear to target the brain's reward circuitry may offer promising treatments for reducing and reversing the desire to abuse alcohol and drugs. All of this is good news and offers new and innovative ways for health psychologists to contribute to the advancements in these areas.

Personal Postscript

CALCULATED RISK: COMPARING THE HEALTH BEHAVIORS AND HEALTH OUTCOMES OF YOUR CLOSE FRIENDS AND YOU

It is quite possible that while reading about risky behaviors in this chapter, you thought about family members or close friends who sometimes engage in one or more of the risky behaviors identified. It is possible, also, that your friends or family members have not experienced negative outcomes as a result of their behaviors. If that is the case, they are quite lucky. Not everyone has the same luck.

Health outcomes vary according to the individual. One person may escape the dangers associated with binge drinking or years of cigarette smoking, but another person may have a bad experience after just one episode. How do you know which experience you will have? The problem is that you have no way of knowing.

So what should you do? Do you gamble and follow your friend's example, expecting the same positive outcome, or do you choose a more careful approach? One thing may help you decide. Rather than talking with your closest friends about their risky health behaviors, talk with another group of people about the same age, people with whom you have little regular contact. Listen to their views on, say, binge drinking or smoking marijuana. Someone from the "new" group may offer a different opinion or a new way of thinking about risky behaviors. Then consider the new information before making a final decision. Different perspectives sometimes help inform our final choices.

Then talk with your friends again. Studies with adolescents show that many overestimate their friends' involvement in risky health behaviors, both with regard to type of activity and frequency. A candid conversation with a friend or an acquaintance might help distinguish between boastful behaviors rooted in fiction and true confessions rooted in fact.

Questions to Consider

1. The new vaping products have made smoking attractive once again, especially to adolescents. Can you use the information on the adverse health effects of these products to craft a persuasive health message to discourage teens from vaping?
2. The new GLP-1 drugs for obesity and perhaps alcohol or drug dependency reinforce the role of the brain and the reward circuitry on addictions and health behaviors. What additional training might health psychologists need in order to contribute to this work?
3. Antiretroviral postexposure prophylaxis (ARTs) have saved the lives of many thousands of people infected with HIV. However, some would suggest that the discovery of ARTs have given some people the impression that HIV is "no big deal." They now believe that HIV is no longer fatal, as long as they can obtain ARTs. Clearly, messages encouraging safer-sexual practices to reduce the risk of HIV needs to change. What would you suggest?

True or False Questions

1. EVALI is the newest vape pod device. True or False.
2. Researchers agree that e-cigarettes are an effective way to quit smoking. True or False.
3. The WHO issues new policy guidelines aimed at ending the promotion of e-cigarettes. True or False.
4. Recreational marijuana use is legal in over 25 states in the U.S. True or False.
5. Fentanyl is a legal drug when used in approved medical settings and according to medical use guidelines. True or False.

Important Terms

acculturation   161
antioxidants   166
atomizer   164
binge drinking   168
buffers   165
carcinogen   175
cirrhosis   169
cognitive-affective theories   165
contingency management   178
conventional commitment theories   165
depressants   174
direct effect   160
dopamine   174
dopamine agonist   180
e-cigarette   163
e-cigarette or vaping product use associated with lung injury (EVALI)   154
electronic nicotine delivery system (ENDS)   164
excessive alcohol consumption   167
fentanyl   178
fetal alcohol syndrome   169
gateway theory   173
glucagon-like-peptide-1 (GLP-1)   178
heavy drinking   168
illicit drugs   173
indirect effect   160
integration theories   166
marijuana   173
mediating factors   160
MPOWER   161
neurons   174
neurotransmitters   174
nudge theory   179
opioids   175
personality trait theories   165
plant phenolics   166
pneumothorax   154
prescription drugs   175
sexually transmitted disease (STD)   180
social learning theories   165
socially normative behavior   159

Risky Health Behaviors: Part II

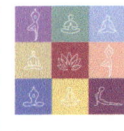

Source: 3xy/
Shutterstock.

Chapter Outline

Chapter Objectives

After studying Part II of this chapter, you will be able to:

1. Define unintentional injuries.
2. Identify the six factors that contribute to motor vehicle accidents.
3. Define graduate licensing or provisional licensing laws.
4. Explain the impact of graduated licensing laws on motor vehicle accidents and fatalities.
5. Identify and define three major types of violence.
6. Describe the effects of violence on individuals and communities.
7. Identify and define the four major eating disorders.
8. Explain the health consequences of anorexia, bulimia, obesity, and binge eating.
9. Explain the potential benefits of GLP-1s for obesity.

DOI: 10.4324/9781003300670-6

OPENING STORY: ON PROM NIGHT: A STICK OF GUM, DISTRACTED DRIVING, AND A FATAL ENDING

Gillian Sabet, the class president of her high school, was driving herself, her boyfriend, and three other teenage passengers to their school prom. According to a CNN story, Gillian's mother reported that while on the way to the prom, one of the four passengers asked for a piece of chewing gum. Gillian had a pack of gum in the driver's seat pocket. As she reached for the gum, she diverted her eyes from the road for the briefest of moments and lost control of the car (Lawrence, 2007). Gillian and her boyfriend were killed in the accident. The three other passengers survived. ■

Accidents involving teenage drivers do not always make the news, but this accident was different. Gillian Sabet, the 16-year-old driver, was not drunk, had not used drugs, and was not speeding. But she was distracted.

This story seems incredible. How is it possible that a very brief distraction – a quick glance to find a pack of gum – could result in a fatal accident? After all, many people do seemingly more distracting behaviors while driving, including changing music selections, looking for coins to pay tolls, reaching for something to drink or even texting. They do not end up in an accident or dead. Why was Gillian's outcome different?

Gillian's situation included several factors that, when combined with the distraction of looking for gum, may have led to the accident. One factor appears to be inexperience. This accident occurred in the U.S., where, in most states, would-be drivers must be at least 16 years of age and have a learner's permit, a precursor to an actual license, before they can operate an automobile. A *learner's permit* allows a new driver to practice driving skills in real settings provided he or she is accompanied by a licensed driver.

At 16, and driving without an adult passenger, Gillian may have obtained both her learner's permit and her driver's license within one year: a nice accomplishment! But such an accomplishment may have a few disadvantages. Being licensed to drive at age 16, Gillian probably had little actual driving experience. Studies of automobile accident rates involving teenagers show that *newly licensed drivers*, that is, drivers licensed for less than one month, and teenage drivers with little experience behind the wheel are less able to detect and avoid oncoming hazards than are more experienced drivers (Committee on Injury, Violence, and Poison Prevention and Committee on Adolescence, 2006; Stanojević, Lajunen, Jakšić, Jovanović, & Matović, 2022). In fact, researchers in Nova Scotia, Canada, found that more driving experience usually means fewer automobile accidents. The Nova Scotia study showed that the rate of automobile crashes for newly licensed teenagers decreases by more than half, from 120 accidents per 10,000 drivers to 50 per 10,000 drivers, after just 18 months of driving experience (Mayhew, Simpson, & Pak, 2003). At age 16, Gillian may have had fewer than 18 months of driving experience. It is possible that with more experience Gillian could have recovered from the hazards posed by a momentary distraction.

A second potential contributing factor to the accident is the driver's age, a factor that is related to inexperience. Age and inexperience are *correlated variables* or, as we explained in Chapter 2, Research Methods, variables that covary. In this case, the variables – driver's age and inexperience – are negatively correlated. As age increases, we find that driving inexperience decreases. Remember that in the opening story, Gillian was only 16; studies show that adolescents 16 to 19 years of age have the highest automobile accident rate of any age group (National Safety Council, 2023).

The presence of other teenage passengers is a third potential contributing factor to accidents. Notice that we specify teenage passengers. What difference does the age of the passengers make? According

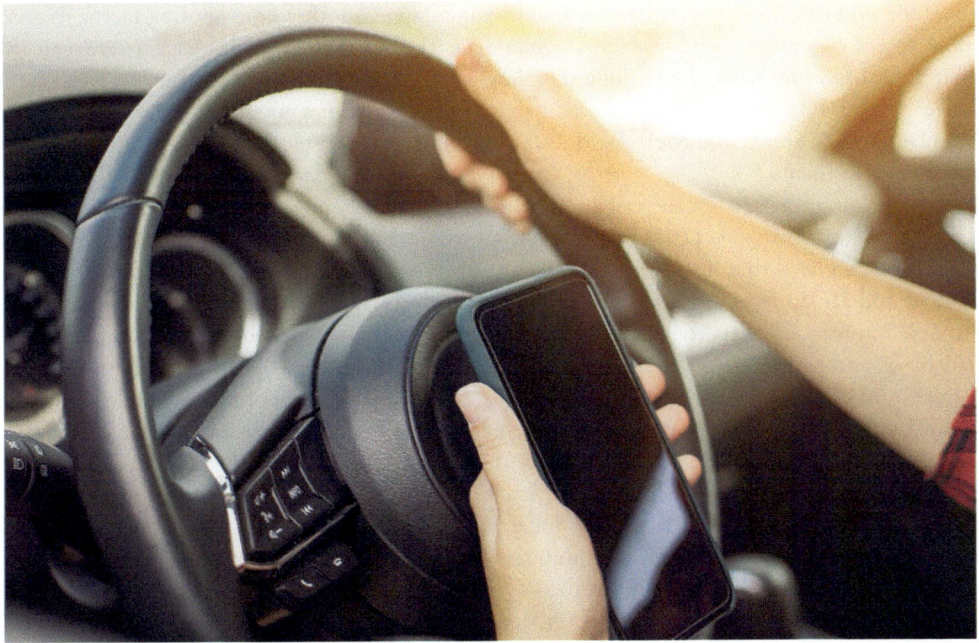

FIGURE 5.II.1 Photo of a female teenage driver and female teenage passenger looking at cellphone while driving.

Source: tong patong via Shutterstock.

to some researchers, it may mean the difference between life and death. Studies suggest that teenage passengers are more likely to engage in behaviors that may distract a driver (see Figure 5.II.1). We saw in the opening story how a minor distraction can prove fatal. Yet research suggests that teens often engage in greater distractions, such as "fooling around," when another teen is at the wheel. Adolescents explain that fooling around behaviors include yelling, loud conversations, arguing, dancing, wrestling or other forms of "horseplay" while in a car (NHTSA 2012a). The behaviors may involve the driver or just other passengers (University of California, Agricultural and Natural Resources, 2007). But even a driver who does not participate in fooling around is prone to be distracted by the action.

As for speeding, here too research suggests that adolescent passengers contribute to the likelihood of this risky behavior. A report by the Committee on Injury (2006) suggests that teen drivers are more likely to speed in the presence of male teenage passengers regardless of whether the driver is male or female. Why do male teenage passengers influence a driver's speed? That is not clear. Perhaps teen drivers are inclined to try to impress or show off their driving skills when males are present. But because most teenage drivers lack experience or well-developed skills, they may overestimate their actual abilities.

Thus, whether distracted, speeding, or just inexperienced, statistics on the rates of automobile accidents by adolescents show that drivers 16 to 17 years of age have a 44% increased risk of motor vehicle accidents and death when accompanied by one passenger under 21 years of age. The risk doubles when two adolescent passengers are present, and quadruples when three or more teens are present (Committee on Injury, Violence, and Poison Prevention and Committee on Adolescence, 2006; Tefft, Williams, & Grabowski, 2012). Gillian was traveling with four other teenage passengers; you do the math.

Newer studies on the dangers of texting while driving add yet another contributing factor to automobile accidents. A recent naturalistic study by the Virginia Tech Transportation Institute (2016) reveals that engaging in ***visual-manual subtasks***, including dialing a cell phone number or texting, or even searching for an object, makes a driver three times more likely to be involved in a crash. Work by Pitt and colleagues (2021) and Delgado, Wanner, and McDonald (2016) put this figure at closer to a fourfold increase in accidents or near accidents.

Admittedly, adolescents are not the only age group that regularly engages in texting while driving. A study by Wilson and Stimpson (2010) places this latest information in context. Their study, involving drivers of all ages, showed that after a gradual decline in distracted driver accidents and fatalities in the U.S. between 1999 and 2005, deaths due to distracted driving, which includes texting, rose beginning in 2005. A total of 5,817 automobile fatalities due to distracted driving were recorded in 2005, up from 4,563 in 1999 (Wilson & Stimpson, 2010). What is more, Wilson and Stimpson (2010) were able to show that the increase in text messaging was strongly correlated with the increased rates of distracted driver fatalities between 2005 and 2008, a finding supported in current studies by Flaherty, Kim, Salt, and Lee (2020).

As for adolescents' role in these outcomes, Wilson and Stimpson (2010) note that drivers between the ages of 16 and 29 accounted for 39% of all distracted driver fatalities in 2008, while those 50 years of age and older were involved in just 27.8% of such incidences. If we focus only on the younger teen cohort, the U.S. National Highway Traffic and Safety Administration (NHTSA) reveals that adolescents between the ages of 15 and 20 constituted 11% of all distracted drivers and 16% of all drivers distracted by cell phones (NCSA, 2023). While adolescents are not the only age group to engage in distracted driving behaviors, we will see that they contribute to this phenomenon at rates higher than their percentage of licensed drivers.

So, what can be done to reduce the rate of distracted and/or risky driving behaviors? And how can health psychologists assist in this process? A first step may be to understand drivers' and particularly adolescent drivers' views about risky driving behaviors. An annual survey by the Automobile Association of America (AAA) Foundation for Traffic Safety (2021) may be helpful. In their 2020 survey of just over 3,700 drivers – 1,036 of whom were 16–18 years of age, the AAA assessed driver's views on distracted, aggressive, drowsy/impaired, and other risky driving behaviors (see Figure 5.II.2). Most drivers clearly identified

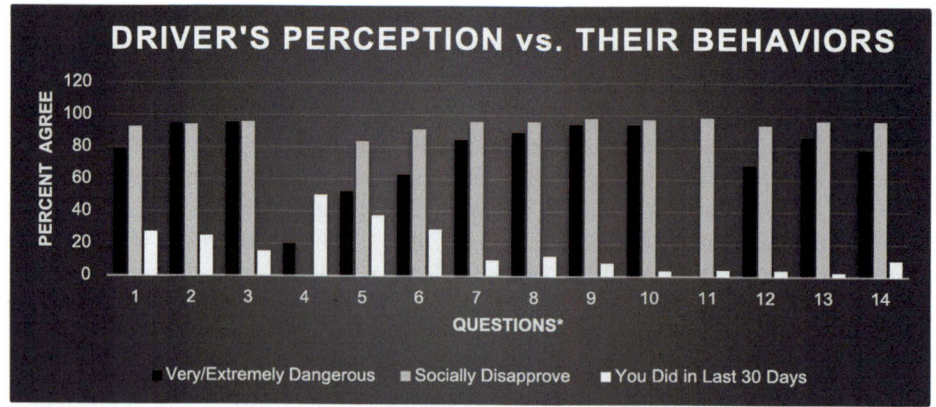

FIGURE 5.II.2 A bar chart compares drivers ratings of 14 risky driving behaviors- including driving while texting, reading a text, speeding, switching lanes, or driving or riding in a car with impaired driver- with the likely opinions of the same behaviors by their closest friends or relatives, and with the driver's actual risky driving behaviors.

Source: Adapted from AAA Foundation for Traffic Safety (2021).

distracted driving (e.g., holding/talking on cell phones while driving, texting, or emailing while driving: questions 1–4), aggressive driving (e.g., speeding on freeways or residential areas, switching lanes quickly: questions 5–8) or impaired driving (e. g., too much alcohol, too tired: questions 9–13) as dangerous. This is good news.

Additionally, they also believed that people important to them would disapprove of these same distracting, aggressive, and impaired driving behaviors. Why is this point important? Recall that in Chapter 3, Theories and Models of Health Behavior Change, we noted that one noteworthy influence on a person's likely behavior is the opinions of their social networks, comprising people whose views are important to them. The question is whether drivers' own beliefs, and those of people who are closest to them, influence their behavior. Turning to Figure 5.II.2 again, we see the answer is, sometimes! Fully 15%–50% of people admitted to some form of distracted driving either a few times, fairly often or regularly. Here it is important to remember, again, what we learned in Chapter 3: Knowledge does not always equal behavior. And the views of those important to the drivers may not always influence behaviors in real time.

Now let's return to the opening story, and ask again, what factors contributed to Gillian's fatal accident? There is no implication of texting while driving, so we can rule that out. But unfortunately, it is impossible to say with certainty which factors caused the fatal outcome. It appears that her assumed inexperience, her age, the distracting request for chewing gum (a visual-manual task?), and the presence of four other adolescents combined to contribute to the fatal outcome.

Indeed, Gillian's story is tragic, but you may be wondering how automobile accidents relate to a chapter on risky health behaviors. We already addressed topics such as substance use and risky sexual behaviors in Part I of this chapter. Here in Part II, we begin with automobile accidents to highlight one often overlooked fact: **unintentional injuries**, injuries resulting from accidents or unplanned events, are a leading cause of injury and death among children aged 1 to 14, adolescents aged 15 to 24, and adults aged 25 to 44 (Centers for Disease Control & Prevention, 2016a; see Table 5.II.1).

TABLE 5.II.1 Leading Causes of Death by Age Group in the U.S

Group	Number of Deaths (2020)	Number of Deaths (2014)	Increase/Decrease (2020 – 2014)
Under 1 year			
Birth defects (congenital abnormalities)	4,043	4,746	–703
Disorders related to premature births (short gestation)	3,141	4,173	–759
Complications: maternal pregnancy	–	1,574	–
Sudden infant death syndrome (SIDS)	1,389	–	–
1 to 4 years			
Unintentional injuries	1,153	1,216	–63
Birth defects (congenital abnormalities)	382	399	–17
Homicide	311	364	–53
5 to 9 years			
Unintentional injuries	685	–	–
Cancer (malignant neoplasms)	382	–	–
Congenital abnormalities	171	–	–
10–14 years			
Unintentional injuries	881	–	–
Suicides	581	–	–
Malignant neoplasms	410	–	–

Group	Number of Deaths (2020)	Number of Deaths (2014)	Increase/Decrease (2020 – 2014)
15 to 24 years			
Unintentional injuries	15,117	11,836	+3,281
Homicide	6,466	4,144	+2,322
Suicide	6,062	5,079	+983
25 to 34 years			
Unintentional injuries	31,315	–	–
Homicide	7,125	–	–
Suicide	8,454	–	–
35–44 years			
Unintentional injuries	31,057	–	–
Heart disease	12,177	–	–
Malignant neoplasms	10,730	–	–
45 to 54 years			
Malignant neoplasms	34,587	–	–
Heart disease	34,169	–	–
Unintentional injury	27,819	–	–
55–64 years			
Malignant neoplasms	110,243	–	–
Heart disease	88,551	–	–
COVID-19	42,090	–	–
65 years and older			
Heart disease	556,665	489,722	+66,943
Malignant neoplasms	602,350	413,885	+188,465
Chronic lower respiratory disease	124,693	–	–
COVID-19		350,831	–

Source: Adapted from data from the Centers for Disease Control (2023j). Leading Causes of Death. WISQARS Leading Causes of Death Visualization Tool (cdc.gov).

In Chapter 3, Theories and Models of Health Behavior Change, we stressed that one goal of health psychologists is to encourage individuals to change the behaviors that lead to preventable injury or illness. Therefore, in addition to our discussion of the causes of unintentional injuries, including vehicle, violence, and suicide in Sections I through III, respectively, we will also examine strategies and techniques for changing the behaviors that increase the risk of unintentional injuries.

Afterwards, we turn to an examination of eating disorders, including anorexia, bulimia, obesity, and binge eating in Section IV. We will explore each of these behaviors by examining the behavioral *antecedents*, factors that influence the behaviors, the frequency of the behavior across age groups and cultures, and the long-term health implications of the behaviors. Finally, we will identify and discuss relevant theories developed by psychologists and other health researchers that may explain the antecedents of risky health outcomes.

Before we begin, just a reminder of the three important points we introduced in Chapter 5, Risky Health Behaviors, Part I. First, a number of risky health behaviors that begin during adolescence continue into adulthood. Thus, we begin with adolescents to explore the origins and possible causes for such behaviors. Second, do remember that the presence of a risk factor or risky behavior does not always lead to an adverse health outcome, although it may increase the chances of a poor outcome. Finally, many studies tend to group together individuals who engage in risky behavior once (or episodically) with repeat or frequent risk takers. Clearly, the probability of an adverse event resulting from risky behaviors will be greater among frequent rather than infrequent risk takers. With this point in mind, whenever possible, we will focus on those behaviors that adolescents engage in more than just once and over time.

SECTION I. UNINTENTIONAL INJURY: MOTOR VEHICLE-RELATED INJURIES

One common cause of unintended injuries is automobile accidents. Global statistics show that injuries, including traffic-related accidents are one of the leading causes of deaths among adolescents 15–19 years of age and young adults 20–24 years (World Health Organization, 2022b). Engaging in risky behaviors such as speeding (aggressive driving), drinking while driving (impaired driving), driving without a license, and driving while texting (distracted driving) are also common causes of motor vehicle accidents for both adolescents and adults.

Adolescent Drivers

Let's put the statistics on accident rates by teen drivers in context taking, for example, data from the U.S. Adolescents (15–20 years of age) made up 7.8% of the U.S. population in 2021, and 5.0% of the licensed drivers. Yet they accounted for 12.7% of all automobile crashes that involved damage to property, and another 12.1% that resulted in injury to another person. Fully 8.6% of these accidents resulted in fatalities (NHTSA, 2023). Hence, there are fewer adolescent licensed drivers than all other age groups, yet they are overrepresented in automobile accidents involving property damage and fatal accidents for their percentage of the population.

Research by Rix et al. (2022), provides real-time data on accident rates for adolescents. They collected simultaneous data on adolescent's risky driving behaviors using a smartphone application, eliminating the need to rely on a person's recall. This application, downloaded by 18 adolescent drivers (ages 16–18) in Pennsylvania, collected six weeks of data on a number of risky-driving metrics. The smartphone devices recorded adolescents speeding 41.5% of the time over approximately 1370 trips (aggressive driving), using a handheld cell phone almost a quarter of the time (24.6% of trips; distracted driving), and braking hard in more than 35% of the trips. Nighttime driving was the least frequent behavior, occurring only during 1.6% of trips. Risky driving behaviors, like distracted driving, when combined with an adolescent driver's age and inexperience – as we also saw in the opening story with Gillian – may explain, in part, the higher accident rates among adolescents,

Aggressive, distracting, and impaired driving are clear examples of risky driving behaviors. Other contributing factors to automobile accidents include nighttime driving, failure to use seat belts, type of vehicle driven, and unlicensed drivers (Committee on Injury, Violence, and Poison Prevention and Committee on Adolescence, 2006; Williams, 2003). In the next section, we briefly explore the impact of the first three on unintentional injuries: the effects of nighttime driving, failure to use seat belts, and type of vehicle.

NIGHTTIME DRIVING Even experienced drivers agree that nighttime driving is challenging, in part because driving hazards are poorly illuminated in the dark (see, for example, Ackaah, Apuseyine, & Afukaar, 2020). For adolescents, however, the usual hazards of nighttime driving often are combined with risky behaviors such as speeding, drinking alcohol, or driving with other teenage passengers (vanBeurden, Zask, Brooks, & Dight, 2005; Villavicencio, Svencara, Kelley-Baker, & Tefft, 2022).

The higher rate of nighttime accidents and fatalities among adolescents is one reason for a health policy instituted in a host of countries for teenage drivers. That policy, instituted first by New Zealand in 1987, is a *graduated license law (GDL)* that issues first-time adolescent drivers a *provisional driving license* under a graduated driving law system that limits adolescents to driving only under specific conditions (Williams, 2017; Sibbald, 2007). Canada, Australia, and, to a more limited extent, selected countries in Europe have also adopted GDLs (Boets, Meunier, & Kluppels, 2016; Truelove, Freeman, & Davey, 2019). In addition, all 50 states in the U.S. as well as the District of Columbia have some form of a graduated license. While the restrictions vary by state (in the U.S.) and country, most GDLs in Australia, Canada, New Zealand, and the U.S. require that all applicants for a graduated license be at least 16 years of age, retain their graduated license for at least 12 months, avoid nighttime driving (between 10:00 pm and 5:00 am or longer), and permit only one young passenger, that is someone under 21 years of age, when driving without an accompanying adult. To obtain a full or unrestricted license, would-be drivers must be at least 18 years of age or older (U.S. Department of Transportation, 2015; Williams, 2017).

In effect, the provisional license provides a test period, an opportunity for the new driver to establish an accident- or incident-free driving record. And to date, studies suggest that provisional licenses for adolescents have been effective. Current findings show that the provisional or graduated licenses helped reduce adolescent automobile accidents and other driving-related incidences. For example, data show that after the U.S. implemented GDLs in 1996, fatal crashes by teens ages 16 and 17 decreased by 74% and 71%, respectively, between 1996 and 2015 (Williams, 2017). Similarly, Moore and Morris (2021) suggest that Australia's version of provisional licenses, known as probationary or P1 license, issued to first time drivers in New South Wales resulted in, on average, 41 fewer hospitalizations per 100,000 first-year drivers and 164 fewer accidents involving property damage per 100,000 first-time drivers.

In essence, the GDLs, which include among their restrictions no nighttime driving, are an example of a health policy that applies to a category of people. It aims to improve health outcomes by limiting adolescents' driving during periods when accidents rates are higher.

SEAT BELTS Why do approximately 90.4% of automobile drivers and passengers in the U.S. use seat belts? (National Highway Traffic Safety Administration, 2022b). The AAA's slogan suggests one reason: "Seat belts save lives." This clever and easy-to-remember slogan helps motorists remember the main message: wear your seat belt and protect your life.

VIDEO #24/60

Chapter 5: Risky Health Behaviors, Part II

·   **Seat Belts: 60 Seconds Driver**

·   *Website: https://www.youtube.com/watch?v=1fFbrPkr1cg*

·   *MB Public Insurance is publicly accessible as they provide educational resources to the public for free regarding safety (www.mpi.mb.ca/Pages/Home.aspx)*

If that slogan does not appeal to you, there are plenty of others. Consider these from the South Carolina Driver and Traffic Safety Education Association (SCDTSEA): "No Belt. No brain." Or what about, "You may think seat belts are uncomfortable, but have you ever tried a stretcher?" Finally, consider this: "A friend is like a seat belt, you may not always need them, but they will be there just in case" (SCDTSEA, 2015). Sports fans may particularly enjoy the clever message shown in Figure 5.II.3. These messages all

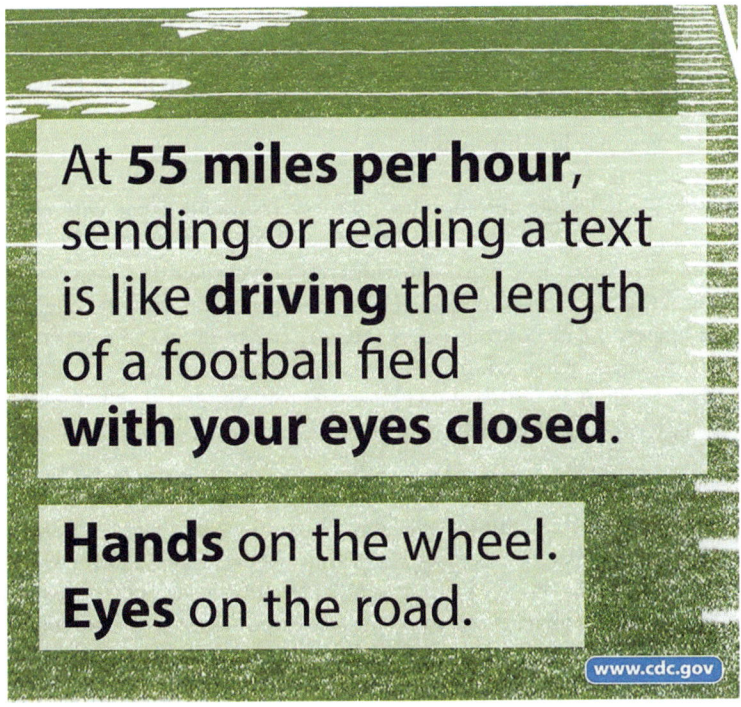

FIGURE 5.II.3 The poster shows an anti-texting-while-driving message superimposed on a gridded football field. It reads: "At 55 miles per hour, sending or reading a text is like driving the length of a football field with your eyes closed. Hands on the wheel. Eyes on the road."

Source: CDC (2022j). Transportation Safety: Distracted Driving. Distracted Driving | Transportation Safety | Injury Center | CDC

have the same intent. Yet, because some are funny, they may be remembered more readily. Using humor to convey a message may help the intended audience not only remember the message, but it may also improve the likelihood of people complying with the message. Health psychologists, take note!

Researchers have shown conclusively that seat belt use reduces the number of fatal injuries due to automobile accidents. Not surprisingly, these findings are universal. Høye (2016) examined the effects of seat belt use in Norway through a meta-analysis of 24 studies beginning in 2000. She found a 66% reduction of both fatal and non-fatal injuries for persons seated in the front seat of a motor vehicle when wearing seat belts. Similarly, passengers in the rear were 44% less likely to suffer fatal or non-fatal injury when wearing a seat belt. Finally, a study conducted in 185 countries, examining four road safety risk factors – speeding, drunk driving, seat belt use, and helmet use – underscores this point. In this study, Vecino-Ortiz and colleagues (2022) concluded that approximately 121,000 lives could be saved per year, worldwide, if seat belts were in use.

Finally, an earlier, classic study by El-Sadig and colleagues (2004) provides unambiguous evidence for the health-enhancing effects of automobile seat belts in the United Arab Emirates (UAE). El-Sadig and colleagues (2004) examined the severity of injuries sustained by adults in automobile accidents before and after seat belt legislation was passed in the UAE in 1999. Before the seat belt legislation, 54% of adults in automobile accidents died after reaching the hospital. El-Sadig and colleagues found that, after the new legislation, the fatality rate associated with automobile accidents dropped to 17% after hospitalization. At the same time, the percentage of minor injuries pre- versus post-legislation increased from 42% to 77% (El-Sadig et al., 2004). Thus, the study showed that seat belt use, a health policy regulation, decreased mortality rates in automobile accidents in the UAE, and improved health outcomes for those with minor injuries since the injuries were not life-threatening.

TYPE OF MOTOR VEHICLE Unlike automobiles, motorcycles do not come with seat belts. In fact, they come with little more than the seat, the motor, the wheels, and a steering device. The structure of a motorcycle – no doors, cushions, or airbags – provides motorcyclists little protection from the impact of other motor vehicles in the event of a collision. The lack of protection may be one reason fatal motor vehicle injury rates are highest for motorcycle riders (NCSA, 2023). In fact, the National Center for Statistics and Analysis notes that, when taking distance traveled into account, motorcycle drivers are more than 24 times more likely to die than automobile passengers (NCSA, 2023). The high fatality rates among motorcycle riders also may explain why emergency department physicians sometimes call motorcycle riders "organ donors."

We stated that motorcycle riding is risky; one behavior that increases the probability of unintentional injuries for motorcycle riders is riding without a helmet. How do we know that? Consider this classic study in the U.S.: In 1997, Arkansas legislators repealed, or withdrew, the state's adult helmet law that required all adult motorcyclists to wear helmets when riding. Coincidentally, as in the UAE example, a group of researchers designed a study to compare motorcycle fatality rates before and after the change in the law. Remember, however, that in this case the law changed from requiring helmets, a health-enhancing behavior, to allowing cyclists to ride helmet-free, a risky or compromising behavior. The result? Researchers found a significant increase in the number of motorcycle fatalities after Arkansas legislators repealed the law. Before the repeal, 39.6% of motorcyclists died as a result of motor vehicle accidents compared with 75.5% after the repeal (Bledsoe et al., 2002). Not surprisingly, the number of severe but not fatal head injuries also increased after the change in the law (Bledsoe et al., 2002). In this example, the repeal of a health policy resulted in poorer health outcomes and underscored the health-enhancing role of wearing helmets when riding motorcycles.

When viewed more broadly, we see that universal helmet laws, that is laws that require all persons to wear a helmet regardless of age, resulted in 36%–45% fewer motorcycle fatalities between 1999 and 2015 in all 50 U.S. states (Notrica et al., 2020). States that passed partial helmet laws, here meaning laws like the one passed in Arkansas that exempts adults from the helmet requirement, reported a 22%–45% increase in fatal motorcycle crashes when compared with states with universal helmet laws.

What is the point of the statistics on unintentional injuries due to automobile and motorcycle accidents? Simply this: Risky behaviors such as driving while drunk, fooling around in cars, texting or e-mailing while driving, failing to use seat belts, and riding motorcycles without a helmet can increase the chance of motor vehicle injuries or death (see Table 5.II.1). These risky behaviors can lead to adverse consequences that are almost entirely preventable.

This information on motor vehicle–related injuries is certainly interesting and highlights the health risks to all drivers, especially teenage drivers, when engaging in risky driving behaviors. But you might be asking, what specifically can health psychologists do to address these issues? The U.S. NHTSA offers a succinct explanation (NHTSA, n.d.). Briefly, the NHTSA notes that because most highway programs aim to change the driving behaviors of motorists, they must try first to understand human behavior, including the inconsistent and at times unpredictable behaviors of drivers (NHTSA, n.d.). They stress that the most effective way to reduce risky driving behaviors is to change the physical and/or social environment, a change that impacts an entire population, not just an individual. By now, you might be thinking that this may be a job for health psychologists. You are right! Additionally, the NHTSA approach might fit well within the social ecological model. Right again.

Universal motorcycle helmet laws and graduated (or probational) drivers licenses are examples of social environmental policies designed to effect change for a population, and by extension, for individuals. For health psychologists, therefore, working with the NHTSA and local communities to encourage adherence to driving policies that foster safer driving will help individuals make and sustain these changes to their driving habits – changes that will result in fewer unintentional motor vehicle accidents, injuries, or deaths.

SECTION II. VIOLENCE

The term violence is a broad concept that includes many different behaviors. For example, most would agree that *homicide*, or the killing of another person, is a violent act. So, too, is a *physical assault*, or a physical confrontation with another person that could include hitting, shoving, kicking, or other physically aggressive behaviors. Violence can also be defined more broadly as the intentional use of force against another person, a community, or even against oneself. According to this definition, suicide is also an act of violence (Corso, Mercy, Simon, Finkelstein, & Miller, 2007).

Homicides

Globally, in 2016, 385,000 people lost their lives due to intentional homicides, with another 85,000 dying as a result of unintentional or accidental homicides (Mc Evoy & Hideg, 2017). This translates to a global homicide rate of 5.15 per 100,000 people. Examples of unintentional injuries resulting from violence are, unfortunately, easy to find. Disputes, angry exchanges, or acts of theft may lead to violence and unintentional acts that injure or kill. And, as the numerous school and community shootings in the U.S. remind us, violent acts often appear suddenly and with little or no warning.

When comparing homicide rates across regions of the world, the Americas, here meaning North, Central, and South America, led with world with 15 deaths per 100,000 in 2021. This translates to 154,000 deaths due to homicides in this region alone (UN News, 2023).

Now, up to this point we endeavored to present statistics, studies, and examples of health behaviors and outcomes drawn from many countries and regions of the world. However, when examining homicides, and specifically those caused by gun violence, we must give special attention to the U.S. Looking only at the U.S., we find that in just one year, from 2019 to 2020, more than 138,600 people died by violence there, and 31.5% were due to homicide (CDC, 2023f). By comparison, in the same year, the death rates due to homicides in Asia, Europe, and Oceania combined reached only 5.8 per 100,000 (UN News, 2023). This compares to the U.S. rate of 7.8 deaths per 100,000 due to homicides (National Center For Heath Statistics, 2021).

To be clear, violence of all types occurs worldwide. But mass shootings of the type that kill more than four persons in a single event (unrelated to armed conflicts), well, that is a phenomenon that occurs disproportionately often in the U.S. and more so than in any other country. Does this seem incredible? Then consider this: Gun violence is so prevalent in the U.S. that the Institute for Health Metrics and Evaluation (IHME), an independent global health research center based at the University of Washington, notes that the U.S. is an outlier when compared with other comparable high-income countries on a measure of gun deaths. Specifically, when comparing all high-income countries with populations in excess of 10 million, the U.S. ranks highest in the rate of gun deaths per 100,000 of population (see Table 5.II.2). The rate of firearm

TABLE 5.II.2 Homicide Rates by Firearms in High-Income Countries: Top 10 Countries

COUNTRY	Rate (per 100,000 population)
U.S.	4.12
Chile	1.82
Canada	0.50
Portugal	0.40
Italy	0.35
Greece	0.35
Belgium	0.34
France	0.32
Sweden	0.25
Netherlands	0.23

Note: Homicide rates in the U.S. are 2.2 times higher than in Chile and 8 times higher than Canada.

Source: Adapted from IHME (2022). On gun violence, the U.S. is an outlier. Accessed online at: On gun violence, the U.S. is an outlier | Institute for Health Metrics and Evaluation (healthdata.org).

deaths in the U.S. (4.12 per 100,000 persons) is more than two times higher than Chile, which ranks second. And the rates for both the U.S. and Chile far exceed those of the eight other high-income countries that round out the top 10 countries on this list.

Again, it is important to stress that deaths due to mass shootings do happen in other countries. Recall that in October 2022, 37 people – 24 children and 13 adults – were killed in a mass shooting at a day care center in Thailand (Satienlerk & Perawongmetha, 2022). And in another part of the world, in July 2011 a gunman killed 69 adolescents taking part in a youth camp on the Norwegian island of Utøya. But these incidents pale in comparison to the multiple mass killings that happen each year in the U.S.

To be specific, in 2022, 42 mass killing incidences in the U.S. claimed the lives of 202 people. One of the most memorable and tragic events that year was the killing of 19 elementary school students and two teachers at an elementary school in Uvalde, Texas. The mass shootings continued the next year. Between January 1 and April 1, 2023 – just three months – 88 persons died in 17 mass killings in the U.S., including four children and two adults at a school in Nashville, Tennessee; nine people at a shopping mall near Dallas, Texas; seven farmworkers in Half Moon Bay, California; and 11 people at a dance hall celebrating the Lunar New Year in California (PBS, 2023).

High school and college administrators in the U.S. also struggle to explain the frequent and apparently random incidences of shootings on school grounds across the nation. These include shootings in high schools in Columbine, Colorado (1999), Jonesboro, Arkansas (1998), and San Diego, California (2001); college campuses in Blacksburg, Virginia (2007) and DeKalb, Illinois (2008); a shooting at an elementary school – Sandy Hook Elementary School – in Newtown, Connecticut (2012); and more recently, at Marjory Stoneman Douglas High School in Parkland, Florida (2018). And they continue. As of June 2023, the U.S. reported 23 school shootings on school grounds while school was in session (Education Week, 2023). Elected public officials seem flummoxed by the multiple shootings in their towns or cities. Clearly, however, these incidences of violence are an indication of a national violence problem in the U.S., one that impacts the nations' emotional, psychological, and physical well-being. We will discuss emotional health more fully in Chapter 6, Emotional Health and Well-Being, but we will also address it briefly here.

PSYCHOLOGICAL EFFECTS OF HOMICIDES

Counting the number of individuals injured or killed is one way to measure the cost of violence. Yet we can also assess the effects of violence by examining the psychological impact on its victims as well as on the observers. Consider this: In a CDC Youth Risk Behavior Surveillance System (YRBSS) Survey, adolescents were asked how often they carry weapons to school. The survey revealed that more than 12,700 high school students reported carrying a weapon to school, and more than 13,000 reported carrying a gun on school property (see Table 5.II.3).

Clearly, a weapon is not an essential school supply. Yet, some students believe that weapons are needed to protect them from unwanted confrontations en route to or from school or even while at school. The YRBSS also revealed a sex difference in the likelihood of carrying weapons to school. They report that males are more likely than females to carry weapons (3.9% vs. 2.1%, respectively), and more likely to carry guns, (5.0% vs. 1.8%; see again Table 5.II.3). It may be no coincidence, given these numbers, that, to date, all initiators of elementary, high school, or college mass shootings have been males.

In the aftermath of so many shootings on school campuses, a number of teachers in the U.S. have expressed a need to protect themselves while at school. For example, in two states, Ohio and Indiana, school boards have enabled teachers, minimally trained in the use of guns, to carry weapons on school grounds. As of 2022, more than 29 U.S. states also permitted non-security personnel to carry guns on school grounds (Mervosh, 2022). At this point, it is reasonable to ask how comfortable and safe students feel when some of their teachers or administrators carry firearms on school grounds. Does this help to foster an emotionally and psychologically safe learning environment, or does it reinforce for students that the school environment is potentially dangerous?

Clearly, carrying a weapon will not necessarily decrease incidences of violence. Nor will it increase a person's perception of a safe environment at school. Although some students carry a weapon to counter unwanted confrontations, others, approximately 10.5% of females, and 6.6% male students in the survey

TABLE 5.II.3 Youth Risk Behavior Survey High School Students and Weapons at School

CATEGORY	Carry Weapons	Carry Gun
SEX	Number (%)	Number (%)
Female	6,113 (2.1%)	6,238 (1.8)
Male	6,505 (3.9%)	6,665 (5.0)
RACE/ETHNICITY		
American Indian/Alaskan Native	107 (3.3)	110 (5.3)
Asian	604 (1.9)	631 (1.0)
Black	2,065 (4.6)	2,214 (5.1)
Hispanic	2,708 (3.3)	2,892 (3.9)
White	6,188 (2.4)	6,072 (3.0)
GRADE		
9th	3,667 (1.9)	3,490 (3.2)
10th	3,245 (2.3)	3,407 (2.8)
11th	3,070 (3.6)	3,054 (4.1)
12th	2,989 (4.1)	3,005 (3.5)

Source: CDC (2023) High School Youth Risk Behavior Survey. Youth Online: High School YRBS – 2021 Results | DASH | CDC

stated that they were concerned about their safety when at school. (CDC, 2023f). What is more, past studies have indicated that when concerned about their safety at school, some students chose to be absent (Kann et al., 2016). Staying home from school will not increase a person's perception of a safe school environment, although it will increase the risk of poor academic performance.

Carrying a weapon and absenting oneself from school are two reactions to violence in the community, here defined as the school community. Both demonstrate fear or apprehension of violent encounters regardless of whether a person has firsthand exposure to violence. And both can undermine a person's emotional or psychological health as a result of exposure to or fear of injury or death due to violence.

We conclude this section by looking again at global statistics to understand the magnitude of the problem in the U.S. A review of the number of school shootings by country from January 2009 thru May 2018 (the last date for which full statistics are available) shows that, unsurprisingly, the U.S. far outranks all other countries, and not in a good way. During this period, the U.S. was in first place with a record 288 distinct school shootings (see Table 5.II.4). Mexico, a distant second, recorded the next highest number of school shootings at eight, followed by South Africa in third place with a total of six distinct school shootings, and a tie for fourth place between Nigeria and Pakistan, who each recorded four distinct school shootings (World Population Review, 2023a). In sum, school shootings are a global problem, but it is an epidemic in the U.S.

Domestic Violence
Generally, the term domestic violence describes actions by one person in a relationship intended to control or dominate another. The actions can be physical, sexual, or emotional, and may include acts of intimidation or threats.

TABLE 5.II.4 Global Data on Mass Shootings 2009–2018

COUNTRY	Number of School Mass Shootings
U.S.	288
Mexico	8
South Africa	6
Nigeria	4
Pakistan	4
Afghanistan	3
Brazil	2
Canada	2
France	2
Azerbaijan	1
China	1
Estonia	1
Germany	1
Greece	1
Hungary	1
Kenya	1
Russia	1
Türkiye	1

Note: U.S. school shootings are 36 times higher than its closest competitor, Mexico.

Source: World Population Review (2023a).

Early research on domestic violence focused primarily on a physically abusive relationship between two persons: for example, spouses or intimate partners (Daughtery & Houry, 2008; Duterte et al., 2008; Marcus, 2008). Today the term is used more broadly to describe abusive relationships between family members or others sharing a living space. It includes elder abuse, here meaning the physical or emotional maltreatment of older persons; child abuse, usually the physical mistreatment of a child by an adult; emotional abuse, including repeated criticism or undermining a person's self-esteem; psychological abuse, including intimidation, threats of harm to oneself or other family members, isolating a person from family and friends, and trauma; and technological abuse, including using technology to threaten, control, harass, or extort another person (U.S. Department of Justice, Office on Violence Against Women, 2023).

VIDEO #25/60

Chapter 5: Risky Health Behaviors, Part II
- *Elder Abuse: Research in 60 Seconds: caregivers and elder abuse*
- *Website: https://www.youtube.com/watch?v=WekgprAsxl0*
- **The Keck School of Medicine of USC website is publicly accessible.** *Keck School of Medicine Home – Keck School of Medicine of USC*

VIDEO #26/60

Chapter 5: Risky Health Behaviors, Part II
- *Child Abuse: Protecting Children from Child Abuse*
- *Website: https://www.youtube.com/watch?v=q8Xg3AlBHZc*
- *The Pan American Health Organization is publicly accessible since the World Health Organization provides it to the public (www.paho.org/en)*

VIDEO #27/60

Chapter 5: Risky Health Behaviors, Part II
- *Domestic Violence: Love Isn't Supposed to Hurt*
- *Website: https://www.youtube.com/watch?v=cmSn3kZDWUo*
- **Florida Coalition Against Domestic Violence is a publicly accessible website with various resources regarding domestic violence and is provided by the state government of Florida (www.fpedv.org/about-us/)**

VIDEO #28/60

Chapter 5: Risky Health Behaviors, Part II
- **Dating Violence: Dating Matters**
- *Website: https://youtu.be/_i8CE029Hh8*
- *The U.S. Centers for Disease Control and Prevention provides information, statistics, and training materials on a range of health issues that are publicly available (cdc.gov).*

Studies examining the psychological impact of domestic violence also examine its effects on others in the home (Lee, Pomeroy, & Bohman, 2007; Ragin et al., 2002; Ward, Martin, & Distiller, 2007). For example, several studies show that infants, children, and adolescents exposed to (although not the target of) domestic violence in the home experience emotional abuse and trauma due to witnessing the violence (Haj-Yahia, Sokar, Hassan-Abbas, & Malka, 2019; Mueller & Tronick, 2019). They may also be at greater risk for physical violence later in life at the hands of an abusive partner (Shields, Tonmyr, Hovdestad, Gonzalez, & MacMillan, 2020; Whitfield, 2003; Whitfield, Anda, Dube, & Felitti, 2003). Another group of studies points to the likelihood of children who, when abused by their parents, become abusive as adults (Greene, Haisley, Wallace, & Ford, 2020; Savage, Tarabulsy, Pearson, Collin-Vézina, & Gagné, 2019; Worley, Walsh, & Lewis, 2004). Even when a child is not raised in an abusive environment, researchers suggest that a pattern of aggressive behavior in childhood is predictive of aggressive behavior in adulthood. A study by Temcheff and colleagues (2008) found that, for males, childhood aggression represented a stable behavioral style that links male peer aggressive behavior to violence toward their spouse and children.

Are there other environmental factors that may predispose someone to abusive behaviors? Perhaps. Some researchers suggest that a higher prevalence of intimate partner violence is found in low- and middle-income countries (Coll, Ewerling, Garcia-Moreno, Hellwig, & Barros, 2020). Indeed, global prevalence data on intimate partner violence by region, for women ages 15–49 who have ever been married or lived with a partner, suggest that this is true (UN Women, 2021). Table 5.II.5 shows that countries in the Oceania region, including Melanesia, Micronesia, and Polynesia, as well as in sub-Saharan and Northern and Southern Africa,

TABLE 5.II.5 Estimates of Regional, 12-Month, and Intimate Partner Violence

Global Region	Violence in Last 12 Months	Lifetime Violence
Melanesia	30	51
Micronesia	22	41
Sub-Saharan Africa	20	33
Polynesia	19	39
Southern Africa	19	35
Northern Africa	15	30
Western Asia	13	29
Southeastern Asia	9	21
Central Asia	9	18
Latin America and Caribbean	8	25
Eastern Europe	7	20
Eastern Asia	7	20
Northern America	6	25
Northern Europe	5	23
Western Europe	5	21
Southern Europe	4	16
Australia and New Zealand	3	23
GLOBAL AVERAGE	13	27
AVERAGE Least-Developed Countries	22	37

Note: Low- and lower-middle income countries report highest rates of interpersonal violence.

Source: UN Women (2021).

have the highest prevalence rates for domestic violence worldwide (UN Women, 2021). But this is not to say that intimate partner violence in high-income countries is not an issue. The CDC reports that in the U.S., clearly a high-income country, approximately 46% of women and 26% of men report sexual or physical violence and/or stalking by an intimate partner each year (CDC, 2022d). Therefore, taken together, globally almost one-third of women, 15 years of age or older, report physical or sexual intimate partner violence in their lifetimes (Coll et al., 2020).

Although health professionals are increasingly attentive to issues of domestic violence, it is unlikely that we will know the true prevalence rates of interpersonal and domestic violence. For many, domestic abuse in any context is an embarrassing experience (Christaki et al., 2023). The victim's shame often prevents him or her from disclosing the experience. Still others fear the threat of retaliation by their abusers in the event that they reveal the truth.

In the U.S., increased media attention to domestic violence through television, radio, and print ads provides information and tangible assistance to people exposed to domestic abuse. Confidential hotlines, counseling services, and domestic violence shelters offer a range of services to help an individual with his or her emotional, psychological, physical, or material needs. In addition, medical staff in many hospital emergency departments screen patients who seek medical care from hospital emergency departments if presenting with questionable injuries. They now routinely ask women whether their injuries were obtained as a result of domestic violence. If women indicate that their injuries are the result of domestic violence, medical staff, working together with social services and domestic violence shelters, can offer domestic violence victims immediate protection, usually by placement in a domestic violence shelter. Such shelters offer the victims a temporary and safe haven from further abuse. Unfortunately, such services are not universally available. Domestic violence shelters in the U.S. are often fully occupied and have long waiting lists.

Other high-income countries also sponsor domestic violence shelters for women. For example, England, Germany, Italy, Spain, and Sweden, each report more than 100 shelters for women in need (McEvoy, 2023). In developing countries, however, shelters may be either fewer in number or considered an unlikely option for women who depend economically on their spouses or family members for survival (Belknap & Cruz, 2007; Khan & Hussain, 2008; Morgaine, 2007).

Dating Violence

New research on the aggressive and abusive behavior between individuals who are not in committed relationships, known as dating violence, has prompted researchers to look more broadly at interpersonal violence. Consider this: The YRBSS high school study revealed that 11.7% of females and 7.4% of males reported being physically hurt by their dating partner (Kann, 2016). What is more, 15.6% of adolescent females and 5.4% of adolescent males reported experiencing sexual dating violence (Kann, 2016). These statistics suggest that interpersonal abuse may go undetected in the early stages of a relationship, a much earlier starting point for violence than previously suspected.

Teens who experience dating violence have reported symptoms of depression or anxiety, may abuse substances like alcohol or drugs, and may even contemplate suicide (CDC, 2023g). Thus, one obvious concern for people, especially adolescents, exposed to dating violence is that such experiences can predispose them to engage in risky health behaviors or become involved in other abusive relationships, both of which may portend poor health outcomes.

Needless to say, this is one area in which health psychologists can play a constructive role. Programs developed to teach teens how to identify and develop healthy relationships at an early age, such as the one developed by the CDC titled "Dating Matters" (CDC, 2023h), aim to prevent adolescents from engaging in or becoming entrapped in negative relationships. These ready-made programs, or others developed by health psychologists, can help individuals, relationship partners, and communities foster and nurture healthy interpersonal relationships.

Self-Inflicted Injuries

SUICIDE Another form of violence that affects the whole community is *self-inflicted injuries*. The most widely recognized forms of self-injury are *suicide* and attempted suicide. Globally, suicides were the 17th leading cause of death, with approximately 750,000 suicides in 2019, or a rate of 9.0 per 100,000 persons (Ilic & Ilic, 2022; see Table 5.II.6).

As in the earlier sections on violence here, too, we see a gender difference. The suicide rate for males (12.6) was more than two times the rate for females (5.4; Ilic & Ilic, 2022). There also appears to be a regional difference in the gender disparity for suicide between males and females. In Europe, males are four times as likely to commit suicide than females. However, a closer look at Table 5.II.6 reveals that the overall suicide rates for males is greatest in Africa followed closely by Europe (18 per 100,000 vs. 17 per 100,000, respectively). For females, however, the highest suicide rates are reported in Southeast Asia (8.1 per 100,000) followed by Africa, a distant second (5.3 per 100,000).

When compared with data from the U.S. we see a similar pattern. In the U.S., suicide is the 11th leading cause of death. Overall, suicide rates in the U.S. increased 30% between 2000 and 2020. Here, too, males are 3.5 times more likely to commit suicide than females (Centers for Disease Control, 2012b; Dattani, Rodés-Guirao, Ritchie, Roser, & Ortiz-Ospina, 2023). In fact, among adults, the highest suicide rates are recorded for men 75 years of age or older. In 2020, this cohort in the U.S. commit suicide at a rate of 40.5 per 100,000 people. In comparison, the highest suicide rate for women was 7.9 per 100,000 and occurred among the 45- to 64-year-old age group (Centers for Disease Control, 2012b; Garnett et al., 2022).

VIDEO #29/60

Chapter 5: Risky Health Behaviors, Part II

*   *Youth Mental Health and Wellbeing: "You Are Not Alone" 60 Seconds*
*   *Website: https://www.youtube.com/watch?v=7vdZx7IBZTg*
*   *The Department of Children and Families of New Jersey is publicly accessible as they are a state agency providing services and resources to the public (www.nj.gov/dcf/)*

TABLE 5.II.6 Global Suicide Rates by Gender and World Regions: Age-Standardized Suicide Rates per 100,000 People

Global Region	Males	Females
Africa	18.0	5.3
Americas	14.2	4.1
Eastern Mediterranean	9.2	3.5
Europe	17.1	4.3
Southeast Asia	12.3	8.1
Western Pacific	9.7	4.8
WORLD	12.6	5.4

Note: Worldwide, males are more than two times as likely to commit suicide than females.

Source: Adapted from Dattani, Rodés-Guirao, Ritchie, Roser, and Ortiz-Ospina (2023).

When we examine the prevalence of suicide by a country's income status, as described in Chapter 2, Research Methods) we find an interesting change from previously reported outcomes. In this comparison, as shown in Table 5.II.7, high-income countries report the highest suicide rates for males (16.5 per 100,000) whereas low-middle income countries report the highest rates for females (7.1 per 100,000). More striking is the fact that the suicide prevalence rates for high-income and low-income females, also shown in Table 5.II.7, are similar (5.4 per 100,000 versus 5.3 per 100,000, respectively). In earlier editions of this text, we included data from the World Health Organization (2016d) that cited higher suicide prevalence rates in developed (high- and upper-middle income countries) than in developing (lower-middle or low-income) countries. Thus, contrary to what we indicated earlier, a country's economic status is not necessarily a factor in suicide rates.

One finding that has not changed over the years, however, is the disparity in suicide rates by age. Suicide rates for older adults remain considerably higher than for young adults. Figure 5.II.3 compares the disparities in suicide rates (adjusted for age) for a sample of six countries: Ghana, India, Japan, Portugal, South Korea, and the U.S. While the age disparities in suicide rates in the U.S. and Japan are small and somewhat irregular, in other countries, such as India and South Korea, there are sizable differences in the rates of suicides between adolescents aged 15–24 and older adults, aged 85 or more (see again Figure 5. II.3). Overall, these global data are largely similar to U.S.-specific data, where individuals 75 years of age or older commit one suicide for every four attempts, a ratio of 1:4. Young adults, however, commit one suicide for every 100 to 200 attempts, a ratio of 1:100 to 1:200 (Centers for Disease Control, 2012b; Goldsmith, Pellmar, Kleinman, & Bunney, 2002; National Indian Council on Aging, 2023).

SUICIDE AND ETHNICITY We conclude this section with one last comparison: suicide rates among ethnic groups in the U.S. Statistics show that the prevalence rate for suicide among Native American and Alaskan Natives is almost twice as high as for other ethnicities. Suicide is the eighth leading cause of death among Native Americans and Alaskan natives of all ages, but it is the second leading cause of death for children and young adults ages 10–34 for these two groups (National Indian Council on Aging, 2023). Clearly, these data represent a departure from the overall suicide statistics for the U.S., which reports higher rates among adults.

The high suicide rates in the U.S. for older males, Native Americans, and Alaskan Natives should prompt us to ask why the rates are much higher for these three demographic groups. Researchers can only speculate based, in part, on information obtained from attempted suicides among individuals from the same group. Such studies find that physical and mental health problems, economic problems, or family and individual crises all contribute to high male suicide rates both in the U.S. and globally (World Health Organization, 2010b).

TABLE 5.II.7 Suicide Rates by Gender and Country Income Status

Country Income Status	Males	Females
High	16.5	5.4
Upper-Middle	10.7	4.0
Lower-Middle	13.7	7.1
Low	15.2	5.3
WORLD	12.6	5.4

Note: High- and low-income countries have comparable suicide rates for both males and females.

Source: Adapted from Dattani, Rodés-Guirao, Ritchie, Roser, and Ortiz-Ospina (2023).

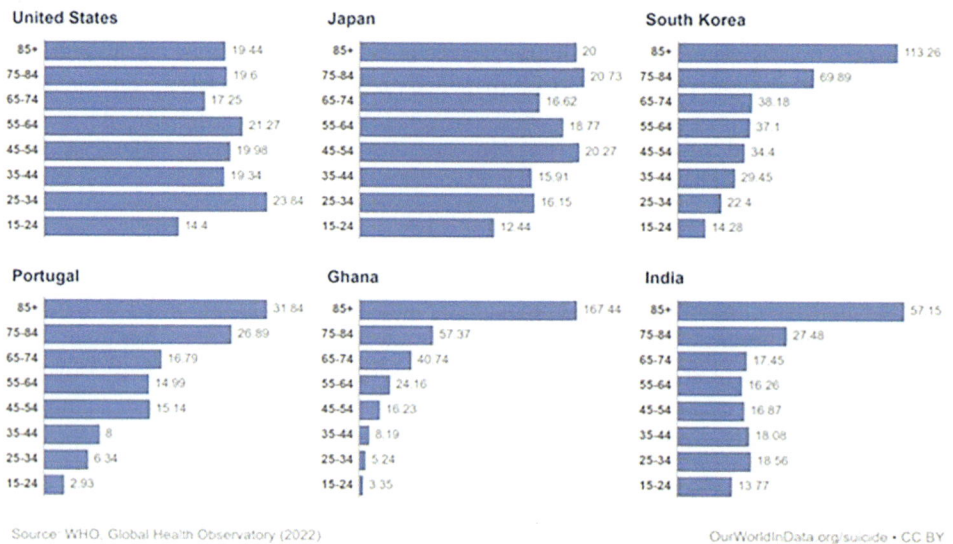

Suicide rate, by age, 2019

Annual number of suicides per 100,000 individuals in each age group. Suicide deaths are underreported in many countries due to social stigma and cultural or legal concerns. This data is adjusted for this underreporting to estimate the actual rate of suicides.

FIGURE 5.II.4 Bar chart comparing the suicide rates by age in six countries: U.S, Japan, South Korea, Portugal, Ghana, and India. Suicide rates are lowest for 15–24 year olds in all six countries, and overall suicide rates increase for each age group (25–34, 45–54, 55–64, 65–74, 75–84 and 85+) in all countries except the U.S. In the U.S. 25–34 year olds have higher suicide rates than all age groups. The U.S. and Japan deviate from a pattern of a graduated increase in suicide prevalence rate by age.

Source: Dattani, Rodés-Guirao, Ritchie, Roser, and Ortiz-Ospina (2023).

For Native Americans and Alaskan Natives, however, current research points to a host of societal problems routed in the colonization and forced removal of Native Americans from their homes. This repeated displacement contributed to extreme poverty, poor education, and a lack of employment options, in addition to social isolation and years of cultural marginalization and historical disenfranchisement (Angelino, Evans, Moore, & Bell, 2023; James et al., 2018; Olson & Wahab, 2006; National Indian Council on Aging, 2023; Yellow Horse Brave Heart, 2003). We must note, however, promising information from the Urban Indian Health Institute suggests that currently, American Indian/Alaskan Native communities are showing a decrease in the rates of suicide and alcoholism – lower, in fact, than some non-Hispanic white communities (Dominguez, EchoHawk, & Liu, 2019). If these findings sustain, it would be a significant and positive change in health trajectories for American Indian/Alaskan Native communities.

As we noted when discussing the impact of gun violence, suicide or self-injury affects more than just the individual. It affects families and entire communities as well. Suicidal acts can cause psychological or emotional health problems for the victim's social network, resulting in emotional and psychological challenges for the family and close friends. As such, although the primary person committing suicide is the recipient of the injury, the act has a residual effect on others. Health psychologists may be helpful in working with communities where the prevalence of suicides is high to develop environmental support systems for the community as well as for the families.

In sum, the statistics on all forms of unintentional injuries, including motor vehicle accidents, violent behaviors, and self-injury, demonstrate that for individuals between the ages of 1 and 44, unintentional injuries pose the greatest health risks. Intervention programs and health policies designed to reduce the adverse consequences of unintentional injuries are growing in number. But as the recent incidences of school shootings in the U.S. show, this is a continuing problem.

SECTION III. EATING DISORDERS

Smoking, alcohol and drug use, and risky sexual behaviors share a common goal for many adolescents: a desire to conform to the perceived social norms of their peer groups. But for many adolescents, the pressure to conform to an idealized thin body image or to emulate popular fashion trends and model-like looks leads to another adverse outcome: eating disorders.

Much of the early research on eating disorders described the problem as a "culture-bound syndrome" rooted in the cultural values and conflicts in Western societies (Prince, 1983). Indeed, many early studies cite examples of high rates of eating disorders occurring most often in the U.S. and other Western countries, including England, Italy, the Netherlands, Sweden, and Switzerland (Hoek, 1991; Lacey & Dolan, 1988; Norring & Sohlberg, 1988; Rathner & Messner, 1993). More specifically, researchers have linked Western culture's idealized thin body type to anorexia nervosa, one of the more prevalent eating disorders in Western societies.

A closer look at the statistics on global rates of eating disorders, focusing for the moment on anorexia and bulimia, offers a more nuanced view of the problem. Table 5.II.8a-c shows rates of anorexia and bulimia as a function of WHO regions of the world, country income status (high, middle, or low), and the

TABLE 5.II.8A Global Estimates of Prevalence of Anorexia and Bulimia (1990–2019) by World Health Organization Region

WHO Region	Anorexia	Bulimia
Americas	813,622	2,208,817
Southeast Asian	806,452	1,948,738
Western Pacific	819,270	1,836,399
European	699,981	1,819,047
Eastern Mediterranean	315,276	1,055,972
Africa	400,093	892,663

Source: Our World in Data. Anorexia or bulimia nervosa estimated cases, 2019 (ourworldindata.org)

TABLE 5.II.8B Global Estimates of Prevalence of Anorexia and Bulimia (1990–2019) by Country Income Status

Income Status	Anorexia	Bulimia
G20 countries[a]	2,703,416	6,719,244
OECD countries	1,295,352	3,308,041
Low income	216,236	451,689
Lower-middle income	1,281,611	3,129,414
Upper-middle income	1,152,800	3,104,653
High income	1,248,866	3,099,357

[a] G20 countries include Argentina, Australia, Brazil, Canada, China, France, Germany, India, Indonesia, Italy, Japan, Mexico, Russia, Saudi Arabia, South Africa, South Korea, Türkiye, U.S., U.K., European Union.

Source: Our World in Data. Anorexia or bulimia nervosa estimated cases, 2019 (ourworldindata.org)

TABLE 5.II.8C Global Estimates of Prevalence of Anorexia and Bulimia (1990–2019): Top 20 Countries

Country	Anorexia	Rank	Bulimia	Rank
India	570,572	1	1,411,201	1
China	467,965	2	1,032,924	2
U.S.	370,503	3	874,568	3
Brazil	153,132	4	375,589	4
Mexico	72,420	12	249,036	5
Japan	126,346	5	235,079	6
Türkiye	45,466	20	214,919	7
Indonesia	101,831	7	211,668	8
Pakistan	88,701	9	201,520	9
Nigeria	90,027	8	194,564	10
Italy	57,131	17	194,518	11
Germany	102,870	6	187,170	12
Australia	51,048	18	180,783	13
Iran	58,350	16	178,660	14
France	74,748	10	178,593	15
U.K.	72,876	11	177,191	16
Egypt	50,811	19	162,627	17
Spain	61,622	13	155,135	18
Russia	58,390	15	151,973	19
Bangladesh	60,947	14	143,679	20
WORLD TOTAL	3,901,694		9,791,067	

Source: Our World in Data. Anorexia or bulimia nervosa estimated cases, 2019 (ourworldindata.org)

top ten countries reporting the highest rates of anorexia and/or bulimia. According to these data, between 1990 and 2019, the Western Pacific region of the world reported the highest prevalence of anorexia, followed closely by the Americas (see again Table 5.II.8a). However, the outcome for the Western Pacific region, which includes 37 countries, is skewed by the rates of anorexia in India, which is ranked first among 20 countries for prevalence of anorexia. Thus, these data would appear to challenge the view that Western countries' values of thinness leads to a higher rate of eating disorders, specifically anorexia, among their population. In fact, looking again at the 20 countries with the highest rates of anorexia or bulimia, India ranks first for both, followed by China. The U.S. and Brazil rank third and fourth, respectively. How would you explain these outcomes?

While current fashion trends and cultural norms are two plausible explanations for eating disorder, we now know that psychological disorders, socioeconomic class, pressures to succeed and to acculturate to the dominant society, and, for some, family dysfunction, may also be factors. Whatever the cause, it has become increasingly clear that people suffering from eating disorders also experience limitations and impairments in their physical, social, and work environments that significantly impact their quality of life (Solmi et al., 2024). As a result, many health professionals now classify these illnesses as severe psychiatric conditions. In this section, we examine four types of eating disorders linked to weight: anorexia nervosa, bulimia, obesity, and binge eating.

Anorexia Nervosa

How much effect does an intense focus on weight have on the physical and psychological health of the individual? In one word, lots!

It may be challenging to think that there are health risks associated with being underweight. After all, much of the research on nutrition and weight in health psychology focuses on the complications resulting from overweight and obesity (Annals of Internal Medicine, 2008; Dixon, Ugwoaba, Brockmann, & Ross, 2020; Meixner, Cohrdes, Schienkiewitz, & Mensink, 2020). But failing to adequately nourish the body can result in significant negative consequences. Some of the adverse effects are evident in individuals diagnosed with *anorexia nervosa*.

ANOREXIA NERVOSA DEFINED To be accurate, anorexia nervosa is a psychological disorder that is characterized by a severe disturbance in eating behaviors (Solmi et al., 2024). The causes of the psychopathology underlying anorexia are thought to include biological factors, environmental factors (family dynamics, cultural and social pressures including social anxiety disorders), developmental factors (struggle for self-control, autonomy, identity), and psychopathological factors, such as an overvaluation of one's body shape and weight (Gailledrat et al., 2016; Grillo, Crosby, & Machado, 2019; Solmi, Collantoni, Meneguzzo, Tenconi, & Favaro, 2018). Although no single cause fully captures the origins of anorexia, recent research suggests that there may be more of a genetic contribution to anorexia than previously thought.

VIDEO #30/60

Chapter 5: Risky Health Behaviors, Part II

- *Anorexia Nervosa: What Causes Anorexia Nervosa?*
- *What Causes Anorexia Nervosa? (YouTube.com)*
- *Website: https://www.youtube.com/watch?v=d-gqIByBNFo*
- **The Eating Recovery Center is publicly accessible to provide valuable information and support related to eating disorders. Eating Disorder Treatment Centers | Anorexia, Bulimia and Binge Eating (eatingrecoverycenter.com)**

A fuller discussion of the role of metabolism and other genetic factors cannot be included here. But briefly, past, and current research suggests a possible connection between some metabolic factors including the role of the hypothalamus (see Chapter 6, Emotional Health and Well-Being). In addition, others suggest that there may be eight genes linked to anorexia (Paddock, 2019). These findings lead some researchers to reclassify this illness as a metabo-psychiatric disorder (Watson et al., 2019; Zhang & Dulawa, 2021).

This probable genetic link does not negate, however, the need to also address the psychological components of this illness. Psychologically, a person who is anorexic has an intense fear of gaining weight that prevents her or him from consuming the nutrients needed to gain or maintain a body weight needed for normal body function. That person's fear of gaining weight, together with an unrealistic body image (imagining her or himself to be fat), and, for women, *amenorrhea*, or the cessation of menstruation, are common conditions that aid in the diagnosis.

Some psychologists believe that an anorexic's misperception of their appearance is due, in part, to poor self-esteem. The origins of poor self-esteem may be within the individual, rooted in a dysfunctional family life, or part of the environmental messages communicated by product advertisers, fashion designers, and female celebrities who reinforce the belief that women must be slender to be attractive (see Box 5. II.1). Negative family relationships, a mother's distorted perception of body size, a mother's body shame, or an individual's perception of parental disapproval also contribute to anorexia (Bennington, Tetsch, Kunzendorf, & Jantschek, 2007; Hudson, Hiripi, Pope, & Kessler, 2007).

Box 5.II.1 Anorexia Taken to the Extreme

In 2006, a 5′8″ Brazilian model, Ana Carolina Reston, died at age 21. She weighed only 88 pounds. By all accounts, Reston died of multiple organ failure, septicemia, and urinary infection (Phillips, 2007). It is also true that she was diagnosed with anorexia nervosa, an eating disorder that is characterized by a dangerously low body weight, a fear of gaining weight, unrealistic assessment of weight, and amenorrhea (Lock & Fitzpatrick, 2009).

Eighty-eight pounds is considered by medical standards to be dangerously underweight on a 5′8″ frame. Using the old weight charts, women who are 5′8″ generally weigh between 126 and 167 pounds. The weight range includes women with small body frames as well as women with medium or larger frames. Thus, according to the old weight charts, Reston weighed only 70% of the lowest acceptable body weight for her height.

If we calculate Reston's weight using the new *body mass index (BMI)*, which measures the proportion of body fat to height, she scored a 13.4. Putting this into perspective, a body mass index (BMI) of 18.5 or less is considered underweight and unhealthy. Normal BMI weight for all heights and frames is represented by a range between 18.5 and 24.9. Whether using the old weight scales or the new BMI scales, Ana Carolina Reston was dangerously underweight.

By depriving the body of food, anorexics also disturb many biological functions. For example, with significant weight loss, the body reduces the production of two hormones needed for reproduction. In women, a significant loss of weight can signal the body to reduce the production of *estrogen*, a hormone associated with reproduction. Similarly, in men, significant weight loss can signal a decreased production of the male hormone *dehydroepiandrosterone (DHEA)*. Other significant physiological changes may include bone loss, extreme sensitivity to cold, bloated stomach, yellowed skin, and thinning hair.

It is important to note that although women report most cases of anorexia, men can also develop this and other eating disorders. In fact, in some studies, men constitute between 10% and 25% of anorexics (Kostecka, Kordyńska, Murawiec, & Kucharska, 2019; Sweeting et al., 2015). In addition, researchers note that men who develop eating disorders are more likely to report dissatisfaction with their body image or to show heightened preoccupation with body image and weight due to their profession. Male actors, dancers, wrestlers, jockeys, and even some athletes are examples of professions in which men pay careful attention to weight and body image (Kostecka et al., 2019).

Because psychological disorders are associated with anorexia, treatment for the disease requires more than just medical attention. An anorexic must address the psychological and emotional problems that contribute to extreme weight loss and the inability to accurately perceive their deteriorating health conditions. Current research suggests a combination of therapies, including cognitive-behavior therapy (CBT; see Chapter 6, Emotional Health and Well-Being), family-based therapy, and nutritional guidance and interventions, can be effective in addressing this issue (Monteleone et al., 2022; Solmi et al., 2024).

It is important to point out, however, that treatment for anorexia and other eating disorders is by no means simple or straightforward. The paucity of information about eating disorders, coupled with the stigma and the shame of carrying this diagnosis, makes treatment challenging (Solmi et al., 2024). Health psychology and clinical psychology are two disciplines well suited to work collaboratively with physicians to address this complex issue.

Bulimia

A second type of eating disorder is *bulimia*, a disorder characterized by binge eating, or the excessive consumption of food. Feelings of guilt, shame, or depression often follow binge eating, which leads to *purging:* vomiting, fasting, or using laxatives to eliminate the food consumed.

BULIMIA DEFINED Bulimics are not easily identified because, unlike anorexics, they do not appear dangerously underweight. But, like anorexics, this disease is now thought to be caused by both genetic and psychological factors. Again, a fuller exploration of the research on the genetic factors that may contribute to illness is beyond the scope of this book. But briefly, the fat mass and obesity-associated gene (*FTO*), which regulates energy homeostasis and food intake, is thought to play a role in bulimia. The mechanisms by which *FTO* appears to influence bulimia is unclear, but it appears to be associated with poor behavioral regulation (Manfredi, Accoto, Couyoumdjian, & Conversi, 2021).

The psychological causes of bulimia can be just as deeply rooted and difficult to treat as anorexia. Psychologically, bulimics, like anorexics, are masking underlying problems with their eating disorders. Researchers continue to explore the psychological causes of bulimia. For the moment, however, the consensus seems to be that family function or dysfunction, self-esteem, emotional problems, psychopathology and, like anorexics, an overvaluation of body shape and weight, may contribute to the development of bulimia (Gailledrat et al., 2016; Grillo et al., 2019; Vázquez-Alonzo, Guzman-Feliciano, De la Cruz-Luna, & García-Ortiz, 2023).

Bulimics are also susceptible to negative physiological health consequences. Consider this: Repeated purging after eating causes an imbalance in the body's electrolytes, necessary elements in the body's fluids containing sodium, potassium, and other elements that stimulate electric charges in the body. The frequent regurgitation of food causes the acidic gastric juices in the stomach to travel in reverse, that is, up through the *esophagus*, the tube connecting the stomach and the mouth. You may know that the body's normal digestive process rarely causes gastric juices to enter the esophagus. Repeated regurgitation that forces the juices of the stomach to reverse and enter the esophagus can cause damage to the lining of the esophagus and tooth enamel, which can result in tooth decay. Frequent vomiting also causes damage to the *colon*, a part of the intestines critical for eliminating waste from the body. Finally, if continually irritated by regurgitation, the colon and esophagus can develop tears or ulcers, a painful outcome that compromises eating and digestive behaviors.

As in the case with anorexia nervosa, family-based therapies for adolescents, and CBT for adolescents and young adults have been employed with some success in addressing the psychological needs of bulimia nervosa (Solmi et al., 2024). But again, this complex issue will require more research and additional, as yet unidentified, therapies.

Obesity

We briefly mentioned obesity in Chapter 2, Research Methods, when identifying the growing number of public health policies to curb obesity in children and adolescents in the U.S. *Obesity* is defined as an excessive amount of fatty tissue that exceeds health limits. The WHO defines overweight and obesity through a measure called the *Body Mass Index (BMI)*, a measure of body fat based on weight and height. *BMI* for adults is calculated by dividing a person's weight in kilograms *(k)* or pounds by the square of their height in meters *(m²)* or feet. Thus $BMI = k/m^2$. A normal or healthy *BMI* ranges from 18.5 to 25.

VIDEO #31/60

Chapter 5: Risky Health Behaviors, Part II
- *Body Mass Index (BMI): What is BMI?*
- *Website: www.youtube.com/watch?v=QIsWHKFTA4M*
- *The Medical University of South Carolina is publicly accessible as it provides free medical-based information and resources to the public. https://muschealth.org/*

VIDEO #32/60

Chapter 5: Risky Health Behaviors, Part II
- **Obesity: Your Weight Mattters Campaign Second National PSA**
- *Website: https://www.youtube.com/watch?v=zOF6geoAF4Y*
- **Other companies can use the Obesity Action Coalition's (OAC) information for free and it is publicly accessible (Home Page – Obesity Action Coalition)**

New data on average rates of obesity across the world shows that obesity rates are on the rise worldwide. As we noted in Chapter 4, Global, Communicable, and Chronic Disease, the increase in the prevalence of obesity is occurring particularly among children, and not just those in the high-income or developed countries. The WHO notes that in 2019 more than 38 million children under the age of five were either overweight or obese (World Health Organization, 2021b), and almost half of this number resided in Asia. What is more, the number of overweight children in Africa has increased by almost 24% since 2000 (World Health Organization, 2021b).

What has caused this surge in obesity rates? New research suggests that obesity may be caused by genetic, environmental, cultural, or psychological factors.

PHYSIOLOGY AND OBESITY New studies investigating a possible genetic determinant of this condition show that pregnant mothers who are diagnosed with diabetes have a higher likelihood of giving birth to babies of higher birth weights who are later found to be obese (Dabelea, 2007). And, as noted earlier in the section on bulimia, some researchers also suggests that the FTO gene, which regulates energy homeostasis and food intake, plays a role in obesity as well (Manfredi et al., 2021; Sheikh et al., 2017).

The most surprising discovery that is reshaping current views on the causes of obesity, however, has been the effects of a new class of drugs, known as *glucagon-like-peptide-1 (GLP-1)* on people trying to lose weight. This new drug, introduced in Chapter 5, Risky Health Behaviors, Part I, was developed and intended for use for people with diabetes, but was also shown to result in weight loss for those prescribed the medication. Scientists believe that this drug mimics the actions of a hormone produced in the body that goes by the same name. Hence, this drug is known as a *GLP-1 agonist* (see Chapter 5, Risky Health Behaviors, Part I).

It appears that GLP-1s contribute to weight loss in three ways. First, the GLP-1 agonist drug binds itself onto and activates receptor cells, in this case cells in the brain, thereby mimicking the effect of the hormone that has the same name. Second, these GLP-1s also appear to interact with the brain's reward "circuitry." Foods, alcohol, and even nicotine for some people trigger spikes in dopamine, a chemical in the brain which encourages greater consumption of that substance (Doucleff, 2023). The GLP-1 agonists reduce those spikes by binding themselves onto the GLP-1 receptors in the brain, maybe even modifying the brain's pleasure pathways, thereby curbing the "cravings" (Ouyang, 2023). Lastly, this drug also appears to slow down the movement of food through the gut, making people feel fuller for longer (Ouyang, 2023).

By all accounts, this is a fascinating discovery, and one that suggests that obesity, like alcohol and drug addiction, may involve a complex interaction with the brain. If so, then behavioral therapies that promote dieting, careful monitoring of food consumption, and increased exercise may be helpful but may not get to the root cause of obesity. If what is involved is a "reward circuitry" issue in the brain, then biological systems and pharmacological agents become central to any effort to address obesity. Thus, in this and perhaps other areas of addiction, health psychologists may need to "retool," learning more about human biology and its effects on behavior.

ENVIRONMENT AND OBESITY This is an interesting finding to be sure. But some researchers argue that a host of environmental factors still play an important role in obesity. For example, Nicolaidis (2019) identifies 16 types of environmental factors shown to influence obesity outcomes. These include the built environment (e.g., schools, elevators, television, smart screens), agroalimentary environments (e.g., pollutants, fast foods, sugary drinks), publicity-marketing (e.g., packaging and media), and sociocultural environments (e.g., low-income, neighborhood and food environment), among others.

LIFESTYLE BEHAVIORS AND OBESITY The increasingly sedentary lifestyles of both children and adults have been documented worldwide. Research has established that adults and children engage in less exercise at home and at school now than in the recent past (Miles, 2008). For children, fewer opportunities to exercise result in more indoor activities that include less movement and possibly more snacking. Similarly, many schools in the U.S. have reduced the number of physical education classes, which compounds the lack of exercise.

The situation is not much better for adults, who also have increasingly sedentary lifestyles. A longitudinal study examining the relationship between adult workers and obesity revealed that job position, stress, and extended and nighttime work hours contribute to increased obesity rates among workers (Griep et al., 2015; Park, Moon, Kim, Kong, & Oh, 2020). The growing rate of obesity is one reason some employers now offer discount memberships to health or exercise gyms or include exercise or fitness rooms in the workplace. Researchers Petridou, Siopi, and Mougios (2019) find that there is sufficient evidence from past studies to conclude that regular and sustained exercise contributes significantly towards fat reduction, maintenance of body weight, and metabolic fitness. The message is clear: Exercise is important to health maintenance.

Finally, health psychologists are also exploring the role of the individual in creating such outcomes. Specifically, health psychologists are examining issues of self-control and feelings of insecurity and inadequacy as psychological factors that may contribute to increased food consumption. Thus, in some instances, emotional or psychological disorders that may contribute to obesity, like anorexia and bulimia, are issues that are well suited to the work of health psychologists.

PSYCHOSOCIAL FACTORS AND OBESITY As mentioned previously, there are many potential physiological health hazards associated with obesity, far too many to review here. Briefly, however, obese individuals are at increased risk for Type 2 diabetes (see Chapter 4, Global Communicable, and Chronic Disease); hypertension, also called high blood pressure; cardiovascular disease (see Chapter 9, Cardiovascular Disease); and chronic health conditions such as arthritis (see Chapter 10, Chronic Pain Management and Arthritis), cancer, gastrointestinal diseases, kidney diseases, pulmonary disease, and even infertility (Annals of Internal Medicine, 2008; Mehler, Lasater, & Padillo, 2003). The physiological consequences of obesity notwithstanding, one additional hazard associated with obesity is social stigmatization (Annals of Internal Medicine, 2008). Research shows that overweight and obese people are frequently stereotyped as lazy, weak-willed, or unintelligent (Puhl & Heuer, 2009). They may be thought of as having poor self-discipline and poor willpower (Puhl & Heuer, 2009). Such stereotypes can lead to discrimination in all settings, including the workplace, educational settings, and even health care facilities (Puhl & Heuer, 2009). For example, overweight and obese children report higher levels of verbal teasing and physical bullying, or exclusion from activities with their peers (Puhl & Latner, 2007). Such treatment may make obese and overweight individuals may prone to negative psychological and emotional health due to the societal response to their physical state.

Even more troubling, however, is that obese persons may be discriminated against while seeking health care (Puhl, Lessard, Himmelstein, & Foster, 2021; Talumaa, Brown, Batterham, & Kalea, 2022). In a study by Puhl and colleagues of just under 14,000 participants enrolled in a behavioral weight management program in one of six Western countries (Australia, Canada, France, Germany, the U.K., and the U.S.), approximately 60% reported a history of weight stigma, and two-thirds of this group reported such stigma from medical doctors. Specifically, these participants reported greater health care avoidance, lower frequency of routine checkups, and less frequent listening and perceived respect from providers (Puhl et al., 2021). Such a response from medical professionals is particularly problematic for overweight and obese people given their additional physiological and psychological health needs.

Binge Eating

Although usually thought to be related to bulimia, binge eating is a different disordered-eating problem. *Binge eating*, as distinguished from bulimia, does not entail the compensatory behavior of purging to avoid weight gain (Solmi et al., 2024). However, researchers support the notion that, like bulimia, binge eating may be introduced in part to help regulate negative affect or negative emotional states such as major depressive, bipolar or anxiety disorders, and even suicide (Welch et al., 2016). Consider this: A study by Clark and Winterowd (2012), examining the relationship between historical loss, racism, acculturation, and emotional distress among 269 self-identified Native American/American Indian women and men, reports that emotional distress, racism (recent, within the past year, and lifetime), and feelings of sadness/depression, anxiety, or shame, related to historical loss of Native Americans/American Indians, were all significantly and positively associated with binge eating. This study would suggest that factors that contribute to binge-eating disorder were, for this study population rooted, in part, in societal or environmental conditions – conditions that may have triggered negative emotional states as well as binge eating.

Other research supports the view that individuals (largely women) who engage in binge eating also do so in response to either negative events or negative emotional states. Yet researchers differ as to the specific intent of the behavior. For example, Peterson and colleagues (2010) suggest that binge eating is evidenced most often by women as a form of harm avoidance, whereas Svaldi, Caffier, and Tuschen-Caffier (2010) suggest that women who binge eat do so to suppress an emotion, most likely a negative emotion.

Whatever the cause or the intent, the outcome is the same. Binge-eating disorder results in increased weight gain, is a contributing factor for obesity, and appears to entail significant negative emotional or psychological states. Consequently, binge eaters are susceptible to the psychological and physiological health problems associated with obesity.

Eating Disorders in Context

We mentioned at the start of the section that one contributing factor to eating disorders is cultural norms: the pressure to adopt and to emulate standards of beauty in the prevailing culture. But as we have noted throughout the text, cultures may differ, and such differences can affect health outcomes. Once again, we see the role of culture as it influences body image and indirectly contributes to behaviors, sometimes unhealthy behaviors that affect health.

Early research on social/environmental factors that contribute to eating disorders focused on the aesthetic preference for and perceived attractiveness of thinness by Western – here meaning European and American – cultures (Calogero, Boroughs, & Thompson, 2007). We now know that the perceived preference for "thinness" and the disordered eating behaviors that are adopted to achieve the ideal body image are evident also in other cultures. Eating disorders appear to be on the rise in western and eastern Asia as well as in the U.S. (Alfalahi et al., 2022; Kim, Nakai, & Thomas, 2020; Smart & Tsong, 2014). Here, as in Western cultures, changes in societal norms, body dissatisfaction, familial expectations, and interpersonal relations are thought to contribute to this increase (Javier & Belgrave, 2019).

We must make one final point. While some studies suggest that all variants of eating disorders are present across the different ethnic and racial groups (Acle, Cook, Siegfried, & Beasley, 2021; Arévalo Avalos et al., 2020), some ethnic groups may express less concern about weight and shape than others. Consider this: Some researchers suggest that, in general, African Americans have a greater acceptance of larger body proportions, are less enamored of thinness, and express lower rates of body dissatisfaction than whites (Acle et al., 2021; Rakhkovskaya & Warren, 2014; Schreiber et al., 1996). These findings might be mediated by the level of acculturation experienced by participants, or just by different standards of beauty.

Summary

In this chapter, we presented Part II of risky health behaviors and the factors that shape adverse outcomes associated with these activities. We explained the effects of unintentional, accidental, unplanned, purposeful, environmental, or culturally induced behaviors and psychopathological behaviors on health outcomes. We explored theoretical explanations for risky activities and reviewed the advantages and disadvantages of strategies designed to limit or eliminate such high risks that lead to adverse health outcomes. We included a brief overview of disordered eating and its impact on health outcomes. Although disordered eating may appear to be unrelated to other types of risky health behaviors, we include it here because eating disorders can jeopardize an individual's physical and psychological outcomes and, according to some, are a form of self-injury.

Personal Postscript

This chapter raises so many issues to consider that are relevant to a college-age population. But if we had to choose just one, perhaps dating violence would be highly relevant. One question that many teens and young adults have is "How do I know if I am in an abusive dating relationship?" This may be difficult to assess at the beginning, but the Centers for Disease Control and Prevention offers some helpful tips through their program "Dating Matters." Although initially designed for pre- and early-teens, it contains information useful to people of any age.

Here are a few things for you and your friends to take note of if you have questions about the behavior of the person you are attracted to:

1. Does the person frequently insult you or verbally put you down, criticize your behaviors or appearance?
2. Does the person frequently yell at you?
3. Does the person push, shove, hit, or act as if they will hit you?
4. Does the person make unfounded jealous accusations?
5. Does the person try to limit your time with friends or family?

These are just a few of the behaviors that, if occurring with regularity, might suggest you should talk with a counselor to determine whether you or your friends are involved in a dating abuse relationship. It may not be the case, but it never hurts to ask.

Questions to Consider

1. More than half of high school seniors text or e-mail while driving. What health policies could communities adopt to stop this dangerous behavior? Could these policies be effectively implemented?
2. Two groups of people are victims of violence: those injured or killed and the witnesses or relatives of those directly affected. How can health psychologists demonstrate to policymakers the impact of violence on all who are directly or indirectly injured?
3. What does the new research on GLP-1s, and the brain's reward circuitry, suggest for addressing issues of obesity and binge eating? How should health psychologists adapt their programmatic and intervention efforts to take these new developments into account?

True or False Questions

1. GLP-1 medications act on the brain's reward circuitry to reduce the desire to eat in large quantities. True or False.
2. Episodes of dating violence have led to new programs designed to teach teens and young adults about forming healthy relationships. True or False.
3. Anorexia nervosa is an eating disorder that affects individuals in Western countries. True or False.
4. U.S. and Mexico are tied for the number of gun shootings on school grounds. True or False.
5. In general, global suicide rates show that suicides are more prevalent among older versus younger persons. True or False.

Important Terms

Emotional Health and Well-Being

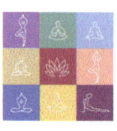

Source: 3xy/
Shutterstock.

Chapter Outline

Chapter Objectives

After studying this chapter, you will be able to:

1. Identify and define four major models of health and well-being.

2. Compare and contrast the concept of well-being in the four models.

3. Define *positive psychology*.

4. Identify three studies that demonstrate the beneficial effects of positive affect on health.

5. Identify and explain two criticisms of the positive psychology movement.

6. Give examples of the real-world application of positive psychology.

7. Describe three major types of traditional medicine.

8. Compare and contrast traditional and Western medicine.

DOI: 10.4324/9781003300670-7

OPENING STORY: ANGELITA

Miguel was getting worried. For the past three months, his wife, Angelita, seemed inexplicably sad. Usually cheerful, talkative, and energetic, Angelita had become increasingly quiet and weepy. She complained of frequent headaches and spent hours alone in her garden. The only activity she seemed to enjoy was cooking. For example, when cooking her favorite foods from her hometown of La Paz, Mexico, Angelita could be heard singing for hours. But lately, during dinner, she was quiet. She would feel her stomach begin to "churn" and then excuse herself from the table.

Miguel encouraged Angelita to speak with her doctor. He hoped that a physical exam would uncover the problem. Angelita's doctor, however, found no viral or bacterial infection and no other physical explanations for the headaches or the upset stomach. The doctor believed that Angelita's symptoms were rooted in emotional problems but was uncertain of the cause. He suggested that she come back in two weeks if there was no improvement in her condition, and he would refer her to someone who could help address what he suspected were emotional problems.

Angelita decided not to return to her doctor. She believed that he had no idea what was wrong and therefore could be of no help. Instead, she phoned her mother, Carmen, and told her about her current health problems. Carmen, who still lived in La Paz, convinced her daughter to come to Mexico for a week of rest and relaxation. In truth, Carmen wanted Angelita to see the village **curandero**, *a traditional healer who practiced a form of medicine called* **curanderismo**, *found in many Latin American countries. Curanderismo is a holistic approach to health that treats a person's material, spiritual, and psychic health in addition to his or her physical needs (Garcia, 2023). Carmen believed that curanderismo was preferable to modern health practices, especially when dealing with emotional or other nonphysical health issues.*

Carmen notified the curandero, and as is the custom, the curandero agreed to visit Angelita at home. He came the day after Angelita arrived and spent several hours talking with her. Angelita remembered that the curandero's father was the village healer when she was a child. It appeared that the healing gift, referred to as "el don," was passed to the son. After talking with Angelita, the curandero gave her an herb tea to drink and rubbed a salve over her temples and forehead. He said he would return to check on Angelita in two days.

On his second visit, the curandero brought more herbs and made another tea. He then asked Angelita about her adjustment to her new home and neighborhood in Nashville, Tennessee. When he learned that Angelita could not find in Nashville the same herbs and spices used for cooking and for teas that she used in Mexico, he gave her extra to take with her when she returned. He also gave her a small pillow filled with strong scents.

Within a week of returning to Nashville, Angelita began feeling better. She seemed happier and appeared more energetic, much like her "old" self. Because she no longer complained of headaches, she was more social and no longer needed long periods of solitude. Angelita called her mother to report the changes, and Carmen immediately relayed the news to the curandero. The curandero replied simply that Angelita needed to reconnect spiritually to her home and culture. He believed that the Mexican herbs he gave Angelita would make her spirit more content while away from her home.   ■

Traditional medicines like curanderismo may have originated several millennia ago, but they are still used throughout the world today (Garcia, 2023). As we saw in the opening story, some people use traditional medicines in addition to or in lieu of Western medical approaches. Recall that Angelita sought the assistance of the curandero only after seeking assistance from her doctor in Nashville. Her mother, however, preferred to use curanderismo as a first or only option.

Using traditional medicines, the curandero determined (or diagnosed, if you prefer) that Angelita's physical symptoms were caused largely by spiritual and emotional health problems, a longing for the familiar. Yet Angelita's doctor in Nashville, who uses Western medical techniques, also concluded that her problem was not physical in origin. In fact, if pressed, the doctor might have suggested that Angelita was suffering from a bout of homesickness, a type of **psychosomatic illness** with emotional or psychological underlying causes. Thus, both traditional and Western medicinal practitioners concluded that Angelita experienced an emotional health problem, even though they differed somewhat as to the cause. Through the opening story we introduce one theme of the current chapter: the contrasting and complementary practices of traditional versus Western medicine. We will explore the similarities and differences between both forms of medicine, focusing specifically on their treatment of emotional health issues.

The opening story also illustrates the effects of emotional factors on overall health outcomes. Specifically, Angelita's story reminds us that emotions contribute to our physical state. Thus, in this chapter we also explore the role of emotional health in overall well-being. In the process, we will identify the contributions of health psychologists to understanding emotions as a health determinant.

We begin our exploration of emotional health in Section I by examining four models used currently in research and practice in the field of health psychology: the biomedical model, the biopsychosocial model, the wellness model, and the social ecological model. The models were developed and tested in the 20th century largely in Western cultures and therefore represent current views of health in some cultures.

In Section II, we explore a new topic called positive psychology. Positive psychology proposes that to understand human outcomes we must identify and examine all contributing factors, positive as well as negative. Included in this concept is a focus on health-enhancing emotional factors that can lead to good health outcomes. According to this view, the positive emotions, experiences, and personal characteristics that contribute to healthy outcomes have been largely overlooked in psychology. Proponents of positive psychology suggest that if we omit the study of "normal" healthy states, we cannot fully understand health.

Finally, in Section III, we explore a sample of traditional medicines, including Chinese traditional medicine, indigenous medicines that include *curanderismo* and *sangoma*, and a brief overview of Native American healing practices. Again, our focus when reviewing traditional medicines is principally to understand the similarities and differences between traditional and Western medicines as well as the relationship between emotions and overall well-being as explained by these two perspectives.

After reading this chapter, you will be able to identify and explain four models of health currently used to diagnose outcomes, to explain the role of emotions on individual health outcomes, to identify the central concepts of positive psychology and its contribution to our understanding of health outcomes, and to compare the treatment of emotional health by Western and traditional medicines.

Consider two important points before proceeding. First, you will notice that some of the health models use the term **well-being** to characterize an individual's overall state of health. As noted in Chapter 1, An

Interdisciplinary View of Health, well-being describes the state of the body (physical), the mind (psychological), the spirit, and social relations (emotions). It offers a holistic view of health similar to the ecological model, with one distinction. The social ecological model does not specifically address spiritual health.

Well-being incorporates many of the same determinants found in the biopsychosocial model. Where applicable, we will use the term *well-being* to characterize a person's physical, psychological, emotional, and social condition. We will add to this concept the effects of the physical environments, health systems, and health policy on health outcomes to explain the social ecological model and its ability to enhance our understanding of well-being.

Second, and equally as important, by using the term *well-being* we are reminded that a thorough study of health integrates the emotional and psychological states of an individual. It further supports the inclusion of health psychologists in the practice of and research on health.

SECTION I. FOUR MODELS OF WELL-BEING

Biomedical Model

The first formal, Western model of well-being, here meaning a model supported by scientific inquiry and empirical study, is the ***biomedical model***. In favor since the early 20th century, the biomedical model proposed that health is the absence of disease or dysfunction. Using this definition as a starting point, *disease* was defined as an abnormality, specifically a dysfunction of or deviation in a body organ or other body structures (Engel, 2002; Wade & Halligan, 2004). Thus, according to the biomedical model, a person who is in good health will be free of any abnormal biological changes in or functions of the body, whereas someone in "bad" or ill health will experience a change in the body system or functions. Furthermore, when diseases occur, this model suggests that locating and eradicating the illness will restore a person to good health.

As we saw in Chapter 1, An Interdisciplinary View of Health, a wholly physiologically based concept of health is consistent with some earlier beliefs. For example, the Cnidians in 500 BCE in Greece and the Roman philosopher and physician Galen in 200 CE believed that physical maladies determined an individual's health status. Research suggests that the early views were enhanced and supported by later studies performed in the 1880s by Robert Koch of Germany and by Louis Pasteur of France (Cantor, 2000; Checkland et al., 2008).

In separate, some say rival, studies, Koch established that "invisible germs carried contagions." In support of that assertion, Koch identified specific microorganisms that caused diseases such as anthrax and tuberculosis (Tan & Berman, 2008). The irrefutable association between a specific organism and a specific disease convinced many Western scientists that illnesses were indeed caused only by microorganisms.

According to some, Pasteur pioneered the use of vaccines to prevent infectious diseases (Pasteur & Chamberland, 2002). However, as we saw in Chapter 4, Global, Communicable, and Chronic Disease, a process known as variolation, widely practiced in China, India, North Africa, and Türkiye and later refined by Jenner in 1796, was a precursor to modern-day vaccines (Boylston, 2012; Ranscombe, 2022; Stewart & Delvin, 2006). These discoveries further supported the germ theory of disease. Thus, it appears that Koch's discovery of the relationship between microorganisms and disease and the practice of variolation, which led to the development of vaccines that protect individuals from such microorganisms (thereby ensuring good physiological health), helped to explain the origins of illness. This work appears to have led to the development of the biomedical model of health (Checkland et al., 2008).

LIMITATIONS OF THE BIOMEDICAL MODEL To be certain, science supports the association between microorganisms and disease, the central tenet of the biomedical model. Unfortunately, the assertion that only physical agents cause illnesses is also a limitation of the model. Other limitations include a problem-oriented approach to health and wellness and a broad, perhaps overbroad, definition of illness. We review each limitation briefly here.

The belief that only physiological determinants cause illness presents, as Engel (2002) suggests, a "culturally specific perspective about diseases," somewhat like a Western-culture version of folk medicine. Past and current models of health, in addition to current research, suggest that microorganisms are only one of several factors that influence well-being. By focusing on the physical causes of illness, the biomedical model overlooks emotional or psychological determinants that also influence well-being. We explain the specific role of non-physiological factors on well-being later in this chapter.

A second limitation is the problem-oriented focus of the biomedical model. It proposes that a change in normal bodily functions that results in a deviation from or dysfunction of the body signals a problem to be rectified. But consider this: Would someone with a hearing impairment or someone who is deaf be considered ill because of his or her "dysfunctional" auditory system? Probably not. Few people equate dysfunction with an illness. Indeed, some individuals who are hearing impaired may characterize their limitations as a disability, but few would consider themselves ill. Yet, according to the biomedical model, a dysfunctional auditory system would be considered an illness.

Even the assumption that physical symptoms are clear indications of an illness or disease can be challenged. Let us return to our opening story. Angelita experienced physical symptoms, prompting her to seek medical care. But, according to the biomedical model's definition of health, she was not ill. There was no underlying viral or bacteriological disease that caused her symptoms. Nothing was broken. Still, it was evident that Angelita was not in a state of well-being. Clearly, she was experiencing some type of health problem – just not the sort recognized by the biomedical model.

In addition, consider this: Some illnesses can occur independent of symptoms. Hypertension, a heart-related disease that we will explore in Chapter 9, Cardiovascular Disease, is nicknamed "the silent killer" because it often develops with no observable, here meaning external, symptoms. Similarly, individuals may often be unaware that they have been infected with a deadly human immunodeficiency virus because it, too, often carries no discernable external symptoms for the first 8 to 10 years. Thus, in some cases, external symptoms of an illness can appear without evidence of an underlying disease (like Angelita's problem). In other instances, a disease may indeed be present (like hypertension or HIV), but show no visible or external symptom, especially in the early stages of illness.

To summarize, the biomedical model defines *dysfunctionality* as an illness and interprets physiological symptoms as signs of the illness. But the biologically based model presents a limited definition of illness that can include a range of dysfunctions not usually classified as an illness. Current research suggests that a more precise yet also in some ways broader definition of health may be more accurate and should include the emotional, psychological, and, for some, spiritual determinants of well-being (Allen, Hatala, Ijaz, Courchene, & Bushie, 2020; Donatuto, Campbell, & Gregory, 2016).

Let us consider one additional point before moving on. It is important to restate that a broader definition of health, one that includes well-being, is not new. Recall that in Chapter 1, An Interdisciplinary View of Health, we briefly reviewed the health practices and beliefs of many cultures, including ancient Greeks (specifically Aesculapius and Hippocrates), Chinese, Native American, and the Sans and Yoruba in southern and western Africa. All of these civilizations embraced a holistic or an ecological view of health that included the emotional, physical, psychological, environmental, and, for some, the spiritual well-being of the individual.

In more recent times, research by Sigmund Freud in the 1890s reaffirmed a broad concept of health, one that included emotional and psychological factors. Specifically, Freud suggested that many of the physical illnesses described by his patients were, in fact, linked to psychological causes. When the psychological problems were addressed, he noted that the physical symptoms were also resolved without direct treatment. Contemporary health and behavioral medicine furthered Freud's version of the mind–body connection by establishing the field of psychosomatic medicine. This new discipline abolished the separation of the mind and body proposed in earlier versions of Western medicine (Mizrachi, 2001) and reintroduced a holistic concept of well-being. Thus, our brief review of health in Chapter 1 that highlighted examples of holistic and ecological health models set the stage for further exploration of the role of emotions in Western medicine. The biopsychosocial, wellness, and social ecological models are examples of such models.

Biopsychosocial Model

Sometimes referred to as a *holistic health model*, the *biopsychosocial model* proposed by Engel (2002) supports the belief, endorsed by many in health psychology, that well-being is determined by biological (*bio*), psychological (*psycho*), and sociological (*social*) factors. The psychological influences on health include emotions, health behaviors, personality traits, and social support systems and their effects on emotional health (Lazarus & Folkman, 1987; Ryan & Deci, 2000; Salovey et al., 2000), while sociological factors include familial, cultural, and community factors. We examine some of the psychological and sociological factors in turn.

PSYCHOLOGICAL FACTOR #1: EMOTIONS We noted earlier that the relationship between health and emotions was proposed many centuries earlier. *Hippocrates*, sometimes called the father of clinical medicine, is often credited with pioneering the interaction of emotions and health in Western medicine. He believed that an imbalance in any one of four bodily fluids, called *humors*, could lead to illnesses (Salovey et al., 2000). The important part is that the illnesses he identified were, in fact, emotional. For example, Hippocrates believed that an imbalance of black bile, one type of body fluid, would lead to sadness or melancholy, while an imbalance of yellow bile, another fluid, led to anger. We will see later in the chapter that traditional medicines also defined well-being as a balance between emotional, physical, social, and environmental forces.

The concept presented by Hippocrates that links health and emotions is supported by current research. We explore this in the following sections, although the details have changed considerably. Current studies show that emotions can affect our physiological well-being through two primary pathways: our immune system and our behaviors.

Emotions and the Immune System Brod and colleagues (2014) suggest that one way that emotions affect our immune system is through the nerve fibers in our bodies. The fibers connect with the *central nervous system (CNS)*, the "control center" for our body or, biologically speaking, the brain and the brain stem (see Figure 6.1). More recently, some researchers have referred to these systems as "affective immunology" (D'Acquisto, 2017).

The nerve fibers act like cables carrying information from our *receptors* (skin, muscles, and other sites) to our CNS. It may help to think of neuron cables as the hardware needed to communicate. The actual message, however, is carried by neurotransmitters that travel within the cables. When sending messages from a receptor site – such as the skin – to the brain, a neurotransmitter is triggered at the receptor site and passed along from neuron to neuron via the axons and dendrites until the message reaches the processing center of the brain. *Dendrites*, from the Greek word *dendron*, meaning "tree," are branchlike structures that

NERVOUS SYSTEM

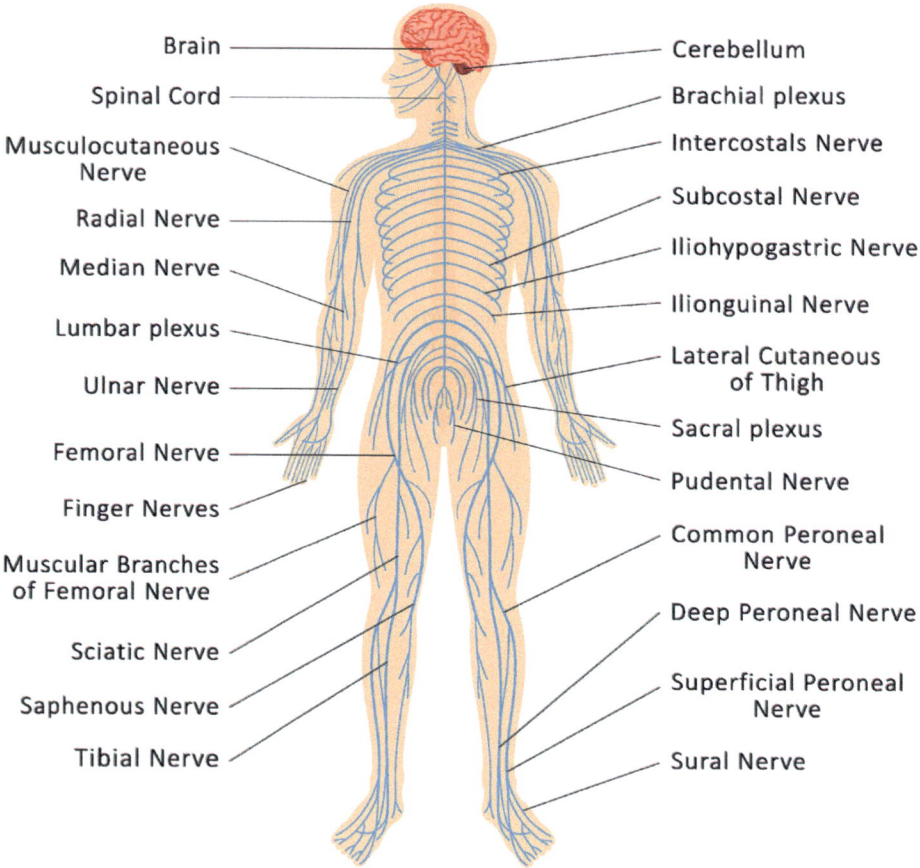

Brain

Spinal Cord

Musculocutaneous
Nerve

Radial Nerve

Median Nerve

Lumbar plexus

Ulnar Nerve

Femoral Nerve

Finger Nerves

Muscular Branches
of Femoral Nerve

Sciatic Nerve

Saphenous Nerve

Tibial Nerve

Cerebellum

Brachial plexus

Intercostals Nerve

Subcostal Nerve

Iliohypogastric Nerve

Ilionguinal Nerve

Lateral Cutaneous
of Thigh

Sacral plexus

Pudental Nerve

Common Peroneal
Nerve

Deep Peroneal Nerve

Superficial Peroneal
Nerve

Sural Nerve

FIGURE 6.1 The figure is an outline of a human body identifying components of the central and peripherial nervous systems.

Source: Alamy ID:2HJKEBX.

extend from the cell body and receive the message from other cells. Once the message is received, the *axon*, another nerve fiber that extends from the cell body, carries the message to neighboring cells (see Figure 6.2).

The nerve cables that carry messages are categorized as either afferent or efferent nerve fibers. The ***afferent nerve fibers*** carry information to the CNS (the brain and the spinal cord) from the receptor sites. For example, if a person touches a sharp object, the afferent nerves may send a sensory signal from the fingers (the receptor site) to the brain or spinal cord for processing and interpretation. The ***efferent nerve fibers***, on the other hand, carry information from the CNS to the periphery of the body to coordinate the response. Using the same example of touching a sharp object, the brain might send a signal of pain or discomfort to the receptor site (hand) that results in the person withdrawing his or her hand from the sharp object.

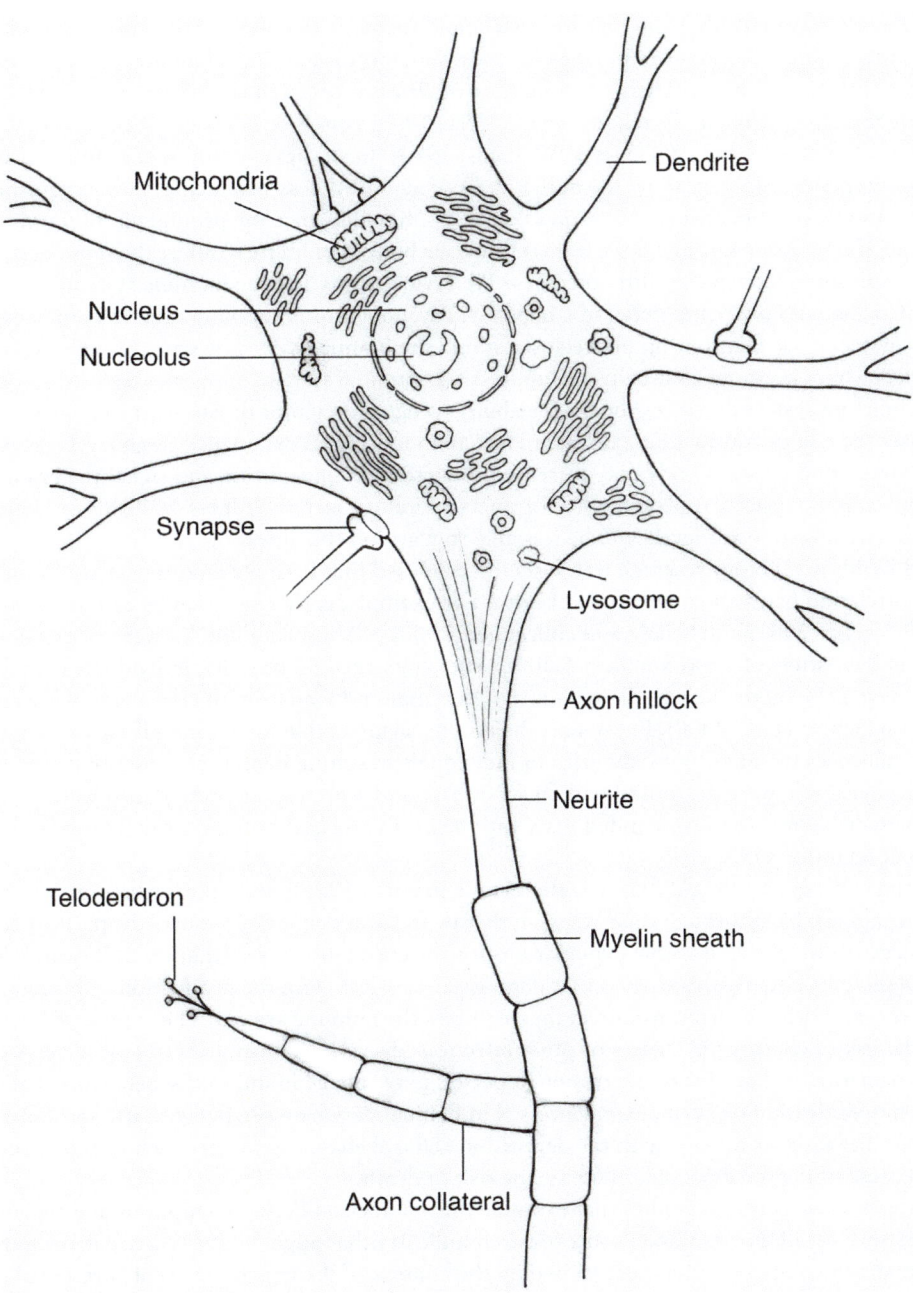

FIGURE 6.2 A drawing of a human cell that identifies the following parts: axon, axon collateral, telodendron, myelin sheath, neurite, axon hillock. In the cell body the following are identified: nucleus, nucleolus, mitochandria, lysosome. Synapse and dendrites are also identified.

Source: CO 172586- Illustration_of_motor_neuron_Sci photolibrary.jpg

Impact of Emotions on Health Now that we understand the basic structure of the body's neurological communication system, we can examine the effects of our emotions on the communication process and hence on our overall well-being. There are a number of classical research studies on stress that help demonstrate this effect (Cohen, Tyrrell, & Smith, 1991, 1993; Dusek & Benson, 2009; Jacobs, 2001; Kiecolt-Glaser & Glaser, 1988; Williams & Williams, 1993). In studies examining the effects of stress on the body's *immune system*, here meaning the body's defense against illness-producing microorganisms, Cohen's 2005 seminal study is foundational. He found that stress may influence the production of *hormones*, another type of chemical message released by cells in our body that, in turn, affect the immune system.

How do hormones influence health outcomes? We review stress and the immune systems in Chapter 7, Stress and Coping, and in greater detail in Chapter 8, Psychoneuroimmunology. For the moment, we note that one example of the relationship between stress and the immune system is seen through the role of *epinephrine*, a stress hormone that helps to suppress the immune system. Suppressing or "turning down" the body's immune system decreases the body's ability to fight foreign or disease-carrying microorganisms and increases the risk of contracting a disease. Thus, if an individual experiences high levels or extended periods of stress, that person's body may increase production of epinephrine and signal the brain to suppress the immune system. A person who contracts a viral or bacterial illness while his or her immune system is functioning at lower levels will be less able to ward off the illness.

Applied health psychology research that tests the proposed link between emotions and illnesses similarly reports a correlation between emotions and health. For example, earlier research by Schulz, Martire, Beach, and Scheier (2005) and Schulz and colleagues (2000) established a link between depression and mortality. In their study of approximately 5,200 participants aged 65 or older, individuals with depressive symptoms were 25% more likely to die within six years than individuals with considerably lower levels of depression (Schulz et al., 2000). In essence, their study suggests that an emotional factor (depression) negatively influences the physiological health of individuals, resulting in an early onset of death. In a related study, individuals who were diagnosed with heart disease and who were depressed also were significantly more likely to die sooner than were individuals with heart disease and no signs or diagnosis of depression (Glassman & Shapiro, 1998).

Shultz and colleagues (2000, 2005), Glassman and Shapiro (1998), and others were quick to note that they cannot establish through their research that depression definitively causes death. Rather, their research suggests one of two possible explanations for the correlations (see Chapter 2, Research Methods). One explanation, as noted previously, is that depression may influence the production of hormones such as epinephrine and other neurotransmitters that suppress the immune system. The suppressed system increases the risk of contracting viruses or other infectious diseases that can lead to mortality. A second possible explanation is that, due to depression, a person may engage in unhealthy behaviors that increase the probability of death. For example, a depressed individual may be more likely to use substances such as alcohol or illegal drugs to cope with the depression. Thus, behavioral factors such as substance abuse, initiated because of depression, could increase the risk of death.

There are, however, current studies that examine this interaction between emotions and the immune system in greater detail. For example, some research indicates that anger – clearly a negative emotion – can also impact the immune system, depending on the context of the triggering event (Brod et al., 2014). One study suggests that anger, triggered in response to a hostile interaction between married partners, can increase inflammatory cytokine interleukin (IL-6) which, we will see a little later, can be detrimental to the body if present long term (Keicolt-Glaser, Gouin, & Hantsoo, 2010). This research illustrates an important link between personal relationships (a social environmental factor), immune systems, and well-being.

The emotion, anger, provokes a physiological response that, if left unchecked, will increase inflammation in the body, a reaction that could lead to a host of physiological symptoms, including fatigue, pain, and psychological symptoms. We discuss this more fully in Chapter 8, Psychoneuroimmunology.

And, just one more fact before we move on. Gouin, Kiecolt-Glaser, Malarkey, and Glaser (2008) also report that people with below-average levels of anger were found to heal significantly slower than others. In essence, suppressing anger can create similar problems with respect to the body's immune system.

Finally, some studies suggest that the relationship between emotions and the immune system response is bidirectional. In essence, these studies found that people with immune system disfunctions also evidence an increase in emotional disturbances, and conversely, people with mental disorders show an increased susceptibility to immune system diseases (D'Acquisto, 2016, 2017). Indeed, Lasselin, Alvarez-Salas, and Grigoleit (2016) further suggest that our immunity is fine-tuned, in part, by our emotions, our personality, and even our social status.

One final note here. Do remember that many of the traditional medicines (e.g., Chinese traditional medicine, Native American medicine, and curanderismo), have long held the belief that emotions play a critical role in our overall well-being. More on that later.

Negative Emotions, Positive Effects Research on emotions and health show that it is also possible for negative emotions to have positive health consequences. In a review of the research on the health outcomes of negative affect, Mayne (1999) found that in some cases negative emotions can activate the sympathetic nervous system (SNS) and thereby *stimulate* the immune system. As Figure 6.1 shows, the *sympathetic nervous system* is part of the *autonomic nervous system (ANS)*, or the part of our body that controls the automatic and involuntary functions that we do not think about but that are essential for living. For example, the ANS controls our heart rate, digestion, and perspiration. Another automatic or involuntary function is the body's physiological response to dangers, emergencies, or foreign organisms that invade the body. The sympathetic nervous system is responsible for mobilizing the body to respond to such dangers. This includes stimulating the immune system. Thus, negative affect, such as fear or fright, can stimulate this system to react to danger, possibly resulting in a positive outcome. We take a more in-depth look at the relationship between our emotions and our immune system in Chapter 8, Psychoneuroimmunology.

Negative emotions can also lead to positive or health-enhancing behaviors. Earlier studies suggest that negative emotions can increase the likelihood that individuals will seek timely medical help. Salovey et al. (2000) and Mayne (1999) found that, when experiencing health problems, negative affect such as anxiety or depression may cause a person to perceive his or her physical condition more accurately and therefore increase the probability of that person seeking medical help.

Yet, other studies suggest a more complex role for negative emotions and help-seeking behavior. Balasooriya-Smeekens and colleagues (2015) suggest, in their review of 33 studies, that worry or anxiety about a health symptom tends to increase help-seeking actions, as shown by cancer patients evidencing a shorter time between cancer discovery and consultation with a health provider. By contrast, they note that fear tends to serve as both a barrier and a prompt to help-seeking behaviors. And, as we have seen before, self-efficacy may play a pivotal role here in motivating behavior. Lee, Hwang, Hawkins, and Pingree (2008) note that high self-efficacy together with negative emotions were positively associated with information seeking among a sample of 122 women diagnosed with breast cancer.

We may be able to translate these findings into less consequential, but still relevant examples. Consider this: An individual with a cold may become increasingly anxious if the cold lingers and produces thick mucus. That person's anxiety, a negative affect, may prompt him or her to seek medical care. In comparison, a person with a positive affect may not accurately assess the severity of the health condition or the fact that medical attention is needed. Someone with the same symptom – a lingering cold and thick mucus – who feels he or she can overcome the problem with sleep and copious amounts of liquids may not seek assistance. The lack of anxiety and the belief in his or her own skills may prevent that person from accurately assessing the severity of the health problem and from engaging in the appropriate health-seeking behavior.

Positive Emotions and Health If negative emotions can lead to both poorer (and in some cases, healthier) outcomes, can positive emotions improve health status? We explore this question in depth in the following section on positive psychology. For now, however, it is important to note that some studies suggest such an association. For example, the role of *positive affect* on physiological health was demonstrated in a classic study by Cohen and colleagues (1991, 1995). In a laboratory-based study, these researchers exposed participants to a common cold virus to determine whether a person's affect influences disease progression. The study revealed that participants with a positive affect, here meaning positive feelings or emotions at the time of exposure to the virus, developed a less severe form of illness than did participants with a negative affect. Similarly, research by Sin, Moskowitz, and Whooley (2015) demonstrated that among 1022 participants with a diagnosis of stable heart disease, those who evidenced high positive affect (502) were more likely to engage in health enhancing behaviors such as exercising, refraining from smoking, and also evidenced no depressive symptoms.

It might be tempting to conclude from this research that people who maintain a positive affect will be less susceptible to severe illnesses, worsening illnesses, or depression. But keep in mind that affect is just one of a number of factors that influence well-being. An individual's physiological state, limitations, dysfunctions, and demographics will contribute also to the likelihood of contracting a disease, to the severity of the illness, and to its progression. In sum, current research shows that Hippocrates' initial premise was correct. Our positive and negative emotions do influence our well-being. He was incorrect, however, when characterizing the process by which emotions contribute to health.

PSYCHOLOGICAL FACTOR #2: HEALTH BEHAVIORS We reviewed a host of health behaviors in Chapter 5, Risky Health Behaviors, Parts I and II, and discussed at length their positive and negative impacts on well-being. We will not repeat the information from Chapter 5 in this section. But it is important to restate what we noted earlier: emotions can and often do influence health behaviors. For example, anxiety, social anxiety, and depression are cited by some as factors that contribute to alcohol abuse or abuse of other substances (Dyer, Easey, Heron, Hickman, & Munafo, 2019; Torvik et al., 2019). Thus, two psychological factors, health behaviors and emotions, can interact to influence health status.

There are also researchers who dispute the association between psychological factors, such as anxiety or depression, and health behaviors like substance use. Some researchers argue that there may be no association between these factors (Dyer et al., 2019) or that while there are mixed results showing an association between depression and substance abuse, there is no such association between anxiety and substance abuse (Hussong, Ennett, Cox, & Haroon, 2017). Translation? "More research is needed!"

SOCIOLOGICAL FACTOR #1: SOCIOECONOMIC CLASS AND INCOME In Chapter 4, Global Communicable, and Chronic Disease, we identified the barriers to health care posed by a lack of access to health insurance or to preventive medical care (Simon, Chan, & Forrest, 2008). What we did not state is that an individual's *socioeconomic class (SEC)* – or the social and economic group that characterizes that person's social position in society – also greatly affects his or her access to care.

Socioeconomic class is a term developed by sociologists that categorizes individuals according to their positions in society as determined by their parents' level of education, parent's occupation, their family's social status, and their family's income and wealth (Hout, Brooks, & Manzay, 1993; Liberatos, Link, & Kelsey, 1988). When evaluating the impact of socioeconomic class on health, researchers often use a simplified categorization scheme based primarily on household annual income levels. We identify the socioeconomic classes in the U.S. as: poor (less than $16,000), working class ($16,000–$35,000), lower-middle class ($35,000–$75,000), upper-middle class ($100,000–$500,000), and wealthy (greater than $500,000; Thompson & Hickey, 2005).

Without a doubt, SEC, defined here by household income, is a sociological factor that affects health by regulating access to medical care, specifically in those countries where access to health is affected by one's ability to pay for needed care. This is not the case in all countries. For example, according to World Population Review, 72 countries have some form of universal health care, here meaning a government-regulated system of health coverage that provides high quality and affordable care to more than 90% of their population (World Population Review, 2023b; see Table 6.1). Certainly, there are significant differences in the implementation of these systems, which we will explain in greater detail in Chapter 12, Health Care Systems & Health Policy. For now, it is only important to remember that SEC is a more significant factor in accessing health care in those countries without some form of universal health coverage.

TABLE 6.1 Countries with Universal Health Care Systems

A	D	K	Romania
Albania	Denmark	Kuwait	Rwanda
Algeria	E	L	S
Argentina	Egypt	Liechtenstein	Serbia
Australia	F	Luxembourg	Seychelles
Austria	Finland	M	Singapore
B	France	Macau	South Africa
Bahamas	G	Malaysia	South Korea
Belgium	Georgia	Maldives	Spain
Bhutan	Germany	Mauritius	Sri Lanka
Botswana	Ghana	Mexico	Suriname
Brazil	Greece	Monaco	Sweden
Bulgaria	H	N	Switzerland
Burkina Faso	Hong Kong (China)	Netherlands	T
C	I	New Zealand	Taiwan
Canada	Iceland	North Korea	Thailand
Chile	India	Norway	Trinidad and Tobago
China	Indonesia	P	Tunisia
Colombia	Ireland	Pakistan	Türkiye
Costa Rica	Israel	Peru	U
Croatia	Italy	Philippines	United Kingdom
Cuba	J	Portugal	
Czech Republic	Japan	R	

Source: https://worldpopulationreview.com/country-rankings/countries-with-universal-healthcare

In countries without universal health care, such as the U.S., the ability to pay for health insurance or to pay a medical provider's fee will influence a person's likelihood of seeking timely health care. Individuals unable to pay for needed health care due to limited income or lack of health insurance may delay seeking care, a decision that could aggravate the health problem. We also explain the effect of socioeconomic status (income) on access to health care in greater detail in Chapter 12, Health Care Systems and Health Policy.

In addition to the inability to pay for care, studies suggest that people in lower socioeconomic groups may express negative affect more frequently than people in other SECs due largely to social environmental factors (Carroll, Smith, & Bennett, 2002). For example, lower SEC individuals are more likely to experience negative emotions, such as depression, that may lead to poorer health outcomes for poor or working poor individuals (Callan, Kim, & Matthews, 2015; Kraft & Kraft, 2023; Kraus, Adler, & Chen, 2013; O'Leary, 2020).

SOCIOLOGICAL FACTOR #2: FAMILY AND CULTURE Familial and cultural patterns of behavior, including diet and orientation to exercise and sports, also contribute to overall well-being. Take, for example, diet. Research on the nutritional practices of Japanese and Korean Americans reveals that many Asian diets minimize the risk of chronic diseases such as hypertension or digestive diseases (Park, Murphy, Sharmay, & Kolondel, 2005; Yang, Chung, Kim, Bianchi, & Song, 2007). Dietary practices in many Asian, specifically East Asian, countries include foods high in fiber, such as fruits, vegetables, and grain products, and low in fats.

Similarly, the Mediterranean diet, here meaning a diet high in fruits, vegetables, fish, cereals, nuts and legumes, moderate consumption of alcohol – specifically red wine – and low consumption of dairy products and red meats, is associated with lower risks of cardiovascular disease and cancer, among other illnesses or death (Aridi, Walker, Roura, & Wright, 2020; Schwingshackl, Morse, & Hoffman, 2019). By contrast, as we also noted in Chapter 4, Global, Communicable, and Chronic Disease, foods with high-fat or high-calorie content, such as pizza, cheeseburgers, and French fries – favorite American fast foods – are linked to chronic diseases, including heart diseases and diabetes (Scott, 2007; World Health Organization, 2002b).

Nutrition and diet are important, but so is exercise. The CDC reports that, for adults, at least 30 minutes of exercise daily, together with a healthy diet, are required to reduce the risk of chronic diseases (CDC, 2023c; Saris et al., 2003). Maintaining a regular exercise regimen is dependent on a number of factors, including past patterns and practices, which takes us back to the role of family or cultural determinants.

To summarize, the biopsychosocial model expands on the definition of health put forth in the biomedical model by including psychological, social, and emotional well-being as part of a holistic definition of health. Yet even with an expanded definition, researchers argue that the biopsychosocial model still places biology at the core of the definition. They contend that, rather than proposing a truly integrative model of health, the biopsychosocial model simply appends the psychological and sociological determinants of health as "add-ons" to the biomedical model (Armstrong, 2002). For this reason, we explore other models that offer alternative concepts of well-being that do not place biology at the center of the definition.

Wellness Model

The biopsychosocial model was the first to include psychological and social determinants as contributors to health outcomes. The *wellness model* includes the same psychological, social, and emotional factors included in the biopsychosocial model, but it adds two new dimensions: quality of life and spirituality.

QUALITY OF LIFE The wellness model defines health according to an individual's assessment of his or her own state of physical, mental, emotional, and spiritual well-being. For example, in a case study by Dinh and Groleau (2008), a Laotian man, Mr. B., summarizes his assessment of his overall well-being using quality of life and spirituality (see Box 6.1). In this study, Mr. B. unwillingly undergoes an emergency amputation of two fingers to protect him from a likely infection. According to the medical doctors on his case, the operation restored him to a state of good physical health. But, according to Mr. B., when surgeons removed his two fingers they also took part of his life and his life force. For Mr. B., the operation that Western medical doctors thought of as a lifesaving procedure diminished his *quality of life* and negatively affected his spiritual and overall well-being.

Box 6.1 Personal Meaning and Health: One Man's View of Wellness

Dinh and Groleau (2008) examine the case of a 49-year-old married Laotian man, Mr. B., living in Canada. According to their case study, Mr. B. was employed as an operator of heavy machinery at a factory in Canada. While at work, Mr. B. caught his glove in one of the heavy machines. The machine severed part of the third and fourth fingers on his left hand. He was immediately taken to the nearest hospital, where he waited approximately one hour before seeing a surgeon.

Mr. B. asked that his fingers be reattached, but the surgeon indicated that the tendons in his third and fourth fingers were dead and that the remaining parts of those fingers would have to be amputated. The surgeon's decision did not seem logical to Mr. B., who demonstrated that he could move the remaining segments of his fingers. The surgeon was not convinced, and three hours later, despite Mr. B.'s protests and pleas not to amputate, the medical staff prepared him for surgery to remove the remaining segments.

In the months after the surgery, Mr. B. received physical therapy to regain strength and movement in his hand. Doctors considered the surgery a success because it saved Mr. B. from probable infection of the hand and ensured that Mr. B. would return to an overall good state of health. Mr. B. did not share the doctor's point of view. Instead, he believed that the surgery "[took] his life."

According to Dinh and Groleau (2008), some Laotians believe that their health depends on the status of 12 souls that comprise a person's life force, known as *H'wen* (Dinh & Gorleau, 2008). The 12 souls correspond to parts of the body. The hands represent one of the souls. When Mr. B. lost his fingers, he lost one of his life forces. Thus, in this case study, Mr. B.'s health, according to the wellness model, was significantly impaired on two fronts: psychosocial and spiritual. First, unable to resume work as a heavy machinery operator, Mr. B. was unable to earn a living and provide for his family. His quality of life was affected by his inability to assume his role as the principal wage earner in the family. Second, the loss of his fingers represented a lost energy force and resulted in diminished spiritual well-being.

When explaining his feelings in French, Mr. B could only say he felt "*triste*," or sad. But, when talking with Laotian friends, his wife, or others who understood the Laotian culture, he explained that he felt indignation and felt unworthy of respect.

Mr. B.'s inability to return to his job affected his sense of responsibility and obligation to his family. His feelings of indignation and of being unworthy of respect reflect the influence of Laotian culture. It suggests a social influence that impacts his emotional state of health and a spiritual influence consistent with his Buddhist beliefs. Mr. B.'s case demonstrates how spirituality, quality of life, culture, and emotional health all contribute to his assessment of his overall well-being. Not surprisingly, he currently views his overall quality of life as poor.

Similar examples of an individual's perception of wellness that departs from a biopsychosocial concept of health are found in the research literature on total knee replacement surgery, an increasingly common surgery for older adults in many Western cultures.

Total knee replacement surgery usually is performed when a person's *knee osteoarthritis*, a form of arthritis in the knee that can become disabling over time, worsens to the point that surgery is recommended to relieve the pain or to correct a functional disability (see Chapter 10, Chronic Pain Management and Arthritis). Interestingly, research by Toye, Barlow, Wright, and Lamb (2006) show that, for most patients, a decision to replace a dysfunctional knee is rarely explained by painful physical symptoms. Instead, Toye and colleagues (2006) found that a patient's feelings of vulnerability because of the unreliable knee, the desire not to depend on others for mobility, and the fatigue associated with an increased effort when performing daily tasks – in other words, quality of life issues – were the driving factors for knee replacement surgery. Thus, Toye and colleagues (2006) suggest that decisions to have knee replacement surgery are based on the value placed on mobility, independence, and improved energy levels rather than on pain or discomfort.

Similarly, Price and colleagues (2018) show that more older adults (those in their 80s and 90s), as well as younger patients, are choosing knee replacement surgery in order to maintain their quality of life. These concepts represent quality of life values that may not be considered important in a biomedical or biopsychosocial model of health but are essential factors in a wellness model.

There is one more thing to consider. Riddle, Jiranek, and Hayes (2014) examined the appropriateness of knee replacement surgeries in the U.S., given research suggesting that such procedures were inappropriate in over 20% of patients worldwide. By inappropriate, they mean that the expected risks of the procedure far outweigh the benefits. (Conversely, *appropriate* means that the benefits of the procedure outweigh the risks). Consistent with global research, Riddle and colleagues found that of 205 patients, knee replacement surgery was determined to be beneficial for only 44% of patients. For fully one-third (34%) of the patients, the surgery was deemed inappropriate, a rate far higher than expected. What does this suggest for the decision to undergo knee replacement surgery? One might suggest that this finding underscores work by Toye and colleagues and Price and colleagues that decisions to have this surgery are based more on quality-of-life factors than medically necessity.

SPIRITUALITY The wellness model also addresses spiritual health, faith, and religion – topics that are not usually included in psychological research. Some scientists consider *spirituality* a pseudoscience or a primitive superstition and therefore not something to be included in rigorous studies that explain individual health outcomes. Recently, however, more researchers have examined the relationship between spirituality and health (see Chapter 7, Stress and Coping). The new research suggests a change among current Western scientists, at least those in the health fields, who believe that spirituality contributes to obtaining optimal health for some individuals (Diaz, 1993; Myslakidou et al., 2008; Seaward, 1991), and especially for those who attend religious services (VanderWeele et al., 2017).

By spirituality, researchers are not necessarily referring to religious dogma. Rather, studies focus on the impact of an individual's philosophy, values, and meaning of life on health status (Laird, Curtis, & Morgan, 2017; Mullen, McDermott, Gold, & Belcastro, 1996). Scientists suggest that spirituality may afford individuals peace and tranquility in the face of stressful events and a sense of meaningfulness that provides them with direction and fulfillment (Laird et al., 2017; Perrin & McDermott, 1997).

As Fardin (2020) notes, religion and spirituality can facilitate mental relaxation, especially in times of crisis, such as the Ebola and the COVID-19 crises. In a review of 11 English- and non–English-language studies, Fardin cited several studies that found beneficial physical and mental health effects of spirituality and religion during such crises. Chaves and colleagues (2015) also suggest that, based on their study of over 600 college students in Brazil, spirituality can be employed as a protective factor to minimize anxiety, arguably reducing another potentially crisis-evoking experience for students.

Finally, some spiritual practices promote healthy behaviors. For example, the dietary practices of Muslims and some Christian denominations include abstinence from alcohol. This can be a health-enhancing behavior, particularly for those who otherwise would be inclined to consume alcohol in excess (see Chapter 5, Risky Health Behaviors, Part I).

Nevertheless, while a number of researchers agree that spirituality does play a role in overall well-being for some individuals, the concept of spirituality presents several difficulties. There is little agreement among researchers on how to define spirituality (Lalani, 2020). And it is often used as a synonym for or expressed in terms of religious faith, practices, or values (Sharma & Singh, 2018; Withers, Zuniga, & Van Sell, 2017). There does seem to be agreement, however, that spirituality is personal and dependent on context (Newlin, Knafl, & Melkus, 2002; Rahimi, Anoosheh, Ahmadi, & Foroughan, 2013). In essence, while there is growing acknowledgment of the contributions of spirituality to well-being, researchers have struggled to empirically identify this relationship. The following study, however, comes close.

Wachholtz and Pargament (2008) sought to explore the effects of four types of meditation techniques – spiritual meditation, internally focused meditation, externally focused meditation, and muscle relaxation – on migraine suffers to determine which, if any, resulted in significantly improved outcomes. Each of the 83 study participants in the migraine study learned and practiced one of the four techniques for 20 minutes a day for a total of 30 days. The results of pre-post test measures (see Chapter 2, Research Methods) revealed that participants who used the spiritual meditation techniques fared much better than those using any of the other three approaches. The spiritual meditation users reported a decrease in frequency of headaches and in negative affect. In addition, they reported an increase in pain tolerance, self-efficacy, and overall well-being (Wachholtz & Pargament, 2008). Thus, this particular study and other on the effects of spirituality on well-being suggests that spirituality offers some individuals tranquility in troubled times, guidance on healthy lifestyles and behaviors, emotional wellness, and an ability to regulate pain levels, all of which contribute to well-being.

VIDEO #33/60

Chapter 6: Emotional Health and Well-Being

- **Migraines: Mayo Clinic Minute – Better tolerated treatment for migraine**
- *Website: https://www.youtube.com/watch?v=J1lfJo0K3Ro*
- *Mayo Clinic is publicly accessible as they offer relevant medically based information on various sources such as YouTube for free (www.mayoclinic.org/)*

We need to make one additional point about the role of spirituality. Consider the case presented in Box 6.2. The late Dr. Paul Farmer, a physician, was reminded that even in Western cultures, individuals combine spirituality with medical science in their efforts to overcome illnesses. From this example and the research, it is clear that spirituality may play a health-enhancing role for many individuals and in many cultures. We will see later that spirituality is also recognized as a central component of well-being in cultures that practice traditional forms of medicine.

Box 6.2 Medicine and Spirituality: A Compatible Combination in Western Medicine?

The late Dr. Paul Farmer was not your "average" doctor. Raised on a boat and on a bus during his childhood, Dr. Farmer's early years accurately could be called atypical. Perhaps his early experience living in nontraditional environments led him to a career caring for the poorest of the poor in Haiti, Peru, Cuba, and Russia (see Figure 6.3).

Dr. Farmer was an infectious diseases specialist, someone who studies and treats contagious diseases. Given his special interests, it is not surprising that Dr. Farmer would travel to developing countries (see Chapter 4, Global, Communicable, and Chronic Disease) in which infectious diseases are quite common. But it was during his work in Haiti that he was reminded of the dual presence of medical science and spirituality in Haitian and Western cultures.

One year, while treating patients in Haiti for tuberculosis (TB; see Chapter 4, Global Communicable, and Chronic Disease), Dr. Farmer designed a study to test an idea debated by his health care staff. He wanted to understand whether the poor health outcomes of impoverished patients like those in Haiti could be attributed to economic conditions and the inability to pay for care or whether their outcomes were rooted in their belief that illnesses had spiritual origins. In Haiti, some individuals believe that illnesses are sent by enemies through sorcery (Kidder, 2003). Dr. Farmer's staff proposed that individuals who believed that illnesses were curses sent by others would be less likely to follow the medical regimen to treat their TB.

To test the idea, Dr. Farmer divided his TB patients into two groups. The medication-only group would receive the necessary treatment for TB, but the medication plus services group would receive the medicine in addition to regular visits from community health workers and cash stipends for childcare and for travel by public transport to the nearest village. Dr. Farmer interviewed all of his patients at the beginning of the study and again one year later. Farmer found that few patients in either group admitted believing that TB was sent to them from an enemy via sorcery. In spite of their denials, Dr. Farmer's results suggested otherwise. One year after beginning the study, less than half (48%) of the medication-only group was cured of TB. By comparison, all of the patients who received medication plus extra services had fully recovered (Kidder, 2003).

As part of the one-year follow-up, Dr. Farmer asked his patients their views on the origins of their disease. He revisited one woman in the medication-plus-services group who, the previous year, seemed offended at his question about her beliefs in the origin of diseases. At the time, she stated that she knew that TB came from "people coughing germs" (Kidder, 2003, p. 35). But one year later, the same woman, now fully recovered from TB, admitted that she knew who sent her the sickness. She vowed revenge on the person.

Realizing that the woman was admitting that she believed in sorcery as a source of the disease, Dr. Farmer asked why she used the medicine to combat TB. The woman's response illustrates the duality of medical science and spirituality in Haiti and, ironically, in the U.S. In Haitian Creole, she responded, "*Cheri . . . eske-w pa ka kom prann bagay ki pa senp?*" (Kidder, 2003, p. 35). Translated, the woman asked Dr. Farmer, "Honey, are you incapable of complexity?"

The woman's question reminded Dr. Farmer of himself and others he knew in the U.S. who held similar complex views on faith and medicine. In fact, there are many examples of such complexities in modern medicine. Chapels in hospitals and chaplains in medical centers are but two examples of the complex relationship between faith and health in modern cultures. Many individuals who seek treatment from health care providers in hospitals also call on their faith, an act that demonstrates their values and belief structures, to guide medical staff and to speed healing and recovery.

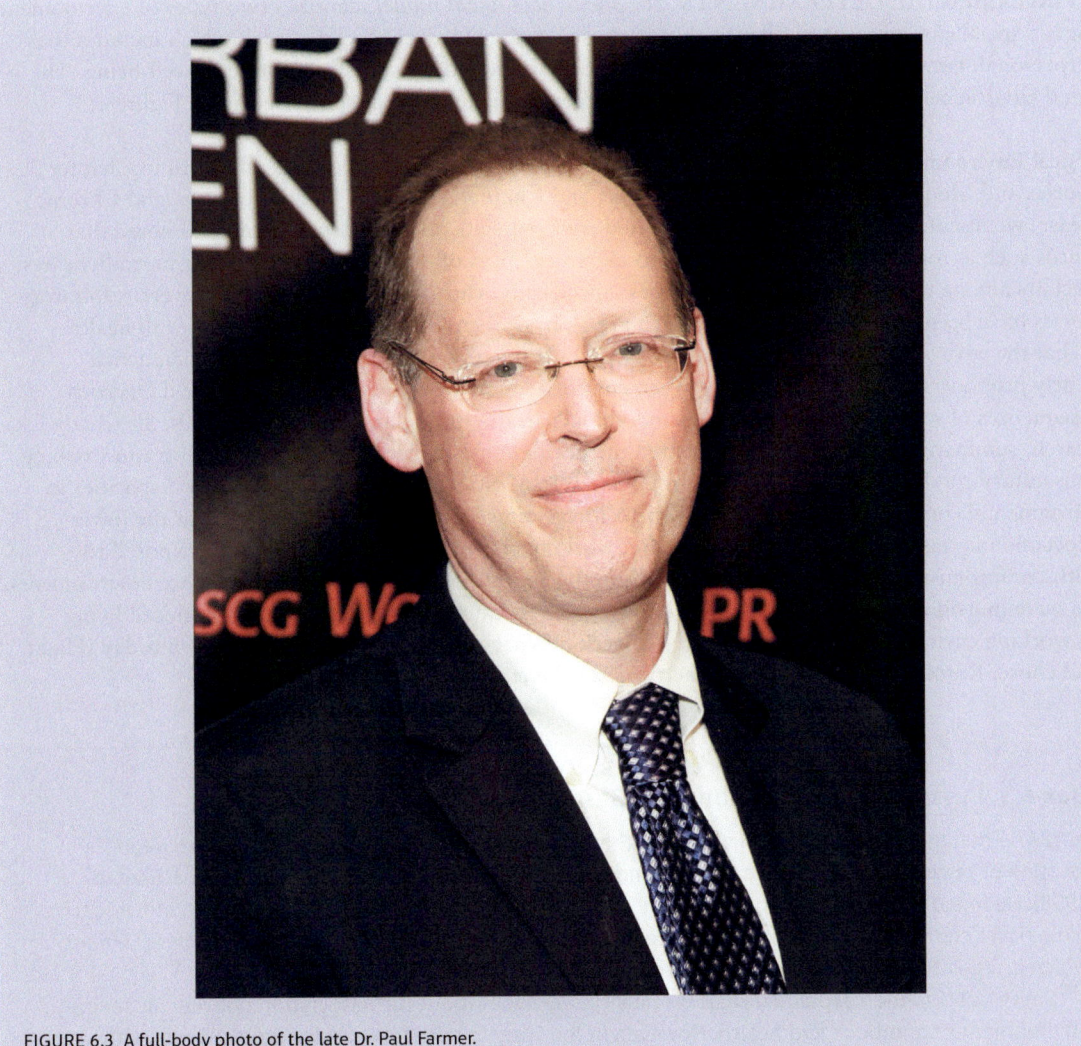

FIGURE 6.3 A full-body photo of the late Dr. Paul Farmer.

Source: UNICEF (2008)/Charles Eshelman via Getty Images.

Social Ecological Model

The biopsychosocial model proposes that biological, psychological, and social factors contribute to overall well-being. The wellness model includes two additional dimensions, perceived quality of life and spiritual health, as essential to overall well-being. Because we have explored the biological, psychological, emotional, and social environmental determinants of health in the previous models, here we focus on three determinants unique to the *social ecological model*: physical and social environments, health systems, and health policy.

ENVIRONMENTAL DETERMINANTS The *social ecological model* identifies two types of environments. First is a social environment, similar to that proposed in the biopsychosocial model, which includes the interpersonal, familial, and cultural factors that affect an individual's emotional state of well-being. The second environment is a physical space and the perceived quality of that space (see again Figure 1.3).

Physical Environmental Determinants When exploring environmental influences on health in Chapter 3, Theories and Models of Health Behavior Change, and Chapter 4, Global, Communicable, and Chronic Disease, we discussed the effects of contaminated environments on overall well-being. We noted that hazards such as toxic waste sites contribute to high incidences of diseases and high infant mortality rates, especially among the poor and working classes. Specifically, we noted that cancers and severe respiratory illnesses have been linked to these sites, which are a physical environmental determinant of ill health.

That the environment can impact health outcomes is not a new discovery. Sir Edwin Chadwick, an early proponent of the association between environment and health, demonstrated the dangerous consequences of some environments on an individual's health in England in the mid-1800s. Sir Chadwick's research, summarized in Box 6.3, documented the health consequences of individuals living and working in unsanitary conditions in urban and rural England. In addition, Chadwick showed that disparities in environmental conditions are correlated with socioeconomic status. He demonstrated that the lower socioeconomic classes, specifically the poor and working classes, were more likely to be exposed to health-compromising environmental conditions in their neighborhoods and their workplace environments, than were individuals in the higher socioeconomic classes. Unfortunately, health-compromised living and working environments for people in the lower SECs are present in most countries even today (Hajat, MacLehose, Rosofsky, Walker, & Clougherty, 2021; Ye et al., 2023).

Box 6.3 Environment, Socioeconomic Class, and Health

In 1847, Thomas Southwood Smith observed that there was an interesting relationship between the location of sewers on a city map in London and the outbreak of fevers in the city (Hamlin & Sheard, 1998). He found what we would probably call a significant correlation between fevers – an individual or biological determinant of health – and the existence of sewers, an environmental health determinant, which is regulated by health policy decisions.

Smith's observation explained what we now clearly know about the association between unsanitary environmental conditions and health. However, in the early to mid-1800s, this argument met with sharp resistance.

Sir Edwin Chadwick, a devout public health advocate, encountered similar resistance when he observed a related phenomenon. Concerned about the living conditions of the working class and the effects of these conditions on their health, Sir Edwin lobbied the English legislative bodies to examine the public health conditions of the poor and working classes in England. In 1832, England was preparing to revisit the Poor Laws, a set of laws designed to provide equitable assistance to the poor to help improve their standard of living. Chadwick was convinced, however, that no significant improvements could be made unless one also addressed the health status and living conditions of the working class.

To this end, Chadwick conducted a survey of adult and infant death rates of the three principal classes in Great Britain in the mid-1800s: the gentry (landowners, aristocrats, and professionals), tradesmen (shopkeepers), and finally the wage-earning working class. He summarized his findings in a report titled *Report from the Poor Law Commissions on an Inquiry into the Sanitary Conditions of the Labouring [Working] Population of Great Britain* (Chadwick, 1842). Two important statistics included in the survey were a comparison of the mortality rates for adults in three socioeconomic classes and infant death rates among these same three classes, as shown in the table.

Adult Mortality and Infant Death Rates, England, 1842

	Mean Age of Death		Infant Deaths
Class	Urban (London)	Rural (Countryside)	Per 1,000 Births
Gentry/professional	44 years	35 years	100 deaths
Tradesmen/shopkeepers	23 years	22 years	167 deaths
Wage/working class	22 years	15 years	250 deaths

The statistics supported Chadwick's hypothesis: The living and working conditions of the three classes explained much of the disparity in mortality statistics. The English wage and working classes in the 1840s could expect, on average, to live only half as long as individuals in the gentry class. In addition, babies born to parents in the laboring classes were 2.5 times more likely to die before age five than infants born to parents in the gentry or aristocratic classes.

Chadwick argued that the wage-earning and laboring classes lived in the most unsanitary conditions and were exposed to the harshest work environments. He believed that these conditions directly contributed to unusually high early adult mortality and high infant mortality rates.

Using these statistics, Sir Edwin convinced the English legislature to pass the Public Health Act and Nuisance Removal and Disease Prevention Act of 1848. Unsatisfied with the weak content of the act, Chadwick continued to advocate for better health conditions for the laboring class.

Both the social ecological model and Chadwick's work identifies the hazardous effects of some physical environments on well-being. In England in the 1800s, many neighborhoods were without sewer or drainage systems. The lack of adequate waste disposal systems (an environmental determinant) resulted in polluted water systems and soiled streets, footpaths, and grounds. Waste disposal systems are usually the purview of municipal or regional governments and are indicative of the health policies of that region. But it is also important to point out that in this case, the water systems were contaminated by waste products generated by individuals and businesses. Thus, individuals also contributed to the environmental hazard.

Health Systems and Health Policy Another unique aspect of the social ecological model is its inclusion of health systems and health policy – specifically the agencies and regulations, respectively – that define the structure of health care and that regulate its services. Both are included as distinct determinants of health outcomes.

As we noted earlier, Thomas Southward Smith found that the absence of sewers and drainage systems in England in the 1830s and 1840s – a health policy decision – was correlated with the frequency of high fevers among residents. Smith's finding is consistent with Chadwick's work, which also attests to the relationship between the physical environmental conditions in poor neighborhoods and the poor health outcomes of its inhabitants. Both Chadwick and Smith understood that health policy initiatives could influence health status and could either enhance or impair the health outcomes of poorer citizens. Their work supports the role of policy as a determinant of health (Gee & Payne-Sturges, 2004).

Consider, also, a current example of a policy issue in the U.S. that had and continues to have a disastrous impact on individual health; the widely publicized Flint water crisis in Flint, Michigan. As we explain in Box 6.4, city officials failed to adequately treat water pipes when changing the city's water sources. The impact of this significant omission will have long-term impacts on the health of the city's residents.

Box 6.4 The Saga of Flint, Michigan

In 2012–2013, the city of Flint, Michigan, sought alternative sources of water that would be less expensive for the city. No crime there. In fact, many would consider such efforts an example of good fiscal policy. So, what was the problem? The issue was that the city of Flint had to build a pipeline to the new water source. So, to save money while the pipeline construction was underway, Flint city officials identified an interim source of water from the Flint River and accessed this water on April 25, 2014, for an interim period projected to last approximately one year (Kennedy, 2016). So, again, what was the problem?

The problem was that the city of Flint failed to treat the new source of water to minimize likely corrosion of the water pipes, a standard procedure when changing water sources. Instead, they opted to take a "wait-and-see" approach (Kennedy, 2016), perhaps hoping that the added expense of treating the water would not be necessary. The result: shortly after the switch, residents of Flint, a low-income city with a majority (56%) African American population, began complaining about the smell emanating from the water and the peculiar color. In August of 2014, *E. coli* bacteria was detected in the water and residents were advised to boil the water before using. The city also increased chlorine levels to address the problem (Kennedy, 2016; See Chapter 2, Research Methods, for the dangers of *E. coli* bacteria). That, however, was the least of the problems.

In February 2015, high levels of lead were detected in the water. In fact, a lead levels test conducted by Virginia Technical Institute (VTI) reported lead levels of 13,500 parts per billion. Lead levels of 5,000 parts per billion is considered hazardous to human health (Kennedy, 2016). The actions afterwards by Flint officials were a mix of denial and cover-up until additional tests by VTI challenged the city's own testing results, noting that VTI's findings characterized the worst water lead levels that they have seen in 25 years (Kennedy, 2016). Additionally, Hurley Medical Center found a twofold increase in the number of children under five years of age with elevated blood lead levels (Kennedy, 2016).

It would be wonderful if, now nine years later, it was possible to report that all is well in Flint, but that is not the case. Once consumed, the effects of lead on the body can have long-lasting impacts. For example, ingesting lead through drinking water has been shown to depress children's growth and cognitive functioning in addition to increasing the risk of mental illnesses such as bipolar and post-traumatic stress disorder (PTSD) in adults (Aschengrau et al., 2012; Cuthbertson, Newkirk, Ilardo, Loveridge, & Skidmore, 2016; Wang et al., 2007).

One last point. Contaminated drinking water and its ill effects is not a regional problem. As illustrated in Chapter 4 Global, Communicable, and Chronic Disease, many countries, including the U.S., struggle with access to safe, clean drinking water. Through its work on drinking-water quality safety, the World Health Organization has demonstrated that worldwide, arsenic, fluoride, lead, nitrate, selenium, and uranium, among other chemicals, are responsible for "large-scale health effects" (World Health Organization, 2011e). They add that interventions, here meaning policy interventions, which improve the quality of drinking water can and do result in significant benefits to health.

Psychological Environment and Health Environment can also be defined as the quality of an individual's physical space as determined by psychosocial variables. For example, overcrowded neighborhoods or communities with high crime rates are psychosocial variables that influence the quality of life and overall well-being.

In Chapter 5, Risky Health Behaviors, we explained how a neighborhood's high crime rate can affect one's health even if an individual is not a victim. For example, people who perceive that their neighborhood is less safe due to crime will be less likely to engage in outdoor exercise in their community. Limited access to exercise will have a direct impact on well-being.

There is another way in which high crime rates can affect emotional health. Consider this: Residents in high-crime neighborhoods may be more anxious about leaving or returning home at night and more apt to listen for threatening sounds from the street while at home. Increased anxiety or greater emotional distress about one's safety or the safety of one's family, even when "safely" at home, may have long-term consequences for well-being. We briefly described the effects of stress on well-being in the previous section and explored the issue more fully in Chapter 7, Stress and Coping.

Workplace Environments as Determinants of Emotional Health Overcrowding and crime are tangible environmental factors that affect psychological health. Yet psychological factors in the environment that also impact health outcomes can be subtle. One example is the effect of the workplace on individuals' physiological or emotional health. Kawano (2008) conducted a study among nurses in Japan to determine whether working in special medical service units, such as the operating room, intensive care units, and surgical or internal medicine units, caused higher levels of emotional distress or physical fatigue among the nurses. The results showed that, in fact, nurses in each of the three special units experienced higher levels of emotional distress than their colleagues in non-specialty units. Nurses working in operating rooms reported higher levels of fatigue, whereas their colleagues in the intensive care units (units that care for patients with critical medical needs) reported higher levels of anxiety. Finally, nurses in surgical or internal medicine units reported higher levels of depression.

These are interesting results, to be sure. But why should one type of medical service cause more fatigue or emotional stress than another? The answer may be clear when we consider what is at stake. The work performed by nurses is vital to returning a patient to a state of overall well-being. In settings like the operating room or in critical care units, unintentional mistakes can seriously impair a patient's health or even contribute to death, a weighty responsibility for any caregiver. Perhaps, then, nurses' higher levels of anxiety or depression reflect their concern about the consequences of an error, the potential for loss of life, and the likely emotional cost borne by them if they were responsible for a mistake resulting in the death of a patient.

Summary

To review, the definition of health has evolved over the past several centuries. The discovery of microorganisms and their role in causing illnesses led Western scientists to focus on the physiological or biological causes of illness and to define health as the absence of disease, as represented by the biomedical view of health. Now, new definitions have led to a shift from the biomedical perspective to a more holistic view of health similar to that espoused by earlier cultures.

Health psychologists, medical sociologists, and public health experts currently argue for a broader definition of health, best conceptualized as overall well-being. The biopsychosocial model was one of the first models to expand the definition of health by adding social and psychological factors to the concept of well-being. The wellness model contributed a spiritual dimension to well-being and redefined wellness as an individual's own assessment of their quality of life, whereas the social ecological model adds the physical environmental determinants and the role of health systems and health policy on individual health outcomes.

In essence, concepts of health and well-being in Western cultures have shifted over time, beginning with the concept of well-being as a mind–body connection, moving to a physiologically based determinant of health, only to return once again to a view of health as a holistic or ecological concept. Still, some health psychologists contend that the definition of well-being is incomplete. Some advocate for a need to examine the positive as well as the negative aspects of well-being in order to provide a balanced perspective of wellness.

SECTION II. POSITIVE PSYCHOLOGY

Positive psychology seems like an odd-sounding "pop psychology" name for a theory. As such, it may be tempting to dismiss the concept as trendy. But, as you will see, it is neither new nor trendy. Positive psychology builds on the wellness model of health and is, according to Seligman (2002), a more complete and balanced perspective of the human experience (Seligman, Steen, Park, & Peterson, 2000). Specifically, positive psychology involves a systematic study of the factors that enhance and maintain an individual's state of well-being.

Defining Positive Psychology

Martin Seligman and Mihaly Csikszentmihalyi (2000) pioneered the concept of positive psychology. In their view, much of psychology focused on issues of mental illness, damage, or dysfunction (Seligman, 2002). According to some, Seligman suggests that psychology's focus on mental illness positioned it as a science of pathology and weakness rather than a science of health, well-being, and strength (Held, 2005).

Consequently, Seligman and Csikszentmihalyi (2000) proposed to correct what they characterized as an imbalance in the field by identifying and explaining the factors that lead to overall well-being, thriving communities, and satisfied individuals and families (Seligman & Csikszentmihalyi, 2000; Seligman, 2019). Seligman, Park, and Peterson (2004) and Peterson and Seligman (2004) proposed that six "virtues," along with 24 signature character strengths (see Table 6.2 and Box 6.5) that represent positive traits, contribute to life satisfaction and a more meaningful life (Park, Peterson, & Seligman, 2004).

Positive versus Negative Psychology?

For some, the term *positive psychology* implies that there is also a "negative psychology." Most likely, Seligman's characterization of some fields as "negative social science and psychology" created the dichotomy that fueled the debate (Held, 2005). Indeed, few would choose to be associated with a discipline

TABLE 6.2 Five Character Strengths Most Strongly Correlated with Life Satisfaction

Strength	Description
Hope	Optimism, future-mindedness, future orientation: Expecting the best in the future and working to achieve it; believing that a good future is something that can be brought about
Zest	Vitality, enthusiasm, vigor, energy: Approaching life with excitement and energy; not doing things halfway or halfheartedly; living life as an adventure; feeling alive and activated
Gratitude	Being aware of and thankful for the good things that happen; taking time to express thanks
Curiosity	Interest, novelty-seeking, openness to experiences: Taking an interest in all ongoing experiences; finding all subjects and topics fascinating; exploring and discovering
Love	Valuing close relationships with others, in particular those in which sharing and caring are reciprocated; being close to people

within psychology, or any field for that matter, which is characterized as "negative." Although Seligman later rephrased his criticism of other disciplines of psychology in terms that are less stigmatizing, the comparison between positive psychology and other areas within the field continues to cause conflicts about the role and relative contribution of – even the need for – positive psychology as its own discipline.

Box 6.5 Seligman's Classification of Character Strengths

Seligman suggests that individuals who strive to achieve six universal virtues, here meaning virtues found in many cultures, religions, and philosophical traditions, and 24 strengths will live a more fulfilled and happy life. The positive effects that result from a happier and more fulfilled life will lead to a greater likelihood of positive, healthy outcomes and overall well-being.

In essence, for Seligman, positive psychology returns the field of psychology to its mission, which is to make normal people's lives more fulfilling and productive (Clay, 1977). His work seeks to understand the factors that contribute to such an outcome. Thus, positive psychology moves away from the biomedical concept of health, which focuses on identifying, isolating, and repairing problems, to a more holistic or ecological perspective regarding human potentials, motives, and capacities but one that explains the positive and negative contributions to overall well-being (Seligman & Csikszentmihalyi, 2000; Sheldon & King, 2001).

It would be easy to become enmeshed in a war of words in the characterization of some areas of psychology as positive or negative. But to do so would miss the principal intent of positive psychology, which is to seek and discover an optimal balance between "positive" and "negative" thinking (Seligman, 2002) and to understand psychological phenomena in their totality (Carstensen & Charles, 2003). In other words, positive and negative influences contribute to the outcomes, states, emotions, and health of individuals. To understand an individual's end state, we need to examine both.

Positive Psychology and Health

After more than 60 years of research using a "disease" model approach to health, Seligman contends that we really are no better at actually preventing negative psychological outcomes or damage than we were when the research began. Rather, he contends that the most effective way to prevent illnesses is to focus on the positive goals of building competencies and on the reinforcing factors that prevent negative events from occurring (Seligman & Csikszentmihalyi, 2000; Seligman, 2019). In this way, positive psychology may be of particular importance to the field of health psychology because it may facilitate a transition from the biopsychosocial to the social ecological approach by examining the multiple contributions, both positive and negative, to well-being.

What are the factors that help build healthier, satisfied, and thriving individuals and communities? According to current studies, personal traits such as an individual's subjective sense of well-being, optimism, happiness, self-determination, and positive emotional states contribute to positive psychology and well-being (Diener, 2000; Diener, Pressman, Hunter, & Delgadillo-Chase, 2017; Ryan & Deci, 2000; Taylor, Kemeny, Reed, Bower, & Gruenewald, 2000; Tenney, Poole, & Diener, 2016). Like all individuals, thriving and happy people exist in a social context that includes other people, places, and institutions. Therefore, positive psychological states are influenced also by social and environmental factors that include interpersonal relationships, social networks (Cohen, 2004; Ray, 2004; Taylor & Turner, 2001), religion and religious faith (Myers, 2000), engagement with others, accomplishments (Seligman, 2019), and external factors, including socioeconomic status (Coburn, 2004).

How do we know that positive psychological states also contribute to our well-being? Well, in addition to the research we presented earlier in this chapter on positive affect, health-enhancing behaviors and well-being, consider for a moment the research on *optimism*, here meaning the view that situations and events will work out for the best, however *best* is defined. Studies on the effect of optimism among cancer patients, for example, have found an association between optimism and better psychological and social adjustment to their illness (Lechner, Carver, Antoni, Weaver, & Phillips, 2006). Researchers have also found that patients who reported higher levels of optimism also reported lower levels of depression or anxiety about the illness (Schnoll, Knowles, & Harlow, 2002). What is more, some cancer patients with an optimistic perspective also believe that they can influence their situation and thereby achieve a better outcome (Balasooriya-Smeekens et al., 2015; Folkman & Greer, 2002; Lee et al., 2008). If optimism has a direct effect on emotional health, and if positive emotional health can directly influence our physiological states, then we may be correct in concluding that positive psychological perspectives indirectly enhance health.

 VIDEO #34/60

Chapter 6: Emotional Health and Well-Being

- **Optimism:** *Mayo Clinic Minute: How optimism improves your health*
- *Website: https://www.youtube.com/watch?v=kYSTcwbz7Qk*
- *Mayo Clinic is publicly accessible since it provides medical-based information to the public at no cost (www.mayoclinic.org/)*

Other studies in the field of behavioral medicine also demonstrate the health benefits obtained from a positive, optimistic state. Ironson and Hayward (2008) and Ironson, Stuetzle, and Fletcher (2006) suggest that optimism, together with active coping strategies and spirituality, predicts a slower progression of HIV disease in HIV-positive individuals. A slower progression of HIV may delay the onset of symptoms associated with the illness as well as slow the debilitating effects of the disease itself. Diener and Chan's 2011 study which suggests that happiness helps to boost the immune system may provide partial explanation for such findings.

The main point of positive psychology is that we understand only part of our human nature if we focus exclusively on pathology, disorder, or dysfunction. To understand the full human experience and how to make people's lives more fulfilling and satisfying, we need to study the "normal," positive, and productive state of human functioning as well as the disordered or damaged states. As we will see in the following section, for followers of traditional and complementary or alternative medicine, an understanding of the positive or normal state is also integral to their health beliefs and practices.

Critiques of Positive Psychology

In principle, positive psychology aims to present a more balanced view of the factors that affect outcomes. There are, however, criticisms of the concept. Seligman (2019) identifies a few criticisms but misses two that appear more robust: the "happiness" approach and the universality of the concept.

HAPPINESS PSYCHOLOGY Remember our earlier caution of not becoming embroiled in a war of words? Some researchers argue that the principal focus of positive psychology is to study what makes people happy. When stated in this fashion, positive psychology seems insubstantial. Yet recent research by Perez-Alvarez (2016) and earlier work by Held (2002) suggests that this critique involves more than just a war a words. They question whether there are more important values than striving for happiness (Perez-Alvarez, 2016). Held (2002) goes further by questioning whether a positive attitude is really necessary to achieve an overall sense of well-being. He asks whether accentuating the positive and eliminating the negative is really beneficial for one's overall physical and mental health. These questions appear to target core components of the theory that must be addressed.

When, however, looking more broadly, the concept of "happiness" also includes research to understand gratitude, forgiveness, awe, inspiration, hope, curiosity, and laughter (Gable & Haidt, 2005; Seligman, 2019). The work of the Truth and Reconciliation Commission in South Africa is one international example of an application of positive psychology in its broadest, and perhaps most applied, sense (see Box 6.6 and Figure 6.4).

Box 6.6 The South African Truth and Reconciliation Commission: Forgiveness in Post-Apartheid South Africa

The full scope of the atrocities committed under the apartheid government in South Africa may never be known. **Apartheid**, a social and political policy of racial segregation enforced by the government of South Africa, was finally dismantled in 1992, but not before tens of thousands of South Africans were killed or severely tortured to protect the apartheid system.

Following decades of forced segregation, forced removals from homes and communities, and restrictions on employment and even on education, South Africa's black, colored, and Indian citizens finally won the opportunity to live without the imposition of socially unjust rules instituted under apartheid. As they embarked on the job of forming a new, democratic government, the country faced the daunting task of healing a nation riddled for decades with the racial animus caused by the apartheid system. Central to that task was finding a way to help foster forgiveness between the races.

South Africa's Truth and Reconciliation Commission was charged with the responsibility of discovering the truth about the thousands of atrocities committed during apartheid while simultaneously moving the country forward in peace. The now late Archbishop Desmond Tutu, the first black Anglican archbishop in South Africa, headed the commission (see Figure 6.4). With his leadership, the commission pioneered a model by which perpetrators of violence and torture could face their victims and their families. By truthfully confessing their crimes, the guilty could seek forgiveness from their victims, and family members of victims could learn the truth about the brutal torture or murder of their loved ones, again from the confessions of the perpetrators of the acts. The act of public confession and contrition was seen as one way to begin the healing process that could allow South Africa's diverse racial groups to survive and to thrive as a nation (Gobodo-Madikizela, 2002, 2003). It was one way to begin to repair the emotional and psychological damage experienced by the nation.

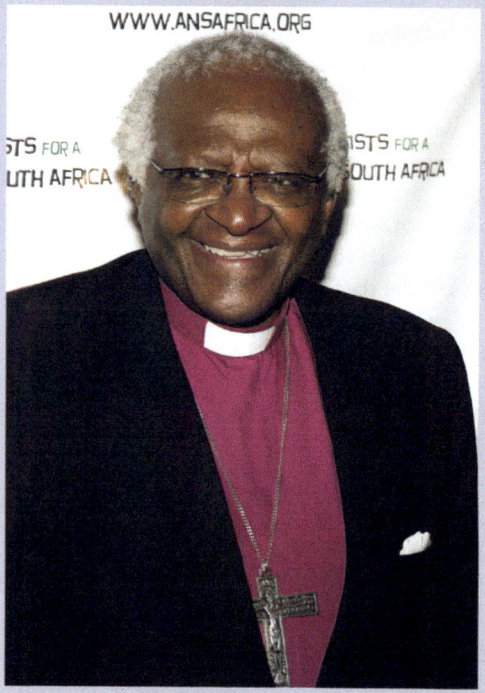

FIGURE 6.4 A headshot photo of the late Archbishop Desmond Tutu, the Chair of South Africa's Truth and Reconciliation Commission. He helped guide South Africans through the Truth and Reconciliation Process in an effort to heal the nation.

Source: Paul Chiasson/Associated Press.

Widely acclaimed as one of the factors that aided South Africa's peaceful transition and positive development in the aftermath of apartheid, the Truth and Reconciliation Commission's approach to conflict resolution and healing has been praised and emulated around the world (Philpott, 2009). More importantly, it was integral to forging a new relationship among ethnic groups that would allow the citizens of South Africa to forgive the atrocities of the past and inspire them to work toward building a stronger and more unified country. Between 1974 and 2010, 40 countries have established truth and reconciliation commissions in order to unearth the truth about atrocities committed in their countries and work towards restorative justice if possible (Amnesty International, 2010). This work seems consistent with Seligman's theme of forgiveness in his positive psychology model.

If positive psychology is defined simply as what makes people happy, it would seem to have limited application to the work in health psychology. The broader implications of "happiness," as seen through the research and work on forgiveness, would support a central role for this field, one that contributes to our understanding of health-enhancing behaviors.

UNIVERSALITY OF POSITIVE PSYCHOLOGY A more compelling criticism of the field is that the new discipline may not be applicable to some people or cultures in spite of its claims of being a universal phenomenon (Aspinwall & Staudinger, 2003). As Diener and Suh (2000) note, in North American cultures there is a strong psychological pressure to be happy. In fact, Diener and Suh characterize it as an inviolable individual right, particularly in cultures with strong beliefs in individualism and self-determination. Critics argue that if, as in some cultures, there is no universal belief in the right of individual happiness then, by definition, positive psychology may not be universal.

The applicability of positive psychology is also challenged when concepts that are interpreted as positive or that elicit positive connotations in one culture have both negative and positive meanings in another. Take, for example, the concept of "sympathy." In Western cultures, sympathy is a positive emotion suggesting the ability to understand another's position. It is one of several strengths that lead to the six virtues identified by Seligman. In Chinese culture, sympathy also has a distinctly negative connotation, meaning to commiserate with or to have sympathy with someone's misfortune (Sundararajan, 2005). Thus, a positive concept in one culture can be linked to both positive and negative concepts in another. The point here is that the notion that positive characteristics are universally seen as positive in all cultures can be easily challenged by examining the understood meaning of words across cultures.

What is more, Confucianism, an Eastern philosophy that emphasizes human morality and moral development of the individual, proposes that negative emotions play an important role in the development of virtue, the underpinnings of happiness and well-being, according to Seligman (Sundararajan, 2005). In other words, Eastern philosophy holds that negative emotions are critical for the full development of the individual. In defense, positive psychology does not deny the existence of negative emotions. But it appears that it fails to consider negative emotional development as integral to positive emotions and outcomes.

We close this section with observations about the role of *pessimism* as an adaptive, and hence positive, approach to select issues or problems. In fact, some contend that pessimism may work to promote problem-solving (Aspinwall & Staudinger, 2003). They note specifically that *defensive pessimism*, a coping strategy that keeps disappointments and expectations in check (Norem, 2001), may be adaptive when responding to negative outcomes. For example, some research suggests that students high in defensive pessimism can enjoy good outcomes more because they are unexpected. Conversely, bad outcomes are not as distressing because they were expected (Gibbons, 2023). Interestingly, this tendency to embrace defensive pessimism does not, according to Gibbons, negatively impact the motivation to learn by students who have been performing well academically (Gibbons, 2022).

Finally, in a current study examining U.K. undergraduate students' stress, coping, course satisfaction, and motivation to learn, defensive pessimism strongly predicted low levels of anxiety among these students (Gibbons, 2023). Thus, defensive pessimism may serve as a coping mechanism when confronting challenging or stress-inducing situations.

One other point. Defensive pessimism may be a particularly advantageous emotion for disenfranchised groups in societies. For such groups, defensive pessimism may help, albeit nominally, to cope with frequent encounters of disappointments and rejections caused, in part, by that group's status in society. For example, minority groups that experience discrimination based on their ethnicity may employ defensive pessimism when involved in social or work settings in the majority culture to minimize the adverse effects of exclusion or other forms of rejection.

And, in an era where older persons worry about aging, other studies have found that when examining older (72- to 98-year-old) persons' optimistic versus pessimistic expectations about their declining health, there was a 313% higher chance of death among those with overly optimistic and unrealistic expectations about their health outcomes (Chipperfield et al., 2019). Those older adults who were what the authors called "realistically pessimistic," as opposed to unrealistically optimistic, evidenced not just a lower risk of death but also fewer depressive symptoms.

Therefore, although Seligman believes that pessimism is maladaptive (Held, 2005), recent studies suggest that it may be an effective method of coping in a number of different situations and for several different populations.

Does positive psychology contribute to our understanding of emotional health? It would seem so, in spite of its limitations. No single model or theory will contain all the elements needed to explain behaviors or outcomes. As we indicated in Chapter 3, Theories and Models of Health Behavior Change, models often borrow concepts to build stronger models. Positive psychology could be an important contribution to existing theories, reminding us that to understand the full spectrum of human behavior we need to identify all determinants that impact well-being.

SECTION III. TRADITIONAL MEDICINES

Models of health developed by modern societies have identified biology, sociology, psychology, emotion, environments, health systems, and health policy as integral to individual well-being. These same factors have also been identified and used in traditional medicines.

According to the World Health Organization (2019b, p. 8), *Traditional medicine* is defined as

the sum total of the knowledge, skill and practices based on the theories, beliefs and experiences indigenous to different cultures, whether explicable or not, used in the maintenance of health as well as in the prevention, diagnosis, improvement or treatment of physical and mental illness.

In a recent speech at the WHO's Traditional Medicine Global Summit, Dr. Tedros Adhanom Ghebreyesus, the WHO's Director-General, confirmed what many already know; traditional medicine is "as old as humanity itself," has a very long history, and is facing a growing demand throughout the world (Ghebreyesus, 2023). As of 2015, traditional medicines were being used by approximately 60% of the world's population (World Health Organization, 2015).

Most traditional medicines share four core principles: a belief in a connection among the individual, the Earth, and a life or energy force; a belief that a person's state of health reflects a balance or harmony of those three connected elements; a belief that treatment for a health problem involves the whole individual (physical, emotional or mental, and spiritual); and a belief in the use of herbal remedies or other practices such as ritual chants, acupuncture, bone setting, or smudging (that is, using smoke from burning herbs to cleanse negative energies around a person; Broome & Broome, 2007; Lam, 2001).

A recent survey conducted by the WHO (2019b) revealed that 170 countries have developed policies, laws, regulations and programs for the use of traditional and *complementary* medicine in their countries. In fact, even the World Trade Organization, an intergovernmental organization that regulates the global rules of trade between nations, recognizes the vital role played by traditional medicines. They note that

> traditional medicine contributes significantly to the health status of many communities and is increasingly used within certain communities in developed countries. Appropriate recognition of traditional medicine is an important element of national health policy.
>
> (World Trade Organization, 2023)

Examples of the critical roles played by traditional medicine can be found in many countries. For example, the South African government integrated the *sangomas*, indigenous healers used by many rural South Africans, into the nation's health care system (Africa First, 2008; International on Line, 2004; World Health Organization, 2003). Now South Africans can choose to receive care from either a Western-trained medical doctor or a *sangoma* and have the cost of care paid for or supplemented by the nation's health care system.

It is important to state that the integration of traditional and Western health practices, as in the case of South Africa, only formalizes a long-standing practice of consulting both Western and traditional medicines. Remember Angelita from our opening story? She consulted a Western health professional but also accepted the assistance of a *curandero*, one type of traditional healer.

One reason people use both health approaches is that they believe that each addresses different health needs. A recent survey of a Malaysian community by Othman and Farooqui (2015) found that of 384 persons surveyed, the majority (almost 80%) reported using traditional or *complementary/ alternative* – here meaning alternative form of medicine not part of traditional or conventional – medicine alongside "conventional" medicines. Fundamentally, many believe that the combined use of traditional/ complementary medicines with conventional medicines will provide a better overall treatment of the disease. Additionally, more respondents (approximately 37%) credit family members or friends with encouraging them to use traditional/complementary medicines rather than other sources, and almost one-third (almost 34%) obtained their medicines from a traditional healer. From these and other studies we see that some people who use traditional or complementary medicines seek to maximize the advantages and minimize the disadvantages of each technique. Interestingly, even some health care providers report consulting both Western medicine and traditional healers for their own health care needs (Bucko & Cloud, 2008; Hon et al., 2005; Lam, 2001; Wong, Lee, Wong, Wu, & Robinson, 2006).

VIDEO #35/60

Chapter 6: Emotional Health and Well-Being
- **Alternative Medicine:** *Mayo Clinic Minute: Meditation is good medicine*
- **Website: https://www.youtube.com/watch?v=nE8MB3wM8Go**
- *Mayo Clinic is publicly accessible since it provides medical-based information to the public at no cost (www.mayoclinic.org)*

Contributions of Traditional Medicine

Would it surprise you to learn that approximately 40% of all pharmaceutical products come from nature and from the knowledge and practices of traditional healers? (World Health Organization, 2023q). This little-known fact is actually taught to children, although they may not be aware of the message at the time. Consider, for example, the Walt Disney movie *Pocahontas*. In the movie, Pocahontas, the daughter of the chief of the Powhatan nation, gives John Smith, an English settler, ground bark from a willow tree to ease his pain from a gunshot wound. The bark contains ***salicylic acid***, an ingredient that controls pain and reduces fever (University of Arkansas, Division of Agriculture, 2007). Native Americans used this natural ingredient. So did the Sumerians and Egyptians 3,500 years ago (World Health Organization, 2023q)! Pharmaceutical companies, the manufacturers of modern medicines, have developed a chemical equivalent of ground willow bark to relieve similar aches and pain. We call it ***aspirin***. Scientists learned to chemically reproduce the same ingredients found in the willow and to mass-produce it for general use.

Today, scientists continue to copy and reproduce for mass distribution the medicinal elements found in plants. Take, for example, the plant *Hoodia gordonii*. "Hoodia," as it is known in the U.S., is a natural plant found in southern Africa used for centuries by the *Sans* people, a nomadic group living in the Kalahari Desert of southern Africa. The Sans use *H. gordonii* to suppress appetite. You may wonder why a nomadic group would want to suppress their appetites. Simply put, the Sans hunt for their food. A hunt for a wildebeest or eland large enough for the needs of the tribe may take several days and may require hunters to be mobile. *H. gordonii* helps the Sans sustain their energy while hunting and minimize hunger so they do not become distracted or too weak to hunt. Like the willow bark, the agents found in *H. gordonii* have been recently chemically reproduced by U.S. pharmaceutical companies and have been sold in the U.S. as "P57," a diet supplement for people who want to lose weight.

Salicylic acid and *H. gordonii* are just two examples, past and recent, of contributions to modern medicine from traditional medical practices. There are many, many more. In the following sections, we explore Chinese traditional medicine (CTM), *curanderismo* (the Mexican folk-healing practice introduced in the opening story), and Native American healing practices – three of the most widely recognized examples of traditional medicines in other cultures. We review them briefly to explore their similarities to and differences with Western medicine practices. Keep in mind, however, that the traditional practices included are a small sample of the total number of such practices, even today.

Chinese Traditional Medicine (CTM)

Chinese traditional medicine (CTM), sometimes referred to as *traditional Chinese medicine (TCM)*, is similar to other folk medicines because it is rooted in the philosophy and the belief structure of its culture. As explained in Box 6.7, CTM consists of three main structures that, together with Chinese philosophy and nature, define an individual's well-being: yin and yang, the five elements, and Qi (pronounced ch'i).

Box 6.7 Traditional Medicines: An Overview

Chinese Traditional Medicine (CTM)

Yin and yang, the five elements, and Qi are the three principal structures of CTM. **Yin** is associated with passive, life-sustaining, conserving energies or latent energies that need to be actualized (Kapke, 2004; Quah, 2003). Yin energies are often associated with darkness and cold (passive, conserving energies) as well as water and females (sustaining forces). With respect to the body, yin is associated with specific organs: the heart, liver, pancreas, kidneys, and lungs. Thus, the yin organs are vital to sustaining life.

In comparison, **yang** energy forces are described as strong forces that cause change. They are dynamic forces that initiate action. The yang forces are usually characterized as male, consistent with the notion of males as active, assertive, or aggressive (Kapke, 2004). Thus, they are associated with light, fire, and heat – all active and potentially destructive forces. In the body, yang is associated with the gallbladder, small and large intestines, and the urinary bladder, which are organs that transmit, transform, and eliminate nonessential items from the body (Kapke, 2004). According to CTM, our health is optimal when yin and yang forces are in perfect balance. When one or the other is out of balance, however, diseases or other ailments may be present. For example, when yin is out of balance for females, a number of symptoms could appear, including irregular menstrual cycles, irritability, early menopause, or other related problems (D'Alberto, 2006).

The five elements – metal, wood, water, fire, and earth – demonstrate the relationship between human beings and nature. Specifically, these structures emphasize the role of harmony between humans and nature and their effect on well-being. Each element has both yin and yang components. For example, water evidences yin properties when it is cool and nourishing. But water also demonstrates yang energy force when it is destructive. Consider this: In a flood, objects in the path of the rushing water can be dislodged, moved, or destroyed by the pressure exerted (Kapke, 2004). Our interactions with the elements, according to CTM, will affect the balance of yin and yang in our bodies. For example, absorbing too much of the sun's rays will burn yin, the cold energy force, resulting in an imbalance and discomfort.

Finally, **Qi** is an energy source that flows throughout the body, similar to the body's circulatory system. The movement of Qi within the body is influenced by seasons and foods that help to facilitate or to impede its flow.

Curanderismo

Curanderos, or the traditional healers for this form of medicine, are believed to have special healing powers. It is a gift (*el don*), not something for which an individual receives formal training, as in Western medicine. Yet, most *curanderos* undergo a period of apprenticeship to learn to use their healing gifts.

Core to *curanderismo* is spirituality and maintaining harmony and balance with nature (Tafur, Crowe, & Torres, 2009). The central role of spirituality is evident in some of the more common illnesses addressed by the healers. These include *espanto*, an extreme fright believed to be caused by a supernatural force, and *susto*, a fright due to a traumatic experience (Lopez, 2005). Both illnesses are described as "soul loss" in *curanderismo* and require spiritual cures. Researchers note that *espanto* and *susto* often lead to emotional and psychological health problems, including depression, apathy, anorexia, and insomnia (Chesney et al., 2005). The spiritual causes attributed to what Western medicine considers mental health issues illustrate one contrast between traditional and Western views of health.

One similarity between *curanderismo* and Western medicine, however, is the presence of specialized practices within *curanderismo*. Like Western health practitioners, *curanderos* may be specialists. For example, herbalists (*yerberos*) focus on the treatment of physical health problems using natural herbs and homeopathic medicines. Thus, stomachaches may be treated with orange leaf tea (*citrus aurantium*), earaches with garlic (*allium sativum*), or sunburns with aloe vera. Illnesses of a spiritual or supernatural origin, however, such as *susto* or *mal de ojo*, the evil eye, would be treated by an *espiritista* who would perform a *limpia* or spiritual cleansing.

Native American Healing Practices

Native American healing traditions were crucial to the survival of the first wave of colonizers to what is now the U.S. In spite of this well-known history, it has taken several hundred years for researchers to document the Native American practices and knowledge of botany to heal both body and mind (Portman & Garrett, 2006).

Currently, there are over 500 Native American nations, so it is not possible to describe each nation's healing practices in detail. However, there are several core principles that apply to many Native American beliefs and practices. First, there are four constructs that are central to the healing traditions: spirituality, community, environment, and self. The core concepts of spirituality, environment, and life force are similar thematically to *curanderismo* and CTM. But as Trimble (2021) points out, spiritual beliefs are at the core of healing practices for indigenous people. This core concept which incorporates relationships with all living beings, is part of an oral tradition that dates back some 8,000 years (Trimble, 2021).

Unique to the Native American practices, however, is a belief in a "circle of life" and in the concept of medicine. The circle of life symbolizes power, peace, and unity (Portman & Garrett, 2006). Each individual holds responsibility for helping to contribute to the circle by living harmoniously with all living elements, and a person's own well-being is inseparable from this responsibility (Trimble, 2021).

What is more, Native American traditions contend that each person holds medicine within themselves. To be certain, Native Americans believe in the healing powers of plants and herbs (or external agents) for holistic health needs. But, as Locust (1985, as cited in Trimble, 2021) states:

> Native American Indians believe that each individual chooses to make himself well or to make himself unwell. If one stays in harmony, keeps all the tribal laws and the sacred laws, one's spirit will be so strong that negativity will be unable to affect it. Once harmony is broken, however, the spiritual self is weakened and one becomes vulnerable to physical illness, mental and/or emotional upsets, and the disharmony projected by others.

In essence, Trimble state, these spiritual beliefs should help individuals and communities to navigate their way back to the circle and a balance. This is not the case with Western medical practices which focus on a specific ill within the body, with less consideration as to whether the whole self is in balance (Trimble, 2021).

According to Chinese philosophers, the yin–yang doctrine explains that all things function in relation to two forces, elements, or principles (Quah, 2003). These forces are in a constant state of dynamic balance, continually interacting to maintain harmony. (Harmony is a core concept in Chinese life; Quah, 2003). Thus, yin and yang are complementary forces; each is needed to complete the other and to achieve and maintain harmony.

The second major structure in CTM is the *five elements:* metal, wood, water, fire, and earth. Each of the five elements is paired with a body organ and a season of the year, demonstrating the close connection between humans and nature. According to this philosophy, a person's health is dependent, in part, on his or her interactions with the physical environment.

The last structure, *Qi*, is a concept taken from Taoist philosophers. Qi is best understood as a substantial energy force that flows within the body, parallel to or as part of the circulation of the blood (Quah, 2003).

TREATING ILLNESSES USING CTM To individuals unfamiliar with Chinese medicine, the philosophy of three forces that work together to influence health may be clear in concept but not in practice. Consider this: Medical providers trained in CTM are taught to probe both the physiological as well as the psychological determinants of health. Thus, instead of searching only for a proximal physical cause of an illness, health providers will explore the relationship among the affected body parts, related areas, emotional states, and physical and social environmental factors to discover the source of the disharmony.

Examining relationships among body, emotions, and nature takes time. A complete exploration of the illness and its related causes may require multiple visits as the CTM provider delves into the patient's emotional health, relationships with others in his or her family, diet, and other aspects of his or her life that may not appear to be the source of the problem but may be related to the disturbance. In this way, the CTM healing process is similar to Angelita's experience with the *curandero* in the opening story.

A principal complaint of individuals who choose the CTM approach for health care is that the process takes longer than when using Western medical methods (Chung et al., 2014). Still, many prefer CTM for specific ills. Chung and colleagues' review of 28 quantitative and qualitative studies revealed that many believed that Western medicine is useful if seeking a quick recovery; however, they preferred CTM care when a quick, Western medical treatment proved ineffective in curing the disease (Chung et al., 2014).

Many individuals, with access to both forms of medicines, believe that there are additional strengths and weaknesses associated with both practices. Western medicine, in addition to being quicker, helps to rapidly control symptoms. When confronting contagious illnesses, Western medicine may be preferred for its ability to not only control the symptoms but also contain the spread of the disease. The disadvantages of Western medicine as Salmon (2022) and Sun and colleagues (2017) show, is that conventional medicines do not adequately address many chronic conditions.

Among users of both CTM and Western medicine, the advantages of CTM include a more effective cure for illnesses, fewer side effects, and a more effective treatment for chronic illnesses. Many prefer it as a treatment for the whole person (Chung et al., 2014; Hon et al., 2005; Wong et al., 2006). Finally, the fact that many users of CTM indicate that family and friends recommend the traditional method suggests that family tradition, culture, and sociological factors also influence the choice of medical approaches (Sun et al., 2017).

In essence, some users of CTM believe that Western medicine is the preferred approach when seeking a quick fix for a medical ailment but favor traditional medicines to treat longer-term, chronic illnesses. Consistent with Chinese philosophy, if illness represents more than just a physical disharmony, then the cure must address all elements, including the energy flow and the individual's interaction with the elements.

Curanderismo

The term *curanderismo* comes from the Spanish word *curar*, meaning to heal (Tafur et al., 2009). Like Chinese traditional medicine, *curanderismo* originated from cultural beliefs. In this case, the most immediate culture of origin is Mexican. However, anthropologists suggest that *curanderismo* has been influenced by the health beliefs and practices of the Greeks, the Moors (Arabs of northern Africa), the Aztec and Mayan empires (Krassner, 1986), sub-Saharan African medical practices (Luna, 2003), as well as a number of European and Native American cultures. Today, *curanderismo* is an umbrella term that refers to many types of treatments and rituals that, melded together over several centuries, represent a form of traditional healing commonly practiced in Mexico (Chávez-Rodríguez, 2021; Lopez, 2005). It is, therefore, an evolving form of medicine, continually expanding and incorporating techniques from other "folk medicines" including *parapsychology* – here meaning psychic experiences including telepathy, clairvoyance, and psychic healing.

Central to the practice of *curanderismo* is the belief that to maintain a healthy body an individual must achieve a balance among biological needs, social-interpersonal expectations, physical and spiritual harmony, and individual and cultural-familial attachments (Del Castillo, Fernandez, & Luna, 2020). It is no surprise, therefore, that the *curandero* in the opening story looked to familial attachments and spiritual unrest as possible causes for Angelita's emotional health problems. In sum, good health, as defined by this practice, is more than freedom from illness.

Note also that, in the opening story, the *curandero* used herbs and teas as part of the healing process. Like Western health providers, many healers also have specialties (see Table 6.3; Torres & Sawyer, 2005). For example, *yerberos* (or *yerberas*, for women) are herbalists who specialize in the use of herbs, homeopathic medicines, and religious amulets, here meaning objects or jewelry intended as protection against evil (Lopez, 2005). Given that the *curandero* in the opening story used herbs as medicinal agents, he may specialize in botanical cures.

It is important to note, however, that unlike CTM, spirituality plays a central role in the concept of health and healing in *curanderismo* (Hoskins & Padrón, 2018). This is seen most clearly in the common types of illnesses addressed through this medicine. For example, there are a number of illnesses that are believed to be supernatural or spiritual in origin. One such illness is *espanto*, often described as a "magical fright" because the cause of the frightened response is linked to supernatural factors. It is also linked with a loss of one's soul and as such is an ailment that is treated with spiritual cures (see Table 6.4).

In sum, *curanderismo* is a form of traditional medicine that evolved from different cultures and is still evolving today. Spirituality and spiritual forces are central to its healing practices, as is a reliance on botany to address physiological and psychological issues (see Figure 6.5).

Native American Health Practices

We must state first that there are over 500 different Native American tribal nations. Consequently, we do not imply in our heading that there is a uniform practice with respect to healing and traditional medicines

TABLE 6.3 Specialties in *Curanderismo*

Specialty	Function
Yerberos (herbalists)	Botanical remedies Homeopathic medicines Religious amulets
Partenas (midwives)	Childbirth
Sobadores (masseuses)	Massages General physical imbalances Sprains Bone setting
Espiritistas (spiritualists)	Faith healers Interpersonal relationships Spiritual health Séance

TABLE 6.4 Commonly Diagnosed Illnesses in *Curanderismo*

Illness	Meaning	Description	Illnesses
Mal aires/Mal viento	Bad air/bad winds	Illness caused by supernatural forces, exposure to sudden change in environmental temperature: cold to hot or vice-versa	Headaches, coldness, diarrhea, vomiting, paleness, fatigue
Mal de ojo	Evil eye	Supernatural or mental illness	Headaches, fever, rashes, death
Espanto/Susto	Magical fright	Illness caused by frightening experiences	Loss of soul, loss of appetite, vomiting, crying, insomnia depression, introversion
Mal projimo, duende, and brujeria	Illness caused by negative thoughts/feelings, negative encounters or witchcraft	Negative thoughts feelings of person(s) about another; negative encounters; manipulation of negative energies causing harm	Negative influences cause mental and physical harm

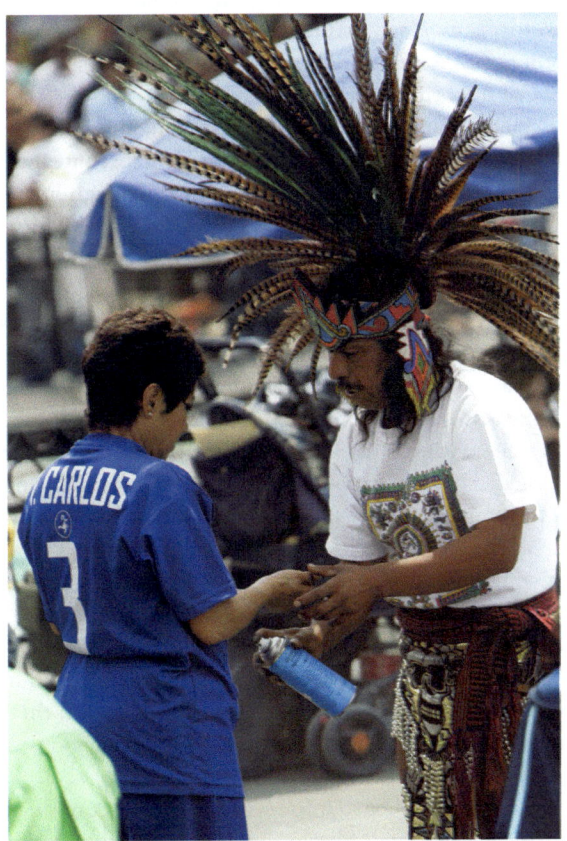

FIGURE 6.5 Photo of a Curandero in a headdress of long feathers, dressed in a shirt and wrap, treating a female patient.

Source: Alamy B1K6YJ.

for all Native Americans. As indicated at the beginning of the section on traditional medicines, here we explore the common themes among the traditional practices of the Nations and compare them to *curanderismo* and CTM, described previously.

Native American healing traditions have been described as a practice that involves traditional medicine practitioners – such as medicine men or women, or shamans – that is intended to restore a person to a healthy state (Walters et al., 2020). The healing process described, however, is a slow process, similar to the slow cures identified in CTM and *curanderismo*.

Principles that are common to all Native American practices are the belief in a higher power called, among other names, the Creator, the Great Spirit, or Great One – a belief in the interconnectedness of the mind, the body, and the spirit, and the belief that well-being characterizes a state of harmony and balance among the mind, body, spirit, and natural environment (Portman & Garrett, 2006). Native American health beliefs hold spirituality as core to the healing process. In this way it is more similar to the views expressed in *curanderismo* rather than CTM.

Four constructs central to all Native American healing practices are spirituality (including the creator, Mother Earth), community (for example, family or tribe), the environment (such as nature, the land), and self (including inner passions, values, and thoughts). It is the balance among the individual, the ecological, and the spiritual that defines, for many Native Americans, "good medicine" (Portman & Garrett, 2006).

Similar to adherents of other traditional health practices, Native Americans believe that a number of forces can cause ill health. Social discord, failure to adhere to tribal and sacred laws (Locust, 1985, as cited in Trimble, 2021), and being out of harmony can disrupt a balance and consequently affect an individual's overall well-being. Among the Lakota, there are six factors integral to obtaining well-being, a concept they call **wigozani**. They note that well-being is obtained through lifelong practice. Furthermore, it is obtained and maintained through an awareness of the sacred, healthy relationships, a consistent practice of prayer, the successful recovery from traumatic experiences, and enacting Lakota values (Noisy Hawk & Trimble, 2019).

There are, however, interesting differences in the healing practices used in this form of traditional medicine. First is the concept of medicine. Although medicinal agents can and do include herbs, teas, or pastes (poultices) – recall the example of the Disney version of Pocahontas earlier in the chapter – Native Americans believe that medicine also exists within each individual. For example, an experience that caused someone to smile and that continues to evoke the same response years later is considered medicine (Portman & Garrett, 2006). Medicine can also be the peacefulness of a moment. In essence, experiences, places, and even individuals themselves have the ability to help restore the balance between a person, the mind, the spirit, and nature.

Cohen (2003) notes interesting differences between Native American and Western medical beliefs. For example, Cohen notes that whereas Western medicine focuses on pathology and curing diseases, Native American practices, like other traditional systems, focus on healing the person and the community. Another distinction Cohen points out is the different approaches to treatment. Western medicine takes what Cohen calls an "adversarial" approach, seeking to destroy the disease. In contrast, the Native American health approach is consistent with "teleological" medicine and seeks learning lessons from the disease: that is, what the person can learn or the message in the illness.

In summary, traditional medicines have existed for centuries. They continue to supply Western medicine with knowledge about the medicinal benefits of herbs and plants, the foundation for many of the prescribed or over-the-counter medicines used today. Traditional medicines retained their holistic and ecological approaches to health, focusing on the well-being of the individual, which includes physical, emotional, social, and spiritual health and harmony with one's environment. They are more consistent with an ecological model of health.

Over time, however, Western medicine's scientific-based approach to health has been refined. It retains the important contributions made by science, but now it is broadening its base to incorporate elements of traditional medical practices into its concept of health and into its treatment approaches.

Having examined "old" and "new" approaches to health, it may seem that there is nothing more to add. However, the research on stress and coping has established clear links between emotional and physical health and also demonstrates the role of social and psychological environmental factors on overall well-being. We continue the exploration of emotional health in Chapter 7, Stress and Coping.

Personal Postscript

Do you sometimes wonder about the best way to treat your chest cold, or whether you really need an antibiotic for your repeated sinus problems? If so, you might be surprised to find that people who "grew up" in a Western medicine culture are increasingly exploring alternative and complementary treatments for many recurrent illnesses.

How do you decide which method is likely to be most successful? There is no one fail-proof system for determining the most effective method. But there are a few questions you can ask to help you decide. Consider the following:

1. Is your medical care provider open to exploring alternative therapies? If not, you may want to consider seeking a second opinion from someone who is knowledgeable about alternative medicines. It would increase your options when deciding how best to treat a medical problem.
2. Is your medical problem recurrent or chronic? Have you tried a number of recommended Western treatments without much success? Perhaps now would be a time to read up on alternative therapies. You may not decide to use them, but you will educate yourself about a range of alternatives that you may consider at a later point.
3. Finally – and this may sound incredible – is there someone in your family who has an excellent reputation for treating some acute (sudden) or chronic illnesses who had no formal medical training? Often we overlook the wisdom and collected knowledge of relatives who have acquired a wealth of information about alternative treatments. Consider obtaining your "second opinion" from that family member.

Questions to Consider

1. Increasingly, alternative, and traditional forms of medicine are being used in lieu of or in conjunction with Western medical practices. What implications does this have for the work of health psychologists?

2. One reason given for excluding spirituality as a variable in health outcomes is the difficulty in measuring that factor. How would you measure spirituality?
3. The role of environment and social policy on health outcomes was explained in a study by Sir Edwin Chadwick in 1842. What examples exist today of the impact of environment and social policy on health?

True or False Questions

1. One reason people choose traditional medical approaches for their health problems is because they are recommended by family members or close friends. True or False.
2. Aspects of the wellness model of health are more closely related to Chinese traditional medicine than to curanderismo. True or False.
3. The biomedical model presents a culturally specific view about disease. True or False.
4. Sir Edwin Chadwick's study of adult and infant mortality rates links these outcomes to race and class. True or False.
5. The Lakota believe that obtaining well-being, or **wigozani**, is a lifelong pursuit. True or False.

Important Terms

afferent nerve fibers 232
apartheid 251
aspirin 256
autonomic nervous system (ANS) 235
axon 232
biomedical model 229
biopsychosocial model 231
central nervous system (CNS) 231
Chinese traditional medicine (CTM) 256
complementary medicine 255
curanderismo 227
curandero 227
defensive pessimism 253
dendrite 231
ecological model 238
efferent nerve fibers 232
epinephrine 234
five elements 258
Hippocrates 231

Stress and Coping

Source: 3xy/
Shutterstock.

Chapter Outline

Opening Story: Sarah

Section I. Defining Stress

Section II. Stress and Illness

Section III. Coping with Stress

Personal Postscript

Questions to Consider

True or False Questions

Important Terms

Chapter Objectives

After studying this chapter, you will be able to:

1. Define *stress* as a stimulus and as a response.
2. Explain the cognitive appraisal process of stressful stimuli.
3. Explain the body's physiological response to stress.
4. Describe the relationship between stress and illness.
5. Identify and describe two cognitive coping strategies.
6. Identify and describe three behavioral coping strategies.
7. Explain the role of positive appraisal in stress and coping.
8. Explain the health psychologist's role in addressing stress and coping.

OPENING STORY: SARAH

Lucinda knew the day would come when her parents would move her grandmother, Sarah, to a nursing home. She just did not expect it to be so soon.

DOI: 10.4324/9781003300670-8

When Sarah was diagnosed with Alzheimer's, Lucinda and her parents decided that Sarah would live with them (Alzheimer's Disease Fact Sheet | National Institute on Aging (nih.gov). Lucinda remembers her parents' excitement as they rearranged the guest rooms to accommodate her grandmother. But in less than one month, the new arrangement led to conflicts and bickering – not with Sarah, but between Lucinda's parents.

Susan, Lucinda's mother and Sarah's only child, believed it was the family's responsibility to care for her mother. But Michael, Lucinda's father, argued that Sarah's presence was causing considerable stress to everyone. In truth, Michael was right. The family spent nights listening to Sarah move about the house. Memories of a two-day search for Sarah, who unexpectedly left the house one night while everyone else was asleep, were still fresh in their minds. For months after the incident, Susan was unable to sleep at night, rising often to check on Sarah.

To add to the challenges, everyone's schedule changed to accommodate Sarah's needs. Lucinda quit her high school cheerleading squad and her job as editor of the school newspaper to care for Sarah after school while her parents worked. Susan stopped accepting consultant jobs after work to be home in the evenings. And Michael reduced his work-related travel to help with some of the caregiving responsibilities. Gone also were the Friday dinner-and-a-movie family nights. Sarah became easily agitated in restaurants and could not sit through an entire movie. As for family vacations, they, too, were a thing of the past.

The changes unexpectedly put a strain on everyone, increasing the amount of tension and bickering over seemingly inconsequential things. After six months of what seemed like endless arguing, Lucinda and her parents sought family counseling. Sarah's presence at the meeting helped the therapist quickly understand the problem. It was also easy to see that the solution to the family's problems lay in finding an acceptable caregiving arrangement for Sarah.

After much debate, Lucinda's parents decided to put Sarah in a nursing home that specialized in caring for Alzheimer's patients. Lucinda and Michael were relieved. They returned to their regular schedules and told the therapist that their lives were almost normal again. But new tensions developed in their interactions with Susan. Susan felt guilty about "abandoning" her mother even though she visited Sarah in the nursing home daily. Unfortunately for Susan, the visits were physically and emotionally exhausting, made even more difficult when Sarah was having a bad day or struggling to remember Susan's name. For Susan, putting Sarah in a nursing home increased rather than decreased her stress.

It may seem that our focus on Susan, Lucinda, and Michael in the opening story is somewhat misplaced. After all, Sarah is the one with the health-related problem.

In truth, however, everyone in the story could be at risk for new health problems after Sarah's arrival. Research suggests that caregivers often experience emotional, mental, and even physical health problems when attending to persons with terminal or chronic illnesses (Perpiñá-Galvañ et al., 2019; Richardson, Lee, Berg-Weger, & Grossberg, 2013; Zhong, Wang, & Nichols, 2020). Caregivers may neglect their own existing health problems and may overlook novel or developing issues created by the emotional and psychological demands of their new role. The opening story with Susan and her family illustrates the problem. The family experienced a number of challenges and emotional conflicts for six months before seeking help.

Because Susan and Michael's problems began when Sarah moved in, it would be reasonable to assume that the difficulties would subside if not cease altogether when Sarah was relocated to a nursing home. But as we saw, that was not the case. Again, research offers an explanation for this outcome. Studies suggest that the decision to find alternative health care and living arrangements for a family member who needs special services can exacerbate existing tensions or cause new ones (Gaugler, Mittleman, Hepburn, & Newcomer, 2009). What is more, disagreements about and lack of support for a decision can create guilt, depression, and anxiety in caregivers (Sury, Burns, & Brodaty, 2013).

It should also come as no surprise that the decision-making process concerning alternative placements for a family member differs by culture. For example, in Chinese families where *xiao*, or filial piety – here meaning a collective moral duty, obligation, or responsibility of children to care for their parents with honor, reverence, and obedience (Chang, Schneider, & Sessanna, 2011; Zhang, 2004) – is widely accepted, placing one's parent in a nursing home may feel like a violation of Chinese filial piety (Chang et al., 2011). A similar sense of guilt and betrayal has been documented also by researchers in other Asian and Western cultures (e.g., Kiwi, Hydén, & Antelius, 2017; Lord, Livingston, & Cooper, 2014; Sury et al., 2013).

Studies also suggest that the decision to place a parent in a long-term institutionalized setting, like a nursing home, impacts men and women differently. They note that for men, the absence of socioemotional support when choosing a nursing facility for family members can cause new tensions and stress, while women cite family conflicts over the decision, rather than the absence of socioemotional support, as the principal reason for increased stress in such situations (Gaugler, Zarit, & Perlin, 1999). Subsequent studies suggest that the quality of a family's relationships prior to decisions to place a parent in a nursing home, in addition to possible negative dynamics between family members, may be the key factors that result in increased emotional stress on all family members (Stone & Clements, 2009). Together, the studies exploring conflicting feelings and guilt about decisions to institutionalize parents may help explain why Susan was conflicted, even guilty, about the decision, even though Michael and Lucinda fully supported the outcome. Susan's feelings sparked conflicts with other family members, which prolonged the stress. Some researchers suggest that unresolved stress could result in psychophysiological illnesses such as chronic headaches, ulcers, or respiratory infections and depression (Madison et al., 2022; Purdy, 2013).

We will explore the complex relationship between stress, the immune system and illness later in this chapter and again in Chapter 8, Psychoneuroimmunology. For the moment, however, it is important to note that according to some health researchers and providers, the proposed relationship between stress and illness demonstrates the need for a holistic approach to health. The opening story reminds us, however, that social environmental stressors also contribute to psychological and physical health problems, making environmental stressors another important determinant of well-being.

We begin this chapter by examining some classic theories of stress. First, we define *stress* in Section I, using the taxonomy proposed by Elliot and Eisdorfer (1982). Next, we briefly review the seminal works of Walter Cannon (1929) and Hans Selye (1946, 1950) that established a physiological basis for stress. To explain Cannon's and Selye's models of stress, we also review the body's physiological response to stressful stimuli, examining the components of the nervous system and the hormones responsible for activating the system when detecting a stressful stimulus. Using Segerstrom and Miller's (2004) meta-analysis of psychological stress and the immune system and Sapolsky's (2004) entertaining description of the effects of short-term versus long-term stress, we then examine current research that proposes revisions to Selye's work. We conclude Section I with an overview of Lazarus and Folkman's transactional model. The transactional model provides another theoretical explanation of stress, but one that focuses on the psychological as well as the physiological processes.

In Section II, we explore causes of stress. We pay particular attention to the role of biological determinants – specifically illnesses, social environmental determinants, and psychosocial factors. We also briefly introduce the field of psychoneuroimmunology, a topic that will be addressed more fully in Chapter 8, Psychoneuroimmunology. We conclude with a discussion of mechanisms and strategies used to cope with stress in Section III. By the end of this chapter, you will be able to define stress as a stimulus, a response, and an interaction of both and explain the body's cognitive, physiological, and psychological response to stressful stimuli. In addition, you will be able to identify potential roles for health psychologists when helping individuals manage daily stressors.

SECTION I. DEFINING STRESS

Undoubtedly, you have heard many people talk about a stressful event: a major exam, an important job interview, or interpersonal relationship challenges with family or friends. The frequent use of the word *stress* suggests that we believe we understand the concept. But do we? We may be very familiar with stressful experiences, but do we understand what causes us to perceive situations as stressful? Furthermore, do we recognize our natural or acquired strategies for addressing stress?

The opening story employed a three-category definition of stress, portraying it as a stimulus, a response, and the interaction of both stimulus and response. The *stressful stimulus* in the story, an event external to the human body that provokes a response, is Sarah. She provokes a response from the family regardless of whether she lives in Susan and Michael's house or in a nursing home. The *stressful response*, that is, a physical or emotional reaction by an individual to the external stimulus, is the conflict, discord, guilt, and depression experienced variably by each member of the family.

Finally, the interaction between the stressor and the response, sometimes characterized as the "interplay and feedback" (Lazarus & Folkman, 1984b), is portrayed by the interaction of the stressful stimulus, Sarah, with other family members. Consider this: Susan's visits with her mother appear to provoke a stressful response. Thus, for Susan, the stress did not dissipate with Sarah's relocation; instead, Susan's stress when visiting her mother appears to provoke additional conflicts with Michael and Lucinda. As some studies suggest, while the physical and objective burdens of care were removed, Susan's *perceptions* of a continuing burden to visit and tend to her mother's affairs may still result in high levels of emotional stress, especially if Michael and Lucinda do not contribute (Stone & Clements, 2009).

Elliot and Eisdorfer (1982) offer yet another way to conceptualize stress. These authors identify five distinct stress categories: acute time-limited stressors, naturalistic stressors, stressful event sequences, chronic stressors, and distal stressors. The first category, *acute time-limited stressors*, describes manipulated or staged events such as public speaking or mental math – activities of short duration, ranging in time from approximately 5 to 100 minutes (Segerstrom & Miller, 2004). The second category, *brief naturalistic stressors*, is familiar to most students because they include things such as academic exams or other short-term, real-life events. Third, Elliot and Eisdorfer (1982) identify *stressful event sequences*. Such events may include the death of a spouse or major human-made or natural disasters that present a number of unforeseen challenges that occur over time. In these stress scenarios, individuals know that the challenges will eventually subside but may not know exactly when (Segerstrom & Miller, 2004). An example might help here. Think, for example, of the multiple disasters that destroyed whole communities across the globe. Need a little refresher? Consider the multiple wildfires that occurred in Canada in 2022–2023 or in Maui, Hawaii, in August 2023. Or perhaps you remember the devastating dam collapses in Derna, Libya, in

September 2023, or the devastating earthquakes southwest of Marrakesh, Morocco, in September 2023 or in parts of Türkiye and Syria in February 2023. What do all of these events have in common? In addition to the fact that they razed whole communities, resulting in the loss of life and upending the lives of many families, they posed significant daily challenges to the survivors. Those who survived these harrowing events know that these daily challenges will eventually lessen, although no one can say when.

Continuing with Elliot and Eisendorf's categories, the fourth stress category, *chronic stressors*, is characterized by the situation presented in our opening story. As caregivers to someone with Alzheimer's, Lucinda, Michael, and Susan experienced multiple daily stressors that continued for months. They had no idea whether these stressors would ever subside. They sought help for themselves and Sarah when they realized that they could neither predict nor cope with Sarah's behaviors and their consequences for the family. Although a change in the living arrangements significantly reduced the stress for Lucinda and Michael, it continued for Susan. And, as mentioned previously, researchers have noted that placement of a family member in a care home does not necessarily remove the emotional stress experienced by the family member who monitors the quality of care given in the nursing homes (Stone & Clements, 2009).

The final stressor Elliot and Eisdorfer identify is *distal stressors*, or experiences of a traumatic nature that took place in the distant past but, because of their long-lasting cognitive and emotional impact, may continue to affect a person's immune system (Segerstrom & Miller, 2004). You may be tempted to ask whether post-traumatic stress disorder is an example of a distal stressor: Hold that thought. We will explore post-traumatic stress disorder later in the chapter.

Whether using three or five categories to define stress, we must consider the stimuli that prompt the response as well as the various responses when talking about stress. Therefore, we begin this chapter by exploring theories that explain our physiological as well as cognitive and emotional responses to stressful stimuli.

Three Theories of Stress

Three theories – Walter Cannon's "fight-or-flight" theory, Hans Selye's general adaptation syndrome (GAS), and Richard Lazarus and Susan Folkman's transactional model – are seminal theories that aim to explain the relationship between stress and illness. Cannon's and Selye's theories focus on the physiological response to stressful stimuli, whereas Lazarus and Folkman seek to explain the cognitive appraisal process in response to stress. All three theories demonstrate the relationship between a stressor and a physiological response that may contribute to illness. For health psychologists, the relationship between an emotional factor (stress) and health and wellness is fundamental to the field, which is another reason to review the pros and cons of each of these theories.

CANNON'S "FIGHT-OR-FLIGHT" THEORY One way to define stress is the body's physical or emotional reaction to an external event. Early research on stress, such as Cannon's *fight-or-flight theory*, did just that, focusing specifically on the body's physiological response to stress-inducing stimuli.

Cannon proposed that stress is best understood as the body's biological activation in response to stress-producing stimuli. Consider the following example: A young woman is walking home from a party late one Saturday night. The walkway is dimly lit. In the distance, she can see the shadow of a person behind a building. At one point, as the young woman continues walking, she sees the person emerge from behind the building, look in her direction, and retreat once again behind the building. How do you think the young woman would respond to the troubling and potentially threatening situation?

Cannon would suggest that the body's biological systems, specifically the sympathetic nervous system and endocrine system, would activate to enable the young woman to exhibit a "fight-or-flight" response to the potential threat.

The Nervous System and Stress In Chapter 6, Emotional Health and Well-Being, we introduced the nervous system. As we indicated then, physiological responses to stress are initiated by a complex communication process that takes place in the *nervous system*, the body's network of cells that communicate information about itself and its environment. The nervous system consists of two principal parts, the *central nervous system (CNS)* and the *peripheral nervous system (PNS;* see Figure 7.1). The CNS is responsible for receiving and responding to information obtained through our *sensory receptor sites*, here meaning the parts of the body responsible for initial sensory perception including the eyes, ears, nose, mouth, and fingers. The CNS uses the vast structure of nerves in our bodies to coordinate the communication between the receptor sites, the spinal cord, and the brain, the processing center for our sensory experiences.

The peripheral nervous system (PNS) contains two substructures, the *autonomic nervous system (ANS)* and the *somatic nervous system (SNS)*. We focus our discussion on the ANS because it is most relevant to our discussion of the body's response to stress. The ANS controls the automatic and involuntary functions that are essential for living. For example, heart rate, digestion, and perspiration are controlled by the ANS.

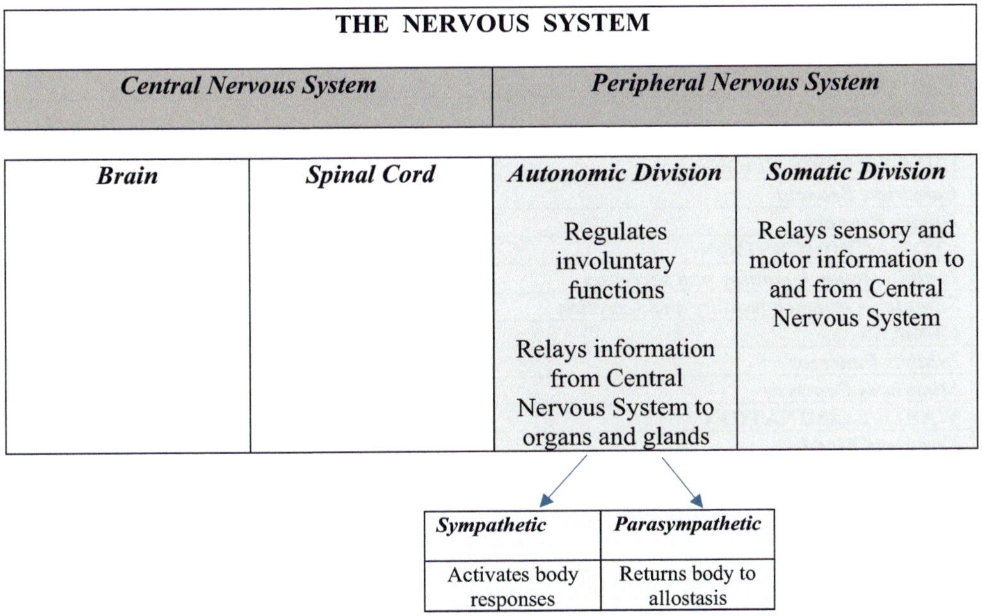

THE NERVOUS SYSTEM			
Central Nervous System		*Peripheral Nervous System*	
Brain	*Spinal Cord*	*Autonomic Division* Regulates involuntary functions Relays information from Central Nervous System to organs and glands	*Somatic Division* Relays sensory and motor information to and from Central Nervous System

Sympathetic	*Parasympathetic*
Activates body responses	Returns body to allostasis

FIGURE 7.1 The nervous system. The chart shows that the nervous system is divided into two parts. The Central Nervous System (CNS) contains the brain and the spinal cord. The Peripheral Nervous System (PNS) contains the Autonomic Divisions, and the Somatic Division. The Autonomic Divisions regulate involuntary functions and relays information from the CNS to organs and glands via the Sympathetic system, which activates the body, and the Parasympathetic system that returns the body to allostasis. Part II of the PNS contains the Somatic Division that relays sensory and motor information to and from the CNS.

VIDEO #36/60

Chapter 7: Stress and Coping

·   **Autonomic Nervous System and Parasympathetic Nervous System: 1 Minute 2 Divisions of the Autonomic Nervous System (ANS)**

·   *Website: https://www.youtube.com/watch?v=dgkHiGZrwd8*

·   *Pathway Education is a neuropsychology YouTube channel that provides educational videos (no website)*

·   **All videos that are publicly posted on YouTube are publicly accessible to the public and free to use. Pathway Education is a neuropsychology YouTube channel that provides educational videos (no website, just YouTube).**

The ANS also contains two substructures, both of which play a role in our body's response to stress: the sympathetic nervous system and the parasympathetic nervous system. The *sympathetic nervous system* activates the body's response to danger, emergencies, or foreign microorganisms that invade the body. Consider this: When encountering a stressor, some individuals may experience a rapid heartbeat, some might sweat under their arms or on their palms, and others may respond with increased respiration (breathing) rate. It is also likely that when responding to stressful stimuli, a person may experience a sensation of "dry mouth" due to the lack of saliva or dilated pupils (see Figure 7.2). Which of these

FUNCTIONS	SYMPATHETIC	PARASYMPATHETIC
EYE/VISION		
Constricts Pupils		✓
Dilates Pupils	✓	
MOUTH		
Inhibits flow of Saliva	✓	
Stimulates flow of Saliva		✓
LUNGS/RESPIRATION		
Constricts Bronchi		✓
Dilates Bronchi	✓	
STOMACH/DIGESTION		
Inhibits stomach motility and secretion	✓	
Stimulates stomach motility and secretion		✓
ORGANS		
Inhibits Pancreas	✓	
Stimulates Pancreas		✓
WASTE/ELIMINATION		
Contracts Bladder		✓
Inhibits Bladder	✓	
EXCITATION/STIMULATION		
Stimulates ejaculation	✓	
Stimulates erection		✓
ENERGY		
Convert glycogen to glucose	✓	
Secrete adrenaline and noradrenaline	✓	

FIGURE 7.2 Parasympathetic vs. sympathetic systems. When activated, the sympathetic system dialates pupils and bronchi, inhibits salivation, stomach motility & secretion, as well as the pancreas and bladder, stimulates ejaculation, converts glycogene to glucose, and secretes adrenaline and noradrenaline. The parasympathetic system reverses these processes to return the body to allostasis.

changes do you think the young woman in our scenario experienced when seeing the stranger dash behind the building? Which have you experienced when stressed? The point here is that when activated, the sympathetic nervous system puts in motion a series of physiological changes that may signal danger and a need to either defend oneself (fight) or flee (flight). We will explain the physiological mechanism that accompanies this sympathetic activation in just a moment.

In comparison, the *parasympathetic nervous system* takes control once the threat has abated. It is responsible for returning the body to its normal or baseline state, often referred to as *allostasis*. Specifically, allostasis refers to the body's ability to maintain its own "steady physiological state" (for example, blood pressure, heart, and respiration rates) through changes in both the environment and in the body's physiology (McEwen & Wingfield, 2007; Romero, Dickens, & Cyr, 2009).

The Endocrine System A second system critical to the body's response to stress is the *endocrine system*, a communication system in the body that sends messages using *ductless glands*, here meaning glands that release *hormones* directly into the body's bloodstream (see Figure 7.3). Hormones, like neurotransmitters (see Chapter 6, Emotional Health and Well-Being), are the chemical messages that facilitate the body's communication process.

The endocrine system has many functions, but one of its responsibilities is to respond to stress. To this end, two glands in the endocrine system, the pituitary gland and the adrenal gland, are principally responsible for releasing hormones in response to stress. The *pituitary gland* is adjacent to the *hypothalamus*, a region in the brain that controls basic human needs such as sleep, hunger, thirst, and sex. The location of the pituitary gland suggests that, even though the brain is part of the nervous system, the endocrine and the nervous systems work together to produce and regulate hormones.

VIDEO #37/60

Chapter 7: Stress and Coping

- **Hypothalamus:** *Hypothalamus in 60 seconds*
- *Website: https://www.youtube.com/watch?v=TmfPGW5p1sU*
- **The Neuropsychiatrist is publicly accessible.**

VIDEO #38/60

Chapter 7: Stress and Coping

- **Pituitary Gland:** *62 SECONDS on REMEMBERING the PITUITARY HORMONES (Easy to remember mnemonics!)*
- *Website: https://www.youtube.com/watch?v=magaTTss0ng*
- **60 Second Medicine is an educational YouTube channel that creates quick and informative about anatomy and medicine.**

The pituitary gland is sometimes nicknamed the "master gland," but this is largely meant to connote the fact that under the direction of the hypothalamus, the pituitary gland produces hormones that stimulate the production of other hormones, which in turn play a role in the body's response to stress. For example, the pituitary gland produces *adrenocorticotropic hormone (ACTH)*, a hormone that is responsible for stimulating the *adrenal glands*, located just above each of the kidneys. As we will see shortly, stimulation of the adrenal glands triggers the release of other hormones critical to the stress response.

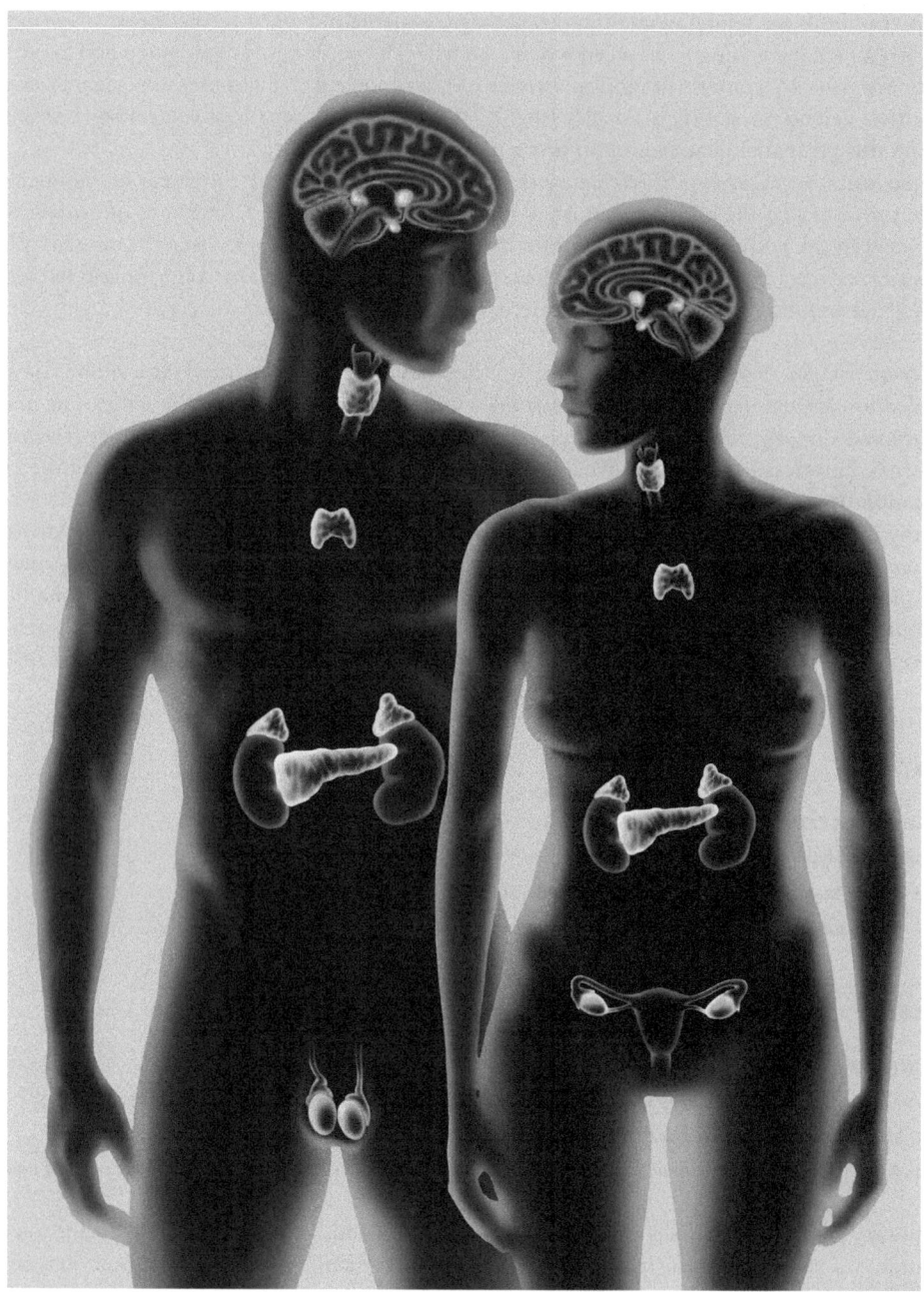

FIGURE 7.3 Major endocrine glands. Two silhouettes, one of a man and second of a woman, shows the location of the glans in the endocrine system, located in the brain, the thyroid, above the kidneys, the pancrease, and the ovaries (in women) or testes (in men).

Source: SciSource_DA9001.jpg

The adrenal glands consist of two components: the adrenal medulla and the adrenal cortex. The *adrenal medulla* is found in the inner layer of the adrenal glands. When stimulated by the sympathetic nervous system, the adrenal medulla produces *catecholamines*, a class of chemicals that contains *epinephrine*, *norepinephrine*, and *cortisol* (Segerstrom & Miller, 2004). You may be familiar with another name for epinephrine: *adrenaline*. If this is familiar, then you know that epinephrine (or adrenaline) helps boost the body's energy level. Thus, when epinephrine is released in the body, the sympathetic system is activating the body in response to a stimulant, possibly a stress-provoking event. In fact, epinephrine is linked so closely with stress that it is sometimes used in studies as a physiological index of stress. When the sympathetic nervous system and adrenal glands interact to cause a reaction, we refer to the combined systems as the *sympathetic-adrenal-medullary system (SAM)*.

The *adrenal cortex* is the outer layer of the adrenal glands. The adrenal cortex, when working together with the hypothalamus and the pituitary gland, forms the *hypothalamic-pituitary-adrenocortical system (HPAC)*, a system responsible for restoring the body to its baseline steady state. This system, when stimulated by ACTH, activates the adrenal cortex to release one type of hormone known as glucocorticoids. In fact, some contend that much of the body's stress response system is mediated by glucocorticoids (Whirledge & Cidlowski, 2010), which include epinephrine, norepinephrine, and cortisol (in humans). We will explore the role of glucocorticoids more fully when reviewing Selye's theory. For now, it is sufficient to keep four points in mind. First, *glucocorticoids* are anti-inflammatory agents that we now know play a complex role in response to stress. Second, glucocorticoids and other stress hormones activate the immune system and immune defenses when the body is exposed to a stressor (Whirledge & Cidlowski, 2010). Third, glucocorticoids also play a role in returning the body to allostasis, or the normal internal set points for the body's blood pressure, heart rate, body temperature, and other internal measures. If the body were to remain in an activated state too long, it could cause damage to the body's organs. For example, as we will see in Chapter 9, Cardiovascular Disease, prolonged activation can stress the heart, causing damage to that organ. In other words, glucocorticoids can play a constructive role in preserving the health of some organs (Dashti-Khavidaki, Saidi, & Lu, 2021). Finally, when experiencing prolonged or chronic stress, the glucocorticoid levels may remain high. These high levels could trigger a suppression of the body's immune system that could expose the body to illnesses such as chronic infections, major depression, or a clogging of the arteries known as atherosclerosis (see Chapter 9, Cardiovascular Disease; Calcagni & Elenkov, 2006). This means that although glucocorticoids protect the body from the short-term effects of stress, prolonged production of this agent may make the body susceptible to illnesses.

Cannon's "fight-or-flight" theory was the first to describe the body's biological response to stress-inducing stimuli, the role of glucocorticoids (including epinephrine, norepinephrine, and cortisol) and the sympathetic nervous system in response to stress (Sapolsky, 2004). Research by Selye showed, however, that the physiological response to stress was actually more complex. But before moving on to Selye's theory, we must note one criticism of Cannon's theory by Shelly Taylor that garnered the attention of many researchers.

Taylor and Master (2011) suggest that the female response to stress does not conform to the fight-or-flight model proposed by Cannon. Rather, she contends that females evidence a "*tend and befriend*" response triggered by the secretion of the hormone oxytocin. According to Taylor, *oxytocin* is the same hormone that stimulates the maternal behavior and milk production needed to nurture an offspring (tending) and the desire to seek social affiliations (befriending). Recent research supports this distinction, suggesting that when stressed, males become more competitive while women are more cooperative and oriented to think of others (Nickels, Kubicki, & Maestripieri, 2017).

Other researchers note that, although interesting, Taylor's gender difference theory misses an important discovery about men. They claim that men do not always respond to a stressor using a fight-or-flight response either. Rather, they suggest that males, especially primates, often display the same "tending" behaviors seen in females (Geary & Flinn, 2002). Eisler and Levine (2002) argue provocatively that "we are not prisoners of our genes." They suggest that cultural institutions and settings, in addition to individual differences, work to heighten or reduce tending-and-befriending behaviors in males and females.

More recent studies focusing on fathers support these findings. Work by Ahnert, Deichmann, Bauer, Supper, and Piskernik (2021) and Kuo and colleagues (2018) focus on the relationship between father's hormone levels and engagement with and childcare of their newborn infant. In one intriguing study by Kuo and colleagues (2018) researchers collected saliva samples to measure father's testosterone and cortisol levels immediately before the birth of their child and again after fathers held the newborn, approximately one hour after birth. A third saliva sample was collected 24 hours later. Additional data on father's self-reported involvement with childcare and play activities (e.g., bathing, dressing, babysitting, and active play) were collected between two to four months later. Kuo and colleagues' findings offer evidence from their 180 participants that father's elevated basal cortisol levels within 24 hours of their child's birth predicts greater parental involvement (tending) in a variety of childcare activities in the following months.

In essence, most researchers conclude that although Taylor raises an important question concerning gender and stress, the findings of studies to date suggest a complex relationship between the two factors because men also evidence "tending and befriending" responses to stress.

We turn now to Selye's discovery that catecholamines (epinephrine and norepinephrine) and the adrenal glands are only part of a rather complicated stress process (Szabo, 1998).

SELYE'S GENERAL ADAPTATION SYNDROME (GAS) Hans Selye's work is considered seminal for its identification of the pathways through which stress elicits physiological reactions in organisms (Selye & Fortier, 1950). Selye's original theory has since been modified, further refining our understanding of the role of stress and the immune system. We review Selye's theory first and introduce the modifications afterwards.

Selye's research initially characterized stress as either a stimulus or an external agent. He later modified this definition to characterize stress as the organism's response to any form of a "noxious stimulus" (Selye, 1936), which he referred to later as the stressor (Selye, 1946). According to Selye, the body responds in the same manner to any stressor (see Figure 7.4). Hence, cold temperatures, surgical injury, or the introduction of intoxicating substances (like drugs or alcohol) would provoke the same three-stage general adaptation syndrome (GAS) response to the stressor (Selye, 1936).

The three stages of GAS – the alarm stage, the stage of resistance, and the stage of exhaustion – describe, according to Selye, not only the body's response to a stressor but also the process by which illnesses can develop when the body tries but fails to cope with the target stressor. In the alarm stage, the organism first experiences shock at the initial impact of the stress-inducing agent. The initial response to the shock may include a lowering of the body's blood pressure or body temperature (Lazarus & Folkman, 1984b). The body then proceeds to the counter-shock phase (still in the alarm stage), in which the organism prepares to respond defensively to the stress-producing agent. At this point, the body may release higher levels of adrenaline and at the same time may increase respiration and blood pressure rates and activate the sweat glands as the body prepares to respond (look again at Figure 7.2).

The second stage, resistance, is best characterized as the body's increased and sustained resistance to specific agent. However, it comes at a price. The sustained resistance to one stressor decreases the body's ability to withstand or defend against other agents (Selye, 1946). In essence, while fighting one agent

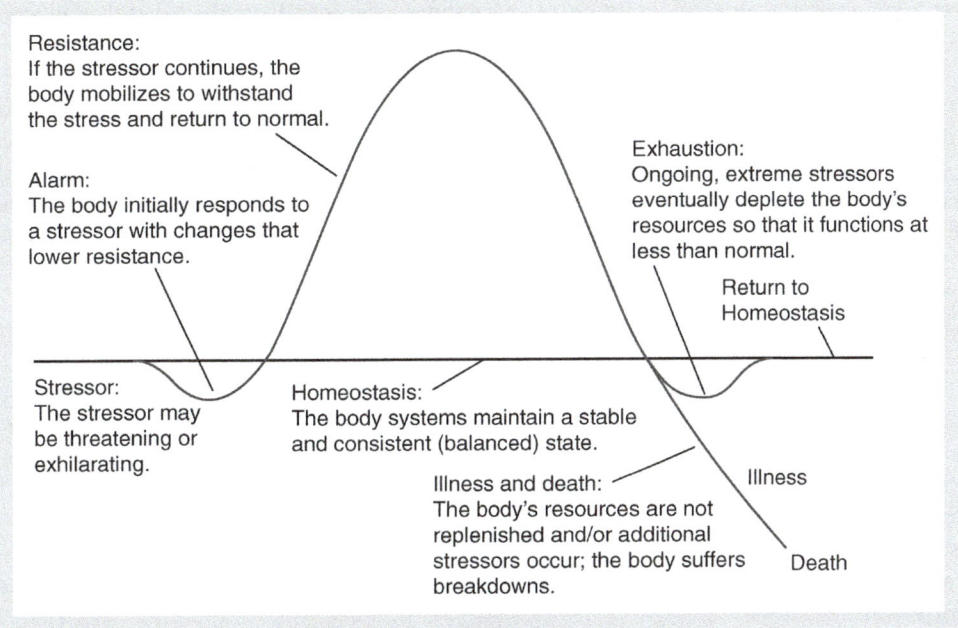

Resistance:
If the stressor continues, the body mobilizes to withstand the stress and return to normal.

Alarm:
The body initially responds to a stressor with changes that lower resistance.

Exhaustion:
Ongoing, extreme stressors eventually deplete the body's resources so that it functions at less than normal.

Return to Homeostasis

Stressor:
The stressor may be threatening or exhilarating.

Homeostasis:
The body systems maintain a stable and consistent (balanced) state.

Illness and death:
The body's resources are not replenished and/or additional stressors occur; the body suffers breakdowns.

Illness

Death

FIGURE 7.4 A bell-shaped curve illustrates Salye's General Adaptation SYndromee (G-A-S). The curve rests on a horizontal line, representing the body's homeostasis (or allostasis). The stressor causes alarm, briefly lowering the body's resistance and causing a dip in the curve belod homeostasis. Resistance to the stressor causes the body to mobilize leading to the high point on the bell curve. The body can either become exhausted by the stressor leading to the downward trajectory of the curve and causing the body to function less than normal (below homeostasis), return to homeostasis – a successful resolution to the stressor – or suffer continued breakdowns leading to illness or death.

Source: Hales (1997).

intensely, the body is vulnerable to attack by other stress agents, which may include a range of factors that could lead to illness. We emphasize here the word *could* because current research suggests that the link between stress and illness is more attenuated. More on this point in just a moment.

The final stage of GAS is appropriately named the stage of exhaustion. How long an organism can withstand and defend itself against a specific stress-inducing agent appears to vary as a function of the individual. In general, Selye notes that prolonged exposure to stressors can cause symptoms similar to those that appear during the alarm stage. Selye notes that in the final stage of exhaustion, organisms will display the nonspecific systemic reactions that were developed during the adaptation stage that it could not maintain. Thus, it is in this stage that the disease of adaptation may form, here meaning illnesses can occur, in part due to the body's inability to defend itself from the specific agent or other stressors (Lazarus & Folkman, 1984b). The illnesses may include hypertension (high blood pressure; see Chapter 9, Cardiovascular Disease) or gastrointestinal ulcers. Even some forms of allergies may be considered diseases of adaptation (Selye, 1946).

Undoubtedly, Selye's work revealed an important association between stress and illness, but his work met with criticism. One critique of the theory is its inability to explain the role of psychosocial factors on illness. Early research by Mason and colleagues (1976) suggests that the body's hormonal response to stress may differ as a function of a specific emotion and even differ by gender. If so, the belief that all stressors would elicit the same reaction would not be supported.

A second criticism, explained by Sapolsky (2004), is Selye's lack of distinction between short-term versus long-term stress on the immune system (see Box 7.1). Briefly, Sapolsky explains that when encountering a short-term stressor, our body activates the immune system. But in the event of prolonged stress, including chronic stressors, the body's immune system is suppressed, thereby weakening its defenses against illnesses. Thus, acute or short-term stress which bolsters rather than suppresses our immune system can be healthy for the body. On the other hand, chronic or long-term stress may introduce health risks.

Box 7.1 Learning about Stress from Other Animals

What can Robert Sapolsky, a professor of biology and neurology who studies primates, tell us about human responses to stress? Probably nothing, you may think. You may assume that stress is unique to the human species and that nothing can be learned from animals. But in his seminal work titled "Why Zebras Don't Get Ulcers," Sapolsky explains the human body's nervous system and its response to stressors in considerable detail and with good comedic timing. It is impossible to summarize the wealth of information contained in his book, so instead we highlight core concepts that help us understand the human response to stress.

We pointed out in the preceding sections that the response to stress is not just emotional; it is also physiological. Sapolsky's work, along with that of other biologists, stress physiologists, and psychoneuroimmunologists, identifies a short-term and a long-term stress response in humans and compares the impact of these two response modes on our immune system. As a result, we now know that the human response to stress goes something like this: During the first few minutes of stress (approximately less than one hour), stressors can activate the body's immune system. Intuitively, this makes sense if you consider what is happening to the autonomic nervous system, more specifically the sympathetic nervous system, when encountering a stressor, but we will explain this more fully in just a few moments. An emergency, a frightening situation, or an alarming encounter starts the sympathetic nervous system pumping, releasing epinephrine and norepinephrine from the nerve endings in the adrenal glands within seconds of the stressor (recall the woman in our example on page 270). In effect, epinephrine and norepinephrine are the "first responders" to stress. But this is just the beginning.

The second responder is an agent called glucocorticoids. Glucocorticoids are steroid hormones that are also emitted from the adrenal glands. This process is a little complex, so bear with us as we explain. As Sapolsky (2004) notes, the "agent" that gets the ball rolling when encountering a stressful event is the hypothalamus: the region of the brain that regulates our basic biological needs and is also next to the pituitary gland (we mentioned previously that they work closely together). The hypothalamus triggers the release of a host of hormones into the hypothalamic-pituitary circulatory system. One such hormone is the corticotropin-releasing hormone (CRH), an agent responsible for signaling the pituitary gland to release the adrenocorticotropic hormone (ACTH; see the section on The Nervous System and Stress in this chapter). When ACTH is released into the bloodstream, it triggers the adrenal gland to release glucocorticoids. Because this process takes time, glucocorticoids are considered reinforcing agents to the first responders. Glucocorticoids hormones are longer-term responders to stressors.

Now comes the tricky part. Glucocorticoids are also associated with a decrease in the formation of lymphocytes, one of two types of cells central to the body's immune system. We explain the immune system in more detail in Chapter 8, Psychoneuroimmunology. For now, just remember that lymphocytes are a type of white blood cell that help attack foreign organisms in the body. And while it is true that glucocorticoids are generally associated with decreased production of lymphocytes, it is also true that the CRH emitted from the hypothalamus plays a dual role with response to stress. This is a major departure from Selye's original theory that suggested that glucocorticoids, which decrease lymphocytes produced in the thymus, are broadly immunosuppressive agents (Segerstrom & Miller, 2004). This assumption by Selye led to the conclusion that a diminished immune response was responsible for higher incidences of infections and diseases, especially among chronically stressed persons (Segerstrom & Miller, 2004).

Later research challenged Selye's immunosuppression model. In fact, current research contends that decreases in the immune function of the body at the first presentation of a stressor would not have allowed the human organism to evolve and adapt in life-threatening circumstances (Segerstrom & Miller, 2004). In other words, how could humans have evolved and survived if stressors immediately triggered an immunosuppressive response? We need to add here that Sapolsky's work with primates helps to underscore this point.

More specifically, work by Dhabhar and McEwen (2001) demonstrates that stressors cause a redistribution of immune cells, specifically the T cells (see Chapter 8, Psychoneuroimmunology). This leads to two potentially different outcomes depending on the nature of the stressor. When examining the impact of stress on mice, Dhabhar and McEwen (2001) found that the presentation of acute (short-term) stressors redistributed the T cells into the skin, resulting in an enhanced immune response. But when presented with a chronic stressor, the T cells were propelled away from the skin, resulting in a suppression of the immune response (Segerstrom & Miller, 2004). Thus, short-term acute stress can stimulate an immune response in the body – in fact, it can enhance cellular immunity even to the point of increasing resistance to squamous cancer cells (Dhabhar et al., 2010). On the other hand, a long-term or chronic stressor does the opposite: It dysregulates, or impairs, immune function (Dhabhar et al., 2010).

Dhabhar (2014) and Sapolsky, Romero, and Munck (2000) note one other important point. While prolonged or chronic stress can cause a suppression of the immune system, the suppression can be a good outcome if the stress abates. With no imminent threat, a suppression of the immune system will result in the immune system returning to its normal level. The problem comes when (1) the stress remains or is chronic; (2) the glucocorticoid levels continue to be elevated; and (3) the sympathetic system remains activated. When any of these three factors occur, the immune system does not just return to allostasis, but it becomes further suppressed; the body's response to the stress is then correctly termed an immunosuppressing physiological response (Sapolsky, Romero, & Munck, 2000).

The bottom line here is that our physiological response to stress is complex. The same agents that are responsible for suppressing the immune system also play a role in activation of the system. The key distinction is time. The duration of the stress will help determine the role of the hormones.

A third criticism is the attenuated link between stress and illness, a point we raised earlier. Sapolsky (2004) advocates for a more careful approach when suggesting that stress leads to illnesses. He notes that studies that suggest such a link make a number of assumptions about an individual's perception of stress and their ability (or inability) to cope with the stressor. According to Sapolsky, before linking a stressor to an illness, we might be advised to determine whether the individual affected has really been stressed by the stressor, to decide whether the identified stress agent actually triggered a stress response, and to ascertain the individual's ability or inability to defend against such agents. Salleh (2008) adds that genetic vulnerability, personality, and support systems also influence a person's susceptibility to stress. And Bieliauskas (2019) agrees that the context in which stress occurs as well as the psychological characteristic of the individual experiencing the stressful situation also influence likely responses.

Other researchers similarly argue for the need to augment Selye's model. For example, Epel and colleagues (2018) suggest that stress is a process involving not just the person, but the other situational factors, including past and present events, as well as the physiological and psychological state of the person. Some would argue that the SARS-CoV-2 pandemic is a prime example of the multiple factors that contribute to stress. For example, a person's concern about their own physical well-being, the multiple warnings about mask-wearing and hand-washing – at least in the early days – and the actions of other family members might cause some during the height of the crisis to experience extreme stress. Others, who feel they can exercise more control over their environment and themselves might not perceive the same level of stress. Thus, these researchers would argue for a transdisciplinary model that takes into account the role of these various factors when measuring stress. Absent this broader perspective that measures individual differences in stress perception, the context in which the stress occurs, and inherent problems associated with a person's accurate retrospective recall of an event, there is considerable room for error when concluding that specific stressors "caused" an illness.

Cannon's and Selye's modified theories form the basis of our understanding of the role of short- and long-term stress on the body's immune system. As health psychologists, however, we are also interested in the psychological response to stress. We turn to Lazarus and Folkman for a fuller understanding of the role of the psychosocial, experiential, and contextual factors on stress.

LAZARUS AND FOLKMAN'S TRANSACTIONAL MODEL (TM) OF STRESS Seminal work by Lazarus and Folkman focuses on the psychosocial triggers of stress – consistent with the *stimulus-organism-response* or *S-O-R* models of stress (Khan & Obhi, 2021), a focus that is missing in Selye's GAS theory. Lazarus and Folkman (1984a) believe that we cannot study a person's response to stress independent of understanding his or her perception of the stress-provoking event (similar to Epel and colleagues and Sapolsky's point noted earlier). To explain a person's perception of the stress process, Lazarus and Folkman developed the *transactional model (TM)*, which proposes that stress is triggered when an external stressor (or event) exceeds a person's personal and social resources to effectively cope with the event. Here, *coping* includes a person's perceived psychological, emotional, and physiological resources.

Central to their theory is Lazarus and Folkman's contention that stress is not a one-time response to a static event. Rather, it involves a person's continuous interactions with and adjustments to the event, somewhat like Selye's revised theory (see again Box 7.1). Recall the opening story: Sarah's family was responding to new, different, and sometimes recurring stressors each day. But many of the stressors appeared to exceed her family's ability to cope with the situation.

We can also apply the transactional model to the example of the young woman walking alone along the dimly lit pathway at night. Recall that the woman saw a person emerge from and then retreat behind a building. Instead of simply asking how her body responds physiologically to the stressor, Lazarus and Folkman ask how the young woman cognitively appraises the stressful event. Equally as important, what does the woman do?

Using the transactional model, we might suggest that before the woman saw the shadow, walking alone at night along a dimly lit walkway did not exceed her personal or social resources. She was comfortable with the setting and confident of her skills. On seeing a person emerge and retreat, however, the woman may have reassessed the situation. She may have perceived that the new factor, a person lurking behind a building, posed a potential threat to her that exceeded her personal resources.

In this situation, the young woman may consider a number of options that will help her minimize the perceived threat. She may begin walking faster and determine whether her increased speed changes the behavior of the person behind the building. Or she may cross the street in an effort to put distance between the threatening situation and herself. Finally, she may use her cell phone to call a friend, requesting that they come and walk with her the remainder of the way home. While considering each possible action, the young woman will reassess the perceived threat. Changes in her behavior and her reassessment are what Lazarus and Folkman mean by "transactions."

Appraisal Process Lazarus contends that transactions are directed by our *cognitive appraisal* of the situation, or the process we use to evaluate the events. Cognitive appraisal involves three components: *primary appraisal*, the initial assessment of the event and determination of the potential harmfulness; *secondary appraisal*, an assessment of our resources and determination of how sufficient our resources are to meet the demands of the event; and finally, *cognitive reappraisal*, the re-evaluation of the event as it develops. In our scenario, the young woman's cognitive appraisal of the initial threat begins with an assessment of the potential harmfulness of the situation (primary appraisal). She then assesses the situation to determine whether her resources are sufficient to address the threat (secondary appraisal). She will reassess the situation (cognitive reappraisal), perhaps more than once, to determine whether it continues to be as threatening as it seemed at first.

In addition, Lazarus's theory of stress and coping assumes two things. First, he contends that situations or events are not inherently stressful. The stressfulness of a situation depends, in part, on our perception (cognitive appraisal) of the event. This means that people will interpret situations differently based on a number of factors including their prior experiences, their own skills, and their level of confidence in addressing such events. Take again the example of the woman walking alone on the dimly lit walkway. She appraised the situation with the person lurking in the distance as stressful – but another woman may not have. Additionally, consider the situation in the opening story. While Susan's family found caring for Sarah taxing, other families may not. Individual differences, or differences in appraisal, will lead to different interpretations of the same situation and possibly different responses. Remember, Sapolsky makes a similar point when explaining why we cannot make causal inferences about stress and illness.

The second assumption posed by Lazarus' theory is that an individual may appraise the same situation differently based on his or her mood, health, or motivation. The young woman walking alone at night may have considered the situation stressful primarily because she was aware that her judgment was impaired by the alcohol she consumed at the party. But had she been returning from a martial arts class, she might have felt less compromised and more comfortable with her resources or her ability to confront a potentially threatening individual.

To summarize, we see that stress is both a stimulus and a response. We also see that there are many different categories of stressors, as shown by Elliot and Eisdorfer (1982). Responses to stress are based in part on our cognitive appraisal of the stressor. Individuals may differ in their appraisal of a situation and, therefore, they may differ in their interpretation of an event as threatening. Within the same individual, there may be differences in the perceived stressfulness of the same situation from one point in time to another, given the individual's own state of mind, mood, or perceived state of health. Finally, the different categories of stressors (e.g., acute time, limited, or chronic) will influence both our perception and our response.

Physiological changes such as accelerated heart rates, dry mouth, and rapid breathing due to dilated bronchial airways (lungs) are but a few of the physical responses triggered by the sympathetic system when we cognitively appraise a situation as threatening (look again at Figure 7.2). No doubt the young woman en route home from the party experienced some combination of these symptoms when seeing the shadow of a person lurking behind a building at night.

But suppose that as the young woman in our scenario continues to walk, the person behind the building emerges. Suppose it is a child walking a small dog on a leash. (Let's suspend for the moment the obvious question of why a child is walking a dog late at night!) In addition, the young woman observes that the dog seems to pull and jerk the child in different directions. What would happen next as the woman cognitively reappraises the situation? Most likely the young woman would determine that the situation is no longer threatening. Now, with no other apparent threat, the parasympathetic system would activate to return the body to its steady state.

SECTION II. STRESS AND ILLNESS

We now know how our body responds physiologically and psychologically to stress, but what causes stress? Simply put, everything! It may seem like an exaggeration, but the statement is largely true. Earlier in the chapter, we stated that individuals will interpret situations differently. A situation that produces stress for one person may not be stressful to another. Therefore, any situation has the potential to cause stress to someone. Yet through research we know that there are some events that commonly cause stress in spite of individual differences in perception. Commonly reported causes of stress are chronic or prolonged illnesses and psychosocial factors including events such as the death of a family member, losing a job, or assuming caregiving responsibilities for someone who is unable to care for him or herself (see this chapter's opening story). Additionally, newer laboratory-based studies suggest that psychosocial stress can be triggered in individuals when they encounter uncontrollable situational demands, or when participants are either unable to avoid negative task outcomes or are subjected to negative judgments (see Khan & Obhi, 2021, for a succinct but thorough review of these studies).

Chronic Illness and Stress

In Chapter 4, Global, Communicable, and Chronic Disease, we defined *chronic diseases* as long-term (three to six months or longer) complex illnesses that can be controlled but not cured. Thus arthritis, diabetes, some forms of heart disease, and migraines are examples of chronic illnesses. A chronic illness requires that the person afflicted, as well as that person's family or others living with him or her, learn to live with the condition over a protracted period of time. It also requires continual adjustment to the changes, challenges, and threats presented by the disease, including changes in physical and emotional conditions, pain and pain management, and the inability to perform normal or expected roles (Benkel, Arnby, & Molander, 2020; Heijmans et al., 2004). While people learn to manage their disease and its symptoms, studies suggest that the uncertainty and the inability to control chronic disease progression can create anxiety and tensions.

In the opening story, Susan, Michael, and Lucinda struggled to cope with Sarah's constant and sometimes unanticipated changes in behavior or ability due to Alzheimer's. The changes caused tensions within the family.

Unpredictable disease outcomes, inability to control disease progression, and the rate of deterioration are commonly reported stressors for people who suffer with chronic illnesses (Benkel et al., 2020). A study conducted in China among 302 patients diagnosed with heart failure found that unpredictable disease outcomes, mediated by perceived stress, negatively affected patients' mental quality of life, with 45.7% of patients reporting poorer mental quality of life and 51.7% reporting poorer physical quality of life (An, Zhang, Wang, Chen, & Fan, 2022).

At this point, it is logical to ask three questions. First, what is unusual about people with chronic illnesses experiencing higher stress than people without such illnesses? Second, is the higher level of stress a problem? And third, what strategies are effective in combatting stress while also managing the chronic illness?

The gradual deterioration in physical or mental abilities due to chronic illness would cause anxiety and distress in many people. Therefore, stress is not an unusual response to such conditions. If elevated stress levels caused no adverse physical consequence, we might not be concerned about their effects either. The fact is, however, that prolonged stress can negatively affect health outcomes in anyone but particularly in people with chronic illnesses. Research shows that people with chronic illnesses who also report high stress levels or prolonged exposure to stressful environments show poorer overall health outcomes than people with similar diagnoses but with significantly less stress (Ahola, Toppinen-Tanner, Huuhtanam, Koskien, & Vaananen, 2009; Kershaw et al., 2008; Lane, Langman, Lip, & Nouwen, 2009; Manderson & Kokanovic, 2009; Morris, Moore, & Morris, 2011). In other words, prolonged stress can exacerbate an existing health problem, causing a further deterioration in health. These findings appear to hold true for many chronic ailments including diabetes, heart disease, high cholesterol, prostate cancer, and even workplace disabilities.

Can Stress Lead to Illness?

In addition to exacerbating pre-existing health concerns, some research suggests that stressful life experiences can precipitate or contribute to new physiological illnesses (Skaff et al., 2009; Stanley & Burrows, 2008). There is, however, one caveat: these stressful events are more likely to lead to physical illnesses when a person is vulnerable to such illnesses.

It is important to remind ourselves that, as Cohen, Murphy, and Prather (2019) state, most people who encounter stressful events do not get sick. However, they note that problematic events that concern interpersonal relationships do have the potential to trigger emotional or physiological responses. For example, conflicts with or the loss of a loved one, including a spouse, close friend, or co-worker, can result in depression, upper respiratory infections, or hypertension, among other ailments (Cohen et al., 2019; Sneed & Cohen, 2014). Additionally, interpersonal situations that result in a loss of social status or social exclusion can also trigger a physical response. And as we explained earlier in this chapter, chronic stressful events, such as those experienced by Lucinda, Michael, and Susan in our opening story, have a greater potential for causing physical ailments (Cohen et al., 2019).

Stanley and Burrows (2008) explore the association among stress, illness, and pre-existing vulnerabilities by examining the relationship between temperament and other inherited characteristics and illness. They cite, by way of example, John Hunter, a Scottish surgeon and scientist in the mid-18th century, who was probably the first to propose that heart ailments could be related to a person's emotional state or personality. Hunter, using himself as an example, suggested that his anxious and argumentative nature (personality) most likely contributed to his experiences of chest pains (Stanley & Burrows, 2008). His supposition was a precursor of the diathesis–stress model of disease.

The Diathesis–Stress (D–S) Model of Disease

Can people be predisposed to illnesses that are triggered by stress? In Chapter 2, Research Methods, we noted that some people were, in fact, genetically predisposed to illnesses. But the ***diathesis–stress (D–S)*** model of disease proposes something more. It states that an individual's biochemical or organ imbalances can predetermine a person's reaction to environmental stressors, which can result in physical symptoms of illnesses (Stanley & Burrows, 2008). In other words, a biological predisposition and an environmental precipitating factor (see Chapter 2, Research Methods) are necessary determinants to cause the onset of a stress-related illness.

The concept of a biological or psychological predisposition to an illness (a *diathesis*), triggered by an environmental precipitating factor (a *stressor*), as postulated by the D–S model has been proposed as a possible explanation for psychopathology such as schizophrenia and depression and for physiological illnesses such as chronic pain. For example, seminal research by Nuechlerlein and colleagues (1992) suggests that known biological markers for schizophrenia (diathesis) are triggered by an environmental stressor that results in manifestations of the illness. Additionally, a unique study by Banks and Kerns (1996) suggests that the diathesis–stress model may explain the relationship between depression and chronic pain. These researchers propose that if depression is a pre-existing condition in someone who developed a chronic pain, then the person's pre-existing psychological state may increase the likelihood of developing major depressive symptoms in response to the ongoing pain. In this instance, depression is the psychological diathesis, and chronic pain represents the stressor. Still others suggest that the relationship between stress and, say, depressive disorders, is reciprocal (MDD; Hammen, 2006; Kramer, 2021), making it difficult to determine the directionality of the relationship. One final point brings us back to emotions. Levenson (2019) argues for the need to explore the role that specific emotions play in the onset of physical illnesses as well as in the bidirectional causal influence in the stress-disease relationship. For example, Levenson states that anger and embarrassment can be tied to cardiovascular diseases and musculoskeletal ailments (Levenson, 2019).

Personality Type, Stress, and Illness

Research on the association between temperament (an inherited quality) and health also led some researchers to propose that personality type may be another predetermining factor for illness. Early research suggested that individuals with type A personalities are more susceptible to illnesses, such as heart problems, than those without such characteristics (Friedman & Rosenman, 1959; Hecker, Chesney, & Frautschi, 1988). You may be familiar with the ***type A personality*** profile – someone who is highly competitive, is high in need of achievement, is impatient, and can appear hostile or aggressive to others. Subsequent studies by Smith, Glazer, Ruiz, and Gallo (2004) and others refined the association between personality and illness. They established that it is the unhealthy elements of the type A personality, such as anger, hostility, and aggression, which are associated with coronary artery disease and decreased longevity, not the personality type itself (Steca et al., 2016).

In addition, consider this: Some professions, such as the finance industry – including the stock exchange and investment banking, law (such as litigation), and even construction, are highly demanding, competitive, and pressurized environments. Several studies support findings that individuals who work in such settings may be at risk for higher incidences of negative health outcomes related to the workplace atmosphere (Reich, 2020; Wu, Hu, & Zheng, 2019). Interestingly, these same professions attract type A personalities. But it is unclear whether it is the work and its related environment or the person that triggers the health consequences. For example, if a person who works in one of these competitive and demanding fields develops a heart-related illness, was the person predisposed to negative health outcomes because of the negative elements of the Type A personality, or did the environment trigger the unhealthy elements of the type A personality, thereby causing the health outcome?

Recent personality studies also contend that if there is any association between personality type and illness, people with *type D* (for distressed) personality characteristics, or people who exhibit generally negative affect (stress, anxiety, hostility, and depression), and social inhibition are more likely to develop heart-related health problems (Denollet, Pedersen, Vrints, & Conraads, 2006; Kupper & Denollet, 2007; Steca et al., 2016). In other words, research would suggest that distressed emotional states, specifically depression, hostility, and anxiety, are more strongly linked to heart problems than personality type or profession.

More research supports the claim that unhealthy elements of a personality can impact health outcomes. For example, Brendgen and Vitaro (2008) conducted a unique study examining the effects of peer rejection on physical health among 157 middle school students (grades 7 and 8) to test the theory that high levels of negative emotionality could result in increased stress that, in turn, could lead to physical health problems. Their results (see Box 7.2) show an association between *negative emotionally reactive* adolescent girls, here meaning girls who were prone to respond to stressful events with anger, sadness, anxiety, or depression, and physical and psychological health problems. No significant difference was found for boys regardless of their level of reactivity.

Box 7.2 Can Social Rejection Make a Person Ill? A Test for the Diathesis–Stress (D–S) Model

No one likes to be an "outcast," rejected from a desired social group. But can such rejection contribute to poor physical and mental health? Brendgen and Vitaro (2008) seem to think so, at least with respect to adolescent girls.

Studies suggest that adolescents who are rejected or intensely disliked by their peers are more prone to evidence mental health problems (Garnett et al., 2014; Mulvey, Boswell, & Zheng, 2017; Russell, Sinclair, Poteat, & Koenig, 2012). An earlier study by Brendgen and Vitaro (2008), designed to examine the role of peer rejection on physical health offers a good example of this phenomenon. They contend that because peer rejection causes considerable stress among adolescents, individuals who experience stress as a result of peer rejection may be at a higher risk for negative mental health outcomes, including anxiety and depression, and frequent incidences of physical health problems.

To test this concept, the authors examined several factors: family adversity (including family structure, parental education, socioeconomic status, and parental occupation), self-reported physical health problems, depression symptoms, and peer rejection (using peer rating of the students they would be most and least likely to invite to a social gathering). Included also was a measure of *emotional reactivity*, a teacher-based rating that assessed a student's temperament, specifically reaction to and anxiety about a negative event (Brendgen & Vitaro, 2008). For example, teachers assessed the student's likelihood to "get irritated easily" or to "cry easily."

Using a group of 157 high school students in Quebec, Canada, the authors studied girls and boys in grades 7 and 8 over two years. When comparing students', parents', and teachers' ratings and also students' health profiles, the authors found that adolescents who were emotionally reactive were more likely to report physical health problems. However, Brendgen and Vitaro (2008) found that such results pertained only to adolescent girls who were moderately or highly emotionally reactive. Girls who were less reactive and adolescent boys regardless of their reactivity level showed no physical or emotional health problems attributable to peer rejection.

What do these findings suggest? Brendgen and Vitaro's findings seem to suggest a link between emotional temperament and physical health for adolescent girls. Specifically, the findings suggest that girls who are predisposed to highly negative responses to stressful situations (remember, we are defining peer rejection as highly stressful) are at higher risk for overall negative health outcomes. These results seem to suggest support for the diathesis–stress model and may hold implications for health psychologists when addressing the health needs of young adolescent girls. Research has long established that adolescent peer groups can affect the emotional well-being of teens. Now it appears that psychosocial stressors from the same adolescent cohorts may impact the physical health of highly reactive adolescent girls as well. If so, health psychologists, with their ecological health training, are uniquely qualified to address such issues.

In addition, a study conducted in northeastern Spain used a Spanish-language version of the Type-D depression scale to compare the depression and anxiety symptoms of four groups of participants: a group of coronary heart disease patients admitted to hospital at the University of Lleida, Catalonia, Spain after a recent cardiovascular incident, and three groups of healthy participants: healthy workers, healthy community volunteers, and professors or service workers at the university. Aluja, Malas, Lucas, Worner, and Bascompte's (2019) findings support earlier research which showed a relationship between Type-D personality and adverse health outcomes. Specifically, Aluja and colleagues found that Type-D participants scored higher on measures of depression and anxiety as well as on the neuroticism-anxiety and aggressiveness-hostility scales. Coincidentally, participants with coronary heart disease also scored higher on neuroticism-anxiety and aggression-hostility. Was this just a coincidence? The researchers did not think so.

To summarize, consistent with the D–S model, some research suggests that an individual's vulnerabilities (biological or temperamental) may predispose him or her to greater adverse responses to stressful stimuli. Such reactions could result in a greater probability of psychophysiological health problems, such as chronic headaches, asthma, skin disorders, and respiratory infections (Madison et al., 2022; Purdy, 2013). But the D–S model, which proposes both an individual and an environmental determinant of stress-induced illness, does not explain the relationship between stress and illness in the absence of pre-existing vulnerabilities.

Psychosocial Events and Stress

The scenario presented earlier in this chapter of a woman walking at night helps explain the cognitive process used to interpret a stressful physical stimulus. But what happens when the stressor is a nonphysical event? Consider, again, the case of Sarah in the opening story. Sarah posed no physical threat to other family members. Yet her story was included in this chapter to illustrate stress.

Sarah's condition caused psychological and psychosocial stressors, here meaning stressors that are both psychological and social in origin, which are capable of producing physical responses. You will recall that, psychologically, Susan (Sarah's adult daughter) experienced sleep disturbances. And everyone except Sarah exhibited heightened irritability, most likely due to the new caregiving responsibilities. Psychosocial stressors included, for example, Susan's ambivalence about putting her mother in a nursing home – a decision that was contrary to Susan's beliefs about her responsibilities as a daughter to care for her mother, a social construct.

Research suggests that physiological symptoms such as an inability to sleep, atypical eating behavior, increased irritability, and exhaustion are common responses to psychosocial or psychological stress (Pawlyk, Morrison, Ross, & Brennan, 2008; Orsal, Orsal, Alparslan, & Unsal, 2012; Rafique, Al-Asoom, Latif, Al Sunni, & Wasi, 2019). For example, Orsal and colleagues (2012) found an association between psychological stress among college students and sleep disturbances. Results from their study with Turkish male and female college students showed that the student's perceptions of the new demands of college, together with additional worries about living away from home, financial worries, and concerns about moral behavior led to higher reports of poor sleep quality among female students. Male students, by comparison, reported no significant impact on sleep quality.

Likewise, research on the association between psychosocial stress and obesity suggests that excessive eating, which can lead to weight gain and obesity, may also be prompted by stress (Strickland, Giger, Nelson, & Davis, 2007; Tobiyama, 2019; van der Valk, Savas, & van Rossum, 2018). Participants in Strickland and colleagues' study (2007) reported that psychosocial factors, such as family responsibilities, workplace issues, and concern about weight, accounted for their tendency to eat frequently or to prefer high-fat and high-calorie foods. By comparison, van der Valk and colleagues (2018) suggest that for some persons, sensitivity to glucocorticoids – which is partly genetically determined – may increase their vulnerability to mental or physical stressors. In short, stress, triggered by psychological or psychosocial causes, or a predisposing genetic factor triggered by stress (think again of the D-S model) can result in physiological health problems or behaviors (such as overeating) that can inhibit good health outcomes.

We close this section on psychosocial stressors with research on the relationship between chronic unemployment, stress, and depression. Of the numerous studies that examine the relationship between employment, income, stress, and depression, one makes the case for the long-term impact of unemployment as a chronic stressor that can affect mental and physical health. Khan and Pearlon (2006) conducted a retrospective analysis of the impact of economic strain over the life course of older adults. Looking at five measures of health, including self-rated health, number of serious health conditions, illness symptoms, functional complaints, and depressive symptoms, they found that the longer a person experienced financial strain in early life, the greater the damage to multiple dimensions of health in later life. One source of financial strain is unemployment. Khan and Pearlon's findings led them to conclude that long-term unemployment can create a chronic stressor that has long-term negative physical and mental health consequences that continue well past the initial presentation of the stressor.

Almost to underscore this fact, a second study by the CDC (Centers for Disease Control, 2013b) reported a dramatic 28.4% increase in the rates of suicide between 1999 and 2010 for men and women aged 35–64 in the U.S. These data are even more perplexing when considering that no other significant changes in suicide rates were reported for other age cohorts. For some researchers, the trigger was the Great Recession of 2008–2009.

You might recall that in 2007, the global economic crisis adversely affected many people. In the U.S., unemployment rates rose to over 10.0% nationally, with some regions reporting almost double that figure among specific populations. Ramchand, Ayer, and O'Connor (2022) note that during this period of the Great Recession a 1 percentage point increase in unemployment was associated with a 1.0–1.6 percentage average increase in suicide rates.

The rest of the world was not as lucky. An analysis of the relationship between unemployment and suicide rates in 63 countries between 2000 and 2011 – a period that includes the Great Recession, suggests that suicide risks associated with unemployment rose 20%–30% (Kawohl & Nordt, 2020). What is more, Kawohl and Nordt note that the increase in suicides occurred prior to the actual rise in unemployment rates.

Such findings have naturally led to concern and speculation about the effects of COVID-19–related unemployment on suicide rates. Using projected job loss data from the International Labour Organization, Kawohl and Nordt (2020) estimate an increase in unemployment-related suicides in the era of COVID-19 ranging from 2,135 to 9,570 per year.

As sobering as these statistics are, some researchers dispute the relationship between unemployment and suicide, suggesting either no relationship, or one that is related to seasonal or regional variations (Ramchand et al., 2022). You can be certain, however, that researchers will continue to investigate to determine whether there is a relationship between suicide rates and unemployment.

Measuring Stress

With so much discussion about stress, it is reasonable to ask: How do we measure it? Of interest here are methods that assess both the situations that create stressful reactions (stressors) as well as the reactions themselves. We begin by examining measures that identify stressors.

SOCIAL READJUSTMENT RATING SCALE (SRRS) The death of a family member, birth of a child, a wedding, a divorce, and major exams are psychosocial events that could provoke a stressful response. How do we know? For the past 60 years, researchers have asked individuals to identify the most and least stressful experiences common to people.

One of the first and perhaps best-known measures of psychosocial stress is the *Social Readjustment Rating Scale (SRRS)* by Holmes and Rahe (1967), also known as the Holmes and Rahe Stress Scale. The 43-item scale includes a list of life events, rank ordered from most to least stressful. Each life event is associated with a *life change unit score*, a measure of the perceived stressfulness of the event, on a scale of 100 to 0. Ratings from thousands of participants produced weighted scores for each psychosocial event, which yielded a rank order of most to least stressful situations that apply to a diverse sample of people. For example, the death of a spouse has a life change unit score (stressfulness score) of 100, suggesting a highly stressful event. Conversely, outstanding personal achievements are assigned a score of 28, or relatively low stress.

In a seminal study to determine the relationship between current psychosocial stressors and future illness, Rahe, Mahan, and Arthur (1970) administered their scale to a group of navy sailors just prior to a six-month cruise assignment. The researchers scored each sailor's response to obtain a life change unit score. Rahe and colleagues (1970) then compared the ratings to sailors' health records six months later and found that the sailors with the highest life change unit scores were more likely to be ill six months later than were the sailors with the lowest scores. These authors believe the results of the study suggest a correlation between the number of stressful experiences, the perceived severity of the event, and overall physical health. They suggest that the number and type of stressful events an individual experiences may be a determinant of health outcomes.

The SRRS does not negate the association between stress, biological factors, and illness proposed by the D–S model. But the emphasis on the role of psychosocial stressors in the SRRS suggests that environmental factors, here meaning stressful events, may also trigger health problems.

CRITICISM OF THE SRRS Criticisms of Holmes and Rahe's scale – specifically, wording problems, lack of differentiation between positive or negative events (spouse stops or starts work is one item with one life change score), outdated events, or an inability to account for individual differences in interpretation or truthfulness – prompted other researchers to refine and improve upon the original scale. For example, some investigators developed scales tailored to specific populations, such as children or college students (see Table 7.1). Do the items in the Undergraduate Stress Questionnaire include some of your major stressors as a college student?

TABLE 7.1 Undergraduate Stress Questionnaire

The following life events were found to be stressful to undergraduate students. How stressful have they been for you in the past month?
1. Death of family member (or friend)
2. Had a lot of tests
3. It's finals week
4. Applying to graduate school
5. Victim of a crime
6. Assignment in all classes due the same day
7. Breaking up with boy/girlfriend
8. Found out boy/girlfriend cheated on you
9. Lots of deadlines to meet
10. Property stolen
11. You have a hard upcoming week
12. Went into a test unprepared
13. Lost something (especially wallet)
14. Death of a pet
15. Did worse than expected on a test
16. Had an interview
17. Had projects, research papers due
18. Did badly on a test
19. Parents getting divorced
20. Dependent on other people
21. Having roommate conflicts
22. Car/bike broke down, flat tire
23. Got a traffic ticket
24. Missed your period and waiting
25. Thoughts about the future
26. Lack of money
27. Dealing with incompetence at the Registrar's
28. Thought about unfinished work
29. No sleep
30. Sick, injury
31. Had a class presentation
32. Applying for a job
33. Fought with boy/girlfriend
34. Working while in school
35. Argument, conflicts of values with friends
36. Bothered by having no social support of family

(*Continued*)

TABLE 7.1 (Continued)

The following life events were found to be stressful to undergraduate students. How stressful have they been for you in the past month?

37. Performed poorly at a task
38. Can't finish everything you needed to do
39. Heard bad news
40. Had confrontation with an authority figure
41. Maintaining a long-distance boy/girlfriend
42. Crammed for a test
43. Feel unorganized
44. Trying to decide on a major
45. Feel isolated
46. Parents controlling with money
47. Couldn't find a parking space
48. Noise disturbed you when trying to study
49. Someone borrowed something without permission
50. Had to ask for money
51. Ran out of toner while printing
52. Erratic schedule
53. Can't understand your professor
54. Trying to get into your major or college
55. Registration for classes
56. Stayed up late writing a paper
57. Someone you expected to call did not
58. Someone broke a promise
59. Can't concentrate
60. Someone did a "pet peeve" of yours
61. Living with boy/girlfriend
62. Felt need for transportation
63. Bad haircut today
64. Job requirements changed
65. No time to eat
66. Felt some peer pressure
67. You have a hangover
68. Problems with your computer
69. Problems getting home from bar when drunk
70. Used a fake ID
71. No sex in a while
72. Someone cut ahead of you in line
73. Checkbook didn't balance
74. Visit from a relative and entertaining them
75. Decision to have sex on your mind
76. Spoke with a professor
77. Change of environment (new doctor, dentist, etc.)
78. Exposed to upsetting TV show, book, movie
79. Got to class late
80. Holiday
81. Sat through a boring class
82. Favorite sporting team lost

Source: Crandall et al. (1992).

Another problem with the SRRS pertains to the limits of using retrospective recall to correctly identify past stressful events. Many studies show that participants perform poorly when attempting to recall past events or to ascertain whether such events were, in fact, stressful (again, see Sapolsky, 2004). Thus, relying on an individual to accurately recall past stressful events or the impact of those events and their subsequent link to an illness is highly problematic.

Daily Life Hassles and Stress

Holmes and Rahe assume that major life events, positive or negative, will affect health. To that end, each of the 43 items on the original SRRS scale represents an event that most people would agree happens infrequently, if ever. For example, the death of a spouse, divorce, marriage, or marital reconciliation usually are one-time or rare events.

Lazarus and his colleagues offer an alternative interpretation of the effects of stress on well-being. They contend that *daily life hassles* are more likely to cause negative health outcomes than are major events (see Table 7.2). They propose that because major stressful events, like marriages, deaths, or divorce, occur infrequently such events cannot explain the frequent incidences of stress individuals claim to experience. For example, when was the last time you or your friends suffered a major personal injury? Now compare

TABLE 7.2 Selected Daily Hassles

Category	*Example*
Household hassles	Preparing meals Shopping Home maintenance
Health hassles	Physical illness Concern about medical treatment Side effects of medicine
Time pressure hassles	Too many things to do Not enough time to do all that needs doing Too many responsibilities
Inner concerns	Being lonely Concerns about inner conflicts Fear of information
Environmental hassles	Neighborhood deterioration Noise Crime
Financial responsibility hassles	Financial responsibilities Concern about owing money Financial responsibilities for someone who doesn't live with you
Work hassles	Job dissatisfaction Dislike of current work duties Problems getting along with fellow workers
Future security hassles	Concern about job security Concerns about retirement Property, investments, or taxes

that to the last time you or your friends received a low score on a test or assignment. No doubt, major personal injuries occur far less frequently than, say, low scores. If stress, a common experience for many, is determined in part by our exposure to stressful events, then events that occur frequently, such as the ones identified by Crandall, Priesler, and Aussprung (1992) for college undergraduates (see Table 7.1), are more likely to create opportunities for stress than are the rare but traumatic major events. For this reason, Lazarus and Folkman (1984a) believe that the frequently occurring daily hassles of life are more likely to explain the numerous stresses cited by individuals. According to Folkman and Moskowitz (2000), if not managed successfully, over time such daily hassles can accumulate and can lead to adverse mental health outcomes.

Returning to the example in the opening story, Lazarus, DeLonges, Folkman, and Gruen's (1985) daily hassles theory would propose that for Susan, Michael, and Lucinda, the daily hassles associated with caring for Sarah may have accumulated to cause high levels of stress for the family. We know from earlier research by Selye (1950) that accumulated stress can result in physiological symptoms and, if uncontrolled, illnesses.

Additional research by Folkman and Moskowitz (2000) further tested the daily hassles theory of stress by examining coping mechanisms. Coping is an important component for understanding the psychological and physiological impact of stress and by extension the impact of stress on overall well-being. We explore coping with stress in Section III.

Catastrophic Events and Stress

Lazarus and Folkman's work notwithstanding, there are times when a single major event produces stress that has an enduring effect on the psychological and physiological health of individuals. Take, for example, man-made disasters such as the destruction of the World Trade Towers in New York City on September 11, 2001. That catastrophic event, along with the attack on the Pentagon and the crash of United Airlines Flight 93, claimed over 3,000 lives and created a stressful environment in New York City, as well as the rest of the nation, for many years. Individuals who witnessed or were directly exposed to the event complained of insomnia, nightmares, and panic attacks, as well as physiological problems such as respiratory distress, chronic respiratory problems, and cancers for years afterwards. Estimates suggest that between 4.7% and 10.2% of the adults in New York City reported some form of health impairment attributable to the stress they experienced from the event. Health professionals have determined that many such individuals were experiencing *posttraumatic stress disorder* (PTSD; Neria, 2009), an anxiety disorder that occurs after witnessing or experiencing a traumatic event.

Earlier in the chapter, we delayed our response to the question of whether PTSD is a distal stressor (Post-Traumatic Stress Disorder – National Institute of Mental Health (NIMH; nih.gov). Current definitions suggest that PTSD may occur after a single traumatic incident or be the result of multiple exposures to trauma, such as the case with military personnel in combat. Exposure to human-made disasters like the events of September 11 or other events related to conflicts or wars, as well as natural disasters such as tsunamis or hurricanes, can lead to emotional and psychological problems that impair an individual's normal functional ability (Makwana, 2019; Putman et al., 2009). And, according to these definitions, such experiences can also lead to behaviors that negatively affect health. For example, traumatic events have been cited as one reason for excessive use or abuse of alcohol or drugs by soldiers returning from war. Using this definition, it is possible that PTSD can occur as a result of a distal stressor.

VIDEO #39/60

Chapter 7: Stress and Coping

- **Posttraumatic Stress Disorder (PTSD):** *AboutFace: Learn about PTSD and how treatment can turn your life around*
- *Website: https://www.youtube.com/watch?v=Eac_CHz8gDo*
- **The information provided by the National Center for PTSD is publicly accessible and available for free (What Is AboutFace? | AboutFace (va.gov))**

But there appears to be some disagreement about the definition of PTSD that is relevant to its classification as a distal stressor. It may come as a surprise that a number of researchers and mental health professionals question the large number of diagnosed PTSD cases. Summerfield (2001) notes that originally, PTSD was defined as an outcome associated with a person's exposure to *one* extreme experience that was not expected to reoccur. Currently, however, PTSD is associated with reoccurring events, including accidents, verbal sexual harassment, or difficult birthing experiences. According to Summerfield (2001), the proliferation of PTSD and its use for a host of experiences may be due, in part, to the lack of specificity of the definition and diagnosis. He contends that the current definition does not allow mental health professionals to distinguish between normal versus pathological distress. If some instances of PTSD are really best described as "normal" distress, then they would not fit well in the category of distal stressors.

One reason for the confusion is, according to North (2009) and Banerjee (2015), a failure to follow standard American Psychiatric Association procedures for validating the diagnostic criteria for PTSD, leading many to question the empirical support for this new diagnosis. Essentially, that means that the scientific "proof" of such a phenomenon is in question. Specifically, North and Banerjee note that although the National Academy of Medicine, an independent, science-based advisor (National Academy of Medicine, 2022) – acknowledges that there is considerable evidence of a clinical description of PTSD, here meaning demographic characteristics and precipitating factors, there is no evidence from laboratory studies, follow-up studies, and/or family studies usually required by the Association to validate this new diagnosis. This is a good time to return to Chapter 2, Research Methods, for a refresher on the relevance and importance of laboratory and follow-up studies to confirm a phenomenon.

Undoubtedly, there are cases of distal stressors that could be diagnosed accurately as PTSD. But if Summerfield's, North's, and Banerjee's analyses are correct, the absence of a clear definition of PTSD, in addition to the lack of evidence for this diagnosis, may lead to the conclusion that a number of such diagnoses arguably are not PTSD.

One last point raised by Banerjee (2015) concerns the applicability of PTSD to non-Western cultures. The concepts and expressions of depression, anxiety, and reactions to trauma are not universally applicable to all cultures. Thus, a diagnosis that is minimally validated in addition to being culturally constrained is of limited value. Therefore, we return to the question of whether PTSD is a distal stressor. Based on the current critiques the answer is: It depends.

To review, stress can have both direct and indirect effects on health. As we saw in Section I, stress can directly affect an individual's physiological, emotional, and psychological response to an event. In Section II, we reviewed the attenuated effects of stress on illness and, conversely, illness as a potential exacerbating factor for stress. In the next section, we examine adaptive (positive) and maladaptive (negative) coping mechanisms employed to reduce the potential adverse consequences of stress.

SECTION III. COPING WITH STRESS

What do you do when you feel stressed? Some people whistle. Others pace, chew gum, listen to music, or exercise. Each of these activities represents ways of coping with situations that exceed our resources (Lazarus & Folkman, 1984a).

The concept of coping used here is a logical extension of the theory of stress explained in Lazarus's transactional model. In the model, stress is a process that begins when external factors exceed, or appear to exceed, an individual's personal or social resources. Coping, however, is a process by which an individual applies cognitive or behavioral responses to stressful situations consistent with his or her personal or social resources.

There are a variety of coping mechanisms people can adopt to address stress. Some are characterized as positive or adaptive actions, those behaviors that help to manage stress and allow us to productively complete our daily tasks. For some people, exercise, listening to music, seeking and obtaining social support, and spiritual practices including prayer are coping mechanisms that assist them in managing stress and responding to stressors. Other mechanisms, such as avoidance, overeating, or risky health activities such as substance use and risky sexual practices, represent negative or maladaptive behaviors that some also employ as coping strategies. We discuss these negative coping mechanisms later in this section. For the moment, it is important to know that these strategies not only fail to address the stressor, but they also introduce additional problems that can create new sources of stress. We cannot review all of the coping mechanisms individuals might use in this chapter. Therefore, we begin by classifying methods of coping and illustrating some of the mechanisms.

Cognitive Coping

Research has identified two principal types of cognitive coping styles: *problem* or *emotion focused* versus *engagement* or *disengagement* focused. As the names imply, problem- or emotion-focused coping includes two levels, problem focused and emotion focused.

PROBLEM- OR EMOTION-FOCUSED COPING When using a *problem-focused* coping strategy, an individual seeks information and generates solutions to address the issue or problem encountered (see Table 7.3). Such a strategy is active and fact-based. It entails planning to resolve the issue, with little time spent on emotional responses. Consider again the scenario presented in the opening story. A problem-focused strategy to address the health care needs of an Alzheimer's patient like Sarah, as well as the health and well-being of other members of the family, could include identifying the source of the problem and the emotional needs of all involved and seeking a solution that will address everyone's needs as best as possible. The family's decision to seek help from a therapist is consistent with a problem-focused approach. Other problem-focused approaches might include a search of the Internet for information about Alzheimer's or for support groups that might provide assistance to family members.

Conversely, the emotion-focused approach to coping entails principally seeking solace or emotional support from others. People who choose the emotion-focused strategy may seek out a family member, friend, or trained professional, such as a health psychologist, to discuss their emotional or psychological pain. They may even obtain a sympathetic audience. In the process, the individual may receive helpful information or guidance; however, that is not the principal intent of his or her interaction. The main goal is to obtain expressive support.

TABLE 7.3 Selected Coping Strategies

Strategy	Description
Problem or emotion focused	
Problem focused	*Principal objective: To find a workable solution to the problem* Seek information Generate solutions Have fact-based approach to solutions Actively engage Have little focus on emotion
Emotion focused	*Principal objective: To find solace and emotional support* Seek comfort Share distress and psychological pain Look for sympathetic audience
Engagement or disengagement focused	
Engagement focused	*Principal objective: To obtain helpful information and support* Seek others to obtain information Share emotional burden Obtain workable solution Look for sympathetic but helpful audience
Disengagement focused	*Principal objective: To minimize emotional discomfort and stress* Address problem without assistance or information Withdraw from problem Avoid problem or efforts to resolve Avoid through substance use Deny problem exists

ENGAGEMENT OR DISENGAGEMENT COPING The second type of coping, engagement or disengagement, also includes two levels. Engagement represents a hybrid of the problem- and emotion-focused coping approaches. It includes both problem-solving and emotional support. For example, an individual who uses an engagement-focused coping approach may initiate conversations about the difficulties of caring for a person with Alzheimer's with another person, perhaps someone experiencing the same problem. Although one outcome of the conversation may be an empathetic connection with the person, the goal is to obtain helpful information.

Finally, as the name suggests, the disengagement approach represents a withdrawal from the problem or a denial of its existence. For example, individuals who use a disengagement-focused strategy may attempt to address the needs of a person with a chronic illness or address their own needs without seeking treatment or assistance from others. Alternatively, some disengagers may become depressed as a result of the stressors or may turn to substance use (drugs or alcohol) to withdraw from the problems altogether (Bourguignon et al., 2020; Helder et al., 2002).

Research suggests that, of the four coping styles, the problem-focused approach appears to be the most effective strategy because effort is expended to address and resolve the source of the stress. On the other hand, the disengagement approach is least effective (Dehelean et al., 2021; Ogoma, 2020). Withdrawal (through denial or substance use) from a stressful event will do little to resolve the issue, although it may temporarily abate the sensation of stress. And as we indicated earlier, if the disengagement approach includes using substances, then this form of coping introduces more potential stressors, including the risk of addiction or physiological health complications.

Finally, it is important to note that studies on coping also suggest that the techniques individuals adopt for a specific illness are related to the strategies they use when dealing with everyday life (Stanislawski, 2019). In essence, coping strategies appear to be linked to an individual's own disposition toward handling stress of any sort and not just the health issue or the problem at hand.

Behavioral Coping Strategies

Cognitive responses to stress may be useful for individuals who prefer such an approach. But not all people prefer cognitive strategies. Some opt for behavioral coping techniques: for example, exercise, music, humor, and spirituality/religious activities. We review these positive behavioral coping methods first, followed by negative behavioral coping approaches. Keep in mind, however, that these are but a sample of the mechanism used to abate stress.

EXERCISE AND STRESS No doubt you have heard someone say, "I'm going for a run to unwind," or "I'm so nervous about my exam; I think I'll go for a swim to help me focus." Maybe you have said similar things yourself. But does exercise really ameliorate stress? A study by Swedish researchers Terjestam, Jouper, and Johannson (2010) sought to test such assumptions. Specifically, these researchers explored whether exercise could positively impact well-being and self-image as well as minimize the psychological distress and stress of students 13–14 years of age. In their study, Terjestam et al. (2010) introduced students to qigong, an ancient Chinese exercise form practiced for thousands of years. Studies suggested that qigong effectively manages stress, reduces psychological symptoms, improves sleep, and reduces incidences of headaches and other body pains (Rodrigues et al., 2021; van Dam, 2020). As predicted, Terjestam and colleagues found that this ancient exercise significantly reduced reports of psychological stress and distress among the experimental group of 13- to 14-year-olds. In contrast, the control group reported reduced well-being.

It is also true, however, that the effects of qigong on stress and well-being could be explained by external factors. Biologically, qigong has been shown to moderate blood pressure, heart rate, and respiration rate (Lee et al., 2000), physiological factors that elevate in response to stress. But it is also likely that, for this group of participants, qigong exercises signaled a reprieve from schoolwork and therefore offered an environmental release from stress (Terjestam et al., 2010). In other words, the impact of qigong on distress and stress is clear; however, the outcomes in this study may have been influenced by both internal (biological) and external (school) forces.

You may recall from Chapter 6, Emotional Health and Well-Being, that some people prefer traditional rather than Western medicine for addressing chronic illnesses. Consequently, you may think that we "stacked the deck" by selecting an exercise associated with a traditional medical practice to demonstrate the positive impact of exercise on health. Rest assured, however, that similar outcomes have been obtained when examining other types of exercise. For example, a study examining the effects of exercise on stress cite the benefits of aerobic exercise on reduced heart rate, muscle tension, and perceived work stress among teachers (Ritvanen, Louhevaara, Helin, Halonen, & Hanninen, 2007). A more recent study using mice also found significant benefits from aerobic exercise. This study by Gioscia-Ryan et al. (2021) found that lifelong aerobic exercising reduces *oxidative stress* – a condition that can result in cell and/or tissue damage – as well as inflammation, thereby helping to protect the vessels in the body that carry blood functioning, which is often adversely affected by aging.

Finally, an interesting study conducted in Iran demonstrated significant benefits of aerobic exercising in nurses. In this study, nurses were randomly assigned to an experimental or control group, with those in the experimental group receiving three, one-hour aerobic exercise sessions per week for a total of eight weeks. The control group received no structured exercises. Mohebbi, Dehkordi, Sharif, and Banitalebi (2019) used the Health and Safety Executive (HSE) questionnaire to measure the stress levels of both groups (experimental and control) before, immediately after the eight-week exercise session, and again, two months after the intervention. While there was no difference in the stress levels of the experimental versus control group at the start of the study, nurses in the experimental group reported significantly lower stress scores immediately after the eight-week intervention. Unfortunately, the follow-up measure conducted approximately two months after the intervention revealed an increase in stress levels among the group receiving the aerobic exercise intervention, essentially erasing the beneficial effects of exercising. In essence, whether using traditional or Western exercise techniques, studies show a role for exercise as a behavioral coping mechanism that effectively ameliorates stress. However, these last two studies also suggest that the exercise intervention must be longterm.

Other stress abatement approaches, like music, seem to have similar beneficial effects.

MUSIC The waiting rooms in doctors' offices, elevators in high-rise buildings, and even some supermarkets share a common practice: They often play "background" music. The music is piped in through the intercom at a low volume. In fact, you may not notice the music when you first arrive. After a few moments, however, you may hear the strands of a melody or perhaps hear a bass line or harmony. Why would these unrelated venues all play music softly in the background? The research on stress and music can explain the practice (What is Music Therapy? | What is Music Therapy? | American Music Therapy Association (AMTA).

With rare exceptions, researchers agree: Music reduces stress and anxiety levels. Research examining the relationship between music and stress falls into three main categories: the relationships between music and physiological indications of stress; music and psychological functioning and stress; and finally, music and performance on specific tasks. Interestingly, whether researching the effects of music on a participant's blood pressure levels, self-reported anxiety, self-reported emotional states, or speed and accuracy on performance tasks, all studies reported that music reduced stress-related responses and improved performance. We will examine all three types of research.

Music and Physiological Health Nilsson's (2009) study on the effects of music on post-operative coronary artery bypass patients shows a clear link between post-operative music intervention and psychological and physiological well-being. In a controlled study, Nilsson put 20 post-operative coronary patients in a music intervention and bed rest condition, while another 20 post-operative coronary patients received bed rest only. She then measured each patient's plasma oxytocin, a hormone that inhibits sympathetic and hypothalamic-pituitary and adrenal activity during stress and helps to regulate cardiovascular activity (Petersson & Uvnas-Moberg, 2007). Finally, she assessed patients' heart rate, blood pressure, and subjective relaxation levels. Her results showed that patients on the bed rest with music intervention had higher oxytocin levels and higher subjective relaxation levels than those in the bed rest–only condition. Not only did patients report being more relaxed, their physiological response as determined by their oxytocin levels also confirmed their subjective assessment.

In a related study, Dai, Huang, Xu, Chen, and Cao (2020) tested the effects of music therapy on the pain, anxiety, and depression levels of patients undergoing coronary artery bypass grafting. Of the three groups in this study (music therapy, rest with no music therapy, and conventional treatment), only the music therapy group reported significantly lower pain, anxiety and depression scores post music intervention. These studies clearly suggest that music has a beneficial effect on both the psychological and physiological health of the study participants.

Music and Emotional Health Do doctors' offices, elevators, and supermarkets create stressful conditions? Yes, for some people. The wait time in a doctor's office can be stressful as people contemplate the many different ailments imaginable while waiting to speak with the doctor. Elevators, too, can be stressful as some people feel uncomfortable in small, enclosed spaces, particularly when the space is crowded with strangers. Finally, supermarkets may not in themselves be stressful, but the process of shopping for groceries while adhering to a budget and managing crowds can create some anxiety. It is common to hear background music playing in all three venues. One reason given for the presence of music is to create a relaxed or relaxing atmosphere for the patient or the customer.

Are all genres of music equally as effective in reducing stress and anxiety levels? Apparently not. Researchers disagree about whether type of music is an important variable in stress reduction. A study by Chafin, Roy, Gerin, and Christenfeld (2004) suggests that only classical music effectively reduces psychological and physiological symptoms of stress. But Labbe, Schmidt, Babin, and Pharr (2008) and Leisuk (2008) disagree, indicating that an individual's preferred music genre will be more effective when attempting to lower his or her specific stress and anxiety levels than will classical music (Labbe et al., 2008; Leisuk, 2008). What do you think? Perhaps the following section on music and performance might help you decide.

Music and Performance An earlier classic, simulated study by Allen and Blascovich (1994) helps put the findings of Labbe et al. (2008) and Lesiuk (2008) in context and also assesses the relationship between music and performance on demanding tasks. Allen and Blascovich's classical study tested the effects of three music conditions on stress reduction: no music, experimenter's selected music type, and participant's preferred music type. It is important to note that the participants in this study were all medical doctors who were also trained surgeons.

Because Allen and Blascovich (1994) could not ethically design an experiment to test a surgeon's skill and accuracy in an actual medical procedure, such as during surgery, they devised a cognitively challenging mathematical task that they believed presented similar cognitive demands as those encountered by surgeons (see Box 7.3). They found that music played during the mathematical task could reduce the surgeon's physiological response to stress in the settings and improve the surgeon's speed and accuracy on the task. They also found that the most effective stress-reducing genre of music is the one preferred by the individual. In light of these findings, should we ask doctors to include *their* favorite CD with the essential surgical instruments? Perhaps, but as with most things, there is a caveat.

Box 7.3 Rockin' and Rollin' in the Operating Room?

"There I was," reported one fourth-year medical student, "assisting in the operating room. It felt great!"

"What were you doing?" asked his roommate, another fourth-year student.

"Holding the arm of the patient while dancing to the music of Usher. I never knew the head surgeon was so cool!"

In truth, very few medical students "dance" with a patient undergoing an operation. But is this story true? Do doctors actually play music in the operating room? This story from a fourth year medical student IS true. And the fact that doctors do play music while operating on a patient was reinforced in a recent *New York Times Magazine* story on bariatric surgery for minors (see Chapter 5, Risky Health Behaviors, Part II). In this true reporting on a procedure for an adolescent at the Texas Children's Hospital, the surgeon, Dr. Rodriguez, began the procedure while listening to music from Bruno Mars and Elton John at a low volume (Ouyang, 2023). So, while surgeons do play music in the operating room, the type of music varies according to the doctor's preference.

Without a doubt, the sounds of pop or contemporary music emanating from an operating room during a procedure may be surprising, even shocking to some. After all, an operation is a serious procedure. So many things can go wrong even with simple, straightforward procedures. Yet research on music, stress, and performance suggests that one way to maximize concentration and improve accuracy is to play background music.

It is necessary to point out that there are a few ethical problems that limit a researcher's ability to conduct a study on the effects of music on a surgeon's performance in an actual operation (see Chapter 2, Research Methods). Therefore, researchers Allen and Blascovich (1994) did the next best thing. They designed an experiment to test the effects of music on three measures of autonomic reactivity – skin conductivity (sweat), blood pressure, and pulse rate – while participants, in this case, surgeons, performed mental arithmetic tasks known to simulate psychophysiological stress.

On the day of the experiment, the surgeon/participants were each placed in a room and told to perform the mental arithmetic tasks under three conditions: no music, experimenter-selected music, and surgeon-selected music, here meaning the type of music identified by the surgeon as the music he or she prefers to play when performing medical operations. The results were overwhelming. Blood pressure, pulse rate, and skin conductivity (sweatiness) were highest in the no-music condition, next highest in the experimenter-selected condition, and lowest in the surgeon-selected condition. All differences were statistically significant (Allen & Blascovich, 1994). In addition, the surgeon's speed and accuracy were better in the surgeon-selected music condition than in the other two.

With such outcomes, many people would eagerly ask their surgeons to play music while operating. But what genre of music should they choose? The study suggests that the stress measures are lowest, and performance is enhanced when surgeons select the music they most enjoy. Allen and Blascovich (1994) noted that, of the 50 surgeon participants, 46 chose classical music, two chose Irish folk music, and two chose jazz. The type of music is immaterial. What matters is whether the surgeon likes it!

A more recent meta-analysis by El Boghdady and Ewalds-Kvist (2020), finds that while music can significantly improve a surgeon's performance, one must consider the potentially distracting effects of loud or "high-beat type of music" that might inhibit performance. So, although "heavy metal" might be the surgeon's favorite type of music, it might be a poor choice here!

HUMOR "Laughter is the best medicine." According to some research on humor, laughter, and physical health, there may be some truth to this saying. Research on humor, defined here as action, speech, or writing that creates amusement, comicality, or fun (Martin, 2001), and on laughter, meaning the behavioral or vocal expression of the humorous experience (Martin, 2001), suggests that there may be health benefits to both. For example, seminal work by Fry (1994) proposed that the physical act of laughing causes changes in the body's physiology, including reduction of muscle tension, increased oxygenation of the blood, and release of *endorphins*, hormones that enhance positive mood states. One concrete example of the health effects of laughter is reported in a study by Tan and colleagues (Tan, Tan, Lukman, & Berk, 2007; Tan & Berman, 2008) in which humor is used as an adjunct therapy for persons with cardiovascular disease. They report that patients who received the combined therapy had fewer incidences of arrhythmia (a fast, slow, or irregular heartbeat), fewer incidences of myocardial infarction (heart attack), and lower blood pressure levels than did patients who received the standard therapy without humor. Similarly, a study by Cha and Hong (2015) examined the impact of laughter therapy on serotonin levels, quality of life, and depression in 64 middle-aged South Korean women. The study consisted of three experimental groups, sorted according to their levels of depression (low, moderate, and high), and one control group. The laughter therapy was conducted 10 times – five times a week for a total of two weeks – for women in the three experimental groups. Cha and Hong found that laughter therapy indirectly affected depression, mediated through significantly higher serotonin levels. Women in the experimental groups were found to have significantly higher serotonin levels than the control group, a positive byproduct of laughter. The highest serotonin levels were found in the more severely depressed women. In addition, depression levels decreased among all experimental (depression) groups, again with the most significant decrease occurring among women in the most depressed experimental group.

These findings notwithstanding, Kuiper and Nicholl (2004), van der Wal and Kok (2019), and others question whether humor and laughter actually improve physical health. They note that the relationship between humor, laughter, and physical health is tenuous at best given the methodological problems in a number of studies that claim to show such a relationship. Rather than show that laughter or humor convincingly improves or changes physical health status, Kuiper and Nicholl (2004) suggest that what is changed is a person's emotional state. More precisely, they argue that humor leads to improved health-related perceptions, or a sense of feeling better. To this end, there are a number of studies that suggest that humor, with or without laughter, enhances positive moods which, in turn, enhances health and may moderate pain perception (Guiliani, McRae, & Gross, 2008; Martin, 2019).

Consistent with this later research, humor has been shown to moderate stress levels in two ways. First, humor serves as an effective coping response to the stressful stimuli, and second, it offers a means of reinterpreting and restructuring the situation so that it is less stressful (Borod, 2006; Mallya, Reed, & Yang, 2019; Martin, 2019; Wu et al., 2021). Consider this scenario: You borrowed your friend's best suit for a very important job interview, which is conducted over lunch. While you are eating, a waiter passes too close to your table and bumps into your arm, causing you to spill the contents of your drink on your lap. Stunned, you say nothing at first, thinking only of your friend's reaction when you tell him of the accident. But suddenly the interviewer laughs as he tells you an amusing story about how he, too, spilled a drink while interviewing with the company's owner, only he spilled his drink on both him and the boss. The humorous story may help you cope with your immediate response to the problem. Admittedly, however, you will still need to address how best to clean soiled clothes and hopefully return a stain-free suit to your friend.

A humorous reinterpretation of situations also reduces stress. Consider another scenario: An accountant was told to resubmit her corrected report with no errors because, as her boss indicated, "Errors leave a bad taste in my mouth." The employee was upset at her carelessness, but as she worked she realized she could not guarantee that the final report was error free. Therefore, she decided to do the next best thing. When she placed her report on her boss's desk, she also gave her boss a cup of his favorite mocha latte. When the boss asked why he'd been given the latte, the employee said, "If you drink the latte while reading the report, there is no chance you will have a bad taste in your mouth."

SOCIAL SUPPORT, THE BUFFERING HYPOTHESIS AND STRESS What effect do social support networks, here meaning social groups or networks of friends, family, and other relatives, have on an individual's overall well-being? According to decades of seminal research, social support from individuals and friends has a direct and oftentimes positive effect on health (Kiecolt-Glaser, Gouin, & Hantsoo, 2009; Putman et al., 2009; Trotter & Allen, 2009).

Much of the early research on the effects of social networks on health indicates that the psychological and material assistance individuals obtain from such networks has a positive effect on overall well-being. We explore the benefits of social support groups for specific health issues such as cardiovascular health, pain, pain management, and cancer in Chapters 9 through 11. Here, however, we note that in addition to numerous studies that show a direct relationship between networks and positive health outcomes, a classic and often-cited study by Cohen and Wills (1985) proposed that such support buffers individuals from the potentially pathogenic influences of stress. Put simply, networks protect individuals from the full impact of a stressful event through a variety of ways.

Because Cohen's study is seminal to this work we review it briefly here. According to Cohen, a person's involvement in social networks will help to buffer or protect him or her from the full impact of the stressor even if that person receives no specific assistance from the network in addressing the stressful situation. Cohen and Wills (1985) suggest that the beneficial effects of involvement with a network include feelings of stability, predictability, and self-worth for the individual. Therefore, although assistance from one's social network that directly relates to a task is always useful, the mere existence of a network is sufficient to buffer the negative impact of a stressor. The recent COVID-19 pandemic and experiences with isolation worldwide is an excellent example of this concept.

Already, there are a host of articles and studies examining the psychological and physical impact of isolation and quarantine requirements enacted in many countries and regions to reduce the spread of COVID-19 – far too many to review here. But with limited exceptions, they all appear to support the finding that social support was critical to individuals' psychological and in some cases physiological well-being (Cao et al., 2020; Rodgers et al., 2020; Szkody, Stearns, Stanhope, & McKinney, 2020).

It is also the case that just the perception of an available network, without consulting with that network, also serves to buffer the individual in stressful settings. Why? According to another seminal study by Cohen and McKay (1984), the support mechanism is mediated in part through one's cognitive assessment of available resources. The knowledge that such resources are available, if needed, may mediate against stress even if no efforts are made to access the network. In essence, Cohen and Wills (1985) suggest that social support networks help to abate stress through direct and indirect support to an individual. Research by Naylor, Baik, and Arkoudis (2018) and Poudel, Gurung, and Khanal (2020) reinforce those conclusions. Support networks, therefore, are one method of coping with stressors.

SPIRITUALITY/RELIGION AND STRESS As we explained in Chapter 6, Emotional Health and Well-Being, a number of studies suggest that spirituality and religious practices may indeed play a role in physical and mental health outcomes (Lima et al., 2020; Shattuck & Muehlenbein, 2020). But as these studies make clear, the relationship is complex.

William James, a leading light in psychology in the U.S., began examining the relationship between religion and human behavior in the early 1900s. He equated the concepts of spirituality and religion when he defined religion as the "feelings, acts, experiences of individual men in their solitude . . . in relation to whatever they consider divine" (James, 1961, p. 42). Some researchers continue to link the two concepts, whereas others see a distinction: they link religion to formal institutions and a more outward-oriented expression of one's beliefs (acts or experiences as defined by James) and link spirituality to a more inward or personal and subjective side of religion (a feeling or a personal belief in the divine; Hill & Pargament, 2003; George, Larson, Koenig, & McCullough, 2000; Sapolsky, 2004). Although there may be objective differences between the two concepts, such differences are not reflected in the current research. Both terms are used almost interchangeably when examining what is connoted to be the effects of one's belief system on health. Consequently, we use both terms when examining the impact of spirituality/religious beliefs on health outcomes.

Why examine spirituality or religion in the context of psychology? Put simply, this is not a new area of research. Miller and Thorenson (2003) comment that throughout the 20th century, psychologists have linked "spiritual" to a person's character, personality, or disposition. This would include a person's social or emotional style such as chronic anger or peace. Roman, Mthembu, and Hoosen (2020) suggest an even more contemporary point of view, noting that spirituality is part of the human psyche. Consequently, it is an integral part of health and well-being for both an individual and their families. Yet as was the case with research on the relationship between humor and health, methodological problems with research that claims to show a connection between spirituality/religion and health, hampers psychologists' understanding of the relationship between these two variables. There are, however, two methodologically sound studies that appear to show support for a link between health and religious activities. In one study, Schneider and colleagues (1995) looked at the effects of stress reduction in hypertension in African Americans and found that transcendental meditation together with a progressive relaxation intervention significantly reduced blood pressure in the study sample of 55-year-old African Americans.

In a related study of social integration and blood pressure, Livingston, Levine, and Moore (1991) found that church affiliation was positively associated with lower systolic and diastolic blood pressure in a sample of African Americans. Admittedly, these two studies examine the relationship between health and religious behavior, in which actions are a proxy for spirituality. Yet they appear to offer sound support for the effect of religious activities on health.

To summarize, research on positive behavioral coping mechanisms focuses on effective strategies for controlling distress in response to an external stimulus. Exercise, music, humor, social support, and religious behaviors are five of a number of largely behavioral coping strategies used by people to respond to stress-inducing events. They are relevant to our understanding of health and well-being. In addition, they are relevant to the field of health psychology because one role of psychologists is to assist people in identifying and adopting behaviors that will enhance their health outcomes and enable them to perform their daily tasks.

People who encounter stress as a regular feature of their jobs may need to find and implement effective coping mechanisms on a daily basis. Consider for a moment air traffic controllers. They are responsible for ensuring the safe conduct of passengers and crew members aboard airplanes. Similarly, nurses and doctors make decisions that have a direct impact on the health of their patients (Lalani, 2020; Roman et al., 2020). Undoubtedly, persons employed in either occupation can experience considerable work-related stress. Thus, people in such occupations need effective coping mechanisms to help them perform their jobs well and to maintain their own emotional health in the midst of crises. Health psychologists can help people in these professions, and others, identify and effectively employ the most effective coping strategies to do both.

Even people in less stressful situations need to employ coping mechanisms on occasion. Not sure of that claim? Consider this: You receive an unexpectedly low grade on an exam. Now think about the various ways you attempt to reduce your anxiety as you examine your test results while sitting among your classmates.

High-Risk Behaviors and Stress

To this point, we have identified two factors that can trigger stress indirectly, thereby causing or exacerbating illnesses. Psychosocial factors (e.g., illness, death, or financial problems) that are largely determined by an individual's social environment can precipitate stress and may lead to illness. In addition, chronic illnesses, like heart conditions or diabetes, can be stressors as individuals and their families attempt to manage the sometimes-unpredictable course of the disease. In this instance, the illness may cause additional stressors that exacerbate the existing illness.

But consider this: Stressful events or situations may lead to risky or unhealthy behaviors that contribute to poor health outcomes. The research on stress and eating, stress and sexual activities, and stress and substance use provide ample evidence of the adverse impact of negative behavioral coping mechanisms on health.

STRESS AND EATING Without exaggeration, there is a large and growing literature that examines the effects of stress on people's eating behaviors. While there is considerable disagreement among researchers about the relationship between the two factors, there is general agreement around some findings. First, researchers tend to agree that, in general, stress can influence the amount and type of foods a person consumes. The recent COVID-19 pandemic provided researchers with ample opportunity to retest this association, finding a strong link between stressful situations and eating behaviors (Cummings, Ackerman, Wolfson, & Gearhardt, 2021; Simone et al., 2021). Furthermore, most studies have found that stress causes people to increase their consumption of sweet or fatty foods, rather than bland or salty foods (Agurto, Alcantara-Diaz, Espinet-Coll, & Toro-Huamanchumo, 2021; Bin Zarah, Enriquez-Marulanda, & Andrade, 2020; Zellner et al., 2006). Finally, researchers generally agree that there is a gender difference in the effects of stress on food consumption. Specifically, women are significantly more likely to increase their food consumption when encountering stressful situations than are men. In addition, in such situations, women prefer foods high in fats and calories (Zellner, Saito, & Gonzalez, 2007).

There is, however, one caveat in these findings. Even for women, the tendency to reach for the high-fat, high-calorie foods is more prevalent among restrained eaters, or people who report frequently monitoring their diet and food consumption. Researchers suggest that stressful events inhibit the ability of such individuals to exercise control over their eating behaviors. As a result, they select the very foods that they normally avoid for weight loss or health purposes (Zellner et al., 2006).

Occasional lapses in one's diet related to stress may not appear to pose health risks. But if Lazarus and Folkman's daily hassles theory is correct, then eating high-fat and high-calorie foods as a coping strategy would be a frequent, not an occasional, occurrence. And as you remember from Chapter 4, Global, Communicable, and Chronic Disease, unhealthy diets contribute to obesity, diabetes, heart disease, and other related health problems. When individuals adopt a negative coping strategy, such as unhealthy eating behaviors, in response to stressful events, then stress is considered an indirect cause of negative health outcomes.

STRESS, SEXUAL BEHAVIORS, AND SUBSTANCE ABUSE Other negative behaviors that may be triggered by stress include risky sexual behaviors such as unprotected sex and substance use. Studies suggest that high rates of violence in one's neighborhood, repeated exposure to discrimination, and high crime rates can create persistent or chronic stressors. To escape from such environments, or perhaps to manage their effects, some researchers contend that adolescents in such environments may engage in high-risk sexual behaviors such as multiple sexual partners or unprotected sex (Arabi-Mianrood, Hamzehgardeshi, Khoori, Moosazadeh, & Shahhosseini, 2021; Brady, Dolcini, Harper, & Pollack, 2009). Although such behaviors may temporarily reduce stress, they also increase an adolescent's probability of contracting sexually transmitted diseases (see Chapter 5, Risky Health Behaviors), including sexually transmitted diseases, or may result in unplanned pregnancies.

Other risk behaviors sometimes associated with stress include the use of substances such as alcohol, cigarettes, or illegal drugs. The practice of using substances in response to stress is common in many cultures, including in the U.S. It is even reflected in conversations. For example, when having a particularly bad day at work or school, when ending a relationship, or when experiencing other emotionally upsetting events, it is not uncommon for people to think of having an alcoholic drink in response to the stress to "drown their sorrows" or "cheer themselves up." In fact, the response is so widely accepted by some that the practice is reflected in cartoons and other forms of humor.

Researchers also document the common reliance on substances when stressed. A study by Brady and colleagues (2009) showed that the accumulation of multiple stressful events, such as parental divorce or an auto accident, prompted adolescents in their study to turn to substances either to escape or to manage the psychological impact of their experiences.

Positive Affect and Stress

So far, we have defined stress as a negative health factor, something to be controlled, reduced, or eliminated. Yet current research suggests that stress can also be a positive experience. How is it possible that something we have treated as an event to be managed, controlled, or eliminated can also be positive? When viewing stress as a negative factor, we are relying on the biomedical model of health in which stress is similar to a disease or illness to be identified, contained, or removed. On the other hand, positive psychology interprets stress as potentially beneficial because a positive affect toward the stressful event may allow for learning or new skill development.

In case this seems counterintuitive, consider the following. Research on the positive outcomes of stress suggests that, during a stressful encounter, there are several important outcomes: how one manages the stressful event, the new skills acquired, cognitive reappraisal of the stressful event, new learning opportunities, and growth experiences that occurs as a result of the event (Jamieson, Nock, & Mendes, 2012; Xu et al., 2020). For example, when approaching a stressor with a positive affect, an individual may be buffered or protected from the adverse psychological consequences of the events. This implies that the attitude one brings to the situation may help to hold at bay the negative reactions, such as anxiety or momentary depression that could result from the problem. Additionally, a positive affect may help to develop new skills or promote individual growth that will be useful when encountering similar events in the future. Some studies of coping, therefore, focus on *positive reappraisal*, or the use of cognitive strategies to see a situation in a more positive light. An expression often used to characterize positive reappraisal is to say, "the glass is half full" instead of "the glass is half empty."

We can apply the positive reappraisal concept to the opening story. Remember that Susan, Michael, and Lucinda decided to place Sarah in a nursing home. But suppose, rather than opt for the alternative living arrangement, Susan decided to view the difficulty with Sarah as a challenge to be resolved. For example, we know that Sarah was easily agitated in restaurants. But suppose Susan discovered that Sarah could entertain herself for hours at home with her Sudoku electronic game board. In fact, Sarah could be so engrossed in the task that she ignored her surroundings and focused only on the game. Using a positive reappraisal, what could Susan do?

One strategy would be to test the effectiveness of the Sudoku game by bringing it along when taking Sarah out with the family for dinner at a small restaurant. Susan may find that the game is sufficient to quiet Sarah, keeping her from becoming agitated by the new surroundings. In the process, the family can enjoy a meal together in a restaurant, one of their favorite family activities.

Research by Folkman and Moskowitz (2000) also applies the positive reappraisal concept. Specifically, they examine the positive reappraisal strategies of caregivers when managing the daily problems associated with the care and management of AIDS patients. The studies found that AIDS caregivers who were able to set and complete a specific goal each day, regardless how small, felt a sense of accomplishment that helped them manage throughout the day. The goal could be an everyday task such as meeting friends, going to the post office, or having a meal, similar to Susan's goal. The ability to complete one task, regardless of how small, demonstrated the caregiver's ability to exert control over a situation that sometimes defied control (Folkman & Moskowitz, 2000). The point here is that the completed task serves as an accomplishment, something that contains positive meaning.

The short-term impact of positive reappraisal in stressful situations is clear. The individual experiences success. For example, Susan, Michael, and Lucinda's ability to enjoy a meal in a restaurant could reinforce their successful control over an otherwise uncontrollable or stressful event.

An interesting additional finding by Folkman and Moskowitz, and one that is particularly relevant to this chapter on stress and health, is that AIDS caregivers in their study who reported small but consistent positive accomplishments also showed better psychological health and adjustment after the death of the AIDS patient than did caregivers who did not use positive reappraisal strategies. Fully three and six months after their caregiving responsibilities ended, AIDS caregivers who demonstrated positive reappraisal strategies were less depressed and had better overall psychological health than non–positive reappraisal strategy caregivers. Thus, positive reappraisal suggests that stress need not be viewed as a negative factor to be controlled and overcome. Rather, positive reappraisal suggests that a positive psychological approach to stress can result in benefits for both the individual and the caregiver and in both the short and the long term.

Summary

In summary, the original and current research on stress considers the beneficial and the detrimental impacts of stress on health. By examining coping strategies, researchers note first that individual responses to situations will vary. An event that is stressful to one person may not produce the same effect on another. As such, the perception of stress as well as the effectiveness of strategies to cope with stress will vary by individuals.

Second, research on coping also illustrates the advantages of a positive psychological perspective to understanding well-being. We explored the contributions of positive psychology in Chapter 6, Emotional Health and Well-Being. The benefits of a positive affect when encountering otherwise stressful events, and positive reappraisal strategies that assist us in interpreting the event, are skills that health psychologists may help individuals acquire to more effectively manage their environments.

Personal Postscript

HOW STRESSED ARE YOU?

Lazarus and Folkman define the daily hassles in life as those little things that can irritate and distress you. We all experience them. Because they are quite common, one way to avoid having such hassles overwhelm us or have a negative impact on our overall well-being is to identify the stressors and then identify, for ourselves, the most effective way to address the problem. This may include the cognitive coping techniques we described, behavioral techniques, or positive reappraisal and positive affect.

To begin the process, included in the following list are items from the Negative Event (Hassles) Scale, a scale adapted from Holm and Holroyd's Daily Hassles Scale (Holm & Holroyd, 1992). Take a minute to look at the items and determine whether any of the items are occasional, regular, or frequent hassles you encounter. Also think about whether they represent no real hassles, minor hassles, moderate hassles, or considerable hassles. Once you have identified the major hassles, the next task is to consider ways of addressing the problem. Remember, problem-focused coping strategies are best for addressing stressful stimulus and for enhancing likely overall health outcomes.

Sample of Negative Events

Inner Concerns

1. Regrets over past decisions
2. Loneliness
3. Fear of rejection
4. Trouble making decisions
5. Concerns about getting ahead
6. Concerns about wasting time

Financial Concerns

1. Not enough money for basic necessities
2. Not enough money for entertainment and recreation
3. Concerns about money for emergencies
4. Concerns about owing money
5. Not enough money for health care

Time Pressures

1. Too many responsibilities
2. Not enough time to accomplish all required tasks

3. Not getting enough sleep
4. Not enough time for entertainment and recreation
5. Concerns about meeting high standards

Work Hassles

1. Job dissatisfaction
2. Hassles from boss or supervisor
3. Don't like current work
4. Don't like fellow workers
5. Problems getting along with fellow workers

Environmental Hassles

1. Pollution
2. Crime
3. Traffic
4. Rising prices of common goods
5. Concerns about news events

Health Hassles

1. Concerns about medical treatment
2. Concerns about side effects of medicines
3. Concerns about health in general
4. Concerns about body functions
5. Physical illnesses

Now that you have identified a number of situations that may cause occasional, regular, or frequent hassles for you, the question is what you can do to reduce your stress in responding to them and to cope more effectively. Part of the answer rests in knowing what strategies work best with you and your system. Simply put, one size does not fit all.

Consider this: If one hassle for you is completing work-related tasks according to a timeline, you may consider ways to make the task less stressful. For example, when working on the task, you may consider playing your favorite music, like the surgeons in Box 7.3. Music helped them relax while performing the procedure and in the process improved both their accuracy and speed in completing the task.

Second, exercise is a known stress reliever. Perhaps you enjoyed exercising in high school or early in your college career. Jogging and swimming are excellent cardiovascular exercises that may help to reduce your stress levels. If, on the other hand, you seek something less intense, yoga, stretching exercises, or meditation may produce the same outcomes for you.

Finally, think about humor. Daily hassles often cause us to lose our ability to laugh. And, as we saw in this chapter, humor can act on the perceptual, physiological, and psychological factors that contribute to stress. Therefore, consider going to the movies or watching one with friends in your dorm room. But be sure to choose a comedy, something with a theme that you find funny. Or attend a comedy club, preferably one that features one of your favorite comedians.

These are just three activities that may help you reduce stress and cope with life's daily hassles. Can you think of others that may work specifically for you?

Questions to Consider

1. People can be buffered from the full effects of stress if they have strong and multiple social networks. But some current research suggests that they adversely affect the mental health of adolescents. Debate this point and consider the effects of these networks on you.
2. Aromatherapy has been found to be ineffective as a stress abatement agent. Yet many claim that it has a calming effect. How would you explain this discrepancy?
3. Is a diagnosis of post-traumatic stress disorder (PTSD) too common? What are the problems with a potential over-diagnosis of this illness?

True or False Questions

1. The hypothalamic-pituitary-adrenocortical system (HPAC) is responsible for restoring the body to its normal resting state. True or False.
2. Glucocorticoids both activate and suppress the body's immune system. True or False.
3. Taylor's "tend-and befriend" theory is widely regarded as an accurate characterization of a gender difference in response to stress. True or False.
4. Lazarus and Folkman's transactional model of stress integrates the psychological, emotional, and physiological responses to stress. True or False.
5. There appears to be a bidirectional interaction between stress and chronic illnesses. True or False.

Important Terms

acute time-limited stressors   *269*
adrenal cortex   *275*
adrenal gland   *273*
adrenaline   *272*
adrenal medulla   *275*
adrenocorticotropic hormone (ACTH)   *273*
allostasis   *273*
autonomic nervous system (ANS)   *271*

CHAPTER 8

Psychoneuroimmunology

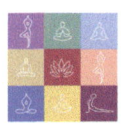

Source: 3xy/
Shutterstock.

Chapter Outline

Chapter Objectives

After studying this chapter, you will be able to:

1. Define and describe psychoneuroimmunology.
2. Define natural, acquired, and cell-mediated immunity.
3. Describe the function of B lymphocytes and T lymphocytes.
4. Define interleukins and cytokines.
5. Explain the relationship between interleukins and cytokines and the immune system.
6. Explain the relationship between stress and the immune system.
7. Explain how social support networks may influence health outcomes.

DOI: 10.4324/9781003300670-9

OPENING STORY: EARVIN "MAGIC" JOHNSON

Earvin "Magic" Johnson has everything: five National Basketball Association (NBA) championships, three Most Valuable Player awards, three NBA Finals Most Valuable Player awards, a winning personality, and a "magic" smile. What more could he ask for?

Actually, the question is what Magic did not ask for. In November 1991, Magic stunned the world when he announced that he was HIV positive. It seemed as if the world stopped and listened. "Sometimes you're a little naïve," he said, "and . . . think it could never happen to you. You only thought it could happen to . . . other people. . . . And it has happened but I'm going to deal with it" (American Rhetoric, 2001, p. 1).

Today, almost 33 years later, Magic seems to be the picture of health. A little heavier than he was in his days as a Los Angeles Laker, Magic is now a business entrepreneur, the principal donor to the Magic Johnson Foundation, a foundation which he created in 1991 to increase awareness of and attention to HIV/AIDS, and a spokesperson for World AIDS Day. He is still strong and active. ∎

No doubt you are wondering why we return to the topic of HIV/AIDS to introduce this chapter on *psychoneuroimmunology.* Consider this: Ervin Johnson has been living for more than 30 years with HIV. But Ryan White, the adolescent introduced in Chapter 5, Risky Health Behaviors, Part II, who contracted HIV from a contaminated blood transfusion, and Arthur Ashe, the renowned tennis champion who contracted the disease in a similar fashion, lost their battles. Why? What explains Magic's longevity and White's and Ashe's early deaths? Why does Magic continue to respond well to treatment for the disease while others, like White and Ashe, did not?

One possible explanation for Ryan White and Arthur Ashe's outcome is that White's hemophilia and Ashe's brain tumor may have weakened their immune systems, increasing their likelihood of succumbing to the disease. Another possibility, suggested by current research, is that the psychological impact of a positive HIV diagnosis, along with an individual's emotional health when coping with the disease and its progression, can influence immune system functions that will affect the physical health of the individual (Chida & Steptoe, 2008; Chida & Vedhara, 2009; Ironson & Hayward, 2008; Kołodziej, 2016; Leserman, 2008). Studies in the field of *psychoneuroimmunology* aim to understand just this phenomenon. Specifically, they seek to understand whether biological, behavioral, psychological, and social factors can contribute to immune system functions and ultimately influence our health outcomes.

Research in psychoneuroimmunology actually began several decades before the HIV/AIDS crisis. Early work by Solomon and Moos (1964) and later work by Solomon (1987) proposed that our psychological states influence our immune functions. Does this sound familiar? If you return briefly to the section on emotional health and physiological outcomes presented in Chapter 6, Emotional Health and Well-Being, and the research on stress and physiology in Chapter 7, Stress and Coping, you will see a number of studies that explore the role of emotions on physiological well-being. But this newer field of psychoneuroimmunology probes a little deeper in an attempt to explain the relationship among mental health *(psychology)*, the central nervous system *(neurology)*, and the immune system *(immunology)*.

Current research suggests that the interface of these three factors may explain disease progressions and outcomes for a number of illnesses, including HIV, cancer, and chronic pain, and even the pain experienced by arthritis sufferers. Thus, by focusing on the immune system, this field may provide a framework for understanding the relationship between biology, psychology, and health (Irwin, 2008; Alessi & Bennett, 2020).

We begin this chapter with a review of the human immune system, focusing on the basic elements of natural, acquired, and cell-mediated immunity in Section I. In Section II we take a closer look at the research on the role of psychological health, including the effects of stress and depression on immunology and on physiological outcomes. We learned in Chapter 7, Stress and Coping, that social support networks and interpersonal relationships play a critical role in mediating stress. Therefore, in this section we look more closely at the relationship between social support networks and psychoneuroimmunology. In Section III, we return briefly to the effects of chronic health conditions on psychological and immunological health, a topic introduced in Chapter 7, Stress and Coping. Finally, we conclude in Section IV with an examination of the role, actual or perceived, of a specific environmental factor, socioeconomic status, on physiological health factors.

One note before proceeding. The human immune system is complex. It involves a large assortment of different types of cell and non-cell components that assume a number of different functions. We cannot provide a full review of this system. Therefore, we focus here on a subset of the immune system which, according to some studies, may have a *possible* association with psychological health. Note the emphasis on the word *possible*. Much of the research in this area is either clinical/observational (Irwin et al., 2019; Irwin, 2008) or correlational. And, as you may recall from Chapter 2, Research Methods, correlation does not mean causation. Thus, while many of the studies that will be presented are intriguing and suggest a possible relationship, we cannot claim a clear causal relationship between psychology, neurologic functions, and immune system responses – at least not at this time.

In addition, and this is something we will see when exploring the relationship between stress and the immune system, people's individual responses to psychological factors vary. As such, it is challenging for researchers to map the precise response of a person's immune system to internal or external triggers. These triggers may elicit varying responses both within and across individuals (see Chapter 7, Stress and Coping). Researchers in this field are careful to state that more studies are needed to better understand the relationship between psychological, neurological, and immunologic factors and their effects on health.

SECTION I. NATURAL, ACQUIRED, AND CELL-MEDIATED IMMUNITY

The Human Immune System

When it is working well, our immune system protects us from a multitude of bacteria, viruses, and microorganisms that are ever present in our world. It does this by protecting our body from foreign substances using *innate, or natural, immunity* and by discriminating successfully between our body's own elements and foreign substances using *adaptive, or acquired, immunity*. For our purposes, we will refer to the two systems as natural and acquired immunity, respectively.

NATURAL IMMUNITY Our body has several first lines of defense against foreign elements. They include the skin, saliva, urinary tract, and mucus, among others. We cannot review all of the body's natural immunities in this text, so we will explore just one: the skin.

The skin consists of two layers. First is the *epidermis*, a thin outer layer that contains tightly packed *epithelial cells* and a waterproofing protein called *keratin*. Together they work to repel germs and other foreign matter from the body's surface and to prevent germs from penetrating the skin. The second layer of skin, the *dermis*, is thicker than the epidermis. It consists of connective tissues that contain blood vessels, hair follicles, and *sebaceous glands*, or glands that secrete an oily substance. The oils help to maintain the pH balance of the skin and to inhibit the growth of *microorganisms*, otherwise known as germs. Many microorganisms will be repelled by the skin; however, openings in the skin from scratches, cuts, or punctures will allow microorganisms to bypass the body's natural immunity. If a microorganism evades the body's natural immunity, the body's acquired immunity will activate to fight the invading germs.

ACQUIRED IMMUNITY The body's acquired immune system is composed of cells and non-cell components that reside in blood and other body fluids. As the name suggests, the acquired immune system learns to recognize and eliminate microorganisms that are foreign to the body. The learning process is what makes the system adaptive because it must recognize and respond to both new and previously presented foreign substances. Adaptive immunity has four main characteristics, as detailed in Table 8.1. First, the *self/non-self process* distinguishes the body's own cells from foreign cells. Second, using *antigenic specificity*,

TABLE 8.1 Brief Summary of the Immune System

Two Types of Immunity	*Description*
Natural (Innate) Immunity	Body's first line of defense against microorganisms Includes: skin, saliva, urinary tract, muscles
Acquired (Adaptive) Immunity	Immunity derived from recognizing and defeating microorganisms that the body has experienced before
Four principal processes	
Self/non-self discrimination	Ability of body cells to distinguish between foreign elements and body's own cells
Antigen specificity	Process of distinguishing among different types of foreign microorganisms and generating a specific immune response to the specific foreign antigen
Diversity	Ability of body to recognize the unique structures of each microorganism
Immunologic memory	Ability to recognize a previously presented antigen when it returns, giving the body the ability to respond more quickly and effectively against foreign microorganisms
Organs and cells	Lymphoid organs (tonsils, lymph nodes, thymus, spleen) that produce white blood cells that fight infection
Main cells	White blood cells or leukocytes that filter microorganisms and help reduce risk of infection
Principal leukocytes	Contain neutrophils and macrophages (phagocytic cells) that collect at the site of an injury of the body to release toxins that produce inflammation and fever that contributes to healing
Polymorphonuclear granulocytes	Comprise 50%–70% of leukocytes but appear to play minor role in immune process
Lymphocytes B cells	Two types that develop and mature in bone marrow: • B memory "remembers" prior invading microorganisms and identifies them when representing themselves; faster recognition aids in the process of destroying foreign antigens • B antibody forms specific antigens to attack invading microorganisms
T cells	Three types born in bone marrow and matured in thymus: • T cytotoxic (TC), or "killer" cells, destroy cells infected with the virus • T helper (TH) help to produce the cytotoxin that destroys invading virus and assists in the maturation of B cells • T suppressor (TS) slows the immune system by reducing activity of TC cells once invading antigens have been eliminated to prevent damage to the immune system
Cell-mediated immunity	Two components: • Humoral immunity: Liquid and non-cellular components (blood, plasma and lymphatic fluid) external to cells. Fights foreign antigens with aid of *B lymphocytes*. • Cell-mediated immunity: Responds to antigens in body by activating antigen-specific TC cells and cytokines, specifically interleukins, a class of cytokines.

the body's immune system distinguishes between different forms of foreign *antigens*, here meaning foreign microorganisms that trigger the immune response in the body. Third, the system uses *diversity*, or the ability to recognize the unique structures of each foreign microorganism. Diversity ensures that the system can identify and target specific foreign organisms. The fourth characteristic is *immunologic memory*, the ability to recognize a specific foreign organism in subsequent exposures.

The four characteristics are one part of the body's acquired immune response. The second component involves the organs and cells that participate in the process. Organs such as the tonsils, the lymph nodes, and the thymus, for example, are called *lymphoid organs* because *lymphocytes*, infection-fighting white blood cells, grow in the organs. Lymphocyte cells can be thought of as the "security patrol" for the body because they search for foreign or infectious microorganisms. They come in two forms: B lymphocytes and T lymphocytes.

VIDEO #40/60

Chapter 8: Psychoneuroimmunology

·   **Lymphoid organs: *How the lymphatic system works***

·   ***Website: https://www.youtube.com/watch?v=f4RQ0UXU50E***

·   ***Nemours KidsHealth is publicly accessible since it provides medical-based information to the public at no cost (https:// kidshealth.org/)***

B Lymphocytes *B lymphocytes*, or *B cells*, form in the bone marrow until mature. B cells have two important immune functions. Some B cells are *antibody-producing cells*. They produce cells that attack specific microorganisms. Other B cells are *memory cells*. They encode information that helps them recognize foreign microorganisms encountered and defeated previously.

VIDEO #41/60

Chapter 8: Psychoneuroimmunology

·   **B Cells: *What are B Cells?***

·   ***Website: https://www.youtube.com/watch?v=xPRAob0xV7I***

·   **The Lupus Research Alliance's information is publicly accessible and shares their research with the public for educational purposes (*Lupus Research Alliance – Lupus Treatment Options | Lupus Research Alliance*)**

Why is it important for B cells to remember previous foreign organisms? Consider this: In Chapter 4, Global, Communicable, and Chronic Disease, we introduced the concept of vaccines (immunizations). We mentioned that when vaccinating children against childhood diseases such as chickenpox, a small amount of the virus is injected into the child. A healthy immune system is able to successfully fight and destroy a small quantity of the chickenpox virus introduced to the body for the first time by a vaccine. After destroying the foreign organisms, the immune system will "remember" the chickenpox virus so that, when it encounters the same microorganism in larger quantities in the future, it will be able to detect, identify, and eliminate it more quickly and efficiently. In essence, the body's memory of the chickenpox virus ensures that, with rare exceptions, the body will respond effectively and quickly and protect the child from the effects of chickenpox.

T Lymphocytes A second type of lymphocyte is *T lymphocytes*, or *T cells*, which form in the thymus (look again at Table 8.1). There are three different types of T cells, all of which perform specific immune functions: T cytotoxic (*TC*), T helper (*TH*), and T suppressor (*TS*).

The *T cytotoxic* cell, or *TC* for short, is known as the "killer" cell. It is responsible for destroying the cells that become infected by a virus. A second T cell is the *TH* or *T helper* cell, which helps the system by producing **cytokines,** or agents that produce antibodies to fight invading viruses. T*H* cells can either help direct the TC cells or help activate the B-memory cells. T*H* cells also display CD4 glycoproteins on the surface of the cell, an element used in the measurement of the strength of the immune system.

Finally, *TS*, or *T suppressor cells*, serve as the "off" switch. They help slow the functions of the immune system by sending messages to reduce the activity of the TC and T*H* cells once the immune system has completed the work of destroying the invading virus.

These three components can provide one measure of the strength of an individual's immune system. The number of **CD4 cells** in the system is one way. Other measures include **cell differentiation, cell proliferation,** and **cytotoxicity** (see Table 8.2). Each of these measures can be obtained from a small sample of blood or saliva.

VIDEO #42/60

Chapter 8: Psychoneuroimmunology

· **T-Cells:** *What are T-cells?*

· *Website: https://www.youtube.com/watch?v=nIQ51gczoCo*

· **The Lupus Research Alliance's information is publicly accessible and shares their research with the public for educational purposes (***Lupus Research Alliance – Lupus Treatment Options | Lupus Research Alliance***)**

Cell-Mediated Immunity The acquired immune system can be further divided into two additional components: *humoral immunity* and *cell-mediated immunity*. Briefly, *humoral immunity* involves the liquid, non-cellular components in the body, specifically blood and tissues like plasma and lymphatic fluid that float outside of cells. In this environment *B lymphocytes* produce the antibodies needed to attack foreign antigens, or microorganisms, which present themselves in this non-cell environment. As such, *B lymphocytes* are said to facilitate the body's immunity in this space.

Cell-mediated immunity, however, relates to the body's response to antigens or microorganisms that invade the cell. This response calls on the *T lymphocytes*, specifically the TC cells, to destroy the antigen. Unlike *acquired immunity*, *cell-mediated immunity* does not involve antibodies. Rather, it combats microorganisms through the activation of antigen-specific TC cells and the release of *cytokines*, proteins produced by the cell which serve as a chemical messenger that affect the interactions and communications

TABLE 8.2 Selected Methods of Measuring the Health of the Immune System

Measure	*Description*
CD4 cell count	Measures the number of TH cells that initiate the process for identifying microorganisms. • Normal CD4 cell count: 500–1,500 • Low CD4 count: 200–499 • CD4 <200 with a positive diagnosis of HIV may be diagnosed as AIDS
Cell differentiation	Percentage of TC, TH, and TS cells produced by the body needed to fight infection
Cell proliferation	Rate of multiplication of each T cell type
Cell cytotoxicity	Cell's ability to kill foreign antigens

between cells and also regulate the response of the immune system (Janeway, Travers, & Walport, 2001; Zhang & An, 2007). One important role of *cytokines* will become clearer when we explore current research on the role of *interleukins*, a class of cytokines produced by T cells. For now, it is only important to know that research on the relationship between psychological health and the immune system suggests that interleukins, including *interleukin-4 (IL-4)*, *interleukin-6 (IL-6)*, *interleukin-10, (IL-10)*, and *tumor necrosis factor-alpha (TNF-α)*, may play a role in regulating the immune system in response to one specific psychological factor: stress (Bremner et al., 2021; Koh et al., 2012).

Summary

We briefly dissected the immune system to explain how it functions. Now, putting it back together we find that we have two primary components of the immune system: natural immunity and acquired immunity. We also have a subdivision of the acquired immune system, which includes humoral and cell-mediated immunity. Natural immunity is readily visible in the form of skin, saliva, mucus, and other elements. It is the body's first line of defense. Less visible to the naked eye, however, is acquired immunity. The acquired system includes a number of organs, cells, and non-cell components. In this system are five types of lymphocytes that serve as the "security patrol" for the body. Included among the lymphocytes are the B lymphocytes that can be either specially programed cells that attach a specific microorganism or "memory" cells that aid the immune system by recognizing foreign microorganisms. The T lymphocytes can be TC cells that function as warriors, attacking and killing the foreign viruses. They can also be TH cells that help stimulate other cells, specifically B-memory and TC cells, to perform their respective jobs. Finally, T lymphocytes can be TS cells that slow the immune system after activation. T cells also produce cytokines, proteins that affect the communication between cells and regulate immune system response. *Cytokines* are part of the cell-mediated immunity. The cytokines in turn produce *interleukins*, which also play a special role in regulating the immune system.

SECTION II. PSYCHOLOGICAL HEALTH AND THE IMMUNE SYSTEM

For more than 30 years, researchers have used academic stress, specifically the type experienced during exam period, to explore the relationship between psychological stress and immunity (Koh et al., 2012; Malathi & Damodaran, 1999, How Does Stress Affect the Immune System? – UMMS Health). Thus, we begin this section on psychological health and the immune system by examining specifically the role of academic stress on immune functioning, a topic which is likely to be of interest to most students.

Many people would agree that medical students are under considerable pressure to perform well on their exams. Elegant studies by Chandrashekara and colleagues in 2007 and Koh and colleagues in 2012 that examined the effects of psychological stress on the immune system of medical students in India and South Korea, respectively, explored this issue more fully (see Box 8.1). Specifically, these studies asked whether objective stressors, which is stress triggered by specific events like an exam or a car accident, are more likely to result in an alteration in immune function than subjective, sometimes called self-reported, stressors (Koh et al., 2012). The findings from both studies were surprising.

Chandrashekara et al.'s study compared subjective, self-reported measures of anxiety with physiological or objective measure of stress for 183 medical students at three different phases in their medical studies: exam session, mid-term session (non–exam takers) and newly admitted students (also non–exam takers). The results showed that for exam-taking students, there was good agreement between their self-assessed levels of anxiety and the objective physiological measure, **TNF-α** levels. **TNF-α** is a cytokine that plays a role in boosting immune system function (see Table 8.3). More specifically, the researchers found that *TNF-α* levels were suppressed (lowered) for exam-taking students who reported high anxiety. Lower *TNF-α* levels suggest a higher risk of infection due to the lower levels of protein in the body, proteins that are needed to boost the immune system. Thus, in addition to showing an agreement between subjective and objective measures of stress, this study also suggests that stress can have a pronounced effect on immunology through the suppression of *TNF-α*, an important protein in the immune system.

But, and this is the important part, there was no significant difference in the *TNF-α* levels of non–exam-taking, high- versus low-anxiety students. In other words, the *TNF-α* levels of non–exam-taking students who rated their anxiety levels as high were not statistically different from that of the non–exam-taking students who rated their anxiety levels as low. These results suggested to Chandrashekara and colleagues (2007) that situational factors – in this case the presence or absence of an exam – may play a significant role in immune system function. In just a moment we will see that the psychological state of the person – here being anxiety level – may be another important factor in immune system response.

Box 8. 1 Is Academic Stress Good for Your Health?

Stress influences the immune system in a variety of ways, but does this extend to academic stress as well? That is to say, does academic stress suppress or activate immune functions?

That is the question addressed by two research teams: Chandrashekara and colleagues in 2007 and later by Koh and colleagues in 2012. In the earlier study, Chandrashekara and colleagues examined the effects of anxiety on immune response, specifically on *tumor necrosis factor-alpha (TNF-α)* levels during psychological stress. *TNF-α* is a key *cytokine* that is believed to play a major role in tumor immunity and immunity against infection (see Table 8.3). Low *TNF-α* levels increase the chance of infection and of a poor response to other stressful situations (Chandrashekara et al., 2007).

Chandrashekara and colleagues selected 183 first-year medical students and separated them into three groups: exam-taking students ($N = 60$), middle-of-term students (non-exam takers, $N = 58$), and newly admitted students (also non-exam takers, $N = 65$). Then, to measure students' stress levels before the exams, researchers administered two subjective – here meaning self-report – measures of anxiety to all students, exam-takers and non-exam takers alike. The two subjective measures were the State Anxiety Inventory to measure how respondents feel "right now," that is to say in the moment, and the student form of the Bell Adjustment Inventory, a scale that evaluates students' home, health, and social and emotional adjustment. The Bell Adjustment scores were also used as an adaptability measure. Adaptability is one estimate of a person's coping skills.

Next, the researchers took blood samples to measure the student's levels of *TNF-α*, **interleukin-4 (IL-4)**, an anti-inflammatory or suppressor cytokine, and **interleukin-2 (IL-2)**, an indicator of T cell activation and inflammation (see again Table 8.3).

The results were both predictable and a little surprising. Predictably, a comparison of the two self-report measures showed that students who scored high on the self-reported anxiety inventory scale were also found to be low in levels of adaptability. Also predicted, exam-taking students who scored high on self-reported anxiety measures had low levels of *TNF-α*, suggesting a higher risk of infection. Thus, among the test-taking group, perceived level of anxiety, as measured by the State Anxiety Inventory, was significantly correlated with *TNF-α*, a key cytokine that plays a major role in immune system response

TABLE 8.3 Summary of Selected Interleukins and Related Cytokines

Interleukin	Function	High Levels Indicate
Interleukin-1B (IL-1B)	Prompts the production of proinflammatory proteins Plays key role in innate immune response Has major role in autoimmune and inflammatory diseases	Boost immune response
Interleukin-2 (IL-2)	Serves as growth factor for B cells Stimulates synthesis of antibodies Promotes proliferation and differentiation of NK cells Is used in immunotherapy for cancer and AIDS treatment Initiates T cell activation and inflammation	Boost immune response
Interleukin-4 (IL-4)	Is an anti-inflammatory cytokine Suppresses immune system Inhibits production of inflammatory cytokines (IL-1, IL-6, TNF-α) Prolongs life span of T and B cells	Suppress immune system
Interleukin-6 (IL-6)	Has important and multiple roles in immune system response Is involved in humoral and cellular immune responses Is involved in autoimmune and inflammatory diseases Enhances B cell differentiation Is involved in Tc cell differentiation	Boost immune system
Interleukin-10 (IL-10)	Prompts immune suppression Inhibits many proinflammatory cytokines Boosts survival, proliferation, and differentiation of B cells Has overall importance in regulating immune system functioning	Suppress immune system
TNF-α	Plays role in tumor immunity and immunity against infection	Boost immune system

(Chandrashekara et al., 2007). In comparison, low-anxiety, exam-taking students were found to have high levels of *TNF-α*, suggesting a lower risk of infection.

As interesting as this first finding was, the surprising outcome was the results obtained from the mid-term and newly admitted students. Each of those groups was also divided into two anxiety groups, low versus high. Chandrashekara and colleagues reported no significant difference in the *TNF-α* levels for low- versus high-anxiety groups in either of those two other clusters of students. That is to say, the *TNF-α* levels were not significantly different when comparing the low- versus high-anxiety mid-term students or when comparing low- versus high-anxiety newly admitted students. For Chandrashekara and colleagues, this suggests that the environmental trigger, here meaning the exam stress, or possibly even perceived stress, influenced the physiological response (i.e., higher *TNF-α* levels) for high-anxiety exam takers only but not for mid-term or newly admitted students. The results of this study strongly suggest that the effects of stress on the immune system response are situation specific and, we would add, also dependent on the psychological state of the individual.

The later study by Koh and colleagues (2012) provides support for these findings, and even goes further. In their study, Koh and colleagues compared the *interleukin-6, interleukin-10* and *TNF-α* levels of 44 medical students at three distinct time periods: baseline, or 10 weeks after the start of classes; stress, or three days before the beginning of exams; and post-stress, or two weeks into the vacation period following exams. Similar to Chandrashekara et al. (2007), Koh and colleagues found that the *IL-6* levels that activate the immune system, also known as a proinflammatory cytokine, were significantly lower during the stress period than during the baseline period. This would suggest that the stress in anticipation of the exams downregulated the immune function, thereby increasing the risk of exposure to infection or illness. In comparison, the *IL-10* levels, an anti-inflammatory cytokine, was significantly higher. *IL-10* inhibits the inflammatory properties found in other interleukins like *IL-6*, needed to combat potential infections. According to Moore, de Waal Malefyt, Coffman, and O'Garra (2001), one way to improve a body's resistance to infections is by reducing the levels of *IL-10*. Thus, when *IL-10* levels are high, as was reported by Koh and colleagues (2012) during the stress period in their study, the medical students were at higher risk for infection.

There is more. Another interesting part of Koh and colleagues' study is what they found in the post-stress or vacation period. First, when measuring the medical student's *IL-6* and *IL-10* levels, they found that exam stress had a prolonged effect. Most telling, the study showed no significant difference in *IL-10* levels drawn during the stress period (3 days before exams) when compared with the vacation (post-stress) *IL-10* levels. The fact that the stress and post-stress *IL-10* levels were comparable could suggest lower resistance to infections during both the stress period and the post-stress or vacation period.

Second, Koh and colleagues also report that although the *IL-6* levels that boost immune function were appropriately higher in the vacation period than in the exam period, the vacation *IL-6* levels were not as high as those obtained during the baseline or pre-exam phase. In other words, the highest *IL-6* levels were obtained in the pre-exam phase, followed by the vacation phase, with the lowest levels obtained in the exam phase. The question here is why are the vacation *IL-6* levels lower than the baseline levels? These measures were taken fully two weeks post exams. One might expect at least a return to normal, or baseline, levels. Instead, this means that the proinflammatory cytokine's levels were downregulated after the stress to a level that was lower than their baseline level – a worrying outcome. If true, this finding suggests that the physiological effects of stress on the immune system may be longer than expected and certainly longer than what we subjectively perceive.

The study by Koh and colleagues (2012) produced results that supported these findings and more (see again, Box 8.1). They measured the effects of three stressors on the production of proinflammatory (immune activating) or anti-inflammatory (immune suppressing) cytokines: end-of-semester examination (an objective stressor); mid-year, non-exam period; and post-exam, vacation period. Like Chandrashekara and colleagues, the study by Koh and colleagues reported a drop in proinflammatory cytokine levels, measured here by **IL-6 levels**, during the stress period. This result suggests a downregulation of immune functioning, hence an increased risk for infection. In addition, the student's **IL-10 levels** were high. IL-10s are another type of anti-inflammatory cytokine that, similar to *IL-4*, serve to suppress the immune system. Thus, high anti-inflammatory levels are another indicator of suppressed immune function.

More interesting, however, were the results of the immune indicators during the vacation period. Here, Koh and colleagues reported lower *IL-6* (proinflammatory) levels in students during the vacation period than in the pre-stress period. Translated, this means that not only were the *IL-6* levels lower in the post-stress or vacation period, thereby suggesting a suppressed immune function, they were even lower than the baseline *IL-6 levels* taken at the beginning of the study, before exposure to the stress period. Based on this outcome, Koh and colleagues suggest that stress may have a prolonged, downregulatory effect on the body's immune response that continues long after the stress has abated. In other words, the suppressed immune response continued well into what should be a relaxing, stress-free vacation mode.

Clearly, these interesting findings may offer important insights into the relationship between stress and immune functions. However, the cautionary note included at the beginning of this chapter should be repeated. Chandrashekara and Koh's studies are both considered correlational studies. Consequently, it is impossible to establish a cause-and-effect relationship between stress, immune system functions, and health outcomes on the basis of these findings.

That said, a number of other observational studies also support the relationship between immune system and mental stress. For example, Anderson and colleagues (2015) report findings that suggest that people with depression may develop *autoimmune disease*, a disease in which the body attacks its own normal cells, mistaking them for foreign microorganisms, while Euesden and colleagues (2017) argue that there is a bidirectional relationship between psychological depression and autoimmune disease (Euesden, Danese, Lewis, & Maughan, 2017).

As is typical in psychological research, there are a number of studies that at best are unable to replicate these findings or, at worst, contradict them. For example, contrary to Koh's and Chandrashekara's studies, work by Goebels, Mills, Irwin, and Zeigler (2000) and Steptoe, Willemsen, Owen, Flower, and Mohamed-Ali (2001) suggest that psychological or perceived stressors do not decrease the production of proinflammatory cytokines, such as *IL-6* and *TNF-α*. Rather, according to these studies, they increase their production, thereby boosting immune function during stress.

It is important to note that findings from Goebels et al. (2000) and other researchers are consistent with the theory that stress is considered an adaptive rsssssesponse (see again Chapter 7, Stress and Coping). According to that theory, stress was necessary for humans to evolve and adapt to life-threatening circumstances in their environment. If stress is truly an adaptive response (and a vital one at that), then, Segerstrom and Miller (2004) ask, why would the best adaptive response to stress be a decrease in immune function? Instead, one would think that the best response to a stressor would be an increase in immune response that would stimulate the system, enabling it to respond more effectively to the stressor.

Dhabhar agrees. He argues that a psychophysiological stress response is a crucial survival mechanism (Dhabhar, 2018). Following this logic, Dhabhar suggests that short-term stressors may prepare the brain and immune system to handle challenges – perhaps that all-important exam or administering critical care to a wounded soldier – similar to how the stressors also prepare our physiological responses to fight or flee (Dhabhar, 2018).

Dhabhar and Segerstrom and Miller make compelling points. How do we explain these different findings? Dhabhar, like Sapolsky (see Chapter 7, Stress and Coping), emphasizes the need to distinguish between the effects of short-term versus long-term stress response in humans. They both argue, rather persuasively, that short-term stress can stimulate the immune system. As shown in earlier work by Dhabhar and McEwen (2001), the presentation of a short-term stressor in mice prompted a redistribution of immune cells, specifically the T cells, into the skin, resulting in an enhanced immune response. But prolonged or chronic stressors do the opposite. They propel T cells away from the skin, causing a suppression of the immune system. Thus, one possible explanation for the conflicting research findings is stress duration. Short term stressors may enhance immune response to allow our system to respond appropriately to the stress, whereas long-term or chronic stressors may do the opposite. What is considered "short-term"? According to Selye, short means about an hour. The three-day run-up to exams experienced by the medical students in Chandrashekara's and Koh's studies clearly exceeded this limit.

Other studies suggest that the variable effects of stress on immune response may be due to environmental factors. For example, Koh and colleagues (2012) and Rojas, Padgett, Sheridan, and Marucha (2002) suggest that in studies examining academic stress and immune response, differences in the form of examination, for example oral versus written, may trigger differences in immune system responses.

Remember we also noted that Chandrashekara's research group (2007) suggests that the effects of stress on immune response are situation specific. Recall that in their study, they found that students who were about to take their medical school exams had higher subjective and objective stress measures than the non–exam-taking students. But, and this is important, these researchers add that their study also found that anxiety levels, an individual variable, played a major role in stress and immune reaction outcomes as well. Thus, they conclude that both situational (environmental) triggers, like exams, and individual stress factors (anxiety) interact to influence immune function. We will focus more on the role of individual factors when we discuss individual differences a little later.

And yet, one other possible explanation for the different study results may be the researchers' decision to use cytokines to measure immune system function. Returning again to Chapter 7, Stress and Coping, we see a number of stress hormones, including catecholamines, cortisol, glucocorticoids, and even white blood cells also play a critical role in immune functions (see again Box 7.1). Studies that choose to examine these agents in addition to or in lieu of the cytokines examined in the studies cited earlier may obtain a somewhat different picture of the effects of stress on immune responses. Furthermore, Chandrashekara cautions that the high variability of cytokine levels in the general population, in addition to their limitations in reflecting the complete status of the body's immune response, pose additional challenges when using this agent to investigate stress and the immune system (Chandrashekara, 2021). Did we mention that the results of these psychoneuroimmunology studies are inconclusive? Perhaps this review of studies suggests why.

Summary

There is no shortage of intriguing but conflicting studies that examine the role of psychological health and immune system functions. We reviewed some of them here. Chandrashekara and colleagues (2007) and Koh's research team (2012) present two studies that argue persuasively that situational and psychological factors can influence immune system response, as demonstrated by the correlation between exam stress and *TNF-α, interleukin-6 (IL-6), interleukin-4 (IL-4), and interleukin-2 (IL-2)* levels. Yet Dhabhar, Sapolsky, Segerstrom and Miller, and others taking a macro look at stress also argue persuasively that decreased immune function in response to stress would be maladaptive. One possible explanation for some of the different outcomes is stress duration. Short-term stress may trigger the immune system in ways that may be adaptive, whereas long-term stress may serve to suppress immune function and be maladaptive. And, according to Selye, long-term is anything longer than one hour!

Individual Variability, Stress, and Immune Function

Chandrashekara and colleagues (2007) study prompts a closer look at individual variability and stress. It encourages us to ask, are all things equally stressful to everyone? More specifically, could individuals differ in their perception of stress? And does our individual perception of a stressful event influence immune system response? Majeed and Naseer (2019) and Ali, Khan, Abbas, Khan, and Ullah (2022) suggests that a person's appraisal of a situation, here meaning the perceived challenge posed by the stressor, may affect a person's cognitive appraisal of the situation and, by extension, their physiological response to the event. Thus, the answer to the first question, according to these two studies, is no. Not all stressors will be perceived as equally stressful because events do not present the same challenges to all individuals.

The answers to the second and third questions are yes. These studies do suggest that people differ in their response to stressors in part based on their cognitive appraisal of the situation. The first proposes what some might consider a controversial finding: workplace bullying may not be perceived as threatening to people with psychological capital or those who view the stress as good stress, or *eustress* (Majeed & Naseer, 2019). The second study by Ali and colleagues (2022), evaluating fear of contracting COVID-19 among working Pakistanis, suggests that people's personal circumstances (e.g., demographics, time spent on social media, those with family members 50 years of age or older or with biological illnesses), in addition to the type of coping styles (see Chapter 7, Stress and Coping), predicted people's stress levels and coping.

You may recall that Lazarus' (1984) transactional model of stress also suggests that the cognitive appraisal process of an event may differ across individuals, a difference that may play a role in stress perception (see again Chapter 7, Stress and Coping). And as we have demonstrated previously, the challenges posed and the individual's response can uniquely combine to present a physiological response in one person that will be different from the physiological response of another.

Consider this: Ever wonder why some people go to the beach to surf in the hours leading up to a hurricane? Surfers may not perceive the high winds and high waves as stressful events. In fact, they may be excited, looking forward to the thrill of riding those waves; hence the call "Surf's up!" For non-surfers, however, the thought of being on the beach before a hurricane may be frightening. The high winds and waves may make them seek shelter from those elements, not more exposure.

Clearly, these perspectives represent two distinctly different cognitive appraisals of the situation. And, if stress can influence immune system response, we would expect that in this situation, surfers' immune response would differ from non-surfers, in part because their cognitive appraisals of the dangers of the weather conditions just prior to the hurricane are vastly different. Thus, applying the work of Lazarus, Sapolsky, Dhabhar, Majeed and Naseer, and others on stress and the immune functions, we might predict that surfers would not show signs of immune system suppression because they do not view the hurricane's weather conditions as stressful. Non-surfers, however, would.

Finally, a person's perceived coping skills may also explain, in part, inter-individual variability in immune system functioning. Recall in Chapter 7 we explored possible differences in the coping skills of a young woman encountering an apparently frightening person/thing when walking alone at two o'clock in the morning (see page 282). In that example, the interpretation of the event as stressful may depend on whether the young woman believed her personal coping skills were adequate to confront the object or person. If the woman was walking alone after attending a party where she had several drinks, she might believe her coping skills to be inadequate for the looming threat. On the other hand, if she were returning home after her martial arts class, she may feel quite up to the task of handling the apparently threatening situation – eustress, as noted by Majeed and Naseer (2019). Thus, a person's perceived coping skills may also affect their perception of stress. And finally, as Koh suggests, both the intensity of the stressful event and the person's perceived coping skills may together account for individual differences in stress perception and immune response (Koh et al., 2012).

Depression and the Immune System

At this point, there appears to be an intriguing yet still ill-defined relationship between stress and immune functioning. Is the same true for other mental health factors? Take, for example, depression, post-traumatic stress disorder (PTSD), or even bipolar disorder. Is there a possible relationship between one or all of these psychological health illnesses and immune functions?

We cited a few studies looking at depressive disorder and stress. We now include additional studies looking specifically at major depressive disorders and the production of proinflammatory cytokines (Grosse et al., 2016; Hoyo-Becerra, Schlaak, & Hermann, 2014; Maes et al., 2012). Some of these studies suggest that the elevated production of certain cytokines, which are found in people diagnosed with major depressive disorder, is indicative of a relationship between depression and immune response (Calcagni & Elenkov, 2006; Hoyo-Becerra et al., 2014; Maes et al., 2012; Song et al., 2015). According to these findings, proinflammatory cytokines prompt symptoms of depression through several mechanisms.

Other researchers suggest that one way in which these cytokines contribute to the development of depressive symptoms is through the stimulation of the hypothalamic-pituitary-adrenocortical (HPAC) system (Song et al., 2015), a system we introduced in Chapter 7, Stress and Coping (see page 275). You may recall from that chapter that HPAC secretes glucocorticoids, a hormone that plays a very complex role in the body's response to stress. To recap: Glucocorticoids, together with other stress hormones, activate the body's immune system. But, as we noted in Chapter 7, Stress and Coping, prolonged levels of this hormone in the body can trigger a suppression of the immune system, leaving the body vulnerable to illnesses. These studies suggest that cytokines stimulate the HPAC which, in turn, initiates an immune system response including a release of glucocorticoids that can trigger depressive symptoms.

Song et al. (2015) even suggests that *seasonal affective disorder (SAD)*, a type of mood disorder characterized by episodes of depression in the winter but normal mood states in summer, may be induced by high levels of proinflammatory cytokines. The bottom line here is that cytokine transmitters can transfer an immune response to the brain that was initiated elsewhere in the body. And, according to these and other studies, such a transfer can lead to depression (Leonard, 2014; Song et al., 2015).

VIDEO #43/60

Chapter 8: Psychoneuroimmunology

· **Seasonal Affective Disorder:** *Seasonal Affective Disorder: How Seasons Change Your Mood | UPMC HealthBeat*

· **Website:** *https://share.upmc.com/2015/10/how-seasons-change-mood/*

· **UPMC HealthBeat audios and videos are publicly accessible (Website Terms of Use | UPMC).**

Are there also links between PTSD and immune system regulation? Generally, researchers agree that PTSD is associated with poorer overall physical health. It is frequently associated with respiratory illnesses, gastrointestinal disturbances, inflammation, and inflammatory and autoimmune diseases (Boscarino, 2004). Yet, some researchers also suggest there is a relationship between PTSD and immune function.

More specifically, the proposed link between PTSD and immune response is suggested in a study by Gola and colleagues (2013). These researchers compared the cytokine levels of 35 severely traumatized PTSD patients with those of 25 healthy patients (the control group). They found significantly higher *interleukin-1B (IL-1B), interleukin-6 (IL-6),* and *TNF-α* levels in the PTSD group than in the controls (see again Table 8.3). What is more, higher *IL-6 and TNF-α* levels were correlated with more severe PTSD symptoms among the 35 patients. According to these authors, the elevated *IL-6* levels may be evidence of a link between PTSD and low-grade inflammation, a link that could suggest a biomarker that associates PTSD with inflammation diseases such as atherosclerosis (Gola et al., 2013).

A second study by Bersani and colleagues (2016) also found an association between higher incidences of chronic viral infections, autoimmune disease, and PTSD. In their study of the role of *natural killer (NK) cells*, lymphocytes that can bind to and kill virus-infected cells without reliance on antigens, Bersani et al., suggest that there was a higher proportion of dysfunctional *NK* cells in the immune systems of the PTSD group. They conclude that such elevated levels of dysfunctional NK cells could result in immune system dysfunction.

These studies notwithstanding, other researchers question the findings that suggest that PTSD patients experience heightened inflammatory states. For example, research by deKloet and colleagues (2007) suggest that while some immune system alterations in his sample of combat veterans may be due to PTSD, other changes are most likely attributable to other trauma that may be associated with deployment to combat, not to PTSD.

What does all this mean? The bottom line is there may be a relationship among psychology, biology, and immunology. But variability in immune system functions, in individual perception, in cognitive appraisal, and other environmental factors indicate that we still have much to learn about the influence of psychological, environmental, and other non-physiological factors on immune system functions. And environmental factors can include, for example, social support networks.

Psychoneuroimmunology and Social Support Networks

Have you ever wondered whether your friends on your social network are good for your health? Researchers do! In a seminal study by Cohen and Willis (1985), researchers asked whether the existence of relationships or the extent to which an individual can receive helpful resources from such relationships, or both, have an impact on an individual's health. In their extensive review of the research of the time, Cohen and Willis concluded that both the existence of relationships and the availability of resources from those relationships enhance an individual's well-being. Specifically, they noted that social support networks can buffer people from potentially *pathogenic*, here meaning disease-producing, responses to stress. In addition, helpful resources associated with these networks can be beneficial, regardless of whether a person is experiencing stress.

Some 40 years after this research, we have additional questions. For example, does this theory still hold? Does this theory also apply to cyber social networks? That is to say, do online networks also buffer people from *pathogenic* stress responses? And do these cyber networks also provide helpful resources?

To address the question, "Does this theory still hold?," we begin by looking at married couples. It is reasonable to assume that most married couples consider themselves social support networks for each other. Therefore, can the interactions of married couples affect the health of one or both people? More specifically, can it affect the immune function of either person?

Consider this: Researchers have established that there is a relationship between marital malfunctioning, here meaning marital conflict or distress, and psychological and physical health outcomes. For example, Liu and Chen (2006) found that marital conflict can result in depressive affect in women. In addition, Henry and colleagues (2015) suggest that marital conflict can cause negative physical as well as psychological health outcomes. Specifically, Henry and colleagues' findings show a relationship between the quality of marital relations and *metabolic syndrome*, a group of health risk factors such as large waist circumference or high blood pressure, which increase the chances of heart disease or other health issues such as diabetes or stroke. Thus, they suggest that marital discord increases the likelihood of metabolic syndrome which may lead to negative psychological health outcomes.

Perhaps the best-known body of research establishing the link between marital quality and health is that of Kiecolt-Glaser and Newton (2001). Their studies show that marital relationships can either positively or negatively influence health status through direct pathways, which is health habits and behaviors, or indirect pathways, here meaning psychological or psychiatric symptoms. Subsequent studies support this finding, showing that, for example, among people over 50 years of age, increases in perceived marital quality resulted in an increase in self-rated health and decreases in disability and in functional limitations (Choi, Yorgason, & Johnson, 2016).

With the link between marital discord and health outcomes established, researchers wondered whether an association between marital quality and the immune system might exist. A study by Whisman and Sbarra (2012) tested such a link and found interesting differences between men and women. In their study of more than 400 couples between the ages of 35 and 84, they found that women, not men, were more likely to show a link between marital quality and their immune systems. While there was no relationship between *IL-6* and marital quality for men, there was a relationship between partner support (a positive marital quality), partner strain (a negative marital quality), and *IL-6* levels in younger women. These findings held for young women even when controlling for different demographic factors including ethnicity, existing health conditions such as obesity, or even health behaviors such as alcohol consumption or smoking patterns. Based on these findings, the authors suggest that *IL-6 levels* may hold important information about some physiological changes for women in relationships (Whisman & Sbarra, 2012).

Additionally, Wilson, Bailey, Malarkey, and Kiecolt-Glaser (2021) also found a relationship between marital satisfaction/support and related biomarkers. In their study, which examined almost 100 couples between the ages of 22 and 77, couples who were less satisfied in their marriage and received what they considered to be low-quality support from their partners were more likely to have higher levels of *TNF-α* (a proinflammatory cytokine) than satisfied couples or younger couples.

Certainly, most people would agree that conflicts and tensions are likely to occur at some point in almost all relationships. If that is the case, then based on the research by Whisman and Sbarra (2012) and Wilson and colleagues (2021), it might be tempting to think that in order to minimize the negative health outcomes associated with relationship conflicts, one might choose to stay single. There is one flaw (perhaps more) in such logic. Although there may be some negative health consequences to relationships with high levels of conflict, other research suggests that there are also negative consequences to loneliness.

Loneliness and Health

Like the research on marital quality and health, several studies report a link between loneliness and poor health outcomes (Hawkley & Cacioppo, 2010).

In two studies exploring the association between loneliness and inflammation, researchers Jaremka and colleagues (2013) examined the relationship between loneliness and stress on inflammation. They first evaluated participants based on the UCLA Loneliness Scale, a common scale used to assess the level of perceived loneliness and isolation. This measure helped researchers sort the participants into two groups, a high-loneliness group and a low-loneliness group. As done in other studies, they drew blood to collect baseline cytokine levels, after which study subjects were given a task designed to induce acute stress. In this case, the participants were instructed to prepare a 10-minute speech on why they would be the best candidate for a job. Then, after presenting the speech orally to a non-responsive (by design) audience, the participants completed an oral math task, again in front of the same deadpan audience. The tasks themselves, preparing a speech and oral math, were designed to be stressful. Performing the tasks for an unresponsive audience intensified the stress.

After completing both tasks, a second blood sample was taken. Results comparing the two blood samples showed that the participants in the high-loneliness group produced higher levels of *IL-6* than those in the low-loneliness group. These results suggest that loneliness is linked to higher production of the proinflammatory, or immune stimulating, cytokine.

Did we say higher proinflammatory (*IL-6*) cytokine? So, high-loneliness results in an increase in the cytokines that stimulate the immune system? Does this mean that loneliness enhances health? Surely, this cannot be correct.

Indeed, it is not. According to Jaremka and colleagues, the lonelier participants were highly *stress reactive*. That is to say, they evidenced a larger proinflammatory response than usual when encountering acute stress, a response that could be interpreted as a show of excessive stress. And, as we know from Chapter 7, Stress and Coping, an excessive stress response is not a health-enhancing response.

Before concluding, we return to one of the topics introduced at the beginning of this section on psychoneuroimmunology and social support networks: online networks and health. Is it possible for a person to engage mainly with online networks and reap the same benefits from those social interactions as from in-person networks?

Social Media and Stress

Before we explore these studies, it is important to note that there have been a number of publications within the past five years, in both the popular press and the research literature, about social media and its negative impacts on children and adolescents (Abrams, 2023; Babic et al., 2017; Benoit, 2018), as well as those claiming no significant impact or improved well-being (Dienlin, Masur, & Trepte, 2017; Valkenburg & Peter, 2007).

Consider the research on the effects of cyber networks like Facebook (now Mega), Instagram, Twitter (now X), Snapchat, TikTok, and others on psychological states, specifically among adolescents. A number of studies report lower levels of life satisfaction and higher levels of depression among adolescents who spend in excess of five hours a night on social networks cites or texting. For example, Kelly and colleagues (2019) report that among U.K. teens 14 years of age, there is an association between depressive symptoms and social media use. This finding was greater for girls than boys. Another study, which reviews three large data bases in the U.S. and the U.K. with a total of over 200,000 teens ages 13–18, similarly reports poorer mental health outcomes for heavy users of social media – here meaning spending more than five hours a day on these sites, versus those who spend less than one hour a day online (Twenge & Campbell, 2019). Specifically, higher social media users were more likely than light users (here meaning less than one hour a day) to report being unhappy, depressed, having suicide ideation, or attempts. Others report higher levels of loneliness overall (Komal & Gurpreet, 2016).

Then, there are the studies that report that computer-mediated communication, regardless of age, results in self-reported declines in life satisfaction, a measure of subjective well-being (Kross et al., 2013). In fact, Kross and colleagues found that this decline in life satisfaction occurred regardless of the size of the network or of the perceived supportiveness of the group. This result was not obtained when participants engaged in direct, that is in-person, interactions.

Finally, McCloskey, Iwanicki, Lauterbach, Giammittorio, and Maxwell (2015) suggest that Meta offers mixed benefits as a cyber social support network. Their study sought to identify and measure the types and levels of social support provided by Meta and to determine which were more closely related to quality of life and depression. They identified four primary types of support: emotional, instrumental, negative, and perceived. In this study, examples of emotional support included getting a number of "likes" or comments on the respondent's Meta page. Instrumental support included receiving tangible assistance such as suggestions or information deemed helpful to the respondent. Negative support was represented through negative responses on Meta or a decrease in the total number of friends. Finally, perceived support was the belief that any assistance believed to be available would be available if needed, although not necessarily tested. (If you are thinking that this research appears to build on Cohen and Willis' 1985 study, you are correct).

Of these factors, predictably, negative social support was positively correlated with depression and negatively correlated with quality of life. Surprisingly, however, emotional support was also positively associated with higher levels of depression and poorer quality of life. In essence, not receiving "likes" on one's Meta page postings or the loss of friends of record seems to suggest a loss and negatively impacts perceived quality of life. Does this mean that Meta use poses risks for a person's psychological health? Again, one study cannot lead to such a conclusion. This study does suggest, however, that elevated levels of emotional social support which rests on whether one receives affirmation on Meta in the form of "likes" or a large number of "friends" predicts higher levels of depression and poorer quality of life when such affirmations are not forthcoming.

Equally as interesting is an alternative interpretation suggested by the authors. They suggest that their findings might also indicate that people who are more distressed or depressed are more likely to access Meta for social support than non-distressed individuals (McCloskey et al., 2015). In other words, it might be the dependence on Meta or other social networking sites as a social support network, rather than the use of this cyber network as an additional support tool, which increases the negative psychological health outcomes of some users.

In essence, there may be a reason to be concerned about the effects of social media on young children and adolescents. Without a doubt, there are a number of studies that suggest that the mental health of individuals 18 years of age or younger has been on the decline, an outcome that appears to coincide with the evolution and increased use of smartphones to access social media sites (Haidt & Rausch, 2023). However, this is a complex issue requiring more research into exactly why social media sites seem to adversely affect some children and adolescents.

One additional point on social media's effects on mental health: Aarts, Peek, and Waiters (2014) and Leist (2013) report that older users, here including adults and particularly those over 65 years of age, report better mental health outcomes as a result of access to cyber networks. Can you propose reasons why social media might be beneficial for older adults?

Rats!

The last word, for now, on the relationship between social support and psychoneuroimmunology is found in research with rats. This research by Cruces, Venero, Pereda-Perez, and Fuentes (2014) and Pisu and colleagues (2013) suggests that the total absence of social networks, in other words isolation, can have a detrimental effect on the immune system (see Box 8.2). Specifically, Cruces and colleagues (2014) report that older rats were particularly susceptible to impaired immune system responses after eight weeks of isolation. Perhaps even more interesting is the finding by Pisu and colleagues (2013) that exposing rats to social isolation conditions for 30 days not only influences the neuroendocrine system, but that this effect can be transferred to the next generation. Thus, according to these intriguing findings, contact with others of the same species may be important for the healthy functioning of adult rats as well as their offspring.

Box 8.2 Rats? Really?

Yes, really!

Researchers have conducted experiments with rats for decades. They have been used extensively in medical research because rats and humans share similar physiologies. Now, however, we see another role for rats. They may help guide our understanding of the relationship between social contact or lack thereof and immune functions. Two studies help explain their role.

One study, by Cruces and colleagues (2014), asks how anxious responses to isolation in the elderly are related to immune system response. To test this question the researchers elected 18 male rats 20 months old (rats live an average of 12–24 months). The rats were randomly assigned to one of two groups: the control group and the experimental or isolated group. Control group rats were housed in pairs in cages, but the rats designated to be in the isolated group were separated and housed alone in cages. To intensify the sense of isolation, a black plastic bag was draped over the cages of the isolated rats. The rats in the control group and the isolated group lived in these cages for a total of eight weeks.

Now the experiment begins. At week four (midway through the experiment) and at the conclusion of the experiment at week eight, researchers weighed both groups of rats and assessed their "anxiety" levels, using a rather unique device known as an elevated plus maze (EPM). Briefly, EPMs are widely used to test the anxiety behavior of rats. The EPM model resembles a three-dimensional plus sign (+) mounted on a round platform that sits approximately 15–18 inches high. The horizontal arms of the plus sign are unobstructed, allowing the rat to travel freely along the horizontal axis. The vertical arms, however, are obstructed. The rat cannot travel in a vertical direction (see Figure 8.1).

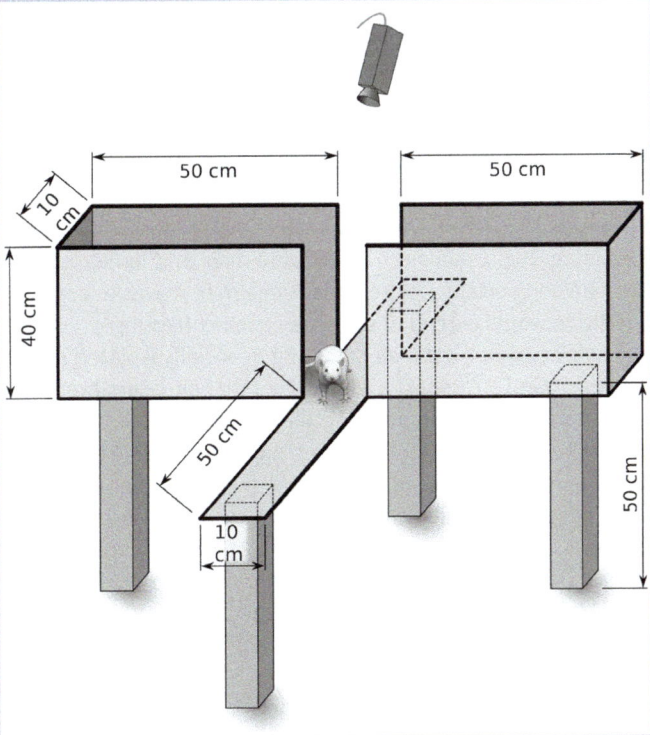

FIGURE 8.1 A drawing of an elevated plus maze (EPM) for a rat experiment. It resembles a three-dimensional plus sign mounted on a platform elivated 15–18 inches from the floor. The horizontal arms of the maze are unabstructed, the vertical arms are obstructed, prohibiting the rat from traveling along the vertical axis.

Source: Adapted from Samueljohn.de, Wikimedia Commons.

In this experiment, weight gain or loss is one indicator of the effects of social isolation stress on the rats. Indeed, at both the four-week and the eight-week periods, the isolation rats showed significant weight loss: a loss of 6.8 grams at week four and a loss of 22.5 grams at week eight. By comparison, control group rats reported weight *gains* of comparable amounts at both week four (2.2 grams) and week eight (2.3 grams).

Measures of anxiety between the two groups also revealed differences. The researchers expected that isolated rats would spend less time in the arms of the EPM, an anxiety response to their 4 and 8 weeks of isolation. Indeed, when left to explore the EPM, isolated rats spent significantly less time in the arms of the maze than did controls.

The link between social isolation and the immune system was found after the rats' spleens were analyzed. The isolated rats were found to have lower natural killer (NK) cell activity. We noted earlier that *NK* cells are needed to kill virus-infected cells. Lower NK activity puts the rats at higher risk for infection or illness. The decrease in NK activity in the isolated rats mirrors what researchers have reported about humans in studies of loneliness and immune system functions (Kiecolt-Glaser et al., 1984).

There is more. The isolated rats were also found to have lower *IL-10* and lower *TNF-α* levels. You will remember from our earlier discussion that *IL-10* inhibits the inflammatory process that is needed to combat infections. Likewise, *TNF-α*, a cytokine, also plays a major role by boosting immunity against infection. The authors contend that lower levels of these two agents suggest an altered immune response that impairs immune system activation.

Additional research by Pisu and colleagues (2013) suggests that not only does social isolation have an impact on the rat's immune system, but they also contend that this effect can affect the offspring of the affected rats. In this study, male and female rats were weaned from their mothers and then socially isolated for 30 days. They were compared with a group of same-sex rats in a control group who were not socially isolated after weaning. The researchers then mated male and female socially isolated rats. They also mated male and female non-socially isolated rats. The aim here was to determine whether the effects of the parents' social isolation would extend in some way to the offspring.

After separation from their parents, the male offspring of socially isolated rats were housed for 30 days and then subjected to several stress test measures before being sacrificed to study the effects on the offsprings' immune system. The results indicated that while there were no differences in emotional reactivity of the rats reared by socially isolated versus group-housed parent rats, there was significant HPAC activity and reduced levels of corticotropin-releasing factor, an agent that plays a critical role in the coordination of a number of systems, including the immune response and endocrine response to stressful stimuli (Hillhouse, Randeva, Ladds, & Grammutopoulos, 2002). These neuroendocrine differences between socially isolated versus group-reared offspring suggest, according to these researchers, that changes in immune system functioning that occur in one generation can be communicated to the next generation.

Could the same findings hold true for humans? Testing the relationship between human social isolation and immune system functioning would be difficult due to ethical concerns (see Chapter 2, Research Methods). However, as we know, one reason research on rats is informative is because their physiology is similar to that of humans (Iannaccone & Jacob, 2009). At this point we can only speculate about the applicability of these findings to humans.

Summary

We began this section examining studies on the relationship between psychological health and the human immune system. We quickly saw that this research covers a wide range of topics including stress, specifically academic stress, individual differences, depression, PTSD and other mental health issues, and social support systems.

For the moment, it appears that stress, depression and other mental health illnesses, social support systems, high conflict-ridden social interactions, loneliness, and yes, isolation, all may have a significant impact on our immune systems and our overall health. Yet research findings to date are equivocal. One thing the studies do suggest: Social support systems are important to our physical and mental well-being. This is the case whether the support network is a "significant other" or a group of family or friends. In addition, studies clearly suggest that social support helps guard against loneliness. And, because loneliness is highly correlated with depression, social support networks offer yet another way to contribute to positive mental health outcomes. The question is what types of networks best contribute to positive mental health. The research suggests that determining which networks work best depends on a number of demographic factors, including a person's age, the frequency and duration of use of online networks, and any existing mental health issues of the user. But we end with the classic line that often appears at the end of research articles: more research is needed in this area.

SECTION III. PSYCHONEUROIMMUNOLOGY AND CHRONIC ILLNESSES

The evidence seems to be mounting. The research we examined so far suggests that there may well be a link between psychology, neurology, and immune system responses. The research we present in this section, which examines the association between chronic illnesses and psychoneuroimmunology, would appear to confirm this assumption. Here, we review a sample of studies that examine separately the relationship between cancer, heart disease and psychoneuroimmunology.

There are a number of reports in the research literature that examine the connection between specific health issues, such as cancer, chronic pain, or other ailments and psychological factors like trait anxieties, stress-prone personalities, and coping styles (Chida, Hamer, Wardle, & Steptoe, 2008; Dahl, 2010; Eckerling et al., 2021; Wang et al., 2023). And, as in the previous sections, there is strong evidence on both sides of the argument: research suggesting an association, including a link to immune functioning, and research that refutes such an association.

At this point, you might be tempted to, figuratively, throw up your hands and say, "Let's wait and have this discussion when the research is more conclusive," or, for some, "Who cares?" Admittedly, the mixed research findings can be dispiriting and a little confusing. The thing to keep in mind is that collectively, this body of research is slowly, ever so slowly, helping us to understand more about the myriad of factors that affect our health. More importantly, this sometimes confusing research is revealing relationships between factors that were previously thought to be unrelated, things like psychological factors and susceptibility to cancer! So, bear with us a little longer as we tease out the possible relationships between psychological factors, chronic illnesses, and immune system functioning.

Cancer and Immune Function

It may seem obvious, but many people who report problems such as pain or who are treated for chronic health conditions also report other conditions such as depression, chronic stress, and fatigue. Research on women who were recently treated for breast cancer seems to support this finding. For example, in a study by Jaremka and colleagues (2013) 200 hundred women, 27–76 years of age, who were between two months and three years post-treatment for cancer, participated in a study to test their self-reported levels of loneliness, depression, and fatigue. But this study included another factor, antibodies for two types of common herpes viruses.

Why would antibodies for two types of herpes viruses, specifically cytomegalovirus (CMV) and Epstein-Barr virus (EBV), be relevant to understanding a link between immune system and chronic illnesses? In Jaremka and colleagues' study, loneliness was associated with higher levels of CMV. Earlier research has already shown a relationship between loneliness, pain, depression, and fatigue. In fact, this relationship is so firmly established that it is now referred to as the pain-depression-fatigue cluster (Jaremka et al., 2013). When Jaremka and colleagues found an association between loneliness and CMV, they concluded that loneliness, a psychological factor, increases the chances of an immune system dysregulation as is evident from the increased antibodies to the CMV herpes virus. Seemingly, once that link is formed, the pain, depression, and fatigue cluster are now possible.

Why is this relevant, particularly for women in the aftermath of breast cancer surgery? Keep in mind that recovery from any illness requires both physiological and psychological healing. When either is suppressed, recovery may be slower or impaired.

Other studies investigating the link between chronic illnesses such as cancer and immune functioning ask whether personality traits may also play a role. Sound odd? It should not. Remember that in Chapter 7, Stress and Coping, we identified several studies that suggested a link between personality and specific chronic health conditions. You may remember, for example, one study that suggested that persons with personality type D, for distressed, were significantly more likely to develop heart-related health problems. This association was thought to be due, in part, to Type D personality's tendency to display negative affect such as stress, anxiety, or hostility (Denollet et al., 2006; Kupper & Denollet, 2007).

Unfortunately, past studies examining the association between personality types and chronic illnesses have been plagued with methodological problems. They have been critiqued for using an overly simplistic design when attempting to examine a rather complex issue. Instead, as Dahl (2010) and others have suggested, what is needed to test this link is a study that examines a connection between biomarkers for personality or other psychological factors and inflammation markers.

To that end, a study by Dhabhar and colleagues (2013) asks whether subjects with high-trait anxiety or stress-prone personalities, such as Type D personalities, might also have lower protective immunity. Sound intriguing? It might, especially if you or someone you know is thought to have a stress-prone personality. It is also intriguing for some scientists who view Dhabhar's research as the type of rigorous study needed to establish or refute a possible link between personality types and cancer.

Dhabhar and colleagues studied rats that were identified *phenotypically* as high or low anxiety. By *phenotype* we mean the observable physical or biochemical characteristics that are influenced both by gender and by environment. In this study the rats were classified as high or low anxiety based on their behavior in two environments, an elevated maze, and a light and dark arena (see Box 8.2). Once classified, the rats were then given three weeks to acclimatize themselves to their surroundings while, at the same time, they were exposed to UV-B light three times a week for 10 weeks. The UV light was intended to promote the growth of tumors. Thus, in this experiment, researchers wanted to determine whether *phenotypically* high- or low-trait anxiety rats would differ in the number of tumors developed, and in the progression of those tumors into *squamous cell carcinoma*, or skin cancer cells.

VIDEO #44/60

Chapter 8: Psychoneuroimmunology

- **Phenotype:** *Genetics in 60 seconds: Genotype vs. Phenotype*
- *Website:* **Genetics in 60 seconds: Genotype vs. Phenotype (youtube.com)**
- **Medicine Can Be Easy is an education platform that makes their information available for students or professionals to study.** *About this site (medicinecanbeeasy.com)*

Dhabhar and colleagues found that the high-trait anxiety group of rats developed more tumors than the low-trait anxiety rats. What is more, they also found a faster rate of progression from tumor to carcinoma cells in the high-anxiety group of rats. The results of this study appear to suggest that high-trait anxiety could be aggravated by environmental stressors and may also contribute to the rate of progression of a tumor from a growth to a cancer cell.

The findings of this study are consistent with research by Chida and colleagues (2008) who also found an association between psychosocial factors, including personality type and cancer. But, as we indicated earlier, not all research supports these claims (see specifically Bleiker et al., 2008; Nakaya et al., 2010).

Heart Disease and Immune Function

For people diagnosed with any one of several varieties of cardiovascular (heart) disease, the diagnosis, not to mention the treatment and recuperation period, may trigger the onset of depression. We explore the topic of cardiovascular diseases in greater detail in Chapter 9, Cardiovascular Disease. For now, just keep in mind that cardiovascular disease refers to a group of disorders of the heart (cardio) or the circulatory system. Studies on the relationship between immune system function and cardiovascular diseases suggest that the strength of this association may be measured also by the changes in specific physiological markers.

One example of research on the link between cardiovascular disease, depression, and immune response is the work by Steptoe, Wikman, Molloy, Messerli-Bürgy, and Kaski (2013). Earlier research has already established a relationship between clinical and sub-clinical, or asymptomatic, depression following a diagnosis of acute (sudden) coronary syndrome (ACS; Thombs et al., 2006). And other researchers have found a relationship between a diagnosis of depression that occurred at the first occurrence of ACS and a reoccurrence of the syndrome or even coronary related deaths (Meijer et al., 2011). But in their study, Steptoe and colleagues wanted to determine whether the magnitude of the inflammatory response to ACS would predict symptoms of depression up to six months after the first, sudden onset of the illnesses. Their research examined the white blood cell counts and the C-reactive protein levels during the coronary event.

Why did these researchers examine white blood cells counts and C-reactive protein levels? White blood cells help fight infections by fighting bacteria germs while also indicating the level of inflammation in the body. C-reactive proteins also serve as indicators of inflammation in the body. As mentioned earlier, high levels of inflammation may suggest an infection in some parts of the body. Thus, Steptoe and colleagues were using white blood cell counts and C-reactive protein to examine the relationship between immune function and depression for persons diagnosed with ACS.

Two findings suggest a link between cardiovascular disease, immune function, and depression. First, Steptoe and colleagues found higher levels of inflammation, signaled by elevated white blood cell counts, associated with ACS diagnosis. Second, their study reported that white blood cell levels were significantly associated with the intensity of depression symptoms three weeks after the initial coronary episode (Steptoe et al., 2013). These two elements are enough to suggest a relationship among the three variables. But there is more. Fully six months after the first acute coronary syndrome episode, Steptoe and colleagues found a relationship between the white blood cell count during the initial episode and cognitive symptoms of depression as measured six months later.

The literature on the relationship between chronic illnesses and depression is robust. But this study by Steptoe and colleagues suggests that the impact of chronic illness also can affect immune response.

SECTION IV. PSYCHONEUROIMMUNOLOGY, ENVIRONMENTAL FACTORS, AND HEALTH

Throughout this chapter we have mentioned that there are some environmental factors that serve as co-determinants with psychology to influence immune system response. In fact, in earlier studies we identified specific stressful environmental factors, such as exams, lack of social support or overexposure to UV light as possible contributors. Now, what would you think if someone told you that a person's perceived social status could also trigger an immune response? It almost sounds too incredible to believe. Yet, it was the subject of several studies.

Before continuing it is important to state that there is sound research that shows that socioeconomic status is related to health. Early research by Adler and Snibbe (2003) has clearly shown that as our socioeconomic status increases (as measured by annual incomes; see again Chapter 6, Emotional Health and Well-Being), so does our health. Conversely, those at the lower end of the socioeconomic scale are more likely to report poorer health outcomes. So, there is a relationship between these two factors. The question here is whether one's socioeconomic status can also affect our immune system functions.

Research by Derry and colleagues (2013), Ghaed and Gallo (2007), and Wang and colleagues (2023) seems to suggest that social status is yet another environmental factor that can trigger immune system dysregulation. A close look at these studies might suggest otherwise. Derry and colleagues' study suggests that people who rate themselves as being in the lower socioeconomic status experience more frequent life stressors. As a result, they contend that these stressors will have an impact on stress-induced *IL-6*, resulting in a downregulation of their immune system. While there is considerable research to support the downregulating effect of stress on *IL-6*, it is not at all clear that the principal contributor to the immune suppression in this study is, in fact, socioeconomic status. This is because Derry and colleagues also include, as part of their study, participants' experience with depression and childhood trauma. Clearly such psychological and environmental factors would be as likely, if not more so, to contribute to immune suppression as one's socioeconomic scale.

Ghaed's study appears to contradict, in part, findings from some earlier studies. Ghaed suggests that a person's subjective perception of their own social status may override the health projections associated with the person's objective social status, as measured by their community of residence, their income, and perhaps their level of education. In Ghaed's study, women's perception of their own social status was significantly higher than that of their community. As a result, they found that the social status of the woman's community was inversely related to measures of anxiety, stress, and blood pressure obtained from the study sample. Specifically, Ghaed and colleagues suggest that if a person perceives their social status to be higher than that of their community, their self-perceived status may be more likely to predict their health outcomes than the actual social status of their community. For example, a person who resides in a working-class community but who perceives their status as closer to lower-middle class will have better health indicators, such as blood pressure and anxiety, than others from the same community whose perception of their status matches that of their community.

Finally, Wang and colleagues found that of approximately 2,100 Chinese adults between the ages of 30 and 79, those who experienced two or more stressful life events had a significantly higher odds of developing cancer. Among the stressful life events included in this study were at least two associated with socioeconomic status: loss of income and living on debt.

While these findings are intriguing, they do not permit a more rigorous examination of the effects of perceived social status on immune system functioning, as do other studies.

Summary

We began this section by noting two important facts. First, there are host of studies in psychoneuroimmunology that suggest that psychological factors, such as stress, depression, and even perhaps PTSD, in addition to environmental factors can regulate immune system functions. Second, and equally as important, the studies conducted to date, while intriguing, are either clinical/observation or correlational, which do not meet the standard of experimental research to show a causal relationship between these factors (see again Chapter 2, Research Methods, for a comparison between correlation and cause and effect).

The studies presented in this chapter are, indeed, fascinating. But until more evidence can be provided that demonstrates a cause-and-effect relationship, the research on psychoneuroimmunology presents interesting prospects in need of further research.

Personal Postscript

"DO I HAVE TO GIVE UP MY INSTAGRAM ACCOUNT TO BOOST MY IMMUNE SYSTEM?"

In one word, no. No one, and probably not even the researchers cited in this chapter, would make such a claim.

What is in question, however, is how much use or reliance on social media cites is healthy. We have no conclusive statement about how much or how little anyone should use their cyber networks to provide the interaction and social support we all need as living beings. The research is not that conclusive.

On the other hand, there have been a number of initiatives that aim to encourage individuals to "unplug." Efforts by local communities, schools and even workplace settings to encourage their constituents to forgo electronics in favor of in-person contact have been growing. This even applies to forgoing email in office settings and instead sending messages through direct, in-person contact.

What should we take from these efforts in different settings? Perhaps the only thing we can infer is that scientists, employers, schools, and even families suspect that using machines as the dominant form of communication between individuals is having a negative effect on many individuals. Note that here we are talking about the impact of this technology as the primary form of communication. The technological advances that enable us to be in contact with people around the globe, or people who are not, for the moment, in our same space are fantastic. But it should not substitute for in-person communication when possible.

The studies cited here do seem to suggest that there are benefits from the in-person contact that are not provided, or even that are negated by reliance on cyber systems of communication.

Questions to Consider

1. Global, technological advances are viewed as essential tools for success and forward progress in developed and developing countries. What limits on their use, if any, might be recommended based on the research on loneliness, depression, and immune response systems on humans and rats?
2. How can health psychologists play a role in the research on the effects of cyber social support networks on individuals?
3. How might health psychologists elevate the importance of healthy interpersonal relationships and interactions based on research in psychoneuroimmunology?

True or False Questions

1. Chandrashekara's study confirms that situational factors play a significant role in our immune system functioning. True or False.
2. The human immune system consists of two systems of immunity: adaptive and acquired. True or False.
3. There are two types of B cells: B memory and B suppressor. True or False.
4. Koh's study suggests that stress may have a prolonged, downregulatory effect on the body, lasting long after the stress has abated. True or False.
5. Dhabhar's study of rats supports the conclusion that there may be an association between psychosocial factors – like personality type – and illnesses such as cancer. True or False.

Important Terms

adaptive (or acquired) immunity   313
antibody-producing cells   314
antigenic specificity   314
antigens   315
autoimmune disease   321
B cells   315
B lymphocytes   314
CD4 cells   316
cell differentiation   316
cell-mediated immunity   316
cell proliferation   316
cytokines   316

Cardiovascular Disease

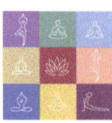

Source: 3xy/
Shutterstock.

Chapter Outline

Opening Story: Tim Russert

Section I. The Heart and Its Functions

Section II. Cardiovascular Disease

Section III. Psychosocial Factors and Cardiovascular Disease

Section IV. Cardiovascular Disease and Health Determinants

Personal Postscript

Questions to Consider

True or False Questions

Important Terms

Chapter Objectives

After studying this chapter, you will be able to:

1. Identify the principal structures of the heart and describe their functions.

2. Identify and describe the four types of cardiovascular disease associated with health behaviors.

3. Identify the six main risk factors for cardiovascular disease.

4. Describe the contributions of carbohydrates, fats, cholesterol, vitamins, and minerals to heart disease.

5. Explain the risks of heart disease for men and women.

6. Explain the risks of heart disease for ethnic groups.

7. Explain the effects of family, community, and environment on risk factors for heart disease.

8. Explain the effect of access to health care on risks for cardiovascular disease.

DOI: 10.4324/9781003300670-10

OPENING STORY: TIM RUSSERT

Television news commentator Tim Russert was known for many things. He was a respected journalist, a tenacious reporter, a challenging interviewer, and the well-regarded moderator of a popular Sunday morning talk show, Meet the Press. *But one thing not widely known was that he had* **coronary artery disease (CAD)**, *a disease caused by* **plaque** *– a composite made up of fat, cholesterol, calcium, and other substances – that builds up in the arteries (National Heart, Lung and Blood Institute [NHLBI, 2023]).*

On June 13, 2008, Tim Russert collapsed at work and later died from a heart attack due to CAD. According to his doctors, Russert had been diagnosed earlier with **asymptomatic** *CAD, meaning that he had experienced no warning signs of his illness. He did not experience pressure in the chest or pain in the shoulders, neck, arm, or back – symptoms that usually accompany CAD – caused by a reduced flow of blood and oxygen to the heart or the brain (NHLBI, 2023). Doctors determined that when Russert collapsed on June 13, part of the plaque buildup in one of the arteries broke off. The dislodged plaque blocked the supply of blood and oxygen from one artery and reduced the flow of blood to the heart. The blockage caused a heart attack and, eventually, Russert's death.*

Russert's sudden death shocked many people. But more shocking was the fact that his CAD was said to be under control. He was taking medication for the disease and even passed a **stress test**, *a test that measures the electrical activity of the heart while an individual exercises on a treadmill or another type of exercise machine (NBC News, 2008). Although not confirmed, we might speculate that Russert was also monitoring his health behaviors: limiting the consumption of foods high in fats and cholesterol and increasing his exercise. Unfortunately, in Russert's case, monitoring, medication, and health behavior changes did not prevent the very thing doctors were working to avoid: a fatal heart attack.* ∎

VIDEO #45/60

Chapter 9: Cardiovascular Disease

- **Asymptomatic:** *Symptomatic vs. Asymptomatic Patients*
- **Website:** *https://www.youtube.com/watch?v=9dexKlQrAxU*
- **Newman Regional Health's information is publicly accessible and available for free.** *Newman Regional Health | Quality Healthcare | Emporia, KS (newmanrh.org)*

Tim Russert's case is sobering. After all, how many times have we indicated in previous chapters that early detection and treatment of an illness, in addition to adopting healthy behaviors, will contribute to good health outcomes?

Without a full medical history, we cannot speculate about the distal causes (see Chapter 2, Research Methods) of Russert's death. But we do know that he was overweight, suggesting that at some point his diet may have contained high levels of fats or cholesterol. Thus, in spite of the fact that Russert was receiving medical care for coronary artery disease (CAD), the medical treatment may not have been sufficient to reverse the effects of years of poor diet, lack of exercise, or other unhealthy behaviors.

Typical of a chronic disease, the behaviors that contributed to the development of CAD in Tim Russert did not lead to death in the short term. Rather, the combined effects over time contributed to a heart attack, which was the proximal cause of death. CAD and other forms of cardiovascular disease associated with lifestyles are, therefore, an excellent example of the health consequences of risky health behaviors. This is one reason that cardiovascular disease is of interest to health psychologists.

This chapter is the first of three that examine a chronic illness relevant to the field of health psychology. In this chapter, we examine diseases of the heart that are highly correlated with health behaviors and lifestyles, including CAD, cardiac arrest, cerebrovascular disease (stroke), and hypertension (high blood pressure).

Before proceeding, it is important to note that most forms of cardiovascular disease are preventable. Why do we refer to these illnesses as preventable? In earlier chapters, we learned that lifestyles and health behaviors will affect health outcomes. Diet, alcohol consumption, use of tobacco, stress and stress management, and physical exercise can singly or in combination increase or decrease the risk of heart disease. And as we will soon see, even the dietary habits of children as young as five years of age, if left unchanged, can predispose them to cardiovascular disease in adulthood. For this reason and others, we view cardiovascular diseases as highly preventable illnesses. The question for health psychologists is how to encourage individuals to adopt and maintain healthy behaviors that limit the risk of avoidable diseases.

We begin the chapter with an overview of the cardiovascular system to identify the important components and functions of the heart and circulatory system and to understand how they work. Next, we use our understanding of the heart and its functions in Section II to examine the development of cardiovascular diseases, such as CAD, cardiac arrests, stroke, and hypertension, which are associated with lifestyle choices. We continue in Section III with an exploration of the risk factors that lead to each of these diseases, including behavioral, genetic, individual, familial, environmental, and health policy factors. Finally, in Section IV, we explore the psychological impact of heart disease on individuals. New research reveals the role of depression in the onset of and recovery from cardiovascular disease. As you may be able to tell by now, these new discoveries of the relationship between emotional health and physiological outcomes identify more ways in which health psychologists can contribute to the health management efforts for individuals and communities.

At the conclusion of this chapter, you will be able to explain the role of the heart in sustaining life, identify and describe the major cardiovascular diseases associated with unhealthy behaviors, describe how various health risk factors negatively affect our heart health, and identify health-enhancing behaviors that minimize the risk of heart disease.

One reminder before we begin: Our opening story introduced Tim Russert, a person who died of CAD. Although cardiovascular diseases of all types can cause death, it is important to keep in mind that these diseases are classified as chronic diseases. As we indicated earlier, chronic diseases are illnesses that may linger for months or years. Although they may contribute to death, they rarely cause immediate death. We do not know how long Russert suffered from CAD. But as we will see later in the chapter, his CAD was probably in formation for several years – too many, in fact, to be reversed by a relatively recent change in diet, exercise, and medication.

SECTION I. THE HEART AND ITS FUNCTIONS

Structure

The heart has been described many ways: a muscular bag made up of two pumps, the body's transport system, and an upside-down pear, just to cite a few. All of these descriptions accurately characterize the heart, including its shape.

The heart is a very strong muscle that is the focal point of the body's circulatory system. It is a vital muscle because the heart circulates blood to all parts of the body. The blood carries necessary "food," here meaning oxygen and other nutrients, needed by other organs and systems to function properly. In addition to carrying "food" to other organs, blood also carries carbon dioxide, a waste product, for the lungs to expel, thus eliminating a substance that is harmful to the body.

How does the heart work? The heart muscle has two sides and a total of four chambers (two per side): the right and left *atria* (the plural of *atrium*) and the right and left *ventricles*. The blood enters the right side of the heart through one of two upper chambers. In general, the right side of the heart receives and transports "used" or deoxygenated blood, from the organs. Other organs in the body extract oxygen (their food) from the blood before returning the blood to the heart.

Figure 9.1 shows that used blood enters the right atrium, is passed to the right ventricle, and then goes through the *pulmonary arteries* to make its way to the lungs. The lungs *reoxygenate* the blood, meaning that the lungs resupply blood with new oxygen. The oxygen-rich blood is then pumped from the lungs into the heart through the left pulmonary veins and enters the heart's left atrium (British Heart Foundation,

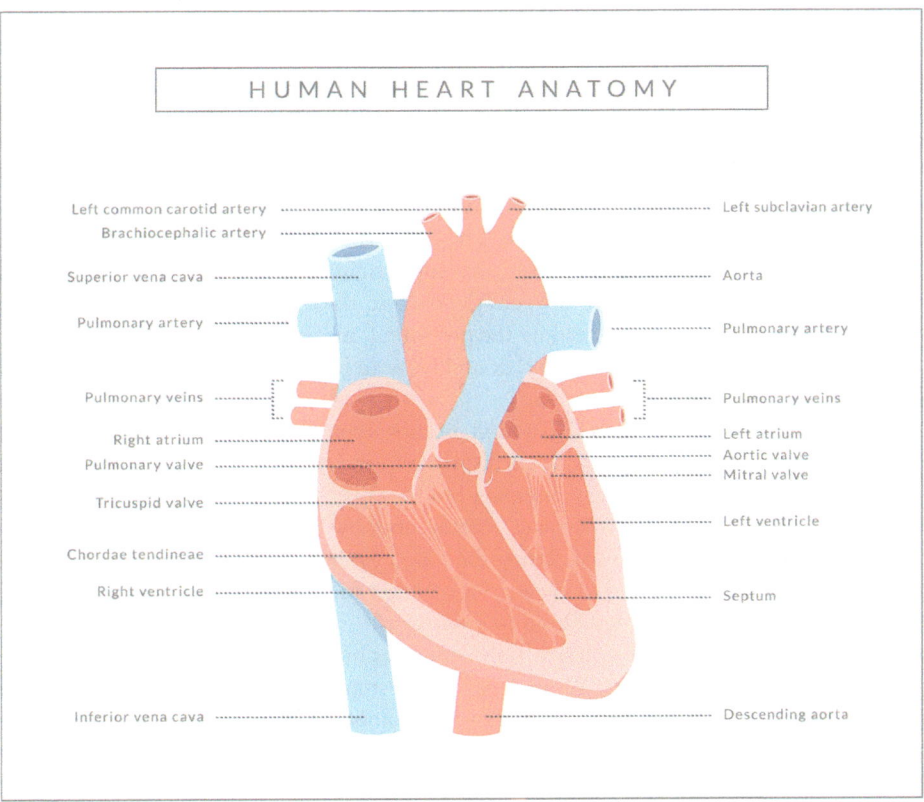

FIGURE 9.1 A drawing of the heart and its chambers identifies the arteries: left common, brachiocephalic pulmonary on the right side, and left subclavian, & pulmonary on the left. Veins include the pulmonary veins (left and right sides). The valves include the pulmonary and tricuspid valves (right side) and the aortic & mitral valves (left side), the right and left ventricle, the septum and descending aorta on the left.

Source: iStock © Henry Rivers.

2021). The blood, now with a fresh supply of oxygen, passes through the aorta to provide oxygen-rich blood to the organs.

One group of critical structures that connects the *arteries*, vessels carrying blood to other organs and *veins*, is the *capillaries*, small blood vessels with very thin walls. The capillaries' thin walls allow oxygen and other nutrients in the blood to pass through the walls to other parts of the body. In addition, capillaries allow waste products like carbon dioxide to pass through their walls into the blood to be carried to the lungs for removal.

Function

The four chambers, the arteries, and the veins are critical structures that facilitate blood flow. Yet as we mentioned earlier, the heart is a complex muscle, and the circulation process involves more than chambers, arteries, and veins. It requires a process to move the blood from one chamber to the next. One function that helps move the blood into the correct chambers is the heartbeat. Consider this: Blood is a liquid. When moving a liquid from one area to another, there is the risk of backward flow. A backward flow of blood would be dangerous to our circulatory system. Therefore, the heartbeat and a system of *inlet valves* that open and close help to direct the blood flow in and around the heart and to prevent backward flow. The heartbeat works with the valves to complete the movement.

You have heard the sound of a heartbeat many times, whether it was your own or someone else's. The sound that characterizes the heartbeat is "lub-DUB." What you may not know is that each part of the sound corresponds to a specific function of the heart. We take a moment to explain the process here because it is important when discussing hypertension, a form of cardiovascular disease, later in the chapter.

The *lub* sound of the heartbeat is produced when either the *tricuspid valve*, one of the inlet valves on the right side of the heart, opens to permits the blood to flow between the right atrium and ventricle, or the *mitral valve*, another type of inlet valve on the left side of the heart, opens to permit the blood to move between the left atrium and ventricle. Remember that on the right side of the heart, oxygen-poor blood is en route to the lungs to be resupplied with oxygen. On the left, the oxygenated blood is moving to other organs in the body. This process, represented by the *lub* sound, measures the *diastolic* blood pressure, or the pressure when the atria and the ventricles relax and fill with blood. It is sometimes referred to as the heart's resting or relaxation state.

The second part of the heartbeat, the *DUB* sound, occurs when the atria and ventricles contract to force the blood out. This process is called systole. It corresponds to the *systolic* measure of blood pressure and measures the heart's pressure when actively pumping blood. This occurs when the *pulmonary valves* on the right side of the heart open and the ventricles contract to move the blood from the right ventricle to the pulmonary arteries, assisting the process of getting the blood to the lungs for oxygenation. On the left side of the heart, the *aortic valves* open, and the ventricles contract to move the blood from the left ventricle to the *aorta*, once again sending oxygenated blood to the organs.

Thus, blood pressure, one measure of heart health, assesses both the heart's resting and working states as blood is moved to and from the heart. We will discuss the importance of blood pressure in the section on hypertension. For now, however, it is sufficient to note that blood pressure is reported using the systolic and diastolic pressure, the amount of pressure exerted when the heart is pumping blood (systolic) versus resting (diastolic).

Summary

In sum, the heart is a complex muscle and critical to the body's circulatory system. It provides oxygen and nutrients (transported by blood) to the body's organs. It also receives the "used" blood from the organs in order to resupply it with needed oxygen.

SECTION II. CARDIOVASCULAR DISEASE

As we mentioned in the beginning of the chapter, the term **cardiovascular disease** refers to a group of disorders of the heart (*cardio*) or the circulatory system. The name for our circulatory system, **vascular**, comes from the Latin word *vasculum*, meaning small vessels. In this case, the small vessels are the arteries, veins, and capillaries that transport blood throughout the body.

To put things in perspective, the prevalence of cardiovascular diseases (CVD) worldwide in 2021 rose to 621 million, an increase of 20 million from the prior year (Journal of the American College of Cardiology [JACC], 2024). Approximately 3% of these cases or 20.5 million resulted in deaths (JACC, 2024).

In general, cardiovascular disease refers to a number of diseases that damage the heart or its vessels as a result of **atherosclerosis**, a Greek word that means hardness (*sclerosis*) of gruel or paste (*athero*). When used in connection with cardiovascular disease, the term *atherosclerosis* describes a process by which deposits of fats, cholesterol, calcium, and other substances called plaque line the arteries (vessels) of our circulatory system and cause the normally flexible arteries to harden (Cleveland Clinic, 2024a; American Heart Association, 2013).

There are three key points to remember about cardiovascular disease. First, plaque narrows the passageway of arteries and reduces the volume of blood flowing to or from the heart. A reduction in blood flow can cause damage to the heart. Remember Tim Russert, from our opening story? In his case, plaque dislodged from an artery, blocked the flow of blood from one artery, and resulted in a heart attack and later death.

Second, a normal artery is flexible, allowing blood to flow easily through the vessel. When plaque forms in the arteries, it hardens the vessels, thereby reducing flexibility and causing another impediment to blood flow.

The final key point is particularly relevant for health psychologists. In the majority of cases, a buildup of plaque is caused by a diet high in fats and cholesterol and low in fiber. In other words, plaque buildup is preventable. And so are heart disease, heart attack, and death associated with atherosclerosis. Motivating individuals to adopt healthy eating habits is one way health psychologists can help prevent cardiovascular disease and possibly death. We review the important elements of a healthy diet in Section III of this chapter.

Although there are six principal types of cardiovascular disease, we will focus our attention on the four most directly linked to lifestyle choices: coronary artery disease, cardiac arrest, stroke, and hypertension.

Coronary Artery Disease (CAD)

Coronary artery disease (CAD), perhaps the most common type of cardiovascular disease, is the leading cause of heart attacks. We explained earlier that CAD is a condition in which the arteries that pump blood to and from the heart muscle become partially or completely obstructed. Less blood flowing through the arteries means less blood for the heart or other vital organs. The reduced volume of blood can damage heart tissues and produce a range of outcomes from chest pain and shortness of breath, often associated with **angina**, to heart attacks, also known as **myocardial infarction**.

We mentioned previously that CAD and atherosclerosis, the condition that causes CAD, are largely preventable. Yet cardiovascular disease is the leading cause of death internationally and in the U.S. (National Safety Council, 2024; World Health Organization, 2024c). How is it possible that a disease that is linked to lifestyles and is very preventable is the leading cause of death worldwide?

As we noted in Chapter 5, Risky Health Behaviors, knowledge of health-enhancing behaviors does not ensure that people will adopt the healthy behaviors. For example, many people know that poor diet, lack of exercise, smoking, and alcohol consumption increase the risks for cardiovascular disease. Such behaviors sometimes are referred to as **modifiable risk factors**. As the name implies, individuals can modify (increase or decrease) their risk of having a cardiovascular disease by changing behaviors: eating high-fiber and low-fat foods, exercising regularly (about 30 minutes a day), avoiding smoking, and limiting alcohol consumption.

It may be difficult to change eating behaviors when fast foods and "junk" foods are widely available, in some cases more available than healthy foods, and promoted as the foods of choice. Likewise, it might be a challenge to discourage excessive video gaming, a sedentary activity that passes for a recreational sport. As we noted when discussing health behavior change models in Chapter 3, Theories and Models of Health Behavior Change, environmental factors like social norms and cultures, in addition to individual differences and familial practices, can reinforce unhealthy diets and behaviors and serve as impediments to change.

It is also the case, however, that many individuals have insufficient knowledge of what constitutes good nutrition, healthy exercise regimes, or the damaging effects of stress on heart health. Clearly, access to information needed to make informed choices will increase an individual's knowledge of the risks of heart disease. But will it increase their likelihood of adopting healthy behaviors? What is important to note here is that many individuals overestimate their knowledge of nutrition and healthy eating behaviors – an error that can increase the incidences of unhealthy behaviors that can lead to heart disease. As for adoption, we will address that a little later. We explore in detail the effects of nutrition on heart health in Section III.

Cardiac Arrest

We first introduced cardiac arrests in Chapter 2, Research Methods. Briefly, a *cardiac arrest* is caused by *ventricular fibrillation*, an abnormal heart rhythm that occurs when the heart fails to pump blood to other organs (Arrogante, González-Romero, Carrión-García, & Polo, 2021; Ragin et al., 2005a). The heart's rhythm is determined in part by electrical impulses that begin with *sinus nodes*, a cluster of cells in the right atrium that serves as a pacemaker for the heart. The nodes send electrical currents through the heart, synchronizing the heart rate and pumping blood to other organs. When the signal is interrupted, the result is a sudden cardiac arrest.

In more than 80% of cases, cardiac arrest is accompanied by a prior history of CAD. The interruption of blood flow to the heart due to CAD can interfere with the heart's ability to send electrical impulses (Mayo Clinic, 2006). Plaque-clogged arteries are the most common cause of obstruction. As we have said numerous times before, plaque buildup is directly related to dietary habits, lack of exercise, smoking, excessive alcohol consumption, and even stress.

It is important to note that the term *cardiac arrest* is not a synonym for a heart attack. A cardiac arrest is a condition that renders a person unconscious and is fatal unless the heart is jolted back into its normal rhythm. Remember that the heart controls the body's circulatory system. When it fails, blood cannot be supplied to the other organs.

Cardiac arrests are not always fatal. If the heart can be restarted in time so that it may resume circulation of blood and oxygen to the body without damage to the brain or other organs, an individual's chances of survival are good. However, time is the key. Although many researchers suggest that a cardiac arrest victim can survive for 10 minutes without medical care, in truth, medical care providers note that after seven minutes without medical attention, a person will suffer irreparable brain damage due to a loss of oxygen to the brain. The chance of surviving a cardiac arrest after eight minutes is poor, an assessment that is supported by research (Cleveland Clinic, 2024d; Ibrahim, 2007).

Without a doubt you have seen, either on television, in movies, or in actual practice, at least one of two processes used to restart the heart of a cardiac arrest victim: *cardiopulmonary resuscitation (CPR)* or *automated external defibrillators (AEDs)*. CPR, most often used by emergency medical technicians and other trained persons, does two things. First, it stimulates the heart of the unconscious person to restart the body's vital circulation process. Second, it provides oxygen to the unconscious person to ensure that the lungs remain inflated, and oxygen can enter the blood. This procedure involves no equipment, just a trained person who knows how to perform what are called "heart massages" and to administer oxygen.

In comparison, automated external defibrillators (AEDs) are portable electrical devices with two pads that send an electric charge to the heart when placed on a person's chest. The charge is meant to mimic the electrical charge of the heart and to restart the circulation process. Studies have shown that AEDs are more effective and work more quickly than CPR in restoring the heart's normal rhythm (Holmberg, Vognsen, Andersen, Donnino, & Andersen, 2017; Ragin et al., 2005a).

It is important to repeat that although the precipitating factor (see Chapter 2, Research Methods) for a cardiac arrest is an interruption in the electrical impulses sent by the sinus nodes, the predisposing factor (again, see Chapter 2, Research Methods) is usually coronary artery disease, a condition that comes about as a result of lifestyle behaviors that increase the risks for heart disease.

Stroke

A third type of preventable cardiovascular disease is stroke, or *cerebrovascular disease*. Cerebrovascular diseases affect the vessels that carry blood and oxygen to the brain (*cerebro*). A stroke can be either an *ischemic stroke*, an interruption of blood flow to the brain, or a *hemorrhagic stroke*, here meaning a rupture of a blood vessel in the brain.

How are strokes related to other cardiovascular diseases that are caused by modifiable risk factors? By now, it is clear that most interruptions in blood and oxygen flow, whether to the heart or the brain, are due to plaque buildup in the vessels or, as in Tim Russert's case, dislodged plaque that impedes blood flow. In the case of an ischemic stroke, the same agent can cause a disruption of blood flow to the brain.

The role of modifiable risk factors may be clear for an ischemic stroke, but how do they apply to hemorrhagic stroke, when a blood vessel in the brain suddenly ruptures? The answer is that this happens indirectly. *Hypertension*, the excessive force of blood pumping through the blood vessels, can prompt a hemorrhagic stroke.

Hypertension

Hypertension, also called *high blood pressure (HBP)*, is a descriptive name that characterizes the effect of the illness on the heart. Hypertension means that the systolic pressure (see page 342), the amount of pressure exerted when the atria and ventricles are contracting to force blood out of the heart's chamber, and the diastolic pressure, the amount of pressure exerted when the atria and ventricles relax and fill with blood, are higher than normal, as defined by medical standards (see Table 9.1). Normal blood pressure

TABLE 9.1 Normal and Abnormal Blood Pressure Ranges

Category	Systolic	Diastolic
Optimal	<120	<80
Normal	120–129	80–84
High normal	130–139	85–89
Grade 1 hypertension (mild)	140–159	90–99
Grade 2 hypertension (moderate)	160–179	100–109
Grade 3 hypertension (severe)	>180	>110

is indicated by a systolic pressure of 120 or fewer millimeters of mercury, and a diastolic pressure of 80 millimeters or fewer of mercury. Mercury, contained in a column, is the substance used in the original blood pressure devices to measure diastolic and systolic pressure readings. The catch here is that the systolic and diastolic pressures cannot be too high. Too much pressure can damage the heart muscle.

VIDEO #46/60

Chapter 9: Cardiovascular Disease

- **Hypertension:** *Hypertension – Amy Erickson, DO | 60 Seconds to Good Health*
- **Website:** *https://www.youtube.com/watch?v=6ugMPYou3-g*
- **The WakeMed Health and Hospitals website is publicly accessible and serves as a valuable resource for health-related information** *(Home | WakeMed)*

It is important to point out that a hypertensive person will show signs of an enlarged heart. Enlarged hearts present new health problems because the heart is no longer able to work as efficiently as it did at a normal size. When the heart muscle is enlarged, it has reached its threshold of efficiency and cannot push blood through the chambers as efficiently as before. The increased pressure readings that signal hypertension indicate greater resistance by the heart when performing its normal functions.

A clue to the dangers of hypertension is its nickname: *the silent killer*. High blood pressure is almost always a disease that escapes detection. One reason is that the symptoms associated with high blood pressure are often nonspecific, meaning that the symptoms are so general that they could be associated with any number of illnesses. It is often the case that an individual with hypertension becomes aware of the problem only when a medical provider measures his or her blood pressure as part of an annual physical or sick visit or when previous exams have indicated a pattern of high blood pressure. If the latter, a collection of symptoms commonly associated with hypertension may occur, including painful headaches, heart palpitations, sudden and unexplained nosebleeds, and a general feeling of ill health. Untreated elevated blood pressure can cause severe damage to the heart, the kidneys, the brain, and the arteries. In the most severe cases, it can lead to sudden heart attack or death.

Hypertension can be assessed using a number of techniques. The most common test involves a *sphygmomanometer*, an instrument that consists of an inflatable rubber cuff and an air valve attached to a meter that measures heart pressure. Physicians use a *stethoscope* with this instrument to listen for the *lub-DUB* sound of the heartbeat to obtain the systolic and diastolic readings. Currently, many physicians use the newer electronic blood-pressure monitors that do not require the use of a stethoscope. Individuals can use modified home versions of blood pressure instruments to obtain a quick blood pressure reading more frequently.

ESSENTIAL AND SECONDARY HYPERTENSION The most common form of hypertension, called *essential* or *primary hypertension*, has no known or identifiable causes. Individuals with essential or primary hypertension have consistently high blood pressure over time, as determined through multiple blood pressure readings over months or years. More than 95% of current cases of hypertension worldwide are diagnosed as essential hypertension. For this reason, researchers believe that one contributing factor for essential hypertension may be genetics (Healthline, 2023). Other potential factors include generalized stress and stressful events occurring over time.

We will explain secondary hypertension more fully in the next section. Briefly, secondary hypertension is caused largely by health-inhibiting behaviors, such as consuming a high-fat, high-calorie diet, lack of exercise, and smoking.

SECTION III. PSYCHOSOCIAL FACTORS AND CARDIOVASCULAR DISEASE

Up to this point, we have identified several nonbiological factors that contribute to the development of cardiovascular disease, including poor diets, lack of exercise, and smoking. We also characterized these as modifiable risk factors because individuals can change their behaviors and, by doing so, modify or reduce their risk of heart disease.

Research shows, however, that there are other psychosocial factors that also contribute significantly to the development of heart disease. The research literature on the relationship of cardiovascular disease and psychosocial factors is too extensive to summarize in this chapter. Therefore, in this section, we highlight the principal findings on the effects of psychosocial factors on one type of heart disease: hypertension.

Stress

In Chapter 6, Emotional Health and Well-Being, and Chapter 7, Stress and Coping, we explained the role of stress on disease. Specifically, we noted that some psychological and biological illnesses are attributable to stress. One such illness is hypertension (Elsaid et al., 2021). Current research suggests that the association between stress and hypertension is strongest when the stressful event is persistent, meaning either repeated exposures, or that the effects of one particular event are long-lasting (Esler et al., 2008; Hassoun et al., 2015; Radi et al., 2005; Schutte et al., 2014; Spruill, 2010). For example, Radi and colleagues' (2005) study of job constraints in approximately 200 French workers revealed that job strain, which they define as a psychologically demanding environment with little ability to affect decisions or outcomes, was associated with high levels of hypertension, especially among women. They note that it is the prolonged effect of psychological stress with little ability to change the environment that increased hypertension rates in the female study participants.

More recent studies by Schutte and colleagues, which followed 107 Africans over five years, found that psychological distress and high scores on measures of nervousness, together best predicted hypertension after five years. And Trudel and colleagues (2019) found that long work hours among white-collar workers predicted masked hypertension – here meaning a blood pressure reading exceeding 135/85 mm Hg when measured on a continual basis over 24 hours. Look again at Table 9.1. Clearly this blood pressure level, which is borderline normal to high, suggests a potential problem.

On the other hand, an intriguing study by Dorn, Yzermans, Guiju, and Zee (2007) demonstrated the association between stress and hypertension from a single stressful event with long-lasting effects. In their study, parents of adolescents who were seriously injured in a large-scale fire experienced stress both at the time of the event and later as they coped with the medical and psychological consequences of the disaster for their children. Dorn and colleagues demonstrated that although only one stressful event occurred, one or both parents of adolescents reported ongoing hypertension due to the long-term effect of stress stemming from the accident. Thus, results from studies like Schutte and colleagues (2014), Trudel and colleagues (2019), and Dorn and colleagues (2007) show that stress experienced over time in response to recurring stress-inducing situations, and the stress experienced as a result of a one-time event, can both lead to hypertension.

Ethnicity

It is the case, however, that some illnesses occur with higher frequency in specific populations. For example, hypertension is prevalent among African Americans. In fact, in 16 studies comparing hypertension rates of African Americans and whites, the majority found significantly higher hypertension rates among African Americans (Kurian & Cardarelli, 2007).

Do significantly higher rates of hypertension among African Americans suggest a genetic predisposition (see Chapter 2, Research Methods) to the disease? Apparently they do not. Although a number of studies have investigated possible genetic links, none has successfully identified specific genes that would explain this difference (Maraboto & Ferdinand, 2020). What these and similar studies show is that, for many African Americans, common cultural behaviors such as preferred foods, individual factors such as weight, and environmental stressors contribute significantly to hypertension. Specifically, findings from a 2018 longitudinal study by Howard, Cushman, Moy, Oparil, Muntner, Lacklandet, et al., which compared non-hypertensive African American and white participants at baseline and again approximately 9.5 years later, found a significant increase in hypertension at follow-up for African Americans versus whites.

What contributed to this difference? Howard and colleagues concluded that there were, in fact, racial differences between African American and white hypertension levels, but this difference could be explained by three factors: the consumption of a Southern diet, higher sodium intake, and lower education levels. This was true for both men and women across racial groups. For women, two additional factors – waist circumference and BMI – also explained the higher blood pressures for African American versus white women after approximately nine years (Howard et al., 2018).

Several of the factors that contribute to higher rates of hypertension for African Americans are related. Consider this: Foods such as baked macaroni and cheese, candied yams, and collard greens seasoned with pork are part of the cultural cuisine for many African Americans. Such foods have a high fat and cholesterol content. You may remember that fats and cholesterol are two substances that contribute to the buildup of plaque in the arteries, a precursor for many types of cardiovascular diseases, including hypertension. The important point here is that it is not ethnicity, per se, that increases a group's risk for hypertension or other heart diseases but the behaviors or the traditions, including culinary delights, associated with specific ethnic groups that put them at higher risk. It is worth noting, however, that such diets also tend to increase weight levels. Hence, a cultural practice can put African Americans at higher risk directly through the food consumed and indirectly through weight gain associated with diet.

When behavioral factors cause hypertension, we refer to the disease as ***secondary hypertension***, suggesting that the illness is the result of other primary behaviors – in this case, high-risk dietary habits that predispose individuals to hypertension.

Perceived Racism

Researchers have been exploring the effects of ***perceived racism***, an environmental factor, on hypertension in several populations, for example among afro descendants in Brazil and African Americans in the U.S. (Faerstein, Chor, Loureiro Werneck, de Souza Lopes, & Kaplan, 2014; Forde, Lewis, Kershaw, Bellamy, & Diez Roux, 2021; Mendes et al., 2018). The term *perceived racism* refers to the belief that another person's actions or words are intended as prejudicial, discriminatory, or demeaning toward people of a specific race or ethnicity. It qualifies as a persistent and stressful factor for the recipients because minority groups are likely to experience racism as both single and repeated occurrences.

Early research by James, LaCroix, Kleinbaum, and Strogatz (1984) examined the reports of perceived racism, job success, and blood pressure among African American men. Although they found no direct association between blood pressure and perceived racism, they reported an interactive effect among racism, coping, and blood pressure. Specifically, James and colleagues noted that men with greater success in their jobs who reported perceived racism at work and who used persistent coping strategies to address the racism in the environment were significantly more likely to have higher diastolic (or resting state) blood pressure than were men who reported no perceived workplace racism.

Contrast this with the outcomes from studies such as Forde et al. (2021). Using a large, multi-ethnic cohort, including African Americans, Chinese, Hispanics and whites, they examined the effects of lifetime perceived discrimination on hypertension over 18 years. As in a previous study by Howard et al. (2014), all participants were non-hypertensive at the beginning of the study. At the final follow-up, Forde and colleagues found that African American participants who reported any lifetime discrimination were more likely to present with hypertension than those who reported no discrimination. This, then, would suggest that there is a direct association between lifetime discrimination and hypertension. Sims, Sims, Glover, Smit, and Odden (2020) go further, suggesting that it is not just lifetime discrimination but even everyday discrimination that contributes to hypertension through cardiovascular reactivity. For example, Lepore and colleagues' (2006) study of cardiovascular reactivity in African American versus white women compared differences in blood pressure and heart rate after no stimulus, after a nonracial or neutral stimulus (a talk about a college tour), and after a perceived racial stimulus (discussion of differential treatment while shopping; a number of African American women would suggest that differential treatment while shopping is a frequent occurrence). The no-stimulus condition was the baseline, the college talks provided the reactivity measure, and the differential treatment condition represented the experimental condition yielding a recovery measure. Lepore and colleagues found that the resting state measures of heart rate and blood pressure for African American women after the perceived racism condition were significantly higher than those of the white female participants in the study.

It is important to note that findings from earlier studies that examine the specific impact of perceived racism on blood pressure appear to yield mixed results (Williams & Neighbors, 2001). For example, in one laboratory-based study, African American participants were exposed to racial stimuli in one of four conditions: videos, films, speech or debate tasks, or harassment from a white experimenter. African American participants showed increased systolic and diastolic blood pressures rates shortly after all tasks (Guyll, Matthews, & Bromberger, 2001). But in other similar studies, no notable changes were associated with perceived racism (Bowen-Reid & Harrell, 2002; Clark, 2006).

One problem with a number of the studies on racism and blood pressure is the difficulty in measuring precisely an individual's reaction to a perceived racial event. This may be one reason why studies such as those by Forde and colleagues assess lifetime perceived racism/discrimination rather than event-specific responses. Still, studies that examine *cardiovascular reactivity (CVR)*, or the body's return to a baseline blood pressure and heart rate at the conclusion of a stressful event, appear to offer reliable measures of the impact of perceived racism on physiological health.

Let's take a moment to put these studies into perspective. We noted in Chapter 7, Stress and Coping, that the body contains systems that help it return to its normal or resting state after stressors. This is true for the heart. After exposures to stress, the heart must be able to return to a normal resting state. A higher than normal diastolic or resting state causes continued stress to the heart and can increase the risk of damage to the heart. Notwithstanding the mixed findings on the association between racism and elevated blood pressure, research suggests that cardiovascular reactivity (CVR) is perhaps a better measure for assessing the effects of racism on blood pressure (Sims et al., 2020). And the studies that suggest that cardiovascular recovery rates remain elevated after a stressful event has ended do seem to suggest that perceived discrimination can lead to early onset and long-term hypertension, particularly for African Americans and afro descendants (Sims et al., 2020).

Personality

Steca et al. (2016) introduced yet another psychological factor thought to be associated with heart disease: type A personality. We first identified the proposed impact of type A personality on stress and illness in Chapter 7, Stress and Coping. Recall that we noted that people with type A personality are described as individuals who are aggressive, ambitious, and impatient and who easily and frequently become angry or hostile (Watson, Minzenmayer, & Bobler, 2006).

Although early research supported the association between type A behaviors and heart disease (Allan & Scheidt, 1992), later research refined the association, showing that it is actually the personality characteristics of anger and cynicism, not personality type, that together predicted a higher risk of cardiovascular disease (Denollet et al., 2006; Kupper & Denollet, 2007). Researchers suggest the expression of anger causes a physiological reaction that increases cardiovascular risks. For example, Williams and colleagues (2000) found that anger can disrupt and dislodge atherosclerosis plaque that can build up in the linings of the arteries. In other words, expressed anger can be considered an acute risk factor that can trigger heart disease.

Summary

The research on hypertension suggests that a number of factors contribute to high blood pressure. Some of the causes are unknown to us and result in essential or primary hypertension. Other factors such as diet, exercise, and smoking are clearly associated with and lead to secondary hypertension (Erdine & Ari, 2006; Sparrenberger et al., 2008). Finally, research indicates that environmental stimuli can also trigger hypertension. This appears to be true whether the trigger is a job-related stressor or perceived racism.

SECTION IV. CARDIOVASCULAR DISEASE AND HEALTH DETERMINANTS

Most researchers agree that there are six principal risk factors for cardiovascular disease: excessive alcohol consumption, tobacco, high blood cholesterol levels due to diet, physical inactivity, overweight/obesity, and diabetes. These factors are often referred to as *moderating risk factors* because, when controlled, they can lessen the risk of contracting cardiovascular disease. We will explore some of these factors in the current section.

In addition, however, other factors – factors that we referred to as health determinants in previous chapters – are often associated with heart disease. They include gender, age, environment, and health systems. In this section, we explore the relative importance of each of these factors when compared with lifestyles. Finally, we will explain in greater detail why race/ethnicity itself is not a risk factor for heart disease and explore the role of health care systems on health outcomes.

Individual Determinants

EATING BEHAVIORS AND NUTRITION   A number of research studies indicate that people may have, at best, a minimal understanding of healthy foods or daily nutritional requirements. This lack of knowledge adversely affects food choices. As Farahmand, Tehrani, Amiri, and Aziz (2012) found, many participants in their study on barriers to healthy nutrition made incorrect food choices based on this lack of knowledge. For example, the women in this study incorrectly assumed that saturated oils were healthier than unsaturated oils (more on that in a moment) and that fried foods were healthy. And while a survey of European consumers showed that individuals do understand what is meant by "healthy nutrition," many consumers are confused by the nutritional recommendations (de Ridder, Kroese, Evers, Adriaanse, & Gillebaart, 2017).

Incomprehensible information labels on prepared and processed foods contribute to this confusion, and can be meaningless, even for individuals with greater-than-average knowledge of nutrition (Fitzgerald, Donovan, Kees, & Kozup, 2019). The capacity for a person to understand the product's contents and to exercise judgment over whether to purchase an item is often compromised by the way in which ingredients are described. In essence, even the most informed consumer may be no match for unintelligible food labels on products (Worosz & Wilson, 2012).

In truth, there are a number of factors that influence a consumer's purchase decisions. The extensive literature on the effects of nutritional labeling identifies a number of individual factors including, literacy levels, motivation, and knowledge, as well as marketing variables, like label design and layout, amount of information, and the inclusion of specific information – such as recommended daily allowance – versus general information, such as "low fat" (Heike & Taylor, 2012; Kemp, Burton, Creyer, & Suter, 2007; Temple & Fraser, 2014). These factors, individually or in combination, often lead consumers to misinterpret information on the food labels. For example, studies suggest that consumers often misunderstand information about trans fats. This may be due in part to confusion about the role of saturated versus unsaturated fats in one's diet, as suggested by Farahmand and colleagues' study (2012), or vague claims of "low fat" as a part of product marketing. A recent study in Brazil by Morais and colleagues (2020), which evaluated consumers' knowledge about nutritional terms often included on package labels, such as "contains gluten," "trans fat free," or "light food," found that consumers knowledge scores were, at best, average, even for those reporting to regularly use nutritional information when purchasing products. Perhaps most surprising was the finding that older consumers' knowledge scores were lower than younger consumers (Morais et al., 2020).

Fortunately, health providers, health policy experts, government, and international agencies have worked aggressively to address this issue. As a result, there have been a number of changes in law and health policy aimed at providing consumers with better nutritional information on food products. Countries including Brazil, Chile, many European countries, Jordan, Mexico, the U.K., and the U.S. (Morais et al., 2020) have introduced *"front-of-package (FOP)" notifications* to "nudge" (see Chapter 5, Risky Health Behaviors, Part II) consumers into making healthier choices.

There are several different forms of FOP. Some include information on specific ingredients, such as saturated fats or sodium. Others place warning labels on foods with very high sodium or fat content, or use a traffic light logo, a universally understood logo, to indicate a product's nutritional content (Temple, 2020). Does the traffic light concept sound familiar? Remember that in Chapter 3, Theories and Models of Health Behavior Change, we mentioned that Kelly and colleagues (1991) used a traffic light logo to inform gay men how to minimize the risk of contracting HIV through sexual activity. Here we see an application of the same logo, but for an entirely different health objective.

The addition of FOP labeling and other "nudges" does not mean, however, that all is resolved. As researchers have noted, manufacturers often have found workarounds using alternative terms for ingredients that disguise the true nature of the ingredients included in products (de Barros et al., 2022). As such, there is still a vital role for health psychologists, particularly in the area of knowledge.

For years, nutritionists and health practitioners used a "food pyramid" to instruct people on the components of a healthy diet. The pyramid was intended, in part, to guide an individual's food choices. For example, the pyramid identified foods that should be consumed in smaller quantities than others due to their high fat and cholesterol content. Yet the pyramids were confusing. For example, an early version of the guidelines indicated that individuals need three to five servings of vegetables a day. Many people had no idea what was meant by a "serving." How much was in a serving? If you have a meal consisting entirely of vegetables, is that one serving or multiple servings?

The revised food pyramid provided clearer guidelines on appropriate and healthy food quantities and food choices. It avoided ambiguity by explaining the quantity of food to be consumed each day using measures that are understood by the average person. For example, it explained that individuals needed 2.5 cups of vegetables per day. A cup of food is more readily understood than a "serving." Clearer, less confusing guidelines increase the probability that individuals understand the information and will use it correctly. In addition, the pyramid explained clearly the types of "good" versus "bad" fats and the role of exercise in preventing weight gain. In essence, the revised pyramid presents a more user-friendly guide to nutrition.

In the U.S., to make this information even more accessible, the U.S. Department of Agriculture issued the "Food Plate," a graphic that apportions the plate with the percentage of proteins, grains, fruits, and vegetables needed for a healthy diet (see Figure 9.2). The message is simple and easily understood from the graphic: Half of our intake at each meal should be fruits and vegetables. Even with this user-friendly graphic, the Food Plate is still an abbreviated guide to nutrition. For this reason, we add a few more details about nutrition here to complete the picture.

Five Food Elements The pyramid categorizes foods into five groups: meats and beans, grains, dairy products, fruits, and vegetables. These are commonly referred to as the *five food groups*. However, these foods can also be explained by their elements, another factor to guide the quantity of each type of food needed to maintain our health. There are a total of five elements: proteins, carbohydrates, fats, vitamins, and minerals. We add to these elements a sixth component: water, an essential ingredient for health.

Proteins *Proteins* are chemical compounds that form the basis of all living organisms. They are essential because proteins help to repair damaged body tissues and to promote new tissue growth. Protein is found in animal products, beans, peas, and some grains. Thus, proteins are contained in the "meat and beans" food group as well as in some of the grains in the "grain" food group. Protein supplies approximately 10%–15% of our energy source. If consumed in excess of the body's needs, however, protein will be stored in the body as fat. Therefore, although protein is needed, it is not needed in large supply.

Carbohydrates *Carbohydrates* are often thought of as one of the "villains" of any diet. Why? Carbohydrates include starches and sugars and are found in foods such as breads, pastas, potatoes, and cereals, among others. The main component of carbohydrates is a sugar molecule; when consumed in excess, carbohydrates are taken in as sugar and stored in the body as fat, an ingredient that is needed only in small quantities. This partly explains why carbohydrates are thought of as villains. Foods high in sugars and starches are so tasty that they are often consumed in excess of the body's needs. This almost ensures added storage of fat in the system.

Current research suggests, however, that not all carbohydrates are bad. In fact, foods such as whole grains, cereals and breads, brown rice (instead of potatoes), whole wheat pasta, and especially beans are good sources of carbohydrates (Harvard T. H. Chan School of Public Health, 2024). Recent studies even suggest that low levels of carbohydrates, especially the "good" carbohydrates, can be helpful and more effective for long-term weight loss than carbohydrate-free diets (Harvard T. H. Chan School of Public Health, 2024). Relevant to our discussion on cardiovascular disease, an earlier study of women's eating habits over 20 years reported than women who consumed a low-carbohydrate, high–vegetable fat diet had a 30% lower risk of heart disease than women who reported a high-carbohydrate, low-fat diet (Hulton, Willett, & Liu, 2006). And a meta-analysis of 12 studies shows that persons maintaining a low-carbohydrate diet for between 12 and 23 months reported lower cardiovascular risks (i.e., lower systolic

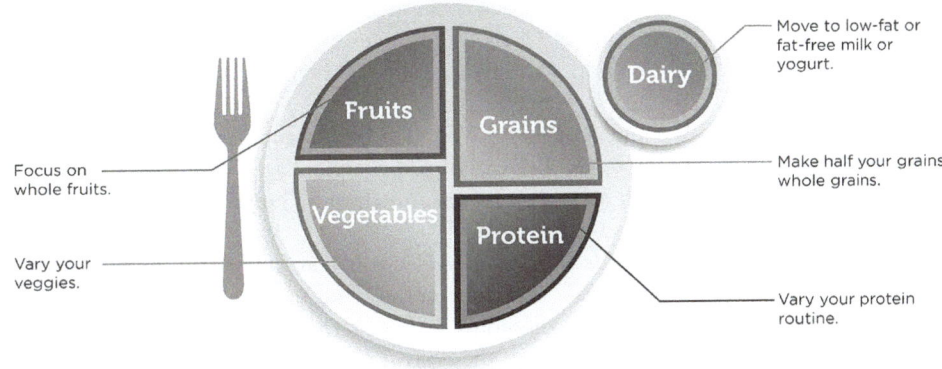

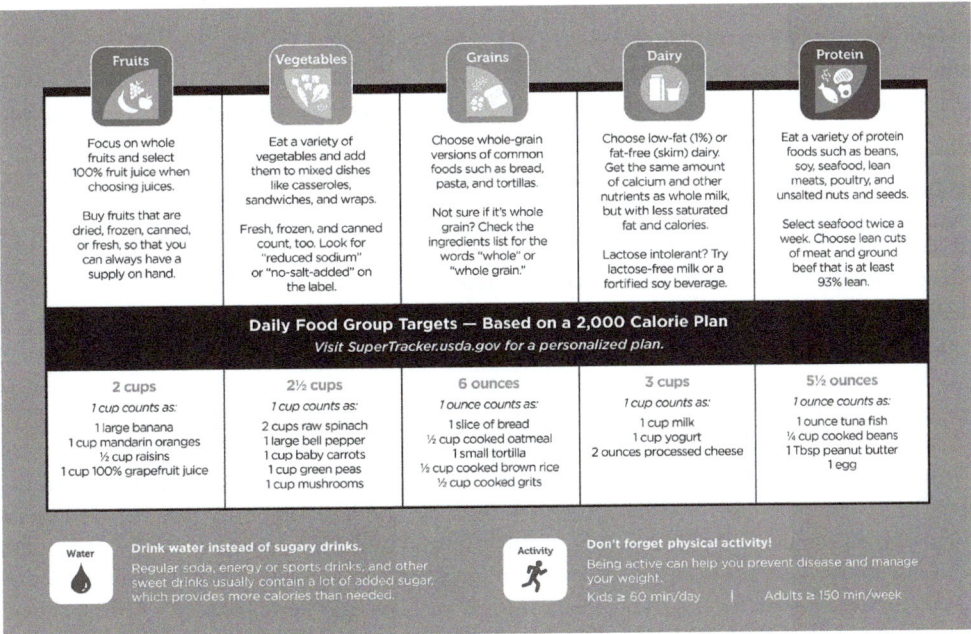

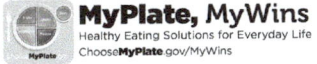

FIGURE 9.2 The new Food Plate. My Plate replaces the old Food Pyramid as a more user-friendly guide for creating nutritious meals. The My Plate figure contains two parts. A round plate is divided to in quarters to estimate fraction of the plate that each of the four types of food should occupy, accompanied by a chart specifying the approximate measurements for each. One quarter of the plate is allocated for each of the following: fruits, (2 cups) vegetables (2.5 cups), protein (5.5 ounces) & grains (6 ounces). An addition smaller plate is for dairy (3 cups).

and diastolic blood pressure and cholesterol, among other factors), than those whose diets lasted less than six months (Dong, Guo, Zhang, Sun, & Chen, 2020). In essence, we do not need large quantities of carbohydrates; however, low levels of good carbohydrates, in combination with other healthy elements, can help protect our heart health.

Other "villains" in diets are *fats* and *cholesterol*. Found in both plants and animals, fats provide energy and also aid the body in repair. But here, as with carbohydrates, there are "bad" fats, which include *saturated fats*, and "good" fats, which include *monounsaturated* and *polyunsaturated fats*. Each of these elements has a direct impact on cardiovascular diseases.

Saturated fats include *trans-fatty acids* (sometimes called trans fats). These facts are a problem for health and hence are thought of as "bad" fats because they tend to raise the levels of *low-density lipoproteins (LDL)* in the system. LDLs are commonly referred to as *artery-clogging cholesterol agents*. They carry cholesterol from the liver to the rest of the body. Excessive amounts of LDL in the system will adhere to the arteries, lining the walls of the arteries with cholesterol. Remember plaque? The substance that clogs the arteries is made from fats and cholesterols, specifically the LDL cholesterol found in trans-fatty acids and saturated fats.

VIDEO #47/60

Chapter 9: Cardiovascular Disease

- **Cholesterol:** *Mayo Clinic Minute: The role of cholestero in heart health*
- *Website: https://www.youtube.com/watch?v=Ih_4BHoZvOU*
- *Mayo Clinic is publicly accessible since it provides medical-based information to the public at no cost (www.mayoclinic.org/)*

VIDEO #48/60

Chapter 9: Cardiovascular Disease

- **Saturated Fats:** *Mayo Clinic Minute: What is a cardiac stress test?*
- *Website: https://www.youtube.com/watch?v=NC4hNOmTRsY*
- *Mayo Clinic is publicly accessible since it provides medical-based information to the public at no cost (www.mayoclinic.org/)*

The problem with trans-fatty acids can be seen more clearly in the following concrete examples: A 2% increase in trans-fatty acids per year – approximately one medium order of fast-food French fries each day for one year – will increase the risk of coronary artery disease by 23%. Furthermore, an analysis of up to six studies examining the impact of trans-fatty acids on 13,000–230,000 participants revealed that trans-fatty acid intake was associated with coronary heart disease deaths (de Souza et al., 2015). On a more positive note, a study in Australia suggest that elimination of trans-fatty acids could result in approximately 2,300 fewer deaths due to ischemic heart disease (Marklund, Zheng, Veerman, & Wu, 2020). These research findings led New York City, Boston, and other cities in the U.S. to require restaurants to eliminate trans fats from all foods.

We indicated that there are, in fact, good fats. These include the monounsaturated fats, which include oils from peanuts, olives, canola oil, and polyunsaturated fats, such as the oils found in sunflowers, corn, and walnuts, and the omega-3 oils found in fish and plants. Monounsaturated and polyunsaturated fats help to decrease the LDL levels in the blood and to increase the level of *high-density lipoproteins (HDLs)*.

The nickname for HDL is the *good cholesterol* or the *garbage truck of the blood system*. Like mono- and polyunsaturated fats, HDL helps to clean the cholesterol from the blood and the walls of arteries, sending them to the liver for disposal.

Fruits and Vegetables The last two elements of the food group, **vitamins** and **minerals**, are contained in vegetables and fruits. Fruits and vegetables are a natural source of vitamins that convert food into energy. Lettuce, spinach, and cruciferous vegetables such as broccoli, cauliflower, bok choy, and cabbage supply vitamin A, C, and E, and minerals such as calcium, sodium, and zinc.

Just how essential are vitamins and minerals to healthy outcomes? Consider this: Studies suggest that individuals who consume at least two and a half to five cups of fruits and vegetables daily are at lower risk for heart disease. Furthermore, a study involving over 30,000 women in the U.K. between 35 and 69 years of age, who were followed for over approximately 17 years, found that eating the equivalent of 80 grams (or just over half a cup) per day of fruits resulted in a 6%–7% risk reduction of deaths due to cardiovascular disease or coronary heart disease (Lai et al., 2015). Therefore, although the expression "an apple a day keeps the doctor away" may not literally be correct, it captures the essence of the beneficial role of fruits and vegetables as necessary to improve health outcomes.

Longitudinal Effects of Eating Behaviors on Health Studies have demonstrated the long-term effects of poor diet and physical inactivity on cardiovascular disease. In particular, two classic studies involving military personnel illustrate the relationship between poor dietary choices and atherosclerosis, even among children.

There is a general assumption that men and women serving in armed forces are at low risk for CAD because of the intense exercise regimen in the military and the need to be physically fit for combat. However, early research by Enos, Holmes, and Beyer (1953) and a later study by McNamara, Molot, Stremple, and Cutting (1971) suggest that even the intense physical training in the military may not counteract the effects of soldiers' poor diet and lack of exercise during their childhood and adolescence.

Enos and colleagues' (1953) study of 300 American soldiers injured during the Korean War revealed a surprisingly high frequency of CAD or atherosclerosis among active military personnel at the time of their injury. They found that of the 300 soldiers surveyed (their average age was 22.1 years), more than 77% had evidence of atherosclerosis and 65% showed signs of plaque buildup, an unexpected outcome given the rigorous physical training in preparation for combat. In a related study of heart disease in the military, McNamara and colleagues (1971) found that 45% of American soldiers in their sample, who had fought in Vietnam, similarly showed signs of atherosclerosis. Although this was a somewhat smaller percentage than that obtained in Enos and colleagues' study, McNamara and colleagues' results confirmed that the risk for heart disease among active military may be higher than expected.

The studies hold several implications for the average citizen as well. First, studies seem to suggest that CAD and atherosclerosis begin forming early in an individual's life. As illustrated by these studies, the high risk of CAD for some military personnel is due to the distal factors of poor diet and lack of sufficient exercise earlier in life. Furthermore, the high rates of atherosclerosis and CAD found in soldiers, due presumably to eating behaviors as children and adolescents, are supported by similar outcomes in studies on nonmilitary study participants (Bashir et al., 2020). Collectively, the studies suggest that nutritional programs, specifically those designed to help maintain healthy heart functions, should include children and adolescents as primary target audiences. Although such programs may benefit adults, introducing such programs to children may help avoid the plaque buildup that creates the conditions for coronary artery disease later in life.

A second and somewhat troubling point of the military studies is that, for individuals with a predisposition to CAD based on lifestyle behaviors, vigorous physical activity without medical supervision and monitoring may be harmful (McGraw, Turner, Stotts, & Dracup, 2008). Indeed, in a study of deaths in the military between 1996 and 1999, 39% of exercise-related deaths were attributed to CAD (Gutmann, Gardner, Potter, & Kark, 2002; McGraw et al., 2008). With the exception of athletes, few people engage in the type of regular and strenuous exercise performed by soldiers. Yet even civilians may unknowingly embark on an exercise regimen that is too strenuous for their preexisting yet undiagnosed heart condition.

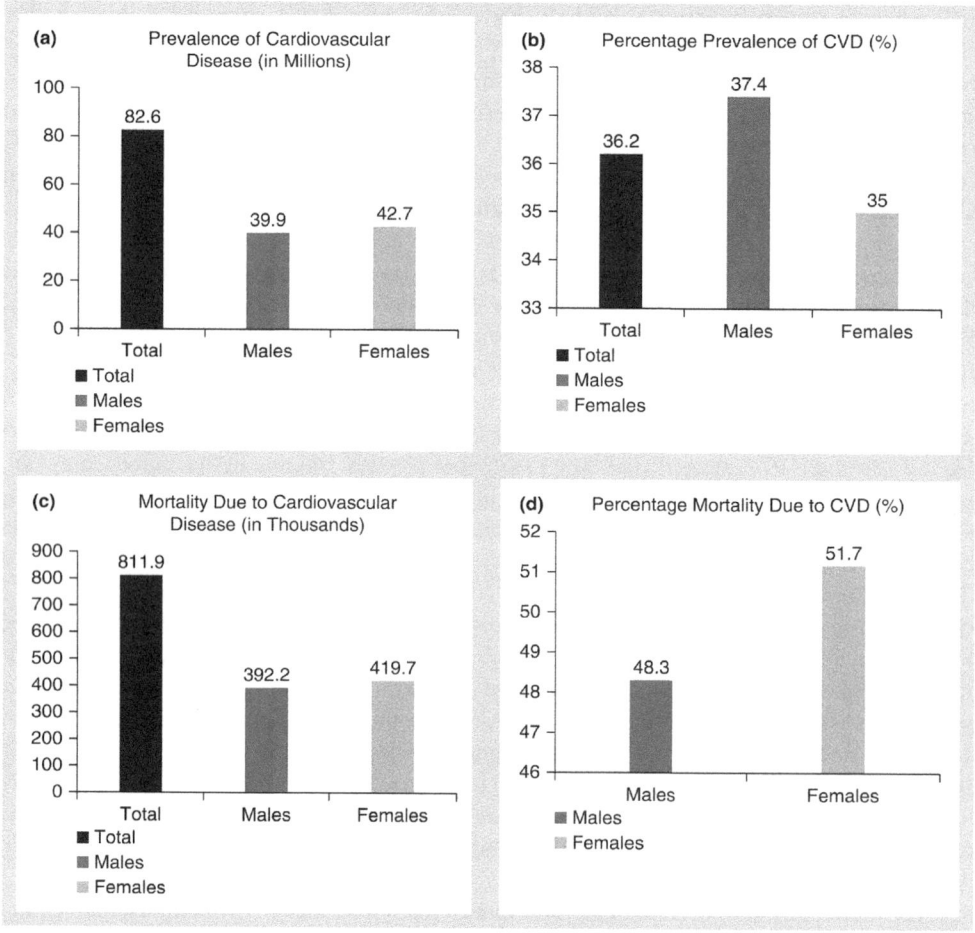

FIGURE 9.3 Actual prevalence of cardiovascular disease by gender. Two bar charts compare the prevalence of cardiovascular disease for men versus women in raw data and percentages, and two bar charts compare the mortality due to cardiovascular disease also in raw numbers and percentages. Raw numbers show women have higher total prevalence than men of cardiovascular disease (42.7 per 100,000 vs. 39.9 per 100,000) but lower percentage (35 vs. 37.4%) whereas women have higher mortality (419.7 per 100,000 vs. 392.2 per 100,000) and a higher percentage (51.7 vs. 48.3%) of mortality.

Source: Based on Roger et al. (2012).

Most researchers would support a program of exercise and diet for individuals at risk for CAD. The key is moderate exercise with supervision to prevent undue stress to the heart. In addition, a physical exam to evaluate a person's ability to engage in rigorous exercise is certainly recommended. Consider this: Routine physicals are usually required for soldiers and even for adolescents who wish to participate in extracurricular sports in their high school or college. However, these findings might suggest that a more thorough exam may be required if atherosclerosis cannot be detected through the routine physicals.

GENDER Which gender is at higher risk for cardiovascular disease? If you guessed men, your answer would be consistent with the outcomes from early research that showed higher rates of cardiovascular disease for men than women (Gillum et al., 1983; Yu, Wong, Lloyd, & Wong, 1995). In fact, during the 1960s and 1970s, the prevailing wisdom was that men were at higher risk for CVD. The findings were so overwhelming that researchers and practitioners focused on developing strategies that significantly decrease the mortality (death) rates of cardiovascular disease for men (Lee & Foody, 2008) and targeted them as study participants. At the same time, women's risk for CVD was not systematically explored. We now know from data obtained through the Framingham Heart Health Study (see Chapter 2, Research Methods) that females have higher prevalence rates than males for most cardiovascular diseases (Rethemiotaki, 2023) and the relative risk of cardiovascular disease morbidity and mortality for women exceeds that for men (Appelman, van Rijn, ten Haaf, Boersma, & Peters, 2015; Möller-Leimkühler, 2007). What is more, current research suggests that there are sex-specific conditions that increase women's cardiovascular risks, including pregnancy-related disorders, premature menopause, and polycystic ovary syndrome – here meaning a hormonal problem in women that may cause irregular or missed periods, among other symptoms (DeFilippis & Van Spall, 2021).

Do you wonder why researchers missed this distinction? One reason for the error is that women either were not regularly included as study participants or were not included in large enough numbers as participants in studies that examined the likelihood of developing CAD. As we learned in Chapter 2, Research Methods, investigators need a representative sample to generalize their findings to the larger population. Due to the overrepresentation of men in earlier studies, the research accurately captured the incidences of heart disease among men but significantly underestimated the incidences of heart disease among women.

Box 9.1 The Red Dress Campaign: Raising Awareness of Heart Disease among Women

The Heart Truth is a national awareness campaign for women about heart disease sponsored by the National Heart, Lung, and Blood Institute (NHLBI), part of the National Institutes of Health. The campaign created and introduced the Red Dress as the national symbol for awareness of heart disease in women in 2002. Seeking to advance the Red Dress symbol, *The Heart Truth* forged a groundbreaking collaboration between the federal government and the fashion industry, an industry intrinsically tied to female audiences (see Figure 9.4).

The purpose of *The Heart Truth* campaign is to give women a personal and urgent wake-up call about their risk of heart disease. The campaign is especially aimed at women ages 40–60, the age when a woman's risk of heart disease starts to rise. But its messages are also important for younger women, because heart disease develops gradually and can start at a young age – even in the teenage years.

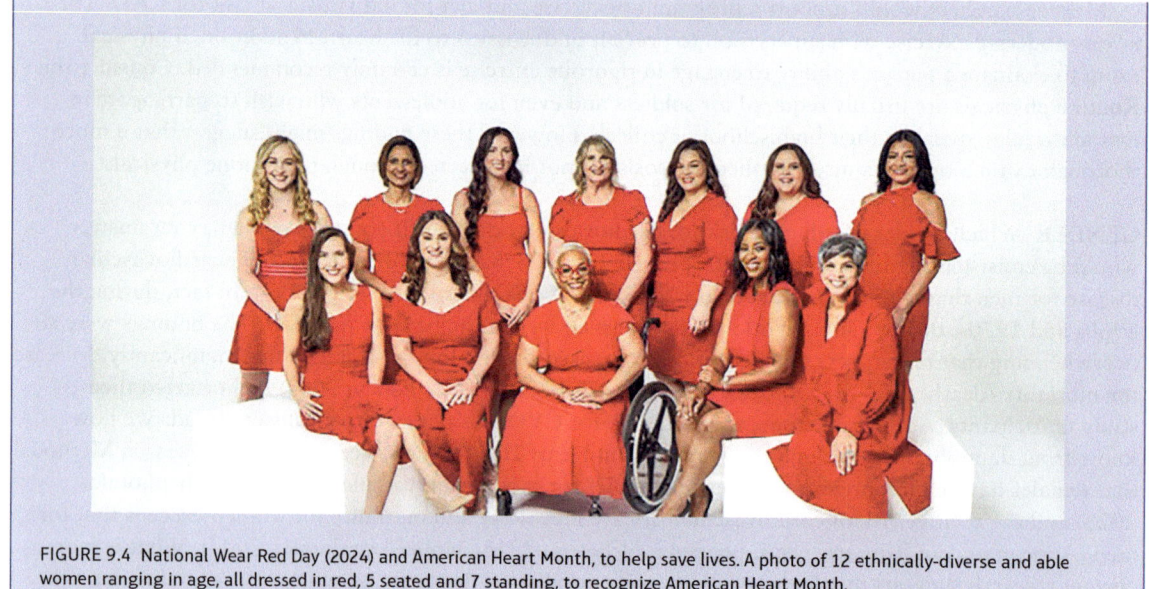

FIGURE 9.4 National Wear Red Day (2024) and American Heart Month, to help save lives. A photo of 12 ethnically-diverse and able women ranging in age, all dressed in red, 5 seated and 7 standing, to recognize American Heart Month.

Source: American Heart Association, Go Red for Women Wear Red and Give | Go Red for Women.

An additional factor that reinforced the mistaken belief that women were less susceptible to heart disease than men was the common belief in many industrialized countries that women did not experience as much stress, especially job-related stress, as men. Here, *job related* refers to paid employment outside of the home. Admittedly, this is a difficult concept to grasp today because changes in employment opportunities for women have, in fact, placed them in a greater variety of paid positions in the workplace. For example, it is not uncommon to see many women employed in managerial and senior management positions that entail high stress, such as chief executive officers of major corporations. Today we even see more women appointed or elected to judicial and political offices, including those as prime ministers and presidents of countries. (We will hold aside for the moment any discussion of the stress related to childrearing and managing a household. Research studies on the stress related to those tasks are far fewer in number.) Not surprisingly, the new studies of cardiovascular disease show that women, too, are at high risk for heart disease in part as a function of more women in demanding and responsible positions in the workforce.

Finally, the symptoms associated with heart disease differ by gender. We explain these differences more fully in the next section. For the moment, it is sufficient to note that differences in symptomology often caused physicians to overlook early signs of heart disease among women. Now that we know that women, too, are susceptible to heart disease and that their susceptibility is comparable to that of men, researchers regularly assess incidences of heart disease and differences in rates of disease in both genders. One surprising results of current studies is that cardiovascular disease is the leading killer of women both in the U.S. and globally (Vogel et al., 2021).

Women and Age We just noted a lower prevalence of CVD for women versus men. But studies confirm that there is an age effect of CVD. On average, heart disease in women first appears at a later point in life than men. Men, on average, report the first signs of cardiovascular health problems in their 40s. The same is not true for women. Only after age 60 do we see rates of heart disease for women that are comparable to or exceed those seen in men (Benjamin et al., 2019). The data on prevalence rates of CVD for males versus females in the U.S. support some of these findings. Table 9.2 compares the prevalence rates for CVD by both gender and age for 2007 and 2016, and shows that in the U.S., men, ages 20–39, reported higher CVD prevalence rates than women in 2007. But that year, women, beginning with ages 40–59 and above, reported higher prevalence rates than men. Similarly, in 2016, women's prevalence rates for CVD exceeded that for men's in the 60–79 and 80+ age cohorts (Benjamin et al., 2019).

One reason for the higher incidences of heart disease in women after age 50 appears to be physiological. Until age 45, women's bodies produce high levels of *estrogen*, a vital hormone for reproduction. Research suggests that estrogen plays two essential roles in women's health. It is crucial for reproduction, but it is also a protective factor that helps minimize the risk of cardiovascular disease for women who are *premenopausal*, that is, women who are still potentially reproductively active. In fact, some research suggests that estrogen also helps to lower the low-density lipoprotein (LDL) cholesterol level in the blood (Aryan et al., 2020). Between the ages of 45 and 55, however, estrogen levels decrease substantially. It is during this time that rates of heart disease show marked increases in women that continue in the succeeding years.

If estrogen protects women from cardiovascular disease, then it seems logical to reason that by replacing the lost estrogen women should continue their trend of lower rates of heart disease. Unfortunately, the research does not support this assumption. Studies testing the effectiveness of *hormone replacement therapy*, a process that restores estrogen to premenopausal levels, have been controversial. However, the current consensus is that hormone replacement therapy is not recommended for the prevention of coronary heart disease (Pinkerton, 2020), primarily because of the risks associated with its use and with risks when discontinuing treatment (North American Menopause Society, 2017).

Gender and Symptoms One additional difficulty in diagnosing heart disease in women is the difference in symptomology between men and women. Studies show that women report different, and in some cases milder, symptoms than men (van Oosterhout et al., 2020). Men generally report tightness in the chest, shortness of breath, and possibly pain in the left arm. These symptoms have come to represent the "classic" indicators of heart disease. We now know that the classic warning signs of heart disease in women are pain in the neck and shoulder, lower back pain, and possibly shortness of breath. Medical providers trained to look for the indications more common among men will miss or misinterpret the symptoms reported most often by women.

TABLE 9.2 Cardiovascular Disease by Age and Gender

Age Group	Gender	Percentage of Population with Cardiovascular Disease 2007 vs. 2016	
		2007	*2016*
20–39 years	Males	14.9	28.9
	Females	9.4	17.2
40–59 years	Males	39.1	56.9
	Females	39.5	51.6
60–79 years	Males	71.3	77.2
	Females	75.1	78.2
80+ years	Males	83.0	89.3
	Females	92.0	91.8

Source: Based on Benjamin et al. (2019).

The delay in recognizing the symptoms of heart disease in women often leads to a delay in diagnosis. And a delayed diagnosis increases the likelihood that the heart disease will worsen, leading eventually to more severe cardiovascular disease and death. Given the assumptions about risk factors for cardiovascular disease, the later onset of heart disease in women, and the difference in illness-related symptoms between men and women, it is not surprising that researchers and medical providers overlooked women as a population at high risk for heart disease. These differences also explain, in part, the higher mortality rate from heart disease for women versus men.

But now that we know that women also are at risk for cardiovascular disease, the question for health psychologists is how to minimize the risk. We know from discussions earlier in the chapter that smoking is one behavior that increases the risk for heart disease. Fortunately for women, cigarette smoking has been called the single most preventable risk factor for heart disease (World Health Organization, 2024). Although studies show that women who smoke are two to four times more likely than men to be at risk for heart disease (American Heart Association, 2024), they also indicate that the health risks decrease *immediately* when women stop smoking.

Findings from a 50-year perspective on smoking-related risks offer even better news. Thun and colleagues (2013) undertook a retrospective study that calculated the death rates and relative risks associated with active cigarette smoking and smoking cessation in three time frames (1959–1965, 1982–1988, and 2000–2010). Their findings suggest both troubling and welcome news. We will discuss the problems first. Thun and colleagues found that females' risk of death from smoking is now almost identical to that of males. In fact, the data suggest that although death rates from lung cancer have stabilized for men, they continue to increase for women. This is in marked contrast to earlier research that showed women to be less likely to die from smoking-related illnesses.

The second stunning finding from Thun and colleagues' (2013) research offers more encouraging news. Put simply, they found that smoking cessation at any age dramatically lowers mortality rates from all smoking-related illnesses. Even more interesting, Thun found that people who quit smoking by 34 years of age can add an average of 10 years onto their life spans. And Thun and colleagues' research suggests that almost all excess risks that are associated with smoking can be eliminated if individuals stop smoking before age 40. Finally, for those people thinking about reducing rather than quitting altogether, Thun's research shows greater health benefits to those who stop smoking by age 40 than to those who only reduce smoking behavior. If there was ever a reason to decide to stop smoking, Thun and colleagues' research might provide that motivation. These findings have been modified but generally supported by current research (Duncan et al., 2019; Lloyd-Jones et al., 2017).

Aging Without a doubt, an individual's age also affects risk for heart disease. As noted previously, older women, that is women 60 years of age or older, are more likely to be diagnosed with cardiovascular disease than older men. In the U.S. the prevalence rates for cardiovascular diseases, including coronary artery disease, heart failure, stroke, and hypertension, increase almost 30% when comparing people in the 40–59 age group with those aged 60–79 in 2007, and approximately 20% in 2016 (Benjamin et al., 2019).

What causes the higher rates of cardiovascular disease among older adults? There appear to be several reasons, three of which we highlight here: the body's aging process, co-occurring chronic diseases, and longer life spans for women. We consider first the body's aging process. Think of it this way: The human body can be compared to an automobile. Although this is not the most elegant example, the body, like most automobiles, is constantly in operation. The older the car, the more likely it is to develop mechanical problems. Similarly, over time, the toll placed on the body by regular daily activities, stressful events, physically or mentally demanding tasks, or health-compromising behaviors such as smoking or excessive consumption of fats, cholesterol, or alcohol will cause damage to the organs. The accumulated damage will result in less effective functioning of the organs including the heart (Laurent & Bautouyrie, 2007; Nicita-Mauro, Maltese, Nicita-Mauro, & Basile, 2007).

In addition to wear and tear, other factors such as co-occurring chronic diseases and medications for non–heart-related illnesses can also impair the heart's functions over time. The impact of these factors can be seen specifically in cardiovascular reactivity (Priebe, 2016). We mentioned earlier that cardiovascular reactivity is the rate at which the heart returns to its resting state. The more quickly it can return to a resting state, the less wear and tear there is on the heart. But other health conditions and medications may slow cardiovascular reactivity, a problem that can, over time, cause excessive wear, possibly damaging heart tissue.

Finally, we noted that women not only have a higher risk of cardiovascular disease than men, but they also have higher prevalence rates for the same disease. One reason for the higher prevalence rate may be the fact that, on average, women live longer than men. Therefore, a third age-related factor for heart disease is that, among older persons, women outnumber men. And among the population of older women, there may also be a greater percentage of women living with CAD.

The aging process, in addition to compromising health behaviors, would seem to paint a somewhat bleak prognosis for the cardiovascular health of older persons. In truth, it is not quite that grim. Many older adults have limited or no heart problems, and others manage their heart disease with appropriate medications and lifestyle adjustments. However, the research is clear about one thing: Adoption of a healthy and nutritious diet, maintaining a moderate weight, engaging in regular exercise, keeping consumption of alcohol moderate (see Chapter 5, Risky Health Behaviors, for a definition of moderate alcohol use), and refraining from smoking will help maintain and restore heart health. This is the first step to improving longevity.

Race/Ethnicity In previous chapters, we identified race/ethnicity as one of several individual characteristics that affect health and health outcomes. But unlike gender or age, there is little evidence in the literature to suggest that people of specific races or ethnic groups are predisposed to heart disease based on genetic or inherited traits. Instead, it appears that high-fat and high-cholesterol diets, smoking, and greater exposure to stressful situations among some ethnic groups contribute to higher rates of cardiovascular disease.

To what extent can research rule out race/ethnicity as a factor in heart disease? Simply put, current research shows that risk factors for heart disease are not race- or ethnic-specific. But many racial and ethnic groups do share risk factors. Consider these two examples: In several studies comparing risk factors for heart disease among African American, Mexican, and Native American populations, researchers found that all three groups shared a number of factors. For example, obesity and hypertension was a shared health outcome between Mexican and African Americans as was smoking among Mexican and Native Americans (Kurian & Cardarelli, 2007; Mensah, Mokdad, Ford, Greenlund, & Croft, 2005). In the majority of these studies, the three groups shared at least two of six risk factors that put them at higher risk for cardiovascular disease.

Because behavioral risk factors account for the preponderance of incidences of cardiovascular disease, studies that demonstrate shared risk factors among ethnic groups help dispel the notion that any single group is predisposed to heart disease because of its ethnicity. Rather, risk factors are directly attributable to health behaviors that are common to many groups. That said, there have been a few intriguing studies that suggest that a specific heart medication is more effective for one ethnic/racial group than another. The heart medication *BiDil* (see Box 9.2) is one such example. These studies, however, are very limited in number and too few to lead to any definitive conclusion.

Box 9.2 Do Some Heart Medications Work Better for One Racial/Ethnic Group Than Another?

Years of research have convinced health researchers and medical care providers that race/ethnicity is not, in and of itself, a risk factor for heart disease. The behaviors associated with some groups may increase risk, but being a member of a specific ethnic group is not a factor.

If that is true, then why did some medical researchers advocate the use of a heart medication specifically for African Americans?

In 1997, the U.S. Food and Drug Administration (FDA) was prepared to withdraw a new heart drug for use on patients who experienced heart failure. They believed that studies did not show conclusively that the drug was effective. Yet the drug appeared to be effective when used by African Americans.

Mindful of the historic legacy and negative repercussions pertaining to medical experimentation on African Americans (see Chapter 2, Research Methods, the Tuskegee study), a number of scientists were leery of efforts to show that the proposed medication, BiDil, was effective on African Americans who experienced heart failure (Saul, 2005). Some disbelieved the claim, whereas others suggested that there was reason to believe that there was no ethnic group difference in the drug's effectiveness.

To test the drug's effectiveness, NitroMed, the manufacturers of BiDil, solicited the help of African American politicians and physicians, including the Association of Black Cardiologists, to co-sponsor a new trial in 2001 to test the effectiveness of BiDil among a study sample of African Americans (Saul, 2005). All participants in the study were African Americans who had a history of heart failure that had been unsuccessfully treated with other heart therapies. The results of the study on the 1,051 self-identified African American heart-failure patients were stunning. They showed that the patients who received BiDil had a 43% decrease in deaths due to heart failure and a 39% decrease in hospitalizations – a significant difference from patients who received the placebo (U.S. Food and Drug Administration, 2005).

The findings were so impressive that the FDA and NitroMed suspended the study and approved the drug for use, in combination with other heart therapies, among African Americans with diagnosed cases of heart failure.

It is not clear exactly why the drug appears to be effective among this group. And others have questioned the methodology of the study, which apparently did not include trials using other ethnic groups. Certainly, the reason for its effectiveness remains an unanswered question. Most researchers contend that the underlying genetic differences among racial/ethnic groups are small, and therefore they would argue against different treatment outcomes based solely on race/ethnicity. However, it is not the first time that a drug has been more or less effective on one group. The FDA has noted that a cholesterol-lowering drug appears to cause serious side effects for Asians, an outcome not obtained when used with other racial/ethnic groups.

The general consensus is that there are few major differences among racial/ethnic groups. Yet on occasion, there may be a drug that appears to be more or less beneficial for a specific group. Initial reports suggest that BiDil may be such a drug for the treatment of heart failure among African Americans.

A second example that highlights the role of risk factors in heart disease is found in the comparison of two samples of populations, both of which are white, but which practice very different lifestyles. Research by Bielak and colleagues (2007) compared the risk factors for cardiovascular disease among the Amish, a population that resides in a rural setting, against an urban/suburban-based population from the Rochester, Minnesota, metropolitan area.

Bielak and colleagues (2007) chose the Amish as one of two groups for their study because the Amish lifestyle in the U.S. is characterized by high levels of physical activity associated with farming and less reliance on modern technologies. For example, they do not use automobiles. In addition, the absence of modern appliances in their homes and on their farms means it takes considerably more physical labor to perform the daily tasks of maintaining both. The Amish were compared with a nonrelated group of whites in Rochester whose urban lifestyle entailed less physically demanding work. The researchers purposely chose a white comparison group to ensure that race did not affect the study's outcomes.

Bielak and his coauthors found that, although the Amish did not engage in health-compromising behaviors such as smoking or drinking as the Rochester group did, they had significantly higher levels of coronary artery calcification than the Rochester group. This was true even though their lifestyles were more physically demanding than the Rochester group. On further analysis, Bielak and colleagues (2007) found that the higher calcification rates of the Amish were due principally to their diets, which contained significantly higher levels of calories, fats, and proteins than that of the Rochester group. The Amish diet is high in energy as is needed for a very physical lifestyle, but it may still cause risk factors for heart disease.

A second and equally interesting finding was that more than one-third of the Rochester group used prescription medicine for lowering cholesterol or blood-pressure levels. Therefore, although the Amish diet led to higher rates of artery calcification, it was not, apparently, high enough to require medication. In comparison, many participants from the Rochester group had already been diagnosed as being at high risk, enough so that they needed medical intervention.

This study by Bielak and colleagues (2007) seems to support the notion that physical exercise may help mitigate the risks of heart disease. But the study appears to suggest that exercise, in combination with low-fat, low-cholesterol diets, could indeed improve heart health and lower rates of heart disease.

Community/Environment

The term *community* can be defined many ways, including through geography (neighborhood, city or region, state or country), close friends and family, work colleagues, or those who share professional or leisure-time interests (Ragin et al., 2008). Indeed, in the current computer age, we can even include cyber communities such as Meta, X, Instagram, Snapchat, and others.

For the purpose of health behaviors, however, we define *community* as the people with whom an individual feels most connected or a place in which an individual feels a sense of belonging. Most individuals identify with multiple communities, including communities of both people and places. For example, for a 10-year-old boy, community could include his family, his closest friends, his Boy Scout troop, his softball team, his school classmates, and his geographic neighborhood. Others may have a larger network of community that would include their religious community, work associates, colleagues from professional associations, and more. The number of communities one associates with is unimportant. More important is the level of influence a community exerts on each individual.

For many people, immediate family members are a very influential community. Immediate family members usually share cultural and behavioral beliefs that may influence health outcomes. Consider this: Thanksgiving is a major holiday in many homes in the U.S. The meal is central to the holiday. At such an occasion, it may be very difficult to avoid Grandma's special gravy for the turkey, Aunt Carole's baked macaroni and cheese with three types of cheese, Uncle Ken's homemade sausages, or, of course, Cousin Sarah's homemade sweet potato pie à la mode. In fact, declining to sample some of these treats might be taken as an insult. Families may unintentionally encourage the consumption of foods that increase risk of heart disease.

We can see the effects of community on health when community is defined as geographic space. In Chapter 5, Risky Health Behaviors, we explored the impact of community violence on overall health. We noted that, in neighborhoods in which violence is prevalent, individuals may not make use of public recreational facilities in their neighborhoods for fear that violent acts by others in the community could increase the risk of injury to themselves or other family members. Children and adults therefore might not engage in activities such as bicycling, rollerblading, or participate in organized sports in local parks such as softball or basketball. And because physical inactivity can increase incidences of heart disease, residents in high-crime neighborhoods may be putting themselves at higher risk of poor health outcomes in an effort to protect themselves from another source of harm.

Health Systems and Access to Care

Several times in this and other chapters, we explored the health profiles of individuals in different communities and countries. Another seminal study also exploring differences in health outcomes of two communities, non-Hispanic whites in England and non-Hispanic whites in the U.S., reveals significant health differences between groups in these two countries that do not appear to be related to age, gender, or education and perhaps only nominally related to socioeconomic class or health-behavior risk factors.

The classic study by Banks, Marmot, Oldfield, and Smith (2006) examined self-report data and biological measures of health for 4,386 Americans and 3,681 English study participants, aged 55–64, from comparable, established databases in both countries. The study examined specifically the prevalence rates for two chronic diseases: heart disease and diabetes. Their findings were surprising. Banks and colleagues (2006) found that, overall, the Americans were less healthy than the English. The American sample reported higher rates of hypertension, heart disease, heart attack, and stroke. They also reported higher rates of other chronic illnesses, including diabetes, lung disease, and cancer.

Having controlled for differences due to age, gender, and education, Banks and colleagues (2006) found that the difference could not be attributed to health behaviors. On average, the English reported higher levels of smoking and drinking behaviors than the Americans. What, then, could account for the difference?

Banks and colleagues (2006) suggest two possible explanations: first, an early onset for disease based on early dietary habits; and second, access to health care. With regard to early onset, these researchers suggest that, as we indicated earlier, diseases that become evident in adulthood may have their origins in childhood. The dietary behaviors one adopts as a child or adolescent can, if unaltered, predispose a person to chronic illnesses.

Second, Banks and colleagues (2006) found an effect of access to care on health outcomes. You may recall that in this and earlier chapters we identified access to health care as a determinant of health status. Why, therefore, are Banks and colleagues' findings considered interesting? Put simply, they found that access to care was not tied to socioeconomic class, at least not in England. Specifically, Banks and colleagues showed that lower- and middle-income Brits have better health outcomes than upper-income Americans. What is more, they found a disparity in health outcomes that favored the English study sample, even though the English study subjects reported engaging more frequently in health-risk behaviors such as smoking and drinking.

What can explain this unexpected finding? The only significant difference between the two groups (English and American) was their access to health care. Put simply, these researchers concluded that long-term and continued access to care contributed to overall better health outcomes for the English over the Americans regardless of either group's socioeconomic status. We review the health care systems of the U.S. and other countries in Chapter 12, Health Care Systems and Health Policy. Briefly, however, in England, people at all socioeconomic income levels have the same level of access to primary care through the National Health Service. It appears, therefore, that when controlling for the effects of individual (e.g., age, gender, education) and social (socioeconomic status) factors and recognizing that the English sample engaged in more risk behaviors associated with smoking and drinking, the only explanation for the better health outcomes for the English sample is a health systems and health policy issue: access to care.

Thus, the important point about Banks and colleagues' (2006) study is that health outcomes can be and are influenced by access to care. This is particularly true when examining issues of heart disease and other chronic illnesses. Banks and colleagues' study, comparing outcomes from individuals exposed to two different health care systems, demonstrates the point.

Personal Postscript

MEASURING YOUR RISK LEVEL FOR CARDIOVASCULAR DISEASE

By now you may have a mental checklist of the behaviors that can put you at high risk for cardiovascular disease. They include diets high in fats and cholesterol, smoking, excessive alcohol consumption, inactivity, overweight/obesity, and diabetes. All of this means little if you do not have a way to measure your current activities against a standard.

The best way to measure your heart risk is through a complete physical exam, which should include a stress test and an electrocardiogram. The stress test will measure your heart's performance while under exertion. For example, walking on a treadmill tests your heart's performance when engaging in physical activity. The electrocardiogram measures the electrical activity of the heart. It measures activity of different parts of the heart muscle. It can help identify any abnormal heart rhythms in need of further examination.

If you are reading this textbook as part of a class assignment, you may wonder why you should be concerned about your heart health. But if you remember the studies we reviewed that examined the long-term effects of diet and physical inactivity on later incidences of atherosclerosis and CAD, you may be able to answer your own question. In addition, the following questions may help you to think about your health behaviors and identify needed changes.

Where do you stand on the following health indicator?

1. Vital measurements
   - Normal blood pressure is 120/80. What is your blood pressure?
   - Desirable cholesterol levels are 200 overall and HDL over 60. What is your cholesterol level?
   - Desirable body mass index is under 30 and ideally under 25. What is your BMI?
2. Physical activity
   - Thirty minutes of moderate to vigorous exercise per day is recommended. This can include walking or any activity that you will maintain. What is your plan in consultation with your doctor?

3. Nutrition
   - Eat at least two and a half cups of fruits and vegetables daily. What is your current consumption? How can you increase your intake?
   - Drink no sugar-sweetened drinks. What do you usually drink? What changes are possible here?
   - Limit snacks high in fats and cholesterol. What are your favorite snacks? What low-fat and low-cholesterol snacks do you like?
4. Smoking
   - No smoking! Immediate effects can be seen in three to five years, especially for women. Are you a smoker? What can you do to limit or end this behavior?
5. Drinking
   - If you drink, consume a moderate amount of alcohol. What is your alcohol consumption pattern? Should you reduce your consumption?

Questions to Consider

1. Many women still believe that breast cancer is the leading cause of death for women. How can health psychologists correct this misperception without minimizing the risks of cancer?
2. How will the new "Food Plate" help individuals manage or change their eating behaviors?
3. Former U.S. First Lady Michelle Obama initiated a "Let's Move" campaign, intended to encourage exercise for people of all ages, but especially children. How successful has it been? Is it able to overcome the fascination with sedentary computer-based activities and the addiction of social media?

True or False Questions

1. A person suffering a stroke can survive for 10 minutes without medical care. True or False.
2. Hypertension's nickname is "the silent killer." True or False.
3. There is a direct, genetic causal link between ethnicity and heart disease. True or False.
4. Heart disease is the second leading cause of death worldwide. Cancer is the leading cause. True or False.
5. Perceived racism can lead to elevated baseline blood pressure, and over time to heart disease. True or False.

Important Terms

angina   343
aorta   342
aortic valve   342
arteries   341
atherosclerosis   343
asymptomatic   339
atrium (atria)   367
automated external defibrillator (AED)   367
capillary   367
carbohydrate   352
cardiac arrest   344
cardiopulmonary resuscitation (CPR)   344
cardiovascular disease   343
cardiovascular reactivity (CVR)   349
cerebrovascular disease   345
cholesterol   354
coronary artery disease (CAD)   339
diastolic   342
essential or primary hypertension   346
estrogen   359
fat   354
front-of-package (FOP) notification   367
hemorrhagic stroke   345
high blood pressure (HBP)   345
high-density lipoprotein (HDL)   367
hormone replacement therapy   359
hypertension   345
inlet valves   342
ischemic stroke   345
low-density lipoprotein (LDL)   354
minerals   355
mitral valve   342
moderating risk factor   350
modifiable risk factor   343
monounsaturated fat   354
myocardial infarction   343
perceived racism   348

Chronic Pain Management and Arthritis

Chapter Outline

Source: 3xy/ Shutterstock.

Chapter Objectives

After studying this chapter, you will be able to:

1. Define and explain chronic pain.
2. Identify and describe four major categories of pain.
3. Identify and describe three factors that explain individual differences in pain perception.
4. Identify and describe the three major types of arthritis.
5. Explain ankylosing spondylitis.
6. Identify and define three pharmacological therapies for arthritis.
7. Define exercise therapy.
8. Explain the benefits of exercise therapy for people with arthritis.
9. Explain the role of psychological therapies for the treatment of arthritis.

DOI: 10.4324/9781003300670-11

OPENING STORY: JUVENILE ARTHRITIS

Caitlin's day began just like all others for the past 11 years. She awoke, and as she got out of bed she felt a familiar pain, stiffness, and soreness in her fingers, toes, elbows, knees, and shoulders (Stahl, 2008). Caitlin has arthritis.

*Aches and pains may seem usual for a person with arthritis; in fact, many older persons experience these symptoms daily. But Caitlin is 14. What is more, Caitlin's problems began when she was only three years old. She first complained of persistent knee pain. Her doctors looked for a host of possible explanations for the discomfort, including a fall from a bicycle, cancer, meningitis, or another infectious disease. But after ruling out these and other possible causes, doctors settled on **juvenile arthritis** – a form of arthritis that affects children usually before age 16 – as the most likely explanation, even if the patient seems a little young (Martini et al., 2022). Like arthritis in adults, juvenile arthritis is caused by inflammation in the joints. Often the cause of the inflammation in children is unknown, but it is thought to be due to an autoimmune disorder. Consequently, children are often diagnosed with **juvenile idiopathic arthritis**, from the Greek words* idios *and* pathos, *meaning a disease of unknown origins (Centers for Disease Control, 2023i; National Institute of Arthritis & Musculoskeletal & Skin Diseases, 2021). In some cases, juvenile arthritis can go into **remission**; that is, show no signs or symptoms of illness. But it is more likely that Caitlin, like other children diagnosed with the disease, will carry it into adulthood.*

Caitlin now manages the ups and downs of juvenile arthritis like thousands of other teenagers with similar diagnoses. At times, she is uncomfortable in the mornings due to the stiffness that comes from lying in one position for a long period. She must remember to take her medications on schedule (a daily activity that is sometimes awkward for her when at school) and try to remember to exercise during the day (a painful task when she is stiff). And not surprisingly, Caitlin admits to being grouchy on occasion because of the discomfort and the sporadic sleepless nights due to joint pain. ■

Caitlin's case calls attention to the fact that there are almost 220,000 children and adolescents in the U.S. with juvenile arthritis, a statistic that reinforces the fact that arthritis is not just an "older person's" disease (Centers for Disease Control, 2023i). This number, which equates to a prevalence of 305 cases per 100,000 from 2007 to 2021 in the U.S., is on the high end of prevalence cases globally, which range from 3.8 to 400 in 100,000 (Al-Mayouf et al., 2021). In total, more than 3 million children and young adults have been diagnosed with some form of arthritis, yet it remains a poorly understood and even less well-researched illness, especially for this age group.

Research on demographic trends in juvenile arthritis reveals that, overall, more female children and teens are diagnosed with the disease. It also appears to be more common among non-Hispanic white children. What is more, the onset for some types of juvenile arthritis can occur in early childhood, between two and six years of age (Arthritis Foundation, n.d-a), as Caitlin's story suggests (National Institute of Arthritis and Musculoskeletal and Skin Diseases, 2009).

The research also shows that children with arthritis experience some of the same sensations of achiness in the *joints* – for example, elbows, knees, and knuckles – as do adults. Complaints of pain and stiffness after prolonged periods of sitting or lying in one position are common to both groups, as is discomfort when engaging in physical activity. Consider this: Fourteen-year-old Caitlin participates in team sports. Before playing, she will take a few minutes to do additional stretching exercises to minimize physical discomfort or stiffness due to the arthritis.

Finally, similar to adults with arthritis, Caitlin will probably experiment with a number of different treatments, including drug, exercise, and psychological therapies. We explain the therapeutic treatments for arthritis later in the chapter. For now, just remember that arthritis is a degenerative disease that gradually erodes bone and inflames tissue. Therefore, people with the disease change therapeutic approaches often to obtain more effective pain relief for their progressive condition. For Caitlin and for many adults, changing treatments to improve pain management is a part of life.

At this point, you may be wondering why we are spending so much time on arthritis in this chapter on chronic pain. After all, there are a host of other illnesses that cause discomfort that, arguably, are more common. But recall that in the beginning of this chapter we noted that more than 220,000 children and adolescents in the U.S. and more than 3 million children and adolescents worldwide are afflicted with some form of juvenile arthritis. Some contend that this statistic alone allows us to classify juvenile arthritis as a common childhood rheumatic illnesses, and one that results in the most common short- or long-term disability (Giancane et al., 2016). Thus, like motor vehicle accidents (which were discussed in Chapter 5, Risky Health Behaviors), arthritis is a frequently occurring yet often overlooked problem that should be addressed in chapters on chronic pain. With that in mind, we will use arthritis throughout this chapter to illustrate the physiological and psychological nature of chronic pain.

We begin the chapter with a brief overview of pain, including a definition of chronic pain, a summary of the physiology of pain perception, and a brief review of the research on individual differences in pain perception. In Section II, we introduce arthritis, an autoimmune disease for which one of the classic symptoms is chronic discomfort, aching, and soreness. Without a doubt there are many other illnesses that include chronic pain as a major symptom, such as cancer and cardiovascular disease. We will briefly examine the relationship between these illnesses and chronic discomfort in our review of the research. We end Section II with a discussion of instruments used to assess pain.

Finally, in Section III, we examine pharmacological and psychotherapeutic pain management treatments. Many new drug therapies and medical regimens have been introduced in the past 20 years to treat chronic pain. That is the good news. The not-so-good news is that because chronic aches and discomforts are influenced also by our emotions and our perceptions, drug therapies alone do not provide effective treatments. We cannot undertake a thorough review of medical treatments for pain in this book. Therefore we will explore a sample of the pharmacological treatments used to address this condition, with particular attention given to treatments for arthritis, thus bringing us back to our initial topic.

We conclude Section III with an overview of non-pharmacological interventions for chronic pain including psychological and alternative therapies. As psychologists, we pay particular attention to the psychological therapies used with drug or exercise therapies because combination therapies appear to be most effective in managing pain and providing maximum pain relief. Treatment regimens for arthritis illustrate that whether used alone or in combination with other approaches, psychological therapies appear to play a major role in successful treatment outcomes. As such, health psychologists can play an important role in pain management.

SECTION I. "THE DECADE OF PAIN"

In the early 1990s, health care providers and legislators in the U.S. called attention to the numerous complaints by patients of undertreatment of pain. The growing awareness of the debilitating effects of poorly regulated pain led, in 1999, to a declaration by the Joint Commission on Accreditation of Healthcare Organizations (JCAHO) that pain management must be a priority for medical practitioners (Joint Commission on Accreditation of Healthcare Organizations, 1999). Shortly thereafter, the U.S.

Congress passed a resolution (Title VI, Section 1603) declaring the period from January 1, 2001, through December 31, 2010, the "Decade of Pain Control and Research" (Brennan, 2015).

The JCAHO position and the health policy put forward by the U.S. legislature came at a time when research on pain revealed that over 80% of all patients in the U.S. listed it as their principal symptom or concern when visiting their primary care provider. This problem, which affects nearly 76.2 million Americans, accounts for more patient visits to physicians than three other chronic illnesses – diabetes, heart disease, and cancer – combined (American Pain Foundation, 2009). What is more, pain management is not just a national issue. Statistics show that collectively, 34% of adults in lower- and middle-income countries report unspecified and persistent pain (Jackson et al., 2016). Zimmer, Fraser, Grol-Prokopczyk, and Zajacova's (2022) analysis of moderate to extreme pain prevalence in adults 25 years of age or older across 52 countries substantiates this claim. Their findings revealed less of a distinction between pain as a function of a country's economic level (see Chapter 2, Research Methods) than, for example, WHO region, demographic characters of individual reporting pain, or contextual country-level factors. For example, Zimmer and colleagues (2022) found higher average reports of pain in the European region (34%) than in the Western Pacific region (21%) and higher reported pain among women, older persons, and rural dwellers (Zimmer et al., 2022).

One difficulty in diagnosing and treating pain is that it is a nonspecific symptom. You may remember that we introduced this concept in Chapter 4, Global, Communicable, and Chronic Disease. Essentially, non-specific symptoms can be widely associated with a host of other primary illnesses, and often defies health providers' best efforts to locate and diagnose the problem. Thus, it is not surprising that chronic pain may go untreated or undertreated. For this reason, health organizations and legislators are playing a critical role in reinforcing the need to include chronic pain as part of a health treatment plan. The World Health Organization and the International Association on the Study of Pain even proposed that chronic pain be considered a disease in its own right (World Health Organization, 2004b). Notwithstanding this elevation of pain as an important medical condition, a problem remains; researchers and health practitioners still struggle to define and accurately measure chronic pain.

Defining Pain

It might be helpful at this point to explain briefly what is meant by pain and pain perception. Our concept of pain has evolved over the centuries. (Given the evolution of the definition of health, as noted in Chapters 1 and 6, this should not come as a surprise!) Early efforts to characterize this ailment were linked to René Descartes. We introduced Descartes in Chapter 1, An Interdisciplinary View of Health, and you may recall that he was a 17th-century mathematician and scientist. He explained his concept of pain and pain perception in his *specificity theory*. Briefly, Descartes proposed that our perception of aches and discomfort is explained by a "linear" sensory projection system. According to this theory, a painful stimulus triggers specific pain fibers and transmits neural signals through designated pathways that lead to a specific pain region in the brain (Melzack, 1993). Unfortunately for Descartes, his theory was discarded when subsequent research revealed that the transmission of pain signals is not quite that simple. The problem is that Descartes' concept is closely linked to a biomedical view of pain, which holds that a specific injury, illness, or damage can be identified, localized, and subsequently treated. About now, you might be saying to yourself, "But in Chapter 6, Emotional Health, we learned that the biomedical model of health is not the best model for addressing chronic and sometimes nonspecific issues such as pain." If you did, great! Many researchers will agree with you. Since Descartes' discovery, researchers have revised their explanations of the pain-perception process, which brings us to our present understanding.

Current theories suggest that there are now four major categories of pain. The first, *nociceptive pain*, is caused by a disease or damage to non-neural body tissues that then activates our nociceptors (Trouvin & Perrot, 2019). Think of it this way. Receptors called *nociceptors* located throughout our body or on our skin send nerve projections to the spinal cord. These projections trigger two actions: a spinal reflex that sends a command to the muscles and a second reflex that sends information about the discomfort to the brain (Sapolsky, 1998). Many times the pain signals originating from these actions subside. When they do not, however, an individual can experience either episodic or continuous sensations of discomfort that may be characterized as chronic pain. Remember that in Chapter 4, Global, Communicable, and Chronic Disease, we indicated that chronic illnesses last more than three to six months and have no cure. Similarly, pain that persists at least three to six months and which abates only temporarily in response to specific but time-limited treatment is classified as *chronic pain*.

VIDEO #49/60

Chapter 10: Chronic Pain Management and Arthritis
- **Chronic Pain:** *Mayo Clinic Minute: Helping older adults manage chronic pain*
- *Website: https://www.youtube.com/watch?v=bUd6i4yGAPY*
- *Mayo Clinic is publicly accessible since it provides medical-based information to the public at no cost. www.mayoclinic.org/*

Nociceptive pain, whether acute or chronic, comes in two forms: *visceral*, involving major organs, and *somatic*, usually involving bones, joints, and muscles. Visceral discomfort is best characterized as a non-localized and episodic pain that principally involves body organs such as the heart or liver. By comparison, somatic pain is typically localized to one area and is usually time-limited. Consider this: Suppose that while hammering a nail you accidentally hit your thumb. The nociceptors sense the blow to the thumb and transmit this information to the brain. The pain is localized, and although it might throb and ache for a little while, it will probably be short-lived.

Notice we said that somatic pain is customarily time limited. That implies an exception. One noteworthy exception is arthritic pain. Although defined as somatic nociceptive pain, arthritic pain is not time-limited. Osteoarthritis, a deterioration of cartilage at the joints that cushions the bones, is an example of somatic nociceptive pain that includes chronic aching, soreness, and throbbing. We discuss osteoarthritis and other forms of arthritis pain later in this section.

The second category is *neuropathic pain*, best described as pain caused by a malfunction of or lesion in our nervous system (Trouvin & Perrot, 2019). It is believed to result from lesions of or damage to the *somatosensory system*, a network of receptors and pathways that transmit sensory information about us and our environment – such as pain, temperature, and position and movement of our body – to our central nervous system. Common examples of neuropathic pain caused by lesions include spontaneous shooting or burning sensations, greater discomfort than normal in response to normally painful stimulus, and sensations of aching, throbbing, or soreness when encountering non-painful stimuli (University of Bristol, 2012). Illnesses such as diabetes, certain types of cancer, or chronic alcohol use can trigger neuropathic pain because of the damage they can cause to the nervous system.

A third category, *nociplastic pain*, was recently added to the definition of pain. In this category, researchers find that a person experiences changes in "cerebral activation" and cerebral connectivity. In essence, this type of pain comes about as a result of altered nociception, but there is no evidence of tissue damage, disease, or lesions that would trigger the pain (Trouvin & Perrot, 2019). People in this category would include those suffering from fibromyalgia, a constant or dull aching musculoskeletal pain that often includes fatigue, and mood or memory problems (Mayo Clinic, 2024), non-specific lower back pain, or other disorders such as irritable bowel syndrome (Kosek et al., 2016).

The fourth and final category of chronic pain is a mixed pain category, a combination of both nociceptive and neuropathic pain (Freynhagen et al., 2019). One example is migraine headaches. All four categories – nociceptive, neuropathic, nociplastic, and combined nociceptive/neuropathic – present challenges for treatment because, as we will see shortly, pain perception also entails a subjective sensory process, here meaning a psychological and an emotional component.

Pain Perception

GATE CONTROL THEORY The complex nature of the pain perception process was further illuminated by groundbreaking research by Melzack and Wall (1965, 2003). Their work, which led to the gate control theory, described pain as a multidimensional and subjective experience.

Melzack and Wall suggest that a gate mechanism located in the dorsal horn of the spinal cord serves as a checkpoint that permits or inhibits the transmission of pain signals to the brain. *Dorsal horns* are sensory nuclei that are found at all levels of the spinal cord. They are responsible for receiving and processing incoming somatosensory information. But in addition to receiving and processing pain signals, Melzack and Wall (1965, 2003) proposed that the dorsal horn also receives input from the brain about the psychological and emotional state of the person experiencing the discomfort. What is more, this psychological information can regulate the transmission of pain signals, influencing a person's perception. This psychological process may, according to Melzack and Wall, help explain individual differences in response to the same painful stimuli.

Individual Difference Factors and Pain

The well-established finding that individuals differ in their perception of and response to pain provides important support for the argument that this phenomenon is a multidimensional and sensory experience. This assertion makes pain perception and management relevant to psychologists because it suggests an interaction between physiology and emotional states. Therefore, we will take just a few more minutes to examine the research on individual differences in pain perception. Specifically, we examine how genetics, emotional and biological factors, personality, race/ethnicity, and gender may influence individual differences in perceptions of discomfort.

GENETIC, EMOTIONAL, AND BIOLOGICAL FACTORS Research on individual differences in pain perception focuses on the role of genetic factors, personality traits such as anxiety, and specific brain regions on our discernment of temperature and pain sensitivity. For example, a study by Solovieva and colleagues (2004) investigating possible genetic links to pain perception suggests an association between the interleukin-1 (IL-1) gene and lower back pain, a common complaint among adults of middle age or older (Moen, Schistad, Rygh, & Gjerstad, 2014).

A seminal research study by Zubieta and colleagues (2001) also supports a genetic explanation for some pain sensations. Their laboratory-based study suggests an interaction between pain and the body's opioid-receptor system. In this study, Zubieta and colleagues tested the pain perception of 20 normal adults. The participants were presented with experimentally induced pain and with a placebo condition. The researchers assessed a participant's discomfort using brain PET scans and the subject's self-reported response to pain questionnaires. Zubieta et al.'s findings suggest that persistent pain resulted in the selective release of endogenous opioids in specific brain regions. What is more, the gender of the subject (a genetic factor) was also found to influence the opioid receptor in the brain, a finding that might explain individual differences – and more specifically, gender differences – in pain perception.

Some researchers specifically examined the relationship between other genetic factors, such as gender and ethnicity, to pain perception (Aufiero, Stankewicz, Quazi, Jacoby, & Stoltzfus, 2017; Mince & Stewart, 2007; Reyes-Gibby, et al., 2012). We explore the relationship between race/ethnicity and pain in just a moment. But here, one area of particular interest is the research that shows gender difference in pain tolerance even among adolescents with juvenile arthritis. In a study comparing abdominal pain and tolerance by age, Rebane and colleagues (2022) found that among young Finnish adults with a diagnosis of juvenile idiopathic arthritis, abdominal pain – a common complaint among arthritis sufferers – was significantly associated with the female study participants. And, although there are a number of studies that report an association between pain perception and gender, some contend that these differences may be influenced by social norms rather than a genetic distinction between the sexes. That is to say, society may permit girls to react to pain more than boys, thus giving rise to the observed gender discrepancy.

Finally, a number of studies have examined the role of biological factors in pain perception. Specifically, some studies demonstrated a relationship between pain unpleasantness, emotional reactivity, and activity in the bilateral amygdala cluster region of the brain. Let's begin with the association between pain perception and emotional reactivity. Research has shown that people who are high in emotional reactivity, as well as depressed individuals and those experiencing periods of depression, are more likely to rate painful stimuli as unpleasant (Berna et al., 2010; Stringo, Simmons, Matthews, Craig, & Paulus, 2008). Such studies also suggest that these individuals are more likely to express greater distress about their future well-being if experiencing discomfort as a result of an illness or injury.

To establish the role of the amygdala and its relationship to pain and emotion, we turn to another study. In a fascinating longitudinal study with 24 participants, Lapate and colleagues (2011) investigated whether individual differences in emotional regulation predicted successful pain regulation. They postulated that because the amygdala is the site for individual differences in the regulation of emotion, it may also be the site for pain processing. Their longitudinal study involved exposing their subjects to emotional-regulation and pain-regulation conditions. In the emotional-regulation condition, participants were shown 84 negative and 42 neutral photos and asked to either decrease their emotional response by reappraising the photos as less negative or to increase their emotional response by reappraising the photos as more negative. For example, in the negative-reappraisal condition, participants were shown a photo of a car accident and asked to reappraise the outcome as more negative; that is, to think that people were injured in the accident. A less negative reappraisal would suggest that no one was injured. Lapate and colleagues (2011) found that participants' ability to successfully regulate their response to negative pictures also predicted successful regulation of pain over two years. Through the use of functional magnetic resonance imaging (fMRI) and behavioral and psychological measures, the researchers demonstrated that these emotion- and pain-regulation skills are shared and are located in the amygdala, thus suggesting a relationship among painful sensations, emotional reactivity, and the brain.

PERSONALITY Work by Bar-Shalita and Cermak (2020) examined the relationship between pain perception and personality. They used the five-factor personality theory identified by McCrae and Costa, which categorizes persons along five personality dimensions: agreeableness, conscientiousness, extraversion, openness, and neuroticism. Bar-Shalita and Cermak suggest that among their sample population of 204 adult males, three of the five personality traits identified by McCrae and Costa – neuroticism, openness to experiences, and extraversion – were pre-existing factors that contributed to adverse responses to pain, or pain sensitivity.

Other studies similarly report an association between pain and personality. For example, work by Croy, Springborn, Lotsch, Johnston, and Hummel (2011) examined the relationship between personality characteristics and a number of sensory thresholds on a German sample of 124 participants. Specifically, they assessed olfactory (smell), gustatory (taste), tactile (touch), and, most relevant for our discussion, pain thresholds. To assess a participant's personality, they also employed McCrae and Costa's five-factor personality theory. In a complementary outcome to that of Bar-Shalita and Cermak, they found that there was a tendency for greater pain tolerance in persons who were rated as conscientious. None of the other personality types showed a high tolerance for discomfort.

We may also be able to demonstrate individual differences in pain perception using a common childhood game. Perhaps you've heard of or played this game as a child. Two people face each other, each of them with hands outstretched. One person, who we will call Person A, places both hands in front with palms facing up. The other person, Person B, places his hands on top of Person A's palms, but Person B's palms are face down. The task? Person A must quickly and without prior notice remove one of her hands and use it to slap one of Person B's hands. Person B must guess which of his hands Person A will try to slap. Person B must then move his own hand in time to avoid the hit. As always, there is a trick: if Person B moves too soon or moves the wrong hand, he will get a penalty slap. So, the bottom line is that Person B must move the correct hand, but only after Person A's hand is in motion and about to make contact with Person B's hand.

If you've played this game, no doubt you've found that some Person B players who guess incorrectly and receive a penalty slap complain loudly that the slap was too painful. Yet others seem almost impervious to the pain. What explains the difference? Admittedly, some players would not want to admit that the slap hurt. Their denial could be due to psychosocial factors like social conditioning, gender roles or, as our previous studies suggest, personality. But for everyone who experienced pain (regardless of whether it was acknowledged), the difference in pain perception is at the heart of our subjective experience of discomfort. As we explained previously, our brains interpret and respond to pain signals. It is this interpretation that influences our perception. There is a difference between the emotional interpretation of pain and the objective pain signal being transmitted to the brain (Sapolsky, 1998). Returning to the hand-slap game, it is conceivable that the actual pain level administered to Person B on one occasion is very slight. But if Person B's emotional response to being slapped is very high, they may perceive even a light slap as painful. Conversely, Person A may have administered a very forceful slap. But if Person B is intent on believing that no slap will make them show pain, Person B may actually interpret the pain signal as less intense.

RACE/ETHNICITY Researchers and some health providers report that another explanation for the individual differences in pain perception and tolerance may be race or ethnic factors. We alluded to this briefly in earlier sections.

In fact, there are quite a few studies that examine differences in discomfort with and tolerance of pain between African Americans, Latinos, and whites. Although some findings suggest no ethnic differences in perceptions of discomfort, others identify racial or ethnic differences in the epidemiology of pain, access to care, assessment and treatment of the disorder, and pain outcomes (Aufiero et al., 2017; Cintron & Morrison, 2006; Kwok & Bhuvanakrishna, 2014).

Consider this: Differences in threshold and sensitivity to experimental pain stimuli among ethnic groups have been reported as early as 1944. An early report by Chapman and Jones (1944) suggested that African Americans showed lower thresholds (here meaning tolerance) for heart pain than did non-Hispanic whites, a finding that was obtained in other studies as well (Rahim-Williams et al., 2007; Sheffield, Kirby, Biles, & Sheps, 1999).

Yet studies examining chronic discomfort or pain associated with chronic health conditions report mixed outcomes when comparing ethnic groups. In some earlier studies, African Americans and Latino patients were more likely than whites to report persistent pain related to cancer (Reyes-Gibby et al., 2012), whereas in a study by Mosher, Duhamel, Egert, and Smith (2011), African Americans and whites report lower cancer pain scores – as recorded using the Brief Pain Inventory Scale – than Spanish-speaking Latinos. We introduce the Brief Pain Inventory Scale in a later section of this chapter, but briefly, it is a measure used widely to assess and measure clinical pain levels.

Subsequent studies either question these outcomes or suggest that the difference in perception may be due – at least in part – to a difference in treatment or pain management rather than pain perception. For example, some studies report that physicians underestimate pain in approximately 75% of African American and 64% of Latino patients, and provide insufficient pain treatment for 31% and 28%, respectively (Kwok & Bhuvanakrishna, 2014). Additionally, in a simulated study of pain perception, Mende-Siedlecki and colleagues (2021) asked study participants to view photographs of African American and white males expressing pain and anger, happiness, fear, and sadness. They found that over 600 study participants were biased in their ability to see and identify pain or sadness on African American male faces when compared with whites. That is to say, participants were better at recognizing painful expressions on white than on African American males. This study, Mende-Siedlecki and colleagues suggest, is relevant to the current research that finds that African Americans' expression of pain are poorly recognized, perhaps due to bias, leading to a greater likelihood of undertreatment (Lee et al., 2019).

Other studies report more complaints of work-related pain by African Americans, which impaired their ability to perform their job responsibilities. Specifically, Allen and colleagues (2012) suggest that in their study, African Americans reported more functional and job-related disability due to knee pain than did whites. One reason for more reports of pain, Allen and colleagues suggest, is that African Americans reported performing more job-related tasks that involved lower-extremity joints than did whites, causing more stress on the knee and resulting in more knee pain. Thus, African Americans employed in jobs requiring more manual labor may report more pain and job impairment because of the nature of the work rather than because of the nature of the impediment.

Additional findings from arthritis research support the notion that types of employment may explain the pain and functional disability difference between African Americans versus whites, rather than ethnic or racial differences in pain perception. For example, research by Bolen and colleagues (2005) reports a higher frequency of severe joint pain and activity limitations among African American and Hispanic adults with doctor-diagnosed arthritis than among other ethnic groups (Table 10.1). Here, too, the research suggests that a significant difference in the physical demands of the work of these ethnic groups could explain the difference in functional disability.

What is clear from recent research comparing pain reports of different ethnic groups is that few studies have identified a biological basis for this apparent ethnic difference. Although some researchers speculate

TABLE 10.1 Estimated Proportion of Adults with Doctor-Diagnosed Arthritis and Arthritis Attributable Activity Limitation in the U.S., 2013–2015

Characteristics	White (%)	African American (%)	Hispanic (%)	Asian (%)	Other (%)
Activity limitations	42.1	49.9	47.7	38.9	51.3

Source: Adapted from Morbidity & Mortality Weekly Report. (2017). Prevalence of doctor-diagnosed arthritis and arthritis-attributable activity limitations: United States, 2013–2015. *MMWR*, 66(9), 246–253.

that ethnic factors could play a role in triggering activity in the nervous centers of the body that modulate pain (Mechlin, Heymen, Edwards, & Girdler, 2010), there appears to be greater support for the belief that social factors, such as limited access to care due to socioeconomic factors, lack of insurance, unequal treatment of pain, provider limitations – including lack of knowledge, training, or inability to accurately perceive expressions of pain by minority patients – and even ethnic differences in coping styles may contribute to ethnic differences in pain expression.

We address issues of patient-provider relations and its impact on health outcomes more thoroughly in Chapter 12, Health Care Systems and Health Policy. But it is important to reemphasize one point here, specifically with respect to pain. Some researchers suggest that attitudes or biases that health care providers hold about their patients may interfere with effective treatment (Diesfled, 2008). Specifically, Post, Blustein, Gordon, and Neveloff (1996) suggest:

> The multiplicity of factors that influence the perception and expression of pain take on special importance in the health care setting, where pain becomes an interpersonal experience between the sufferer and reliever. How pain is signified by the patient and understood by the provider determines in large measure how it is valued and, ultimately, how it is treated.

Remember our introduction to this section on pain? The health policy regulations by JCAHO and the U.S. Congress were designed to address such examples of the undertreatment of pain. What this explanation from Post and colleagues suggests is that health providers are a critical component in the experience, measurement, and treatment of pain.

We explore other disparities in pain treatment in the following section on arthritis. Before we do, we add one more point. Researchers have also noted differences in pain-coping strategies. Some studies, such as the one conducted by Ferreira-Valente and colleagues (2022), which reviewed 24 studies examining the association between religiosity/spirituality and coping with pain, shows that for some there is a strong association between these factors. For example, several studies they reviewed found an association between spirituality and a positive attitude, a reconceptualization of the illness as a chance, religious coping, and religious or spiritual well-being. Other research examined coping strategies employed by different countries, cultural or ethnic groups. For example, Sharma and colleagues' (2020) review of existing studies found a difference between three lower-middle income African countries and France in pain coping strategies for persons experiencing lower back pain. They note that in Tunisia, Morocco, and Côte d'Ivoire, individuals turned to prayer, social support, and diverting their attention from the pain as coping mechanisms. Studies in the U.S. suggests that African Americans are also more likely to rely on support systems and religious coping (prayer) to manage pain. In comparison, whites are more likely to implement techniques such as ignoring the pain, belief in a greater ability to control the pain themselves, or greater faith in Western medicines, whereas Asian patients might disguise their pain, believing it represents "bad karma" (Kwok & Bhuvanakrishna, 2014). Researchers suggest that the differences in strategies may be learned within ethnic groups or cultures and that such differences may affect an individual's awareness of and level of comfort with pain.

Changing Characteristics of Pain

We have identified a number of factors that affect our perception of pain, but there is one more: time. The sensation of pain may differ over time. For example, chronic lower back pain is a common complaint among adults 45 years of age or older (see Figure 10.1). The Health Statistics: National Health Interview Survey (2017) estimates that just over 30% of people ages 45 and older report frequent occurrences of lower back pain (again, see Figure 10.1). Yet pain experienced over weeks or months can appear to be different each day. For example, a person complaining of chronic lower back pain may characterize it as dull but persistent one day and as sharp but intermittent on another. The original source of the pain remains unchanged, yet the perception can change based on a person's subjective assessment of the sensation at the time. Factors that may influence the variable perception include a person's psychological state, mood, and general affect.

The variable manifestations of lower back pain may also contribute to a health care provider's inability to diagnose the problem correctly or lead them to conclude incorrectly that the pain has no identifiable physical cause. They may also deduce that the pain is minor, perhaps resulting from a minor injury, and will cease eventually or that the individual's reports of pain are unreliable. The medical provider's difficulty in diagnosing the cause of the pain or prescribing effective treatment is understandable. But such challenges almost assuredly mean that individuals will experience continued discomfort. In fact, health data for the U.S. show that 57% of older Americans report pain that has endured for more than one year, whereas approximately 37% of younger adults reported similar pain duration. What is more, previous notions that pain and disability caused by injuries are short-lived and will stop once the injury heals are now widely discredited. Instead, researchers find that injury-related pain and disability rapidly decrease in the first three months. After that time, however, progress on both fronts is slow. In many cases, an individual may never be fully free of pain due to injury or return to full and normal functional ability (Tunks, 2008).

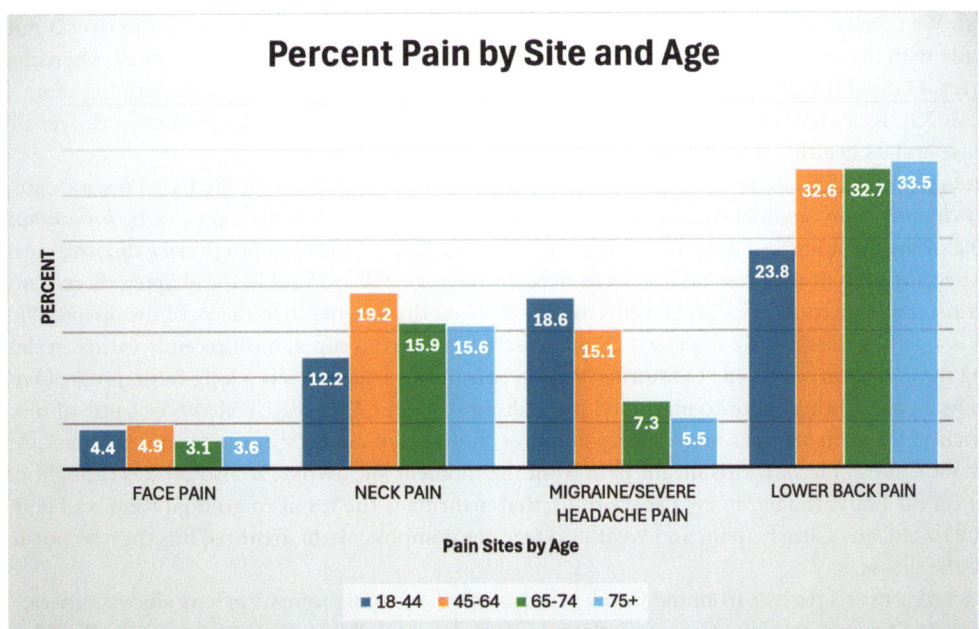

FIGURE 10.1 A bar chart compares experiences with face, next, migraine/severe headache and lower back pain for three age groups: 18–44, 45–64, 65–74 and 75 and over. All Four groups reported more back pain (approximately 24%, 33%, 33% and 34% respectively) than any other type. Reports of face pain were similar for all three groups (ca. 4–5%), neck pain was greater for 45–64 year olds (19%), and 18–24 year reported greater migraine/severe headache than the other groups (19%).

Source: Adapted from Health Statistics: National Health Interview Survey (2017) Table A-5. Migraines and pain in neck, lower back, face, or jaw among adults aged 18 and over, by selected characteristics: United States, 2017 (cdc.gov).

In essence, pain can be an enduring problem. The chronic and unremitting nature of this condition together with subjective perceptions form several reasons why pain is interesting to health psychologists. And because chronic pain will certainly affect a person's overall well-being and perceived quality of life, it is also an example of a physiological health problem that has a direct impact on an individual's emotional and psychological health.

Finally, pain and pain management are also relevant topics for health psychologists when addressing the needs of people with terminal illnesses. Most health care professionals would agree that one goal of health providers when caring for terminally ill patients is to provide *palliative care*, or maximum relief from pain, suffering, and stress due to the illness. The goal is to improve an individual's quality of life for as long as possible. We review selected issues concerning palliative care and end-of-life care in Chapter 13, The Health Psychologist's Role: Research, Application, and Advocacy. For now, it is sufficient to note that end-of-life care presents a host of medical, psychological, and ethical challenges for health care providers, challenges that include chronic pain management.

SECTION II. PAIN AND ARTHRITIS

Now that we have described the physiology of pain and the myriad of factors that may influence pain perception, we turn our attention to examining pain in the context of a disease: arthritis. We began the chapter with a story about Caitlin, a 14-year-old girl diagnosed with juvenile arthritis when she was three years old. We noted that Caitlin was only one of almost 220,000 children in the U.S. and over 3 million worldwide with the disease. This may seem like a large number of sufferers, but it is small when compared to the over 44 million U.S. adults and over 595 million adults worldwide diagnosed with the same illness (IHME, 2023). Research on the characteristics and forms of arthritis for adults presents a clearer picture of the disease and its health outcomes.

For adults, three characteristics define arthritis. First, arthritis is a physiologically based disease caused either by *degeneration* (gradual wearing away or erosion) of the bones near the joints, or by *inflammation*, a swelling of the tissue surrounding the bones and joints. Second, arthritis is a *progressive disease*, meaning that the degeneration or inflammation worsens over time. As we will see later in the chapter, there is no cure for arthritis, nor have treatments proved effective in reversing the degenerative effects of the disease. Finally, arthritis is a chronic disease. We discussed chronic diseases numerous times, most recently earlier in this chapter. Applying the definition of chronic to arthritis, we can conclude that arthritis is a long-term, progressive disease that can be a contributing factor to mortality. It is a distal (Chapter 2, Research Methods) cause of mortality.

For many, the term arthritis immediately conjures thoughts of aches, stiff joints, and soreness. Again, think about Caitlin. Her arthritis meant pain from the moment she awoke. It also evokes thought of wear and tear on the body. In fact, many people think that arthritis is the result of gradual wear and tear on the body due to old age. Clearly, pain and wear and tear are components of arthritis, but they do not fully describe the illness.

The word arthritis derives from the Greek words *arthro*, meaning joints, such as elbows, knees, shoulders, and fingers, and *itis*, meaning inflammation – hence, inflammation of the joints (Pisetsky, 2007). Yet even this is a limited definition. *Arthritis* refers to any painful joint conditions or disease-causing inflammation, pain, and stiffness in the joint or in connective tissues (Harvard Medical School, 2024; Pisetsky, 2007). Therefore, arthritis can describe inflammation of the joints, as is common in rheumatoid arthritis, but it also may refer to the degeneration of the joints commonly found in osteoarthritis. As with juvenile arthritis, the term arthritis is an umbrella term that we use here to describe a painful joint condition due to one of a number of underlying conditions. We begin by examining rheumatoid arthritis.

Types of Arthritis

RHEUMATOID ARTHRITIS (RA) Research on *rheumatoid arthritis (RA)* is still evolving; however, RA is classified at present as a chronic, inflammatory, autoimmune disease for which the exact cause is unknown (Radu & Bungau, 2021; Tedesco et al., 2009). It is considered an inflammatory disease because one characteristic of RA is swelling (inflammation) of the joints and of the *synovium*, the thin layer of tissue that covers the joints.

VIDEO #50/60

Chapter 10: Chronic Pain Management and Arthritis

· **Rheumatoid Arthritis: *Mayo Clinic Minute: What's rheumatoid arthritis?***

· *Website: https://www.youtube.com/watch?v=fNlu2rW9PkY*

· *Mayo Clinic is publicly accessible since it provides medical-based information to the public at no cost. www.mayoclinic.org/*

We also refer to RA as an *autoimmune disease* because it appears that RA is triggered by the body's immune system. We explored the body's immune system in Chapters 6–8 (Emotional Health and Well-Being, Stress and Coping, and Psychoneuroimmunology). The immune system is also relevant to understanding arthritis because inflammation is the body's normal response to injury. You will recall from those chapters that when the body detects an infection or experiences damage to tissue, white blood cells are sent to the affected areas to attack and destroy foreign organisms. The inflammation is an autoimmune system response, designed to protect the body. RA, however, triggers inflammation in the absence of infection or injury. It is a *false alarm* that causes an immune system malfunction, resulting in unnecessary inflammation in addition to possible damage to tissues, blood vessels, and other organs, as well as pain, stiffness, and swelling of the inflamed joints (Pisetsky, 2007; Scherer, Häupl, & Burmester, 2020; Tedesco et al., 2009).

Like other forms of arthritis, rheumatoid arthritis is a progressive disease, meaning that the inflammation, tissue damage, and functional limitations usually become worse over time. In advanced stages of the disease, the joints and the surrounding areas may become deformed, as shown in Figure 10.2.

In addition to the physiological damage, studies show that RA also affects psychological health. The physiological damage to the joints often results in physical disabilities. Inflamed, swollen, and stiff joints reduce an individual's ability or desire to perform tasks that involve the affected joints. For example, arthritis of the hand and finger joints can cause stiffness that limits a person's ability to bend his or her fingers or grasp objects securely (see Figure 10.3). As a result, it can limit a person's ability to perform simple tasks that we take for granted, such as using utensils to eat.

People with RA often identify emotional and psychological health problems as part of the disease. This includes depression, excessive worry, avoidance behavior, and helplessness (Lwin, Serhal, Holroyd, & Edwards, 2020). How frustrating and, perhaps embarrassing, would it be for you if eating took much longer and resulted in spillage or dropped food? How often might you avoid foods that spill easily or even avoid eating to limit the embarrassment to yourself or feelings of helplessness?

People who suffer from RA may face such challenges on a daily basis. It is not difficult to imagine that the aggravation or, as Lazarus calls it, the "daily hassles" (see Chapter 7, Stress and Coping) caused by the physical limitations can result in feelings of incompetence or helplessness when an individual is unable to independently perform routine hygiene or self-help activities that he or she successfully performed in the past. Thus, as we indicated earlier, *functional limitations* or inability to perform daily tasks independently can contribute to depressive symptoms.

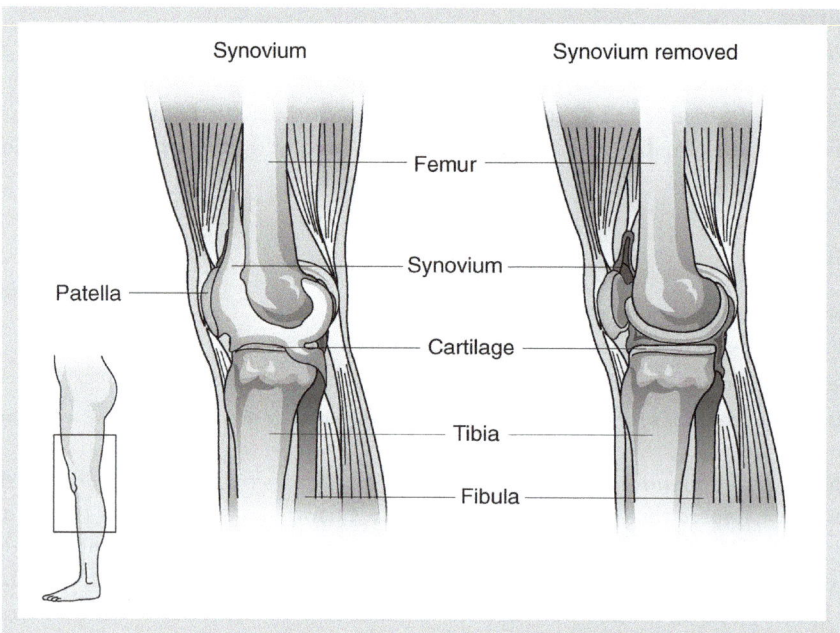

FIGURE 10.2 Effects of rheumatoid arthritis. A cross section of a human leg just above and below the knee shows a normal the femur, synovium, cartliage, tibia & fibula, and these same sections in a person with rheumatoid arthritis. The synovium of the rheumatoid leg is deformed and cartilage is missing.

Source: U.S. National Library of Medicine & National Institutes of Health (2010).

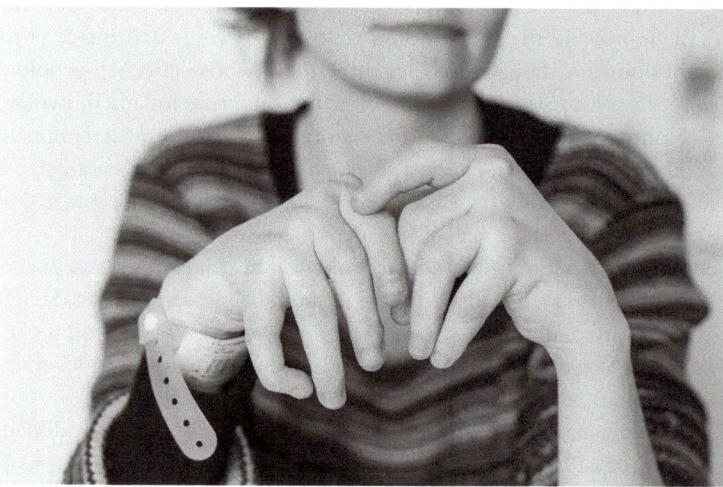

FIGURE 10.3 A photo of a older woman's hands affected by late-stage rheumatoid arthritis. Both hands show swollen knuckle joints and the index fingers on both hands are at an approximately 20 degree angle.

Source: Paul Conklin/PhotoEdit, Inc.

ANKYLOSING SPONDYLITIS (AS) A specific type of RA that affects the spinal joints is *ankylosing spondylitis (AS)*. Also of Greek origin, the word *ankylos* means bent, and *spondylitis* means inflammation of the spinal column. Today, the diagnosis of AS does not suggest a bent, inflamed spinal column but a rigid or stiff spine. The disease usually causes the spinal column to fuse, limiting an individual's ability to pivot or turn his or her neck, or pivot at the waist, a movement that people without AS do effortlessly and without thinking. It may also cause a stooped appearance if the spinal column fuses or stiffens sometimes in a bent or curved position in accordance with poor body posture (Robinson, van der Linden, Khan, & Taylor, 2021; see Figure 10.4).

AS is largely genetic in origin. Many individuals with AS also carry a gene – the **HLA-B27 gene** – that appears to be a marker that predisposes individuals to AS. Remember, however, that having a predisposition does not mean that a person will, in fact, develop the disease or its associated symptoms. In this case, the HLA-B27 gene indicates that a person is more likely than those without the marker to be at high risk for AS.

Research also reveals that AS is closely associated with specific ethnic/racial groups. Studies of individuals with the HLA-B27 gene reveal that approximately 90% of Northern Europeans who are diagnosed with AS and 80% of Mediterranean individuals with AS carry the gene. However, only about 50% of African Americans with AS also have the marker (Khan, 2006). Interestingly, current research indicates that the AS prevalence in the Chinese population is 0.2 to 0.42%. However, among people in China with AS, the HLA-B27 prevalence rate is between 88.5% and 89.4% (Zhang et al., 2022). Thus, it appears that HLA-B27 is highly prevalent in people with AS in China.

Consistent with the characteristics of RA, AS is a progressive inflammatory disease that advances over time. It first appears during adolescence, usually in individuals 15 to 24 years of age (Khan, 2006). Unlike

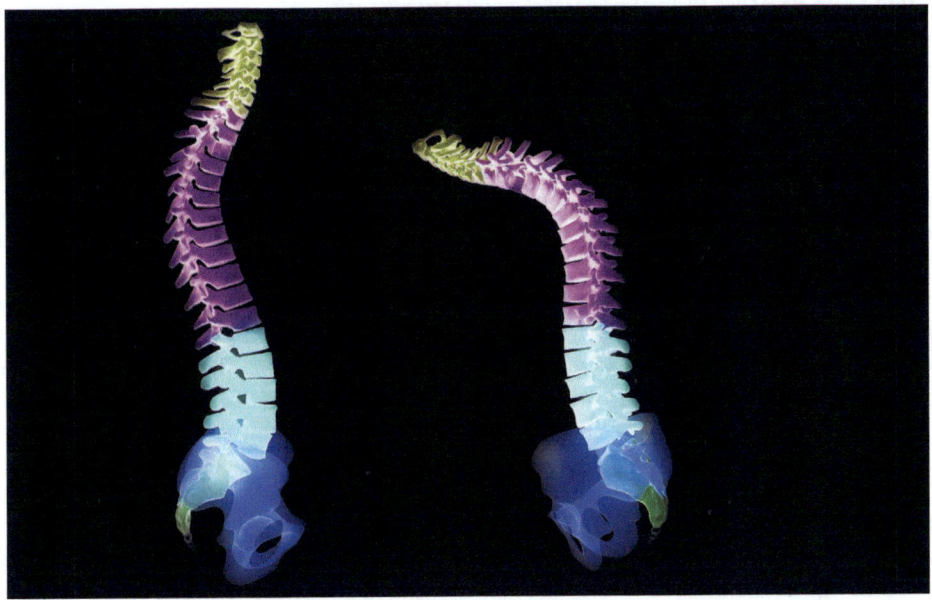

FIGURE 10.4 A normal spine (left) versus one that is affected by ankylosing spondylitis (right). The Ankylosing Spondylitis spine is shorter due to its curvature at the top, an almost 70 degree curve.

Source: Getty Images MedicalRF.Com #56778118.jpg

RA, which occurs more frequently in women than in men, AS appeared to be more prevalent in males (Khan, 2023; Hamilton-West & Quine, 2007). But here we sound another cautionary note. Like the early research on cardiovascular disease in Chapter 9, Cardiovascular Disease, early studies on AS tended to focus primarily on men and led to the conclusion that the disease was more prevalent in males. Recent research has expanded the disease classification and revealed that the disease is roughly equally prevalence in both males and females (Khan, 2023). We include AS in this chapter primarily because it is an interesting genetic version of RA that, in spite of its origins, responds well to psychological therapy when added to medical regimens. We will explain the effects of psychological therapy on arthritis more fully in Section III.

OSTEOARTHRITIS (OA) Approximately 600 million people globally suffer from some form of Osteoarthritis (GBD 2021 Osteoarthritis Collaborators, 2023). *Osteoarthritis (OA)* is the oldest known form of arthritis and was commonly associated with wear and tear on the body. Now, however, it has been reclassified as a disease that affects the entire joint, including the bones, joints, and tissues (Arthritis Foundation, n.d-b). Even the *cartilage*, the part of the joint that cushions the end of the bones and enables easy movement of the joints, is worn away. As a result, *bone spurs* may form. These spurs rub against each other, causing pain and further deterioration of both the cartilage and bones (Arthritis Foundation, n.d-b; Pisetsky, 2007). The erosion process is one reason OA is considered a *degenerative joint disease*, here meaning one that causes the permanent deterioration of cartilage.

VIDEO #51/60

Chapter 10: Chronic Pain Management and Arthritis
- **Osteoarthritis Pain:** *Mayo Clinic Minute: Finding relief for osteoarthritis pain*
- *Website: https://www.youtube.com/watch?v=tva_EQrmOhw*
- *Mayo Clinic is publicly accessible since it provides medical-based information to the public at no cost (www.mayoclinic.org/)*

What causes OA? Like RA, the cause of degeneration is not well understood. Researchers suggest that several factors may play a role in the development and progression of OA, including genetic abnormality, developmental defects, or trauma that alters or disrupts the body's normal biomechanics, including a breakdown of the cartilage and tissues in the joints (National Institute of Arthritis and Musculoskeletal and Skin Disease [NIAMSD], 2023).

OA is most commonly reported in the hand, knee, hip, or foot joints. Unlike RA, which often affects multiple joints simultaneously, OA usually affects a smaller number, perhaps one or two joints. Most often OA targets the larger joints, such as the knee or hip (Pisetsky, 2007). These joints can be repaired by surgery that replaces the kneecaps or hip joints with artificial devices.

GOUT *Gout* is an increasingly common disease that is more prevalent in men than women and the prevalence rates increase with age (Dehlin, Jacobsson, & Roddy, 2020). Currently, the global prevalence rate ranges from 1% to 6.8% (Dehlin et al., 2020).

Researchers suggest that gout is caused by crystal deposits in joints and tissues (Doherty, 2009). Sometimes called "gouty arthritis," it is also strongly associated with the environment, behavior (i.e. dietary factors and obesity), and genetics (Dehlin et al., 2020; Doherty, 2009).

Let's look at diet. A buildup of *uric acid*, a by-product of foods eliminated from our bodies as waste products, becomes lodged in the joints and causes inflammation, redness, and soreness (National

Institute of Arthritis & Musculoskeletal & Skin Diseases, 2006). Behaviors such as overeating, excessive consumption of red meat, and excessive alcohol consumption (especially beer) are known contributors to gout (Annemans et al., 2008; Fields, 2024). As such, some types of gout are preventable with changes in diet, a health behavior or lifestyle issue. Is it no surprise, then, that health psychologists are well suited to help people with gout adopt new, healthier behaviors that will significantly affect their gout?

Some research suggests that gout may also be caused by genetic factors. Genetic disorders associated with an overproduction of uric acid, though rare, have been found primarily among males and within families (Doherty, 2009; Fields, 2024).

To review, arthritis is a painful disease that causes inflammation and deformities in joints, appendages, or even the torso, as in the case of ankylosing spondylitis. It is not a life-threatening disease and rarely is a proximal cause of death. It is, however, a painful, chronic condition that has a significant impact on daily functioning, psychological health, and overall well-being. For many arthritis sufferers, addressing this health condition means primarily reducing the pain to manageable levels to improve overall quality of life and daily functioning.

Measuring Pain

So far we have reviewed the physical, psychological, and psychosocial etiology of pain. We have examined one illness for which aching, soreness, and other discomforts are the core symptoms. And we noted in all of these discussions that researchers and practitioners face challenges when assessing and measuring pain. That brings us to our current discussion of pain measurement. Efforts to more effectively study, diagnose, and manage pain have been hampered by four factors: accurate measures of pain, the changing characteristics of pain, pain management versus pain elimination, and gender and cultural differences in the classification of pain. We address each of these issues in the following sections and illustrate how they apply to chronic arthritis pain.

PAIN INSTRUMENTS We noted earlier that pain is a challenging concept to measure. It is influenced by an individual's subjective perception of discomfort, by their accurate or inaccurate recall of the pain and its location, and by a provider's assessment of the physiological symptoms. If you add to these points the fact that pain is a private and internal sensation that cannot be observed directly and that it may include changing symptoms, then you may understand why pain is sometimes considered an elusive health problem (Heir, Ananthan, Kalladka, Kuchukulla, & Renton, 2023; Ghazisaeidi, Muley, & Salter, 2023; Gregus, Levine, Eddinger, Yaksh, & Buczynski, 2021).

Pain is best understood as the interaction of a painful stimulus (biological or environmental) experienced by the body, the characteristics of the individual experiencing pain, such as his or her age, gender, and coping strategies, and the social and environmental circumstances, such as cultural upbringing, that may proscribe an individual's perception of or response to pain (Tran, Koven, Castro, Goya Arce, & Carter, 2020). But measuring these individual factors and their interaction is complicated by the absence of comprehensive assessment instruments. Earlier, we identified some experimental measures used to identify genetic, biological, or brain indications of pain. Unfortunately, these measures are intended for use in laboratory studies. They are not easily administered in nonlaboratory settings.

Some of the studies cited earlier used self-administered surveys to corroborate genetic or biological measures. When assessing pain in a health psychologist's office, a medical provider's office, or another non-laboratory setting, practitioners and researchers most often choose from one of over 80 pain-assessment measures currently in use. Many of these measures are self-assessment instruments. These measures focus largely on one dimension: either a pain intensity or duration dimension or a measure of a specific type of pain (Hjermstad et al., 2008). Although pain and intensity are important components, research shows that eight additional factors (in addition to intensity or duration) may present a fuller understanding of the phenomenon: temporal pattern, treatment effect (including relief/exacerbating factors), pain quality, location, interference, affect, pain history, and beliefs about pain (including attitudes, coping, and beliefs about causes and consequences of pain; Hjermstad et al., 2008). Presently, few assessment instruments include all ten factors. For this reason, a health provider's ability to fully characterize an individual's pain is limited often to one assessed factor and the individual's own descriptive abilities.

SELF-ASSESSMENT MEASURES Researchers and practitioners must employ some method to assess the level of discomfort caused by chronic pain. One approach therefore is to use one of three types of self-assessment measures: verbal or written questionnaires, behavioral observations, or visual analogue pain ratings. *Verbal or written questionnaires* allow respondents to characterize their pain (dull, sharp, throbbing), describe its duration (minutes, hours, weeks), rate its intensity, usually on a scale of 1 to 10, and explain any functional limitations resulting from the pain. The Brief Pain Inventory (see Figure 10.5) is an example of an assessment instrument that focuses primarily on level of severity of pain as well as related functional limitations. Respondents rate their level of pain and their functional ability using a number of Likert scales (see Chapter 2, Research Methods). For example, one question on the scale asks, "Please rate your pain by circling the one number that best describes your pain at its LEAST in the past 24 hours." Responses to this question range from "No pain" with a corresponding score of 0 to "Pain as bad as you can imagine" with a score of 10 (Cleeland & Ryan, 1994).

By comparison, Melzack's (yes, the one who gave us the gate control theory) McGill Pain Questionnaire (1975) uses 102 items to assess pain along three dimensions: the sensory quality of the pain (cool, cold, or hot), the affective qualities of pain (pain or exhaustion), and the subjective intensity of the experience (pain that is annoying, intense, or unbearable). Individuals rate their pain experience by selecting the appropriate word or by indicating pain intensity on a scale of 1 to 10.

To be sure, both the Brief Pain Inventory and the McGill Pain Questionnaire provide subjective assessments of pain and pain tolerance. But an individual's perception of pain will influence his or her likely participation in activities of daily living or dependence on others for assistance. What is more, as we indicated earlier, a person who perceives himself or herself to be dependent on others due to chronic pain may feel helpless or become depressed as a result of the inability to function independently. For these reasons, some of the pain questionnaires also assess an individual's psychological state. For example, the Brief Pain Inventory includes three questions intended to assess an individual's emotional state. Although more would be preferred, the questions can identify psychological health issues due to pain that will contribute to a person's overall sense of well-being.

OBJECTIVE OBSERVATION MEASURES A second technique for assessing pain obtains *behavioral observations* of an individual's functional ability in one of two situations: during a health care visit with a medical or other health care professional or during the execution of daily activities as observed by relatives, friends, or caregivers. When conducted as part of a health care visit, the observed individual performs assigned tasks that test the flexibility or maneuverability of the affected joints. For example, when assessing the pain levels associated with arthritis, health care providers document the limitations of movement and any associated expressions of pain using a standard assessment form, such as the Patient Evaluation Conference System Form (Harvey & Jellinek, 1981), to score the person on his or her functional and psychological status. The assessment measures physical mobility, activities of daily living (hygiene, dressing, etc.), use of devices (crutches, cane, or wheelchair), pain behavior, and psychology, among others.

1903

PLEASE USE
BLACK INK PEN

Date: ☐☐ / ☐☐ / ☐☐☐
(month) (day) (year)

Subject's Initials : _____

Study Subject #: ☐☐☐☐

Study Name: _____

Protocol #: _____
PI: _____
Revision: 07/01/05

Brief Pain Inventory (Short Form)

1. **Throughout our lives, most of us have had pain from time to time (such as minor headaches, sprains, and toothaches). Have you had pain other than these everyday kinds of pain today?**

☐ Yes   ☐ No

2. **On the diagram, shade in the areas where you feel pain. Put an X on the area that hurts the most.**

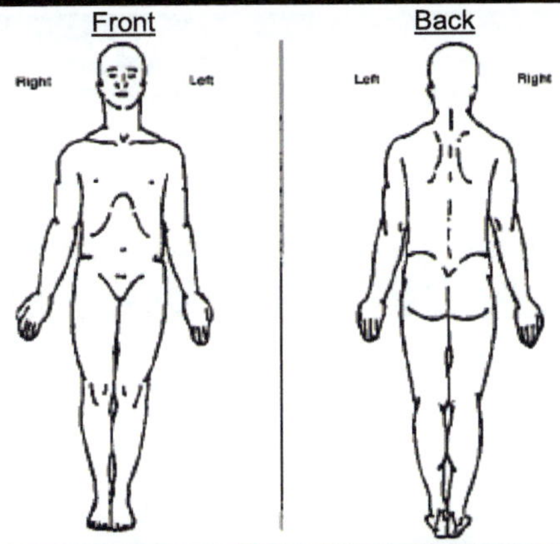

Front   Back

Right   Left   Left   Right

3. **Please rate your pain by marking the box beside the number that best describes your pain at its** worst **in the last 24 hours.**

☐ 0   ☐ 1   ☐ 2   ☐ 3   ☐ 4   ☐ 5   ☐ 6   ☐ 7   ☐ 8   ☐ 9   ☐ 10
No   Pain As Bad As
Pain   You Can Imagine

4. **Please rate your pain by marking the box beside the number that best describes your pain at its** least **in the last 24 hours.**

☐ 0   ☐ 1   ☐ 2   ☐ 3   ☐ 4   ☐ 5   ☐ 6   ☐ 7   ☐ 8   ☐ 9   ☐ 10
No   Pain As Bad As
Pain   You Can Imagine

5. **Please rate your pain by marking the box beside the number that best describes your pain on the** average.

☐ 0   ☐ 1   ☐ 2   ☐ 3   ☐ 4   ☐ 5   ☐ 6   ☐ 7   ☐ 8   ☐ 9   ☐ 10
No   Pain As Bad As
Pain   You Can Imagine

6. **Please rate your pain by marking the box beside the number that tells how much pain you have** right now.

☐ 0   ☐ 1   ☐ 2   ☐ 3   ☐ 4   ☐ 5   ☐ 6   ☐ 7   ☐ 8   ☐ 9   ☐ 10
No   Pain As Bad As
Pain   You Can Imagine

Page 1 of 2

FIGURE 10.5 Brief Pain Inventory (Short Form). An outline of a human figure (front and back) is used on the Brief Pain Inventory to identify the site of pain on the body.

Source: Cleeland & Ryan (1994). www.npcrc.org/files/news/briefpain_short.pdf

1903

Date: [ ] [ ] / [ ] [ ] / [ ] [ ]
(month)   (day)   (year)

Subject's Initials : _____

Study Subject #: [ ] [ ] [ ]

Study Name: _____

Protocol #: _____
PI: _____

Revision: 07/01/05

---

7. What treatments or medications are you receiving for your pain?

8. In the last 24 hours, how much relief have pain treatments or medications provided? Please mark the box below the percentage that most shows how much relief you have received.

0%	10%	20%	30%	40%	50%	60%	70%	80%	90%	100%
☐	☐	☐	☐	☐	☐	☐	☐	☐	☐	☐
No Relief										Complete Relief

9. Mark the box beside the number that describes how, during the past 24 hours, pain has interfered with your:

A. General Activity

☐ 0   ☐ 1   ☐ 2   ☐ 3   ☐ 4   ☐ 5   ☐ 6   ☐ 7   ☐ 8   ☐ 9   ☐ 10
Does Not Interfere   Completely Interferes

B. Mood

☐ 0   ☐ 1   ☐ 2   ☐ 3   ☐ 4   ☐ 5   ☐ 6   ☐ 7   ☐ 8   ☐ 9   ☐ 10
Does Not Interfere   Completely Interferes

C. Walking ability

☐ 0   ☐ 1   ☐ 2   ☐ 3   ☐ 4   ☐ 5   ☐ 6   ☐ 7   ☐ 8   ☐ 9   ☐ 10
Does Not Interfere   Completely Interferes

D. Normal Work (includes both work outside the home and housework)

☐ 0   ☐ 1   ☐ 2   ☐ 3   ☐ 4   ☐ 5   ☐ 6   ☐ 7   ☐ 8   ☐ 9   ☐ 10
Does Not Interfere   Completely Interferes

E. Relations with other people

☐ 0   ☐ 1   ☐ 2   ☐ 3   ☐ 4   ☐ 5   ☐ 6   ☐ 7   ☐ 8   ☐ 9   ☐ 10
Does Not Interfere   Completely Interferes

F. Sleep

☐ 0   ☐ 1   ☐ 2   ☐ 3   ☐ 4   ☐ 5   ☐ 6   ☐ 7   ☐ 8   ☐ 9   ☐ 10
Does Not Interfere   Completely Interferes

G. Enjoyment of life

☐ 0   ☐ 1   ☐ 2   ☐ 3   ☐ 4   ☐ 5   ☐ 6   ☐ 7   ☐ 8   ☐ 9   ☐ 10
Does Not Interfere   Completely Interferes

FIGURE 10.5 Continued

The functional assessment conducted by family, friends, or a caregiver, identifies any diminished capacity on tasks of daily living. This includes, but is not limited to, preparing a meal, playing a game, various writing tasks, and attention to ongoing events such as a television program or current events. Recall that in Chapter 7, Stress and Coping, we read that Lazarus and Folkman (1984b) theorized that diminished functional capacity created the type of daily hassles that may lead to depression. Thus, according to their theory, a functional assessment of an individual should include an assessment of his or her psychological state.

VISUAL ANALOGUE MEASURES Finally, as a third technique, researchers may choose to use *visual analogue measures* to rate pain severity. Scott and Huskisson (1976) popularized visual analogue measures in the 1970s. The typical scale includes a straight, vertical line capped at each end with words that describe pain severity. For example, Huskisson chose "pain as bad as it could be" to appear at the top of the vertical line and "no pain" to appear at the bottom (Scott & Huskisson, 1976). Here individuals are instructed to place a mark along the vertical continuum to indicate the pain level experienced as a result of a specific injury or illness. One property of all three types of pain assessment instruments described here is that they all measure an individual's tolerance for pain.

To review, pain may be assessed using one or more of three principal techniques: self-reported questionnaires or interviews, behavioral observations conducted by health care providers or individuals in frequent contact with the observed individual, or visual analogues. Research suggests that pain reports are, for the most part, subjective and vary as a function of gender and ethnicity. As we mentioned before, it is the case that self-reported pain from some ethnic groups is frequently underestimated and undertreated, and in those instances, additional measures should be adopted to confirm and, for the individual, reaffirm their experiences with pain.

Pain Management versus Pain Elimination

Much of the research on chronic pain focuses on two main processes, *pain management* and *pain elimination*. Research and intervention efforts emphasize pain minimization or management. There is no proven, effective treatment that offers total and complete relief from pain related to chronic disorders (Crombez, Eccleston, Van Hamme, & De Vlieger, 2008; De Oliveira et al., 2020; Friedrichsdorf & Goubert, 2020; Fregoso, Wang, Tseng, & Wang, 2019). In addition, as Tunks (2008) points out, injury-related pain also focuses on management because often such injury-related discomforts linger well beyond the point of treatment, in some cases, for years afterward. Consider this: There are millions of high school, college, and professional athletes. These athletes suffer sports-related injuries often – so often, in fact, that there is a special branch of medicine known as sports medicine. Initially, some sports injuries may be treated with drug therapies. Others require surgery to repair torn or broken elements, and still others are addressed through some form of physical therapy, such as exercise and strength-building techniques. Whatever the therapy, you can be sure that the injury itself, as well as the process of repair, will entail some level of pain: pain at the point of injury, discomfort during the repair and healing process, and possibly intermittent or persistent aching and soreness once the injury is resolved.

Severe athletic injuries will require more than medical and exercise treatments. For some individuals, healing from sports-related injuries will also include psychotherapy. Consider another example: A baseball pitcher or a champion butterfly swimmer who injures his or her *rotator cuff*, one of four muscles in the shoulder, will experience severe pain and be unable to rotate the arm as needed to perform his or her sport. The damage may be severe enough to warrant surgical repair. However, even after surgery and physical therapy, the pitcher or competitive swimmer may face additional challenges. In some instances, surgery and physical therapy will be sufficient to return the athlete to full or near full form. But in other instances, the damage may be too severe. Even though surgery may repair the shoulder muscle sufficiently to allow the pitcher or swimmer to perform most daily activities, it may not permit the type of repetitive motion and strenuous exertion required in either sport. In such cases, the individual must learn more than how to cope until the shoulder muscle heals. The athlete may need to learn to cope with feelings of loss, disappointment, or dismay as he or she adjusts to a life without a favorite pastime or a preferred career.

VIDEO #52/60

Chapter 10: Chronic Pain Management and Arthritis
- **Rotator Cuff:** *Learn About Rotator Cuff Damage*
- *Website: https://www.youtube.com/watch?v=vEtxetU3dJc*
- **The Mayo Clinic is publicly accessible to provide accurate and reliable details about various medical conditions (***Rotator cuff injury – Symptoms and causes – Mayo Clinic***)**

There is little doubt that such a change will present significant psychological health consequences in addition to likely ongoing challenges to pain management. It is in such situations that health psychologists can assist people with their feelings of loss and perhaps depression following their inability to resume their activities. Using coping strategies, cognitive-behavioral therapies, or other psychotherapeutic techniques described in Chapter 7, Stress and Coping, and Chapter 11, Cancer, health psychologists can aid athletes in adapting to their new limitations. They may find productive ways to use their limited athletic skills or adopt new interests. Whatever their choice, they will find that the healing process requires both physical and psychological adjustments.

SECTION III. PHARMACOLOGICAL AND PSYCHOTHERAPEUTIC MANAGEMENT OF PAIN

In this section, we continue our discussion of pain management by exploring a sample of medical, psychological, and alternative therapies to address arthritis pain. The methods used to treat most forms of arthritis include pharmacological measures (drugs), exercise, and, more recently, psychological and alternative therapies. But as we noted earlier, treatments for the pain associated with arthritis have met with very mixed results. A discussion of the full range of medical treatments available to treat arthritis is beyond the scope of this book. Rather, in this section, we explore a limited number of pharmacological therapies with specific references to arthritis outcomes. We also examine how psychological and alternative (sometimes called complementary) therapies, either independently or together with pharmacological treatments, improve pain management.

Medical Therapies for Arthritis

Medically, health care providers use one of three types of treatments, either alone or in combination with other therapies: nonsteroidal anti-inflammatory drugs (NSAIDs), which are drugs that reduce the pain and inflammation associated with arthritis; opioid analgesics, narcotic substances generally used to treat non-cancer pain; or the newest agent in the arsenal of NSAIDs, anti-tumor necrosis factor (anti-TNF) drugs.

NONSTEROIDAL ANTI-INFLAMMATION DRUGS (NSAIDS) Aspirin is the mildest *nonsteroidal anti-inflammatory drug* available to control mild, arthritis-related symptoms of inflammation and pain. When taken in low doses, aspirin is a relatively safe medication. However, to relieve the inflammation and stiffness associated with arthritis, aspirin must be taken frequently and in high doses, a dosing practice that can cause other health problems (Fiala & Pasic, 2020). Research has shown that aspirin in high doses causes disruptive effects on the urinary and digestive tract and can result in stomach ulcers, a limitation of an aspirin regimen for arthritis. An ulcer is essentially a hole in the stomach's lining. Ulcers present a problem because the hole allows the gastric juices from the stomach to irritate other body systems. If severe, the hole may not be repaired but only treated with medication and a restricted diet. Such a diet would exclude aspirin and other medications that similarly can irritate the stomach. Therefore, a high-dose aspirin therapy needed to control arthritis pain and inflammation has risky side effects, can limit the effective use of other medications, and must be used only with medical supervision.

Other NSAIDs that are also effective in reducing inflammation include *ibuprofen*, a generic drug more commonly known by the brand names Motrin, Advil, or Excedrin. Ibuprofen, regardless of the manufacturer, can also cause stomach distress and thus poses similar risks to those of aspirin regimens. Somewhat stronger NSAIDs include *naproxen* – brand name Aleve – and *ketoprofen* – brand name Acton (Khan, 2006). Naproxen and ketoprofen are believed to be more effective because they block the body's natural production of *COX-1* and *COX-2*, enzymes that help protect the stomach lining (COX-1) and that produce inflammation (COX-2).

The advantage of non-aspirin NSAIDs is that they appear to be more effective than aspirin in minimizing pain. They also may cause fewer gastrointestinal or digestive problems, bleeding, stroke, or renal damage (Bjordal, Klovning, Ljunggren, & Slordal, 2007; Davis & Robson, 2016). Yet they are considered inadequate pain relievers because they do not totally relieve pain and stiffness. In fact, individuals who use NSAIDs report relief from 80% of pain at best (Khan, 2006), adequate to allow someone to resume daily functions while tolerating a reduced level of pain. What is more, NSAIDs do not appear to slow or reverse the progression of the disease. They are therefore moderate pain relievers that manage symptoms and minimize pain but do not address the underlying disease.

OPIOID ANALGESICS *Opioid analgesics*, commonly known as opioids, are a second type of drug therapy that researchers and practitioners believe to be more effective than NSAIDs in alleviating pain. We discuss opioids in Chapter 5, Risky Health Behaviors, Part I. The most potent pain relievers known to medicine, opioids are often called the "gold standard" for treating severe pain (Size, Soyannwo, & Justins, 2007). This powerful pain-killing substance was used as early as 4000 BCE when the Sumerians of Mesopotamia (current-day Iraq and parts of Iran) discovered that opium could suppress pain and put an individual in a calm, somewhat sedate state of consciousness.

We will not repeat the pros and cons of opioid uses here and refer you to Chapter 5, Risky Health Behaviors, Part I for a full review.

ANTI-TUMOR NECROSIS FACTOR (ANTI-TNF) DRUGS The newest NSAIDs drug treatment for arthritis, *anti-tumor necrosis factor drugs*, also has positive and negative effects. Anti-TNF drugs are unique because, unlike other *pharmacological therapies*, they significantly reduce pain and stop the progression of the disease. Far more effective than other NSAIDs and free of the addictive properties of opioid analgesics, anti-TNF drugs work quickly and are effective in a variety of arthritic conditions, including ankylosing spondylitis, the genetic form of arthritis mentioned earlier. Current versions of this drug are known as *adalimumab* (brand name Humira), *infliximab* (brand name Remicade), and *etanercept* (brand name Enbrel).

By now you may be asking, "What is the catch?" If anti-TNFs are the most effective treatment for arthritis, why are they not the drug of choice for arthritis? There are several "catches." First, TNFs fight the body's natural inflammation process. We mentioned earlier that inflammation is a natural immune system process for fighting infections. Anti-TNFs lower the body's natural production of inflammation, leaving an individual vulnerable to infections, and thus increase the probability of illnesses. Nevertheless, because anti-TNFs are effective in stopping the progression of the disease, many physicians recommend these drugs while monitoring carefully the user's immune responses.

A second "catch" is the administration process: These drug must be given by injection. Although adalimumab and etanercept can be injected at home by an individual, infliximab is taken intravenously, meaning an injection by needle into the veins, a procedure that must be done by a medical provider. This means that either the user must be comfortable with self-administered injections, or plan regular trips to their provider for treatment. If self-administered at home, the user faces the added issue of how to dispose of the syringes responsibly.

Finally, anti-TNF drugs are expensive. The full retail cost (assuming no health insurance supplement) of a year's supply of either drug in 2019 ranged from approximately $57,000 to $70,000 in the U.S. (San-Juan-Rodriguez, Piro, Good, Gellad, & Hernandez, 2021). Clearly, without health insurance in the U.S. to offset the costs, anti-TNF drugs may be unaffordable. We explore the role of health insurance companies in providing or restricting access to medicines in Chapter 12, Health Care Systems and Health Policy.

In sum, drug-treatment approaches to arthritis have a number of limitations. Only opioids control pain totally, but the addictive properties of opioids make them an unacceptable long-term treatment option for chronic arthritic pain. NSAIDs, although safer, are less effective for pain management and carry high risks associated with gastrointestinal distress. Anti-TNFs, the newest drugs available, carry higher risk of susceptibility to infection and are likely to be unaffordable without health insurance. It is no surprise, therefore, that researchers and physicians look to additional therapies to treat arthritis.

Alternative Therapies

EXERCISE THERAPIES In earlier chapters, we indicated that exercise is an effective treatment for some illnesses. We noted the beneficial effects of exercise for cardiovascular health (see Chapter 9, Cardiovascular Disease), stress reduction (see Chapter 7, Stress and Coping), and emotional health and overall well-being (see Chapter 6, Emotional Health and Well-Being). Exercise is beneficial for individuals with arthritis also but for somewhat different reasons.

The inflammation and stiffness that result from arthritis can make movement of the affected joints very painful. As arthritis sufferers know, exercise will minimize pain and improve functionality in the long term. Therefore, we have a dilemma: How do we convince someone to engage in daily exercise regimens that will be very painful in the short term but beneficial in the long term? And how do we make exercise a sustainable behavior that individuals will continue for the rest of their lives?

This is precisely the type of problem best suited to the work of health psychologists. Exercise therapies for individuals with arthritis are one form of behavioral intervention designed by health psychologists. The therapies may be one-on-one interventions administered by a *physical therapist*, an individual trained in techniques that provide maximum movement and flexibility. Individual therapies may be customized to work on specific regions of the body and to improve specific motor functions. They usually include stretching and weight-bearing exercises to improve both mobility and strength. Alternatively, therapies may be conducted in a group exercise program that aims to improve range of movement or to target specific regions of the body that are often cited as painful or problem sites. The goal of individual as well as group exercise-therapy programs is to increase an individual's range of movement while decreasing his or her pain levels.

For health psychologists the goals of such programs are somewhat different. They too want to increase movement and decrease pain. They also seek to motivate individuals to do something that is not immediately gratifying and that will increase their pain burdens in the short term but which will have long-term benefits. In many ways, the problem is analogous to healthy eating intervention programs introduced in Chapter 9, Cardiovascular Disease. Such programs identified the difficulty of convincing individuals with cardiovascular disease to forgo the sweet, starchy, and high-fat foods that are tasty and easy to obtain, substituting them with high-fiber foods that may be less appealing but that will improve cardiovascular health in the near future. Likewise, research by health psychologists on chronic arthritic pain show that although long-term adherence to an exercise regimen is one of the best methods for reducing the pain, stiffness, and inflammation caused by arthritis, the exercises are initially painful and may be a disincentive (Gyurcsik, Cary, Sessford, Flora, & Brawley, 2014; Iversen et al., 2016).

With few exceptions, studies on exercise therapy for arthritis show that individuals report significant decreases in pain after short-term exercise regimens (Karlsson et al., 2020; Siddall et al., 2022). However, longer regimens that involve more strength training are better. For example, studies of individuals enrolled in Pilates and aerobic exercise classes show that participants were as likely to report significant improved movement in both Pilates and aerobic exercises, but pain was best alleviated with Pilates. And comparisons between high-versus low-intensity exercise programs revealed that high-intensity exercise programs were effective while low-intensity exercise programs were not only less effective than high-intensity ones, but they were also no better than the no-exercise group (McDermott et al., 2021; Yentür, Ataş, Öztürk, & Oskay, 2021).

Other research report on the benefits of yoga and pain remediation. A study by Tekur, Singphon, Nagendra, and Raghuram (2008) found that participants in a one-week intensive residential yoga program reported significant reduction on disability measures when compared with those assigned to the physical exercise group. The yoga group, which received instruction in physical posture, breathing practices, and the philosophical concepts of yoga, also reported greater flexibility of the spine and spinal extension than the control group. Similarly, Tilbrook and colleagues (2011) report better functioning for the yoga group participants in their study than for those treated to a non-exercise, usual-care program. However, Tilbrook's findings remind us of the difficulties in sustaining such outcomes. Their post-test assessments of both groups found better functioning for the yoga group than for the usual-care group at three, six, and 12 months after the 12-session program. However, when assessing self-efficacy, another important criteria for improved functioning, the yoga group and the usual-care group reported similar levels 12 months after the program.

One impediment to the success of such exercise programs is barriers to participation. If normal movement is painful, it will be challenging to convince people with arthritis that more intense movement or exercise will hurt less in the long run. Tilbrook's study reported that only 60% of the participants attended at least four of the 12 yoga classes. Therefore, in spite of the fact that the yoga group demonstrated measurable improvement in functioning ability over the control group, 40% of the yoga group missed eight or more classes. To overcome such barriers, health psychologists can match individuals with exercises that appeal to their interests. For example, people who usually enjoy recreational or competitive swimming may be more likely to participate in water aerobics programs, something they can enjoy while reaping the therapeutic benefits of exercise at the same time. Likewise, individuals who enjoy exercising with free weights might find that working with a physical trainer on a program of strength building may have a similar appeal.

The goal of exercise programs is to connect people with arthritis or other forms of chronic pain to a program that is both therapeutically beneficial and enjoyable. By matching an individual to his or her preferred physical activity, health psychologists may be more likely to improve retention rates in programs and to obtain good immediate and long-term outcomes. As we noted in Chapter 3, Theories and Models of Health Behavior Change, psychological theories or models, together with social-marketing techniques, may offer health psychologists tools to encourage initiation of exercise regimes and to improve adherence in the long term.

Psychotherapeutic Treatments

Drug and exercise therapies each provide limited relief for the pain and discomfort of arthritis. But the perception of pain, the frustrations associated with limitations of movement and their consequences for daily functioning affect the psychological well-being of persons with arthritis. What is more, researchers have shown that an individual's psychological state can and does affect their disease progression. Therefore, it is logical that therapies that address the psychological effects of the disease must be included as part of a holistic health approach to chronic diseases.

PSYCHOLOGICAL INTERVENTIONS It bears repeating that arthritis is a physiological illness. However, the inability of drug and exercise therapies to address the psychological factors that also affect arthritis offers a strong rationale for including psychological interventions in all arthritis-treatment plans (Turk, Swanson, & Tunks, 2008). Such arguments have been proposed by a number of researchers. For example, recently Dixon, Keefe, Scipio, Perri, and Abernethy (2007) examined the effectiveness of psychological therapies on arthritis management and outcomes. These researchers conducted a *meta-analysis*, a review of the findings of relevant studies, of the psychological interventions used most often as part of a combination therapy for individuals with arthritis. Their study revealed five frequently used treatments: cognitive-behavioral therapy for pain-management/pain-coping skills training, biofeedback, stress management, emotional disclosure, and *psychodynamic therapy*. Of the five modalities, they found cognitive-behavioral therapy (CBT) to be the most frequently used and most successful technique in addressing arthritic pain.

Cognitive-Behavioral Therapy (CBT) *Cognitive-behavioral therapy (CBT)* involves four key components: education, skills acquisition, skills consolidation, and generalization and maintenance (Turk et al., 2008). The aim of CBT is to help individuals remove self-imposed inhibitions to independent functioning based on their fear of pain and feelings of helplessness (Turk et al., 2008). If this seems similar to the concept of self-efficacy introduced in Chapter 3, Theories and Models of Health Behavior Change, it is. CBT encourages individuals to realize that they can manage their pain independently by mastering their pain, their fear of pain, and their feelings of frustration and hopelessness.

Turk and colleagues identify assumptions about the cognitive-behavioral approach which further illustrate the relationship between this approach and Bandura's model. Most noteworthy is their assertion of reciprocal determinism (Turk et al., 2008). Do you remember this from our discussion of Bandura? Turk and colleagues, like Bandura, propose that behavior is reciprocally determined by the individual and by the environment (see Chapter 3, Theories and Models of Health Behavior Change; Figure 3.1).

In addition, Turk and colleagues assert that in the cognitive-behavior process people are mentally engaged in the management of their problems. They are active, not passive, processors of information. As such, their active thought processes can affect their mood and their physiological processes and can have social consequences (Turk et al., 2008). Turk and colleagues also propose that people can learn more adaptive ways of thinking, feeling, and behaving. This too is suggestive of Bandura's model. Bandura proposed that one of the ways we learn is through our engagement in our world. This learning can be direct, vicarious, persuasory, or inferred (see Chapter 3, Theories and Models of Health Behavior Change). In essence, the cognitive-behavioral approach to the management of physical ailments borrows extensively from earlier theories that outline processes for learning and shaping our behaviors as well as our behavioral responses to our environment.

There is one additional important note specific to CBT. Although CBT is recognized as the most successful form of psychological intervention for the management of arthritis pain, it can and often does include elements of other psychological techniques, such as stress management, biofeedback, and hypnosis (Turk et al., 2008).

Biofeedback A second commonly used psychotherapeutic approach to pain management is *biofeedback*, a self-regulatory technique in which individuals learn to voluntarily control their responses to pain to minimize its sensations (American Psychological Association, 2024). The goal is to teach people to control the physiological process and to re-regulate the autonomic nervous system (Turk et al., 2008). You may remember from Chapter 6, Emotional Health and Well-Being, that the autonomic nervous system includes two subsystems, the sympathetic nervous system and the parasympathetic nervous system, both of which are essential in our response to stress. Some researchers contend that stress is another major contributing factor to arthritis pain. Therefore the biofeedback approach uses *stress management* techniques to manage pain. The assumption is that management of pain will lead to improved control of arthritic pain symptoms (Dixon et al., 2007).

Emotional Disclosure The third technique, *emotional disclosure*, is used less frequently than either CBT or biofeedback. Emotional-disclosure therapy is based on the assumption that current and past unresolved issues create stressors that are poorly managed. It supports the notion that stress contributes to arthritic pain. Like biofeedback, therefore, emotional disclosure includes stress management as a critical component in minimizing the pain of arthritis.

In emotional disclosure, individuals talk or write about traumatic experiences and associated emotions over three or four consecutive days. Researchers believe that by releasing suppressed feelings about traumatic events, people with arthritis also obtain relief from the stress and other related pain that aggravates arthritis.

Emotional-disclosure therapy has been tested on individuals with RA and those with ankylosing spondylitis. Findings suggest that both groups report an improvement in immune functions and lower levels of pain and disease progression than individuals in control groups who were not given emotional-disclosure conditions (Hamilton-West & Quine, 2007).

Emotional disclosure may be conceptually similar to psychodynamic techniques that also seek to address unresolved conflicts that contribute to pain (Palmieri et al., 2022). There is one main difference in the two theories: Psychodynamic therapies assume that the underlying emotions contributing to the arthritic discomfort are unknown, whereas in emotional disclosure the traumatic events may be known but not discussed or resolved previously.

In general, whether using CBT alone or in combination with other psychological techniques, researchers found that individuals using psychological interventions report improvements in pain coping, pain self-efficacy, anxiety, depression, and physical and psychological disability (Dixon et al., 2007; Palmiere et al., 2022). In essence, psychological interventions contribute significantly to the emotional and physical well-being of individuals with arthritis and are a necessary component of care for chronic arthritis. It goes without saying, therefore, that health psychologists can and have made significant contributions to the treatment and management of arthritis through the psychological intervention techniques that now are a standard part of many treatment regimens for arthritis.

In sum, arthritis is a chronic condition that affects quality of life and overall well-being. Although it is a physiological condition, a significant component of treatment for arthritis is pain management. In fact, the pain associated with arthritis is often cited as the most irritating and troublesome part of the disease. Pharmacological (drug) and exercise treatments alone are insufficient remedies for the pain caused by arthritis. Current treatments recommend an interdisciplinary approach that includes medical, exercise, and psychological interventions.

The three-therapy approach to arthritis does not mask the fact that no current treatment can eliminate arthritis pain entirely. The point here is that the combination-therapy approach can and does reduce pain levels more effectively than any single therapeutic technique. Remember that absent a cure for arthritis, the goal remains to reduce pain levels so that arthritis sufferers are able to function independently.

We need to add one more point: A number of studies suggest that several psychosocial factors also appear to manage arthritis. These include coping strategies, gender, and social support. To conclude this section, we review the effects of these factors on chronic pain, specifically arthritic pain.

COPING STRATEGIES *Coping strategies* are not meant to solve a problem but to help an individual manage the consequences of the problem. Yet studies that examine coping strategies of men and women show significant differences in their choice of techniques that directly impact pain. Specifically, research findings appear to suggest that women use less effective coping strategies, resulting in perceptions of greater and less-controlled pain.

In Chapter 7, Stress and Coping, we explored theories on coping styles. Therefore, we will only briefly review coping strategies here. The research on coping suggests essentially two principal cognitive coping styles: problem- or emotion-focused versus engagement/disengagement. *Problem- or emotion-focused coping* includes two levels, problem focused and emotion focused. Problem-focused coping involves seeking information to generate solutions to address the issue or problem. Conversely, an emotion-focused coping approach seeks solace or emotional support from others for emotional reasons.

The second type of cognitive coping, *engagement/disengagement*, also includes two levels. Engagement is a hybrid of the two levels in the problem- or emotion-focused coping approach. It includes both problem-solving and emotional support. Finally, as the name suggests, disengagement is best characterized as withdrawal or a denial of the problem. For example, individuals with arthritis who experience a pain flare-up and who use a disengagement coping strategy may continue with their activities, tolerating the pain as best they can but not seeking treatment or acknowledging that the pain is related to arthritis. Other disengagers may resort to substances (drug or alcohol) to disengage from the pain. Researchers have demonstrated that, of the four coping styles, the problem-focused approach appears to be the most effective strategy for addressing a problem, whereas, predictably, the disengagement approach is the least effective (Lazarus & Folkman, 1984a).

In a study testing coping strategies among adults with osteoarthritis pain, France and colleagues (2004) found a gender difference in pain-coping strategies that resulted in a difference in perceived pain. These researchers compared postmenopausal women and similarly aged men and found that women were more likely to use emotion-focused strategies than were men. Moreover, individuals who used the emotion-focused approach were significantly more likely to report more arthritis pain and a lower pain tolerance than were individuals who used another strategy.

Research on coping also suggests that the coping techniques individuals adopt for a specific illness are related to the coping strategies they use when dealing with everyday life (see again Chapter 7, Stress and Coping). In essence, coping strategies appear to be linked to an individual's own disposition toward handling stress of any sort and are not limited to approaches to address pain or to one's gender.

SOCIAL SUPPORT Researchers agree that individuals are able to achieve better overall outcomes when they receive support from others. The most beneficial form of support is *tangible assistance*, such as materials or help with issues that directly address the problem. For individuals with arthritis, tangible support could include help with daily tasks such as cooking or getting dressed or assistance with transportation – getting to a doctor's office or to the bank – when needed. Other forms of support include information, guidance, or emotional support. Although all forms of support are helpful, research suggests that tangible support that assists an individual in accomplishing specific goals is most beneficial.

Although both genders benefit from social support, research suggests that women with arthritis who receive strong social support are less likely to experience depressive symptoms. Consider this: Women often report feelings of guilt when they are unable to perform household or family responsibilities due to the restricted movements associated with arthritis. To illustrate this point, researchers Hwang, Kim, and Jun (2004) offer transcripts of interviews in a case study of five Korean women with RA that revealed many expressions of guilt or anxiety because they were unable to attend to their children's needs or to perform household tasks as expected. In addition, Hwang and colleagues (2004) report that in more traditional societies women with RA who do not receive strong social support from their spouses are not only at greater risk of functional disabilities over time but also at greater risk of depression.

Such outcomes appear to hold for women in general. Other researchers similarly suggest that women's feelings of anxiety or guilt due to their inability to perform their expected family roles often lead to depression (Escalante, del Rincon, & Mulrow, 2000). As noted previously, arthritis sufferers' inability to perform simple daily tasks for themselves or for others, such as dressing, cooking, and eating or feeding others or involving themselves in social activities, also leads to a sense of helplessness that can promote depressive symptoms (Mella, Bertolo, & Dalgalarrondo, 2010).

Social support for the management of osteoarthritis and rheumatoid arthritis has also been linked to improvements in an individual's coping process and daily functioning as well as his or her perceptions of pain over time. In a study of 78 individuals with RA, researchers found that both coping styles and social support predicted overall well-being. Patients who reported passive coping strategies to deal with pain, here meaning avoiding or restricting activities due to pain, reported greater functional disability over three years (Evers, Kraaimaat, Geenen, Jacobs, & Bijlsma, 2003). In addition, those with fewer social support networks, here meaning fewer support groups, or individuals who could not count on others for emotional support when facing physical challenges also showed greater functional disability and poorer pain tolerance when followed up three and five years later (Evers et al., 2003). Similar findings by other researchers strengthen the claim that social support, in addition to coping strategies, contributes to better health outcomes and overall well-being of arthritis sufferers (Rat et al., 2021).

It is important to observe that cultures may help shape the coping strategies individuals choose. Women may be supported in their use of emotion-focused coping because seeking solace and emotional support for problems is consistent with the roles assigned to women in many societies. On the other hand, emotion-focused coping is not encouraged among men. Men may receive messages that society expects them to work through the pain and stiffness, neither focusing on nor calling attention to their limitations and discomfort. Individuals who receive such messages may perceive greater pain and less tolerance associated with the illness and evidence less effective management of their arthritis than others who take a more problem-centered coping style.

The social support literature leaves little doubt that assistance of whatever sort and from a variety of support groups is an essential element in the effective management of the illness and the mental health status of individuals with arthritis. In addition, these findings demonstrate a need for health psychologists to participate in developing interventions and therapies for arthritis management. What is more, health psychologists must pay particular attention to the needs of each individual they aim to serve. For example, group-structured interventions may offer support for individuals with limited personnel or financial resources. In addition, exercise-therapy groups, discussion groups that address relationship issues, and arthritis self-management techniques may be particularly helpful as part of the disease-management process for individuals needing more social and emotional support (Barlow, Cullen, & Rowe, 2002).

The psychosocial impact of arthritis underscores the need for psychosocial therapies as part of a comprehensive process of treating and managing arthritis (Dixon et al., 2007).

Caregivers, Pain Management, and Psychological Distress

There is one additional topic we must address when examining the psychological effects of chronic pain. An increase in functional disability and dependency on others, together with chronic pain, is dispiriting to many individuals. Research on chronic pain indicates that depression, worry, avoidance behavior, and a sense of helplessness are common psychological reactions for people with chronic pain (Samwel et al., 2009). Like those with other chronic conditions, people who suffer from chronic pain do not suffer alone. Family members and caregivers of chronic pain sufferers also experience psychological and emotional health problems when caring for someone with a chronic condition. Consider this: A study by Simon, Kumar, and Kendrick (2009) measured the psychological distress of live-in caregivers of stroke victims (see Chapter 9, Cardiovascular Disease) in England to determine whether the role of caregiver to first-time stroke survivors would increase levels of psychological distress among the caregivers. These researchers measured the caregiver's psychological health and social well-being before the stroke victim was discharged from the hospital, six weeks after discharge, and again 15 months after the stroke. They found that not only was caregiver distress commonly reported among the 105 people sampled but that it started quite early in the care process.

What is more, when comparing the psychological health and social well-being of caregivers with a matched sample of noncaregivers near the same time period, caregivers were two and a half times more likely to evidence significant psychological distress (Simon et al., 2009). They even found gender differences in caregiver distress: Women were more likely than men to develop stress in anticipation of the caregiving role. Men, on the other hand, were more likely to first evidence stress when the caregiving responsibilities began.

Research by Ho, Chan, Woo, Chang, and Sham (2009) similarly reports that caregivers suffer negative psychological health. In their study, 246 caregivers of elderly persons were compared with approximately 490 non-caregivers. These researchers found that caregivers reported more doctor visits to tend to their own health needs than did non-caregivers. Caregivers were also at higher risk for anxiety, depression, and reported increases in weight loss. And once again, females seemed to fare worse than males, reporting greater incidences of chronic disease and insomnia.

The research on caregivers clearly shows that chronic illnesses affect more than the person who is afflicted. The task of providing ongoing assistance and aid to someone with a chronic illness, including chronic pain, can cause emotional, psychological, and physical harm to the caregiver. This research suggests that it is as important to address the health needs of the caregiver as those of the person afflicted with the illness when examining chronic health problems (see Chapter 6, Emotional Health and Well-Being).

INTERVENTIONS FOR CAREGIVERS To this end, there is hope for caregivers. Research on interventions for caregivers report a number of strategies that have been used with varying levels of success. For example, Folkman and Moskowitz (2000) examined the emotional and psychological health of caregivers for people with late-stage AIDS. The slow physical deterioration and social stigma still experienced by some people with HIV/AIDS presents additional psychological stressors for both the sufferer and his or her caregiver. Folkman and Moskowitz found that caregivers who were able to set and accomplish small, goal-specific tasks each day – for example, to mail a package at the post office or purchase needed groceries at the supermarket – were more likely to report better overall psychological health in the short term and in the longer term once their responsibilities ended.

Similarly, other studies examining interventions for caregivers report less long-term psychological distress when caregivers employ psychotherapy or psychoeducational interventions. We explain these interventions in more detail in Chapter 11, Cancer. For now it is important only to note that social support assistance, such as respite care that allows the caregiver time away from care responsibilities or specialized care training, proves helpful to a caregiver of persons with chronic or debilitating diseases (Pinquart & Sorensen, 2005). Arthritis, a chronic but not life-threatening illness, can present similar challenges for caregivers.

Personal Postscript

Many times, family members comment that parents, grandparents, or aunts and uncles are often "grouchy" or in a bad mood for no apparent reason. If you have made similar observations, you may wonder why also. Are these relatives just grouchy people, or is something wrong?

Chances are that if any of the relatives are experiencing a form of arthritis there will be times when the pain and discomfort make them very uncomfortable. Certainly you would agree that when a person is uncomfortable, it is very difficult to be pleasant.

If you suspect that a parent or relative suffers from arthritis, there are a number of things you can do to help without calling attention to their illness or discomfort. Consider the following suggestions:

1. Invite your relative to join you on an outing that will provide that person with a low-stress form of exercise. Bicycling, swimming, and even walking are excellent forms of exercise that help to move and stretch the painful joints.
2. Offer to draw his or her bath. Soaking in a warm bath provides relief to the inflamed and swollen joints.
3. If your relative has been given an exercise regimen by a physical therapist, offer to do the exercises with him or her. Having someone as an "exercise buddy" can make the task more enjoyable.
4. Offer to help with tasks when the inflammation or pain is particularly bothersome.

There will be times when the relative refuses your offers. In fact, he or she may do so the first several times. But just knowing that someone has offered support and understands his or her disease will provide emotional comfort even if your relative does not accept your assistance.

Questions to Consider

1. Consider this: Many Western nations are seeing an increase in the average age of their population. What might this portend when considering the role for health psychologists in the next 10–20 years?

2. Research in biology and neurology are showing us the role that each of these areas contribute to our overall well-being. What does this suggest for the educational needs of the next generation of health psychologists?
3. What would you recommend to address the apparent conflict between an attempt to treat pain more aggressively and the growing use and abuse of opioids?

True or False Questions

1. Neuropathic pain is a malfunction of our nervous system. True or False.
2. Physicians often have a difficult time diagnosing pain because the intensity and location of pain on the body may change from day to day. True or False.
3. Rheumatoid arthritis is triggered by the body's immune system. True or False.
4. Ankylosing spondylitis is a form of arthritis only found in Europeans and white Americans. True or False.
5. Gout is caused by crystal deposits in tissue. True or False.

Important Terms

adalimumab 391
ankylo 383
ankylosing spondylitis (AS) 383
antitumor necrosis factor (anti-TNF) drugs 391
arthritis 370
arthro 380
autoimmune disease 381
behavioral observations 386
biofeedback 395
bone spur 384
cartilage 384
chronic pain 373
cognitive-behavioral therapy (CBT) 394
coping strategy 396
COX-1 inhibitor 391
COX-2 inhibitor 391
degeneration 380
degenerative joint disease 384
dorsal horns 374
emotional disclosure 395

Cancer

Chapter Outline

Opening Story: Misinformation, Disinformation, or Misrepresentation?

Section I. Defining Cancer

Section II. Risk Factors for Cancer

Section III. Cancer Treatments and Prevention

Section IV. Medical and Psychological Treatments

Personal Postscript

Questions to Consider

True or False Questions

Important Terms

Chapter Objectives

After studying this chapter, you will be able to:

1. Define benign and malignant tumors.

2. Identify and define the four major types of cancer.

3. Identify and give examples of five risk factors for cancer.

4. Compare mortality rates for cancer with those of other major illnesses.

5. Describe how nutrition and exercise help prevent cancer.

6. Identify the benefits of and barriers to breast self-examination.

7. Explain the benefits of psychotherapeutic interventions for cancer treatment.

8. Explain the benefits of problem-focused coping as a psychological intervention for cancer management.

9. Explain the benefits of social support as a psychological intervention for cancer management.

DOI: 10.4324/9781003300670-12

OPENING STORY: MISINFORMATION, DISINFORMATION, OR MISREPRESENTATION?

February 5, 2015: The Toronto Star, *the most-read newspaper in Canada (Vox, 2015), published online a front-page story titled "A Wonder Drug's Dark Side" (Washington Post, 2015). The article reported the stories of five young women who suffered side effects after receiving the two-shot* **human papillomavirus (HPV)** *vaccine by* **Gardasil**, *one of several approved vaccines to protect against the sexually transmitted HPV, a virus linked to cancers of the cervix, penis, vagina, and throat, among other areas.*

The article noted that adverse events were experienced by several dozen women who received the vaccine. The authors focused specifically on the experiences of five women who reportedly experienced muscle pain, swelling, heart attacks, and/or egg-sized lumps on the feet, and other symptoms (Vox, 2015; Washington Post, 2015). A 14-year-old girl even died two weeks after the second shot of the vaccine (Vox, 2015).

Interestingly, the reaction to this story from medical experts was fiercely negative. They strongly condemned the article for misrepresenting the data. The publisher of the Toronto Star, *John Cruickshank, acknowledged that the headline was wrong and that there was no evidence to link the adverse outcomes to the Gardasil vaccine (Young, 2015). Even the* Toronto Star's *public editor, Kathy English, admitted that the Star did not give "proper weight" to science in this article (Young, 2015). Two weeks after the article was published, the* Toronto Star *retracted the story. It is no longer available online.* ∎

There is so much to unpack here that it is difficult to know where to start! We will certainly address the issue of data interpretation, misinterpretation, and responsible reporting. And you can be sure that we will answer the burning question, why did the paper retract a true story about adverse effects experienced by five women, not to mention the death of one woman? But first: context. We must explain the relationship between the **human papillomavirus (HPV)** and cancer.

HPV is actually a group of over 200 related viruses (National Cancer Institute, 2021). The virus is largely transmitted through sexual contact and transmission can occur soon after intimacy (WHO, 2022c).

To be clear, *HPV* infections are common. In fact, they are so common that Canada (the country where the dozens of reportedly adverse events occurred) estimates that approximately 70% of their population will contract *HPV* (Public Health Agency of Canada, 2020). Similarly, the U.S. CDC suggests that almost everyone in the U.S. will get an *HPV* infection at some point in their lives (CDC, 2021).

Globally, the WHO estimates that as of 2017, approximately 11.7% of women tested positive for *HPV* of the cervix, with the highest prevalence rate reported in women 25 years of age or younger (WHO, 2017). The prevalence rates for men were equally alarming. Reported as ranges, the WHO found the prevalence of *HPV* for "low-risk men" to be between 1% and 84%. The rate for "high-risk men" was between 2% and 93%. Here, high-risk men include those who attended sexually transmitted infection clinics, who were HIV positive (see Chapter 5, Risky Health Behaviors, Part I) and the male partners of women with positive *HPV* results (WHO, 2017).

The logical question at this point is: If *HPV* is so common, what is the concern? The answer lies in the distinction between "low-risk *HPV*" versus "high-risk *HPV*" strains. Generally, the majority of *HPV* infections are low risk, asymptomatic, and will resolve without treatment (WHO Weekly Epidemiological Record, 2017). For example, two varieties of the virus – *HPV6* and *HPV11* – cause approximately 90% of all *genital warts*, which are small, flesh-colored bumps that some describe as "cauliflower-like" in appearance. Yet, they are considered low risk because they are rarely associated with cell abnormalities that cause cancer (New Zealand HPV Project, 2022). On the other hand, high-risk *HPV* strains, like *HPV16* and *HPV18*, can cause *oropharyngeal cancers*, here meaning cancers of the tonsils or other oral or throat areas, and *anogenital cancers*, those found on the cervix, vagina, penis, vulva, and anus (Kombe Kombe et al., 2021). What does this mean? Basically, anyone – not just women – who becomes infected with a high-risk strain of *HPV* may be at risk for developing pre-cancerous lesions.

Cervical cancer is ranked the fourth most common cancer for women (see Figure 11.1b). Studies confirm that *HPV16* and *18* contribute to approximately 70% of all global cervical cancers (approximately 60% for *HPV16* alone; WHO Weekly Epidemiological Record, 2017). More alarming, the death rate associated with cervical cancers is high. In Canada, of the estimated 1,350 women who contracted *HPV* in 2020, approximately 410, or just under one-third, are projected to develop *and* die from cervical cancer. What is more, the WHO reported that of the 630,000 global incidences of *HPV*, 530,000, or 84%, were linked to cervical cancer. Of those cases, 260,000, or almost 50%, resulted in death (WHO Weekly Epidemiological Report, 2017).

Cervical cancer prevalence and mortality rates present disturbing statistics, but other *HPV16*-related cancers cannot be ignored. The global prevalence rates of cancer of the vagina (43.6%; see Figure 11.2a), is surprisingly consistent across four of the five geographic regions of the world: Europe (47.4%), Oceania (includes 14 countries in Central and South Pacific; 46.2%), the Americas (42.2%), and Asia (39.4%). Likewise, statistics on *HPV16*-related cancer of the anus (71.4%) are similar across three geographic regions of the world: the Americas (74.3%), Europe (73.4%), and Asia (67.3%; see Figure 11.2b). This is also the case for *HPV16* related penile cancer (worldwide, 22.8%; Africa, 26.3%; the Americas, 23.8%; Europe, 23.4%; see Figure 11.2c). More variable are the rates for vulvar cancer (worldwide, 19.4%; Africa, 58.3%; Oceana, 27.3%; The Americas, 26.5%; Asia, 18.1%; and Europe, 13.8%). Taken together, these data illustrate the global impact of *HPV*. More importantly, they underscore the point that sexually transmitted *HPV* is a global health issue for both men and women.

With these data in mind, we return to the story reported in the *Toronto Star* featured in this chapter's opening story.

Data Misrepresentation or Just Missing Information?

Without a doubt, news articles such as the one in the *Toronto Star* would make any parent, or teen for that matter, think twice about getting the *HPV* vaccine, even with the data on *HPV* related cancer rates and deaths. Who would want to risk significant discomforts or death from a vaccine? And information from a trusted source – the *Toronto Star* – increased the credibility of the story, at least for the public. So, why did medical experts and the paper's editors take issue with this report?

We present a thorough analysis of the problems with the article and the probable reasons for its retraction in Box 11.1. But to summarize briefly, there were four major errors. First the article omitted critical, scientific information – an omission that could lead readers to believe that the vaccine was dangerous when numerous studies show that it was not. Second, the article failed to mention the hundreds of thousands of teenagers successfully vaccinated in Canada without incidence. Third, numerous studies

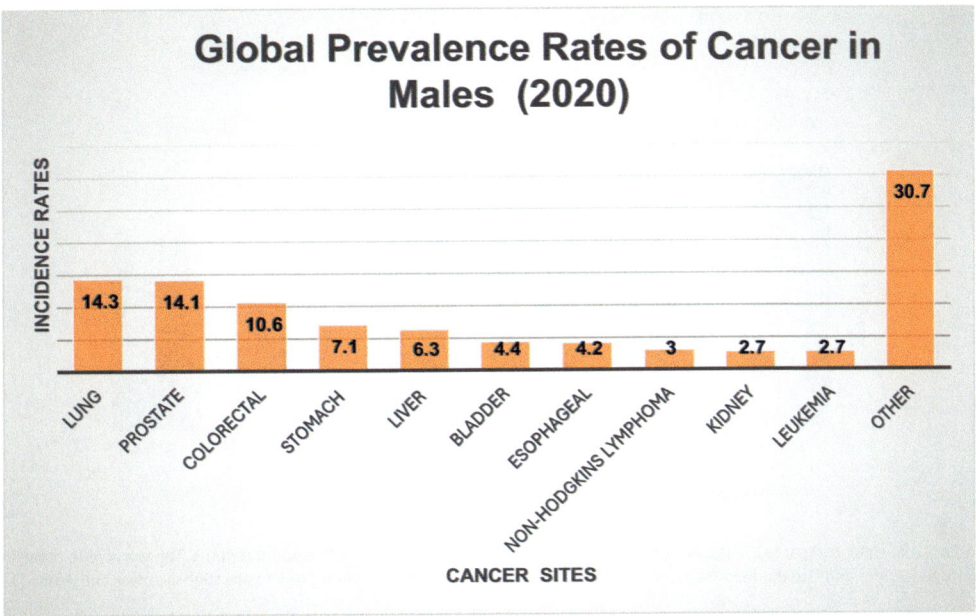

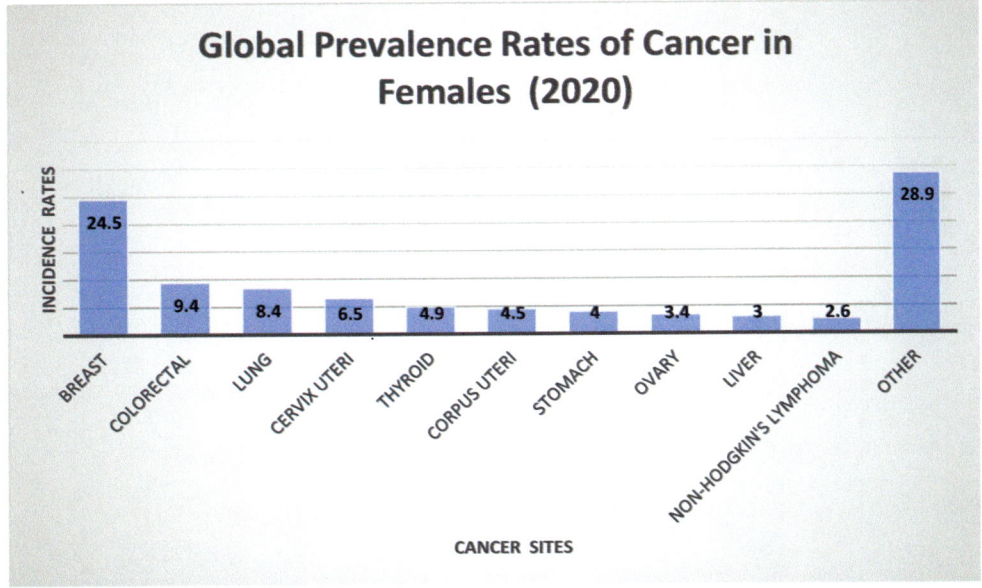

FIGURE 11.1a and 11.1b A bar chart compares the global prevalence of cancer in women as of 2020. Highest specific sites include: Breast (24.5%), colorectal (9.4%), lung (8.4%), cervix/uteri (6.5%), thyroid (4.9%), corpus uteri (4.5%), stomach (4%), ovary (3.4%), and liver (3%). A second bar chart compares the global prevalence of cancer in men as of 2020. Highest specific sites include: lung (14.3%), prostate (14%), colorectal (10.6%), Stomach (7.1%), liver (6.3%), bladder (4.4%), esophagus (4.2%), kidney (2.7%), and leukemia (2.7%).

Source: Adapted from Sung et al. (2021).

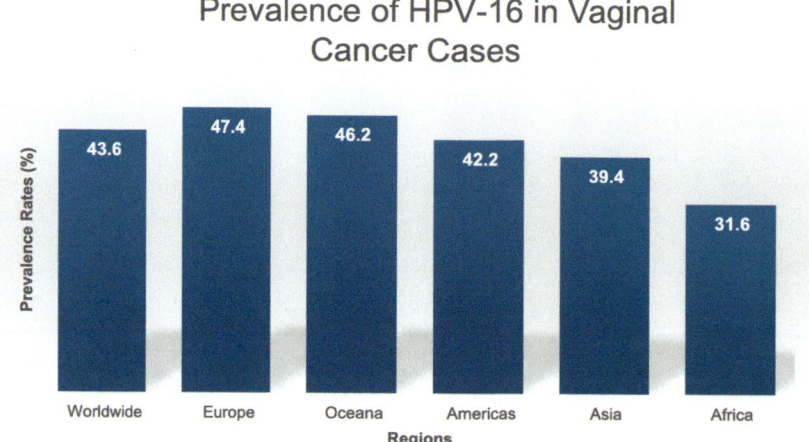

FIGURE 11.2a A bar chart compares the global HPV-16 related vaginal cancer cases across five world regions. The worldwide prevalence rate is 43.6%. Europe (47.4%) and Oceana (46.2%) exceed this rate, the Americas (42.2%) and Asia (39.4%) are slightly lower and Africa (31.6%) is lowest.

Source: Adapted from Bruni, Albero, Serrano, Mena, Collado, Gómez et al. (2021).

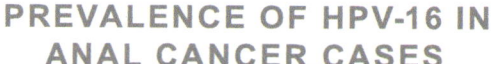

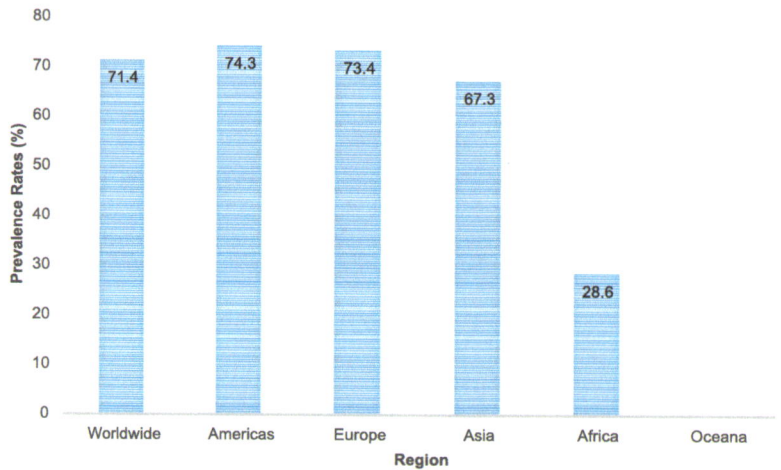

FIGURE 11.2b A bar chart compares the global HPV-16 related anal cancer cases across five world regions. The worldwide prevalence rate is quite high (71.4%). The Americas (74.3%) and Europe (73.4%) exceed this rate, Asia (67.3%) is lower and again Africa (28.6%) is the lowest.

Source: Adapted from Bruni, Albero, Serrano, Mena, Collado, Gómez et al. (2021).

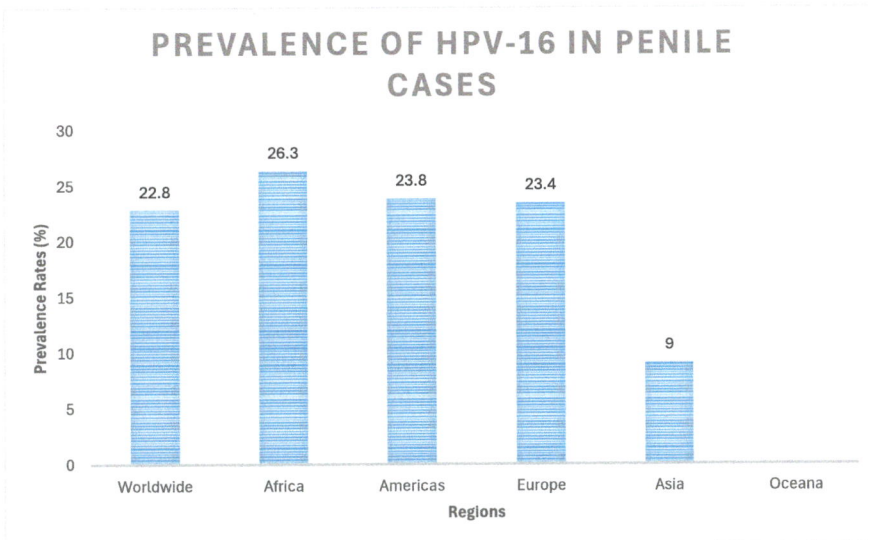

FIGURE 11.2c . A bar chart compares the global HPV-16 related penile cancer cases across five world regions. The worldwide prevalence rate is low (22.8%). This time, Africa reports the highest rate. (26.3%). The Americas (23.8%) and Europe (23.4%) also exceed the worldwide rate, Asia (9.0%) is the lowest.

Source: Adapted from Bruni, Albero, Serrano, Mena, Collado, Gómez et al. (2021).

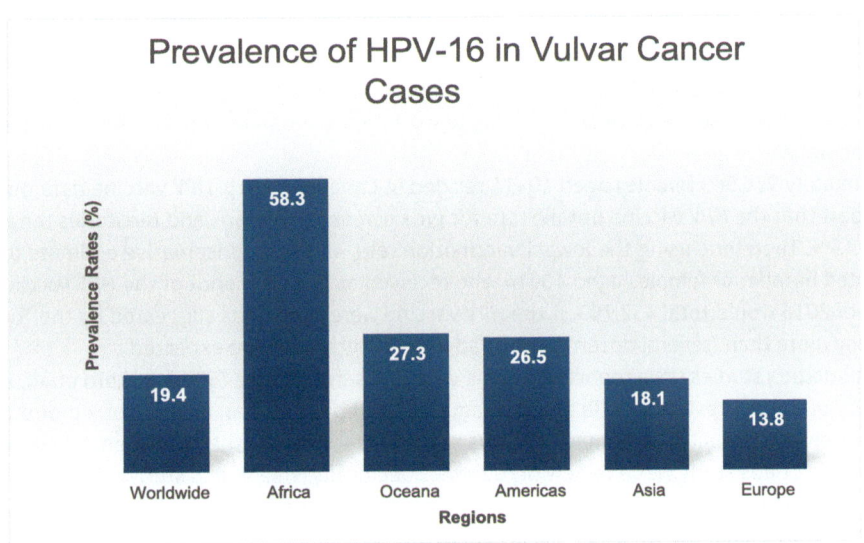

FIGURE 11.2d A bar chart compares the global HPV-16 related vulvar cancer cases across five world regions. The worldwide prevalence rate is low (19.4%). Here, too, Africa reports the highest rate (58.3%). Oceana (27.3%) and The Americas (26.5%) follow. Asia (18.1%) and Europe (13.8%) are lower than the worldwide rates.

Source: Adapted from Bruni, Albero, Serrano, Mena, Collado, Gómez et al. (2021).

have reported on this vaccine's strong safety record (Shimabukuro et al., 2019). And finally, the emotional appeal and use of personal stories are often used in social media sites and other publications to promote negative messaging about vaccinations (Teoh, 2019). It certainly attracted interested readers, but it may have solidified the false impression that the vaccine is dangerous when, in fact, the safety data on the HPV vaccines is among the best (Steben, Norris, & McFadyen, n.d.). These are the "headlines," but do read Box 11.1 for all the details!

Box 11.1 An Incredible Misleading Article about the HPV Vaccine

The *Toronto Star* is not the first paper to publish a sensational and misleading article about a critical health issue. Fortunately, the editors decided to retract the article. Nevertheless, it provides a great opportunity to examine how media sources can misinform the public on a health topic of interest to health psychologists. So, let's begin.

There were several problems with this article. First, the article omitted critical, scientific information – an omission that could lead readers to believe that the vaccine was dangerous. First, recall from Chapter 4, Global, Communicable, and Chronic Disease, that vaccines are designed to either prevent or lessen the severity of specific diseases. But, as we also learned in Chapter 4, no vaccine is 100% safe. All vaccines carry a risk of side effects. While deaths caused by vaccines are a serious problem, there was no evidence that the *HPV* vaccine caused the death of the vaccinated women as reported in the article. This is an important point and one underscored by the publisher, John Cruickshank.

A second critical point, however, is that the article failed to mention the hundreds of thousands of teenagers successfully vaccinated in Canada without incident. We focus on Canada since the story reported on an incident in that country. So, consider this: In 2007, Canada introduced a voluntary, school-based *HPV* vaccination program for girls, ages 9 to 14. By 2013, all Canadian providences and territories had initiated vaccine programs for girls. (For boys, a similar program was introduced in 2013.) Because all of Canada had active *HPV* vaccine programs for girls by 2015, the year the article was published, we will use the data on girls only to explain the problem of misrepresented data in the *Toronto Star* story.

Approximately 926,560 females aged 10–14 resided in Canada in 2015. *HPV* vaccine data published in 2016 report that the *HPV* vaccine uptake rate for girls across the regions and territories ranged from 46.7% to 93.9%. Therefore, using the lowest vaccination rate, 46.7% (a conservative estimate to be sure), the estimated number of females aged 10–14 who received at least one shot of the *HPV* vaccine by the beginning of 2016 would total 432,703. If the *HPV* vaccine were as risky as suggested by the *Toronto Star* article, many more than "several dozen" serious adverse events would be expected.

Third, numerous studies have reported on this vaccine's safety record (Shimabukuro et al., 2019). For example, an "umbrella" review by Villa and colleagues (2020) produced an analysis of a group of studies which, themselves, conducted systematic reviews of other studies published between 2006 and 2018. In essence, Villa et al.'s study was a review of reviews. Specifically, Villa et al.'s study (2020) examined 30 reviews of studies in over nine countries, including Canada. The number of vaccinated individuals in the umbrella review totaled more than *five million*. No deaths attributed to the *HPV* vaccine were reported in Villa et al.'s review of reviews. Additionally, the occurrence of other adverse events was not statistically significant when comparing *HPV*-vaccinated individuals versus a placebo group (see Chapter 2, Research Methods). Given this information, what conclusions would you draw when comparing the findings, reported in the umbrella review of more than five million vaccine recipients, with the "several dozen" reported adverse *HPV* vaccine events in the opening story? Do note that placing the claim of "several dozen" adverse events in the Toronto Star publication in quotation marks is not intended to disparage this claim. Rather, it is meant to emphasize this rather imprecise data point.

It is important to restate that serious adverse events should *never* be ignored. In this case, however, the *Toronto Star* omitted important context. They failed to compare the number of adverse events to the total number of adverse-free vaccine cases (at a minimum, over 400,000) in Canada.

Finally, the emotional and heart-rending reporting by the *Toronto Star* certainly attracted interested readers, but it may have left the false impression that the vaccine is dangerous when, in fact, the safety data on the *HPV* vaccines is among the best (Steben et al., n.d.). Researchers have found that the use of personal stories and emotional appeals are often used in social media sites and other publications to promote negative messaging about vaccinations (Teoh, 2019). The story's headline, "A Wonder Drug's Dark Side," is provocative and perhaps biases the reader even before reading the story. Appeal to emotions, like that found in the *Toronto Star* article, might encourage readers to refuse the vaccine, choosing instead to risk contracting a high-risk variant of *HPV*, a disease clearly linked to a range of cancers for both men and women. By comparison, a focus on facts and logic is often used when promoting positive messaging. The downside, however, is that accurate facts and logic can seem boring.

Vaccine Acceptance

By this time, you may be thinking, interesting! But what does this have to do with health psychology? Simply put, health psychology can and does play a critical role in advancing health-enhancing behaviors. We mentioned this in Chapter 4, Global, Communicable, and Chronic Disease. One such behavior is being vaccinated to protect against diseases shown to cause serious illness or death.

Without a doubt, new medical approaches and vaccines will face careful scrutiny, including opposition by the public as they evaluate their benefits and limitations (see Chapter 4, Global, Communicable, and Chronic Disease and the COVID-19 vaccine). What is interesting is that this still applies to the HPV vaccine, even though it has been in existence and administered for more than 15 years. One reason for the continued resistance to the vaccine is parents. When considering the vaccine for their children, some parents worry that the vaccine might encourage early sexual activity. Simply put, vaccinating one's 9- or 10-year-old daughter or son to protect them from a sexually transmitted disease is, for many parents, unthinkable and contrary to their parenting practices and values (see Box 11.2). Yet it is here that health psychologist can play a pivotal role by addressing parent's concerns, beliefs, and values and developing messages that address the concerns of many different groups (see Chapter 3, Theories and Models of Health Behavior Change, specifically Social Marketing). Increasingly, psychologists – specifically health psychologists – are working with medical doctors to address the emotional, psychological, and physical health of individuals while addressing their concerns about the suggested medical regimens and their personal values and beliefs (Fleury, Imboua, Aube, & Farand, 2012; Solana, Pirrotta, Ingravalle, & Fayella, 2009).

Box 11.2 Your Challenge: Convince a Parent to Vaccinate Their Primary School Child from a Sexually Transmitted Disease

Finally, there is good news in the war on cancer. Researchers discovered that *human papillomavirus (HPV)–related cancers* can be **prevented** by a new vaccine. This is so important it needs to be repeated. The *HPV* vaccine is not a cure. That is to say, it is not a treatment that is applied after an individual has been diagnosed with the disease. Rather, it prevents individuals from contracting the disease in the first place. It works in the same way that childhood immunizations protect children from diseases such as measles, mumps, and chickenpox.

This discovery marks the first time in the history of cancer research that scientists have developed a vaccine to prevent the onset of a cancer. The vaccine was first tested for effectiveness on women. Results indicated that the vaccine is very effective in preventing *HPV* infection and protecting against cervical cancer for five years after the vaccine (Cutts et al., 2007; Stanley, 2008). At present, approximately 49% of adolescents in the U.S. have been vaccinated (World Health Organization, 2022c). This compares less favorably with Canada where the vaccination rate is approximately 87% (World Health Organization, 2022c). Globally, while approximately 42% of WHO member states have officially incorporated HPV vaccines into their routine immunization schedule (see Figure 11.3 and Table 11.1), only 12% of 15-year-old girls have been vaccinated (World Health Organization, 2022c).

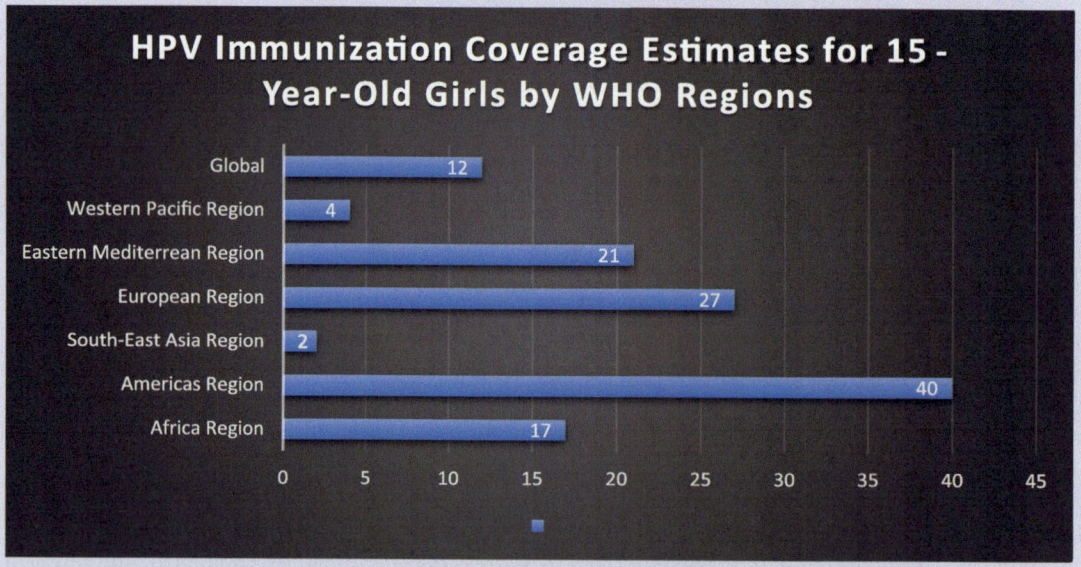

FIGURE 11.3 Although 42% of WHO member states have included HPV vaccines into health regimens, only 12% of girls 15 years of age have been vaccinated.

Source: WHO (2022c).

TABLE 11.1 HPV Immunization Coverage Estimates for 15-Year-Old Girls by WHO Region and Country

Africa Region

Country	% Immunized	Country	% Immunized
Cote d'Ivoire	13	Rwanda	68
Ethiopia	76	Senegal	31
Kenya	16	Seychelles	24
Liberia	18	Uganda	30
Malawi	77	United Republic of Tanzania	58
Mauritius	74	Zambia	69

The Americas Region

Country	% Immunized	Country	% Immunized
Argentina	46	Guatemala	20
Bahamas	4	Guyana	25
Barbados	7	Honduras	47
Belize	11	Jamaica	3
Bolivia	24	Mexico	5
Brazil	72	Panama	44
Canada	87	Paraguay	37
Chile	74	Peru	16
Colombia	34	Saint Lucia	74
Costa Rica	77	Saint Vincent & the Grenadines	12
Dominica	76	Suriname	4
Dominican Republic	7	U.S.	49
Ecuador	36	Uruguay	25
Grenada	32		

Southeast Asia Region

Country	% Immunized	Country	% Immunized
Bhutan	81	Maldives	68
Indonesia	7	Sri Lanka	51

European Region

Country	% Immunized	Country	% Immunized
Andorra	77	Malta	85
Armenia	8	Netherlands	63
Bulgaria	2	North Macedonia	30
Denmark	70	Norway	90
Estonia	55	Portugal	78
France	33	Republic of Moldova	40
Georgia	22	San Marino	50
Germany	43	Slovenia	59
Iceland	91	Spain	79
Ireland	77	Sweden	82

Source: Adapted from World Health Organization (2022c).

Vaccinations against HPV in the U.S. are encountering resistance, however. Because HPV is a sexually transmitted disease, researchers and health care providers strongly recommend that girls and boys receive the vaccine before they become sexually active. Current statistics suggest that a significant minority of adolescents are sexually active by age 13. Therefore, health care providers recommend that girls and boys between the ages of 9 and 14 years be vaccinated.

To that end, researchers and health care providers globally have engaged in an active public health campaign to convince parents to vaccinate their 9- to 14-year-old daughters and sons against the virus. For example, campaigns in the U.S. and Canada inform parents of 9- to 14-year-old children about the risks posed by HPV. They also aim to increase awareness of the vaccine as an effective protection from a disease that infects more than 37,000 men and women in the U.S. annually (CDC, 2022d).

Here's the problem: Most parents of 9- to 14-year-old adolescent girls discourage their daughters from becoming sexually active. Some studies suggest that parents are concerned that by giving pre- and early teens a vaccine against HPV, a sexually transmitted disease, they may send a message to their daughters promoting promiscuity (Davis, Dickman, Ferris, & Dias, 2004).

Research by Beavis, Krakow, Levinson, and Rositch (2018) reveal additional reasons that parents of female children refuse the vaccine (see Table 11.2). Parent's reasons vary somewhat according to the sex of their child. Parents of male children identify a lack of necessity for the vaccine (22%), the fact that their doctors have not recommended the vaccine (17%), a lack of knowledge on the part of the parent (14%), and safety concerns (14%) as their top reasons for refusing. With female children, parents cite largely identical reasons but in a different order: concerns about safety of the vaccine (22%), the lack of necessity of the vaccine (20%), and parent's general lack of knowledge about the vaccine (13%).

TABLE 11.2 Parent's Reasons for Refusing HPV Vaccine by Adolescent's Gender

Reasons for Refusing (%)	Parents of Male Children (%)	Parents of Female Children (%)
Safety	14	22
Lack Necessity	22	20
Lack Knowledge	14	13
No Doctor Recommendation	17	10
Not Sexually Active	9	10
Gender	2	–

Source: Adapted from World Health Organization (2022c).

Researchers have shown that strong and high-quality recommendation by a teen's medical provider positively influences parent's decision to authorize the HPV vaccine (Gilkey & McRee, 2016), an interesting outcome given that lack of doctor's recommendations is a key reason that some parents of adolescent boys cite for refusal (Beavis et al., 2018). Clearly, medical providers may be missing an opportunity to increase uptake of the vaccine, particularly among adolescent boys.

We could spend chapters teasing apart each of the reasons for HPV vaccine refusal and how to address them, but if we have learned anything from the reactions to the COVID-19 vaccines, we know that **how** one communicates health information may be as important as what is communicated (Thomson et al., 2018). We also learned from Chapter 4 that there is no "one-size-fits-all" strategy for effective vaccine communication. The message and how it is delivered must be tailored to the needs and interests of the intended audience. Here, health psychology can and does play a critical role in advancing health behaviors.

One more point. We cannot overlook the impact of health care providers' knowledge of and opinions about the vaccine on vaccine uptake. Rosen, Shephard, and Khan reviewed 60 qualitative and quantitative studies assessing health care provider's knowledge, attitudes, and practices regarding the HPV vaccine. The findings were sobering. Providers' knowledge about the facts concerning the HPV vaccine ranged from poor (17% correct responses) to excellent (93% correct). Their personal beliefs and attitudes about the vaccine, vaccine safety, and efficacy were found to influence their intention to administer or recommend the vaccine to their patients. Finally, provider's intention to recommend the vaccine varied widely depending on the patient's gender or age. Fully 59%–79% of providers reported an intention to recommend the vaccine for female patients, whereas between 7% and 84% reported an intention to recommend to parents of male patients. What is more, they were more likely to recommend the vaccine for girls and boys between 13 and 17 years of age and between 18 and 26 years of age (Rosen, Shephard, & Khan 2018). A number of providers considered the vaccine "optional" for 11- to 13-year-olds (Rosen et al., 2018; Washam, 2005). Remember, researchers found the average age of initiation is 13 years. Do you see a problem here?

We will identify more cutting-edge research aimed at treating or reducing cancer mortality rates in more detail in the following section. For the moment, however, it is important to restate that for some cancers, like *HPV*-associated cancers, an individual's own behaviors may increase their individual risk of contracting the illness. Therefore, efforts to address lifestyle behaviors – something that health psychologists routinely address – is also important to efforts to reduce cancer prevalence rates.

We will also see in the subsequent sections that increasingly, research and medical treatments have led us to reclassify many cancers as chronic, rather than terminal, illnesses. After more than 60 years of research, medical science has developed life-prolonging and in some cases lifesaving treatments for many forms of cancer. As a result, the diagnosis of many forms of cancer no longer means imminent death. Instead, many individuals live one or two decades after receiving a cancer diagnosis, sometimes dying of other, wholly unrelated causes. Thus, we include cancer as the third of three chronic diseases for review.

Improved cancer survival rates also allow researchers more time to learn about and understand cancer: the causes as well as effective prevention strategies and treatments. Therefore, in this chapter, we focus our discussion of cancer on the same three areas: the causes of cancer, its prevention, and its treatment. As in the preceding chapters on cardiovascular disease and chronic pain and arthritis, we will continue with a review of basic information about the disease, its definition, and its origins in Section I. Like arthritis, cancer is an umbrella term used to describe a collection of diseases. There are many different types of cancer. In Section I we will focus on the five most frequently occurring forms of the illness: lung, prostate, breast, colorectal, and cervical cancers.

In Section II, we explore risk factors for cancers. In particular, we discuss the role of gender, genetics, race/ethnicity, environment, and health-risk behaviors (individual behaviors) on cancer. We will also explore the interaction of some of these factors because two or more factors may collectively increase the relative risk of cancer to individuals.

In Section III, we explore cancer treatments. The diagnosis, treatment, and management of cancer have physiological as well as psychological implications not just for the individual with cancer but also for his or her family and friends. We examine the effects of depression, one of many possible psychological reactions to the disease. Specifically, we explore the impact of depression as a deterrent to improved health outcomes after treatment and as a possible contributing factor to the illness. Finally, we discuss the vital role of social support and support networks in cancer treatment. Here we will see that again, health psychologists can and do play a significant role in cancer treatments.

SECTION I. DEFINING CANCER

Like arthritis, the term *cancer* represents a number of diseases. In fact, some cite over 100 different types of cancers that are usually named for the organs or tissues where they form (National Cancer Institute, n.d.).

Cancer is a collection of cells that reproduce in an uncontrolled, or some say "rebellious," manner, forming a mass of cells. In our discussions of the immune system in Chapters 6–8, we noted that cells are the essential ingredients for life. They reproduce in the body as needed to perform the myriad functions we require to live. Normally, cell reproduction is controlled and regulated by the body, producing only the type and number needed. Cancerous cells, however, occur as the result of unregulated or uncontrolled cell reproduction. In other words, something went wrong.

VIDEO #53/60

Chapter 11: Cancer

- **Definition of Cancer: *3D Medical Animation – What is Cancer?***
- **Website: *https://www.youtube.com/watch?v=LEpTTolebqo***
- ***BioDigital is publicly accessible. It is an interactive 3D platform that teaches anatomy, diseases, and treatments through interactive learning. BioDigital | Interactive 3D Anatomy – Disease Platform***

Although scientists have identified a causal agent for some types of cervical, vaginal, penile, and throat cancers (see page 404), the exact cause of most other cancers is difficult to determine. Research has shown that chemical agents (tobacco smoke, asbestos, or formaldehyde), biological agents (viruses like HIV and HPV, bacteria, or parasites), environmental factors (ultraviolet light and radiation), and genetic factors may contribute to abnormal or uncontrolled cell growth (American Cancer Society, 2008; Blackadar, 2016; Moadei & Harris, 2008; World Health Organization, 2008a). In addition, some individual health behaviors also increase the risk of cancer. These include poor nutrition, smoking, obesity or overweight, physical inactivity, exposure to sexually transmitted diseases, and engaging with multiple sexual partners (Blackadar, 2016; Moadei & Harris, 2008). The WHO estimates that over one-third of deaths from cancer are caused by poor health behaviors including tobacco use, poor dietary habits – here meaning low intake of fruits and vegetables – excessive weight as measured by body mass index, alcohol consumption, and infrequent physical activity (WHO, 2022d).

Some of the health behaviors associated with cancer should sound very familiar because they contribute to other illnesses as well. With that in mind, you should understand why health psychologists would be interested in helping individuals to adopt healthy behaviors that also reduce the risk of some cancers.

Tumors

When cells reproduce in an uncontrolled manner, they form a *mass* or *tumor*. Two types of tumors are possible, benign and malignant. A *benign tumor* is a large mass of overgrown cells. The important point about benign tumors is that they are not usually life-threatening. Although they may grow in size, they do not reproduce, nor do they spread to other parts of the body. In most cases, benign tumors can be removed safely and without damage to other body tissues or organs.

MALIGNANT TUMORS Malignant tumors are life-threatening. They consist of a large mass of cells that grow and multiply uncontrollably and interfere with other body organs and functions. They are also cancerous. Undetected, the tumors can *metastasize*, or spread to other parts of the body, making it virtually impossible to locate or to remove all of the tumors. A cancer that has metastasized is unlikely to be contained or effectively treated, so the outcome usually is fatal.

CATEGORIES OF CANCER BY TYPE OF TISSUE (HISTOLOGICAL) Cancers are categorized in two ways; by where in the body the cancer originates (primary site) or by the type of tissue where the cancer developed (histological; National Cancer Institute, n.d.). An extensive review of both cancer categories is beyond the scope of this book. Therefore, we will limit our discussion to the histological category of cancers.

The four principal categories of histological cancer are carcinomas, sarcomas, leukemia, and lymphomas. *Carcinomas* are cancers derived from epithelial cells. Epithelial cells are found in many parts of the body, including skin, glands, and organs such as the liver or bladder. The skin and breasts, for example, contain large quantities of epithelial cells that are susceptible to cancer.

One common form of carcinoma is the *non-melanoma* cancers: *basal and squamous cell carcinomas*. *Basal* and *squamous cell* carcinomas most often start in parts of the body subjected to prolonged and unprotected exposure to harmful ultraviolet sun rays. Globally, these types of skin cancers are the most common *and* the most frequently occurring skin cancers (American Cancer Society, 2022; Sung et al., 2021). Yet they are the least deadly forms of cancer. They rarely spread to other parts of the body and if caught early can be treated effectively (American Cancer Society, 2022). The highest incidence rates of non-melanoma skin cancers are reported in high-income countries including Japan, and specifically among the white populations in Australia, New Zealand, North America, and Northern and Western Europe (International Agency for Research on Cancer, 2014; Sung et al., 2021).

Other forms of carcinomas include breast, liver, bladder, and prostate cancer. We will discuss some of these forms of cancer more fully in the following section. For now, it is important to note that the mortality rates associated with each of these four carcinomas exceed those for skin cancer even though the incidence rate for these four carcinomas are much lower than skin cancers. Carcinomas illustrate one property of cancer: The most frequently occurring form of the disease is not necessarily the deadliest.

SARCOMAS *Sarcomas* that develop in soft tissue are called soft-tissue cancers and can occur in a number of sites in the body, including fat, muscle, nerves, tendons, and other tissues that support organs (University of Minnesota, 2008). There are more than 50 types of soft-tissue sarcomas (Cancer Australia, 2022). Sarcomas can also form in the bone and those are referred to as bone sarcomas. Sarcomas often spread to other places in the body. Therefore, they usually form malignant tumors.

Sarcomas can be caused by genetic diseases, exposure to chemicals such as herbicides or arsenic, and some infectious viruses such as the virus that causes Kaposi's sarcoma, a type of sarcoma that is associated with HIV in some countries. There appear, however, to be other causes of sarcoma that are as of yet unidentified (International Agency for Research on Cancer, 2014).

LEUKEMIA *Leukemia* develops in blood-producing tissues, most commonly in the bone marrow. ***Bone marrow*** produces most of the body's blood cells, including all of the red and most of the white blood cells (Cleveland Clinic, 2024c). The disease known as *leukemia* is best characterized as an uncontrolled growth of white blood cells. Although the uncontrolled growth of cells is in itself a problem, *leukemia* presents additional problems because the cells produced as a result of the disease are abnormal, sometimes characterized as "immature" cells.

You will remember from Chapter 8, Psychoneuroimmunology, that white blood cells are critical to the body's immune system. To review, the white blood cells include the T cells, responsible for killing microorganisms or producing the antibodies that fight microorganisms, and B cells, a second type of white cell that also produces antibodies to attack microorganisms. *Leukemia* produces an abundance of white cells, but they are abnormal. They are unable to perform the protective function of the body's more mature white blood cells. Because of a smaller than needed supply of mature white blood cells, the body's immune system weakens over time, leaving the body vulnerable to infections.

Leukemia generally is a rare disease; however, globally, it is the most common form of cancer among children less than 15 years old, accounting for approximately 30% of all childhood cancers (Namayandeh, Khazaei, Najafi, Goodarzi, & Moslem, 2020). A review of global leukemia statistics for children 0–14 years of age by Namayandeh and colleagues (2020) shows that in 2018, the highest incidences of leukemia for children were found in Malaysia (8 per 100,000), the Republic of Moldova (7.2 per 100,000), and Singapore (2.8 per 100,000). By comparison, the highest mortality rates for the same disease and population were reported in Malaysia (4.2 per 100,000), Honduras (4 per 100,000) and Sri Lanka (1.4 per 100,000).

The research on childhood leukemia suggests that several factors contribute to its occurrence, including genetic predisposition, nutrition, drug use, infections, and environmental factors (Bunin, 2004; Schüz, Morgan, Böhler, Kaatsch, & Michaelis, 2003). New research suggests that childhood leukemia may also be associated with socioeconomic status, delayed exposure to common infections, as well as changes in reproductive behaviors (International Agency for Research on Cancer, 2014). As we will see later in this chapter, an environmental contributor to leukemia, especially for children under five years of age, is exposure or proximity to nuclear power plants (Kaatsch & Mergenthaler, 2008; Kaatsch, Spix, Schulze-Rath, Schmiedel, & Blettner, 2008). We will explore the effects of environmental factors on cancer in more detail in the following sections.

People with leukemia may be treated with bone marrow transplants from bone marrow donors. Similar in concept to blood donation, donors agree to the removal of a small portion of their marrow, which is injected into the individual with leukemia. The transplanted marrow helps to replace the diseased cells, here meaning cells damaged by cancer.

Although the disease is rare, the mortality rates associated with leukemia are high. More than 70% of individuals in need of bone marrow transplants are unable to find suitable nonrelated donors with compatible bone marrows (Institute for Justice, 2013). Within families, approximately 40% of whites but only 2% of African Americans find matches from their own siblings (Institute for Justice, 2013; Nosheen, 2009). This fact helps to explain the high mortality rates associated with this infrequent but deadly form of cancer.

LYMPHOMAS The fourth category of cancers, ***lymphomas***, are malignant and form in the lymphatic system. Recall from Chapter 8, Psychoneuroimmunology, that the lymphatic system consists of lymph vessels (glands) and organs that produce white blood cells needed by the body's immune system (see Table 8.1, Chapter 8, Psychoneuroimmunology). The white blood cells, called lymphocytes, which serve as the "security patrol" for the body, produce the T cells and B cells that search for and destroy invading microorganisms (see Chapter 8, Psychoneuroimmunology). Put another way, they defend against infection.

When the white blood cells in the lymph glands, called *lymphocytes*, become abnormal, they are unable to effectively destroy invading viruses or other infections. What is more, abnormal lymph glands cannot perform their second function, preventing infections from spreading to other parts of the body. Like the immature cells developed as a result of leukemia, abnormal lymphocytes also leave the body vulnerable to infections or other illnesses.

Lymphomas are usually classified as either *non-Hodgkin's lymphoma* or *Hodgkin's disease*. Non-Hodgkin's lymphoma is frequently a fatal form of lymphoma because the tumors are usually malignant. And although the incidence rates for non-Hodgkin's lymphoma are low, the mortality rates associated with the disease are high. By comparison, Hodgkin's disease is less severe. Although it also infects the lymph glands, it is less likely to spread to other organs. Therefore, it is more easily controlled and treated.

To summarize, benign tumors are not cancer forming and are not life-threatening. Malignant tumors are often cancerous and have varying mortality rates depending on the type of cancer. Generally, basal cell carcinoma, the most frequently occurring form of cancer, has the lowest mortality rate, whereas other forms of cancers, such as leukemias and lymphomas, are less commonly occurring but have higher mortality rates.

Global Cancer Incidences and Mortality: Developed versus Developing Countries

In Chapter 4, Global, Communicable, and Chronic Disease, we noted that chronic diseases disproportionately affect people in developing countries. Lack of access to health care for many in developing countries often results in higher death rates for illnesses that are curable or easily controlled in developed countries. Cancer is an example of a disease with poor outcomes in developing countries. Tables 11.3a and 11.3b help illustrate this point.

While the prevalence and mortality rates for some cancers is high for both developed and developing countries, incidence and mortality rates differ as a function of income and gender. Let's begin with the similarities. For males in both developed or high/upper middle-income and developing or low/low-middle income countries, the most frequently occurring (i.e. highest incidences) cancer is lung cancer. It is also the leading cause of cancer deaths for both groups (see again Table 11.3a). In addition, prostate cancer is the second most frequently occurring cancer for males by country income status, but it is not ranked second as a cause of cancer death. For both groups, liver cancer is the second leading cause of cancer deaths. After this point, however, we see differences in the incidences and mortality rankings for cancer by country status. For example, colorectal cancer is the third most frequently occurring cancer and the third leading cause of death among high/upper-middle income countries. For low/low-middle income countries, however, lip/oral cancer is the third most frequently occurring cancer, while stomach cancer is the third leading cause of cancer deaths.

Similar disparities in cancer incidence and mortality rates are reported for women. In high/upper middle-income countries, breast, colorectal, and lung cancers are the top frequently occurring cancers. As for mortality, they also represent the top three ranks, just in a different order (see Table 11.3b). For low/lower middle-income countries, however, breast, cervix uteri, and colorectal cancers respectively are the three most frequently occurring cancers, but here, breast, cervix uteri, and ovarian cancers are the leading causes of cancer mortality. Thus, women in low/lower-middle income countries experience higher cancer mortality rates associated with female reproductive organs than do women in high/upper-middle income countries. See again Table 11.3b.

TABLE 11.3a Global Incidences and Mortality Data for Cancer by Gender and Country Status: Males, 2020

Cancer Sites	High/Upper Middle Income				Low/Lower Middle Income			
	Rank	Incidence	Rank	Mortality	Rank	Incidence	Rank	Mortality
Lung	1	1,268,289	1	1,037,597	1	167,018	1	150,558
Prostate	2	1,251,977	5	295,237	2	160,914	6	79,640
Colorectal	3	941,410	3	441,355	4	124,064	7	74,046
Stomach	4	616,343	4	413,704	6	103,015	3	88,965
Liver	5	512,952	2	463,573	5	119,145	2	113,749
Bladder	6	383,942	9	127,711	10	56,677	12	30,984
Esophagus	7	331,634	6	293,410	7	86,607	4	80,803
Kidney	8	239,504	12	96,986	13	31,613	14	18,567
Non-Hodgkin's lymphoma	9	238,235	10	107,720	9	65,748	9	39,297
Pancreas	10	235,605	7	220,496	14	27,126	13	26,222
Leukemia	11	202,551	8	127,720	8	66,837	8	50,023
Brain (central nervous system)	12	126,771	11	103,135	12	41,512	10	35,091
Lip/oral	13	118,775	14	44,305	3	145,348	5	80,693
Larynx	14	103,944	13	50,864	11	56,228	11	34,441

Source: Adapted from World Health Organization (2022e).

TABLE 11.3b Global Incidences and Mortality Data for Cancer by Gender and Country Status: Females, 2020

Cancer Sites	High/Upper Middle Income				Low/Lower Middle Income			
	Rank	Incidence	Rank	Mortality	Rank	Incidence	Rank	Mortality
Breast	1	1,758,823	2	446,312	1	501,304	1	238,280
Colorectal	2	764,758	3	360,428	3	100,432	5	58,902
Lung	3	701,386	1	546,136	4	96,040	4	61,013
Thyroid	4	396,260	19	19,220	9	52,486	18	8,514
Corpus uteri	5	358,908	13	79,521	8	58,186	15	17,781
Cervix uteri	6	319,464	7	162,412	2	284,399	2	179,268
Stomach	7	306,765	4	213,031	6	62,712	7	52,901
Ovary	8	218,089	8	141,407	5	95,736	3	65,748
Liver	9	214,736	6	196,675	7	58,514	6	55,878
Pancreas	10	212,457	5	199,361	17	20,344	14	19,702
Non-Hodgkin's lymphoma	11	192,179	12	84,629	13	47,900	11	28,369
Leukemia	12	153,559	10	96,116	12	51,367	9	37,606
Melanoma of skin	13	141,924	18	20,959	19	8,776	19	3,693
Kidney	14	137,562	14	51,362	16	22,412	16	12,390
Esophagus	15	133,701	9	121,097	11	52,016	8	48,635
Bladder	16	114,374	15	44,602	18	17,971	17	9,518
Brain/CNS	17	109,518	11	87,629	14	30,197	12	25,390
Lip/Oral	18	61,265	17	22,275	10	52,210	10	30,453
Gallbladder	19	47,010	16	32,938	15	27,861	13	21,483

Source: Adapted from World Health Organization (2022e).

Individual health behaviors, including diet and nutrition, may explain some of the between-country differences in types, prevalence, and mortality rates of cancer. We explore the effects of health behaviors on cancer more fully in the following section. But for the moment, the point here is that a country's income status impacts the type and mortality rates of many cancers.

SECTION II. RISK FACTORS FOR CANCER

Cancer and Gender

Do women have higher incidence and mortality rates for cancer than men? Educational campaigns in the U.S. in the early 1900s suggested that women were, in fact, at higher risk (Reagan, 1997; Wood, 1924).

As early as 1913, public health officials and other health organizations in the U.S. produced and distributed public service advertisements, mainly print and radio advertisements, to educate the public about cancer, a newly discovered and somewhat feared disease. Many of the early ads either identified women as a high-risk group for those cancers or identified women as the caregivers, responsible for overseeing the health and welfare of their family.

Some researchers contend that many men and women interpreted the ads to say that women were at higher risk for cancer than men (Reagan, 1997). In fact, the belief that cancer largely affected women was so pronounced that, in the early 1950s, the American Cancer Society changed their educational campaign to emphasize that men, too, were at high risk for cancer (Reagan, 1997). But decades of misperception were difficult to correct. Even today, women continue to misperceive their risks of cancer. For example, American women still overestimate the mortality rates for breast cancer compared with, say, heart disease. A quick reminder is needed here. Heart disease is, and remains, the leading cause of death worldwide for men and women (see Chapter 9, Cardiovascular Disease). Today's misperceptions may be due in part to the effective marketing campaigns that stressed women's risk for breast cancer.

So, what is the truth? Statistics do show a gender difference in cancer incidence rates as well as incidence and mortality data between genders; however, men, not women, have higher relative cancer risks. Figure 11.4a and 11.4b, along with Tables 11.3a and 11.3b, illustrate this point. Whether considering overall global rates or disaggregating the data by country status (high/upper middle vs. low/lower middle), men's incidence rates of cancer exceed those of women in all comparable categories.

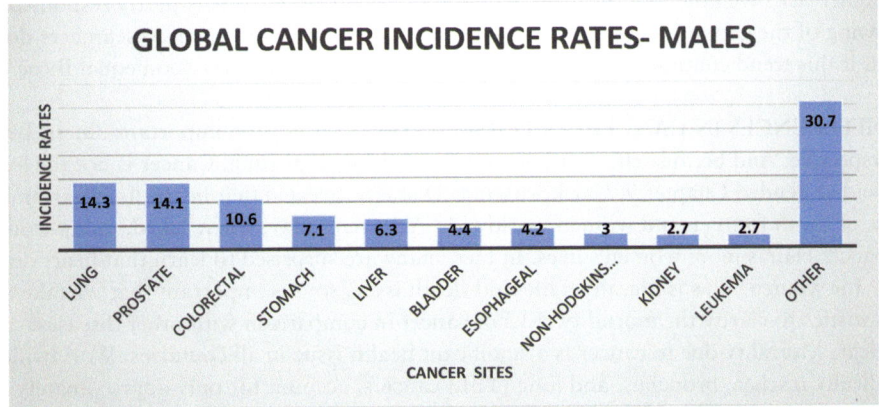

FIGURE 11.4a Global cancer incidence rates for males are higher than those for females in all comparable categories.

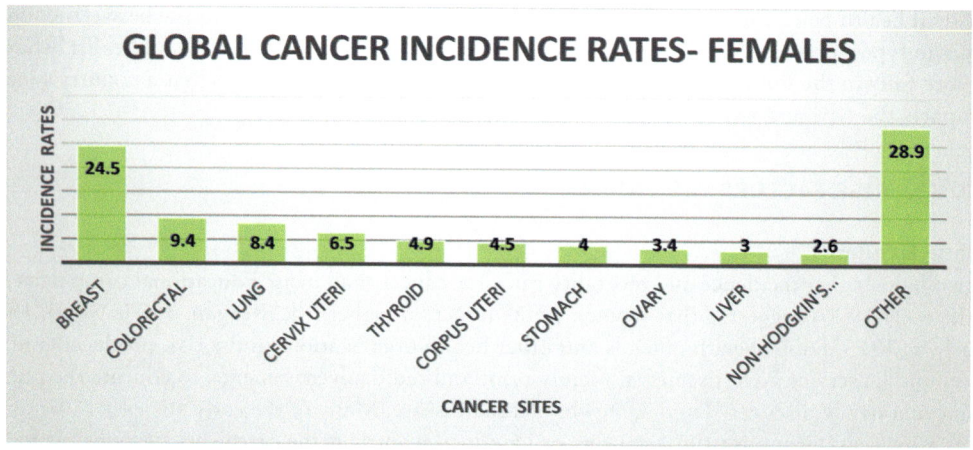

FIGURE 11.4b Global cancer incidence rates for females are lower than those for males in all comparable categories.

Source: Adapted from WHO (2022e).

Historically, one reason for the dramatic difference between men and women has been the relationship between smoking and lung cancer. We will examine the impact of smoking on cancer later in this chapter. For the moment, just remember that before the 1960s, few women smoked or smoked regularly. Therefore, the incidences of cancer linked to smoking were higher for men than for women. After 1960, the number of female smokers and their frequency of smoking increased substantially. Their increased smoking behavior led to an increase in the incidence rates of cancer in women as well as an increase in cancer-related mortality.

To review, the answer to the question posed at the start of this section is no, women do not have a higher relative risk for cancer than men. Efforts to educate the public, and especially the U.S. public, about the new disease in the early 1900s appear responsible for the misperception in the U.S. The newest data on cancer incidence and mortality rates show that overall, there is a gender difference, but that it is men, not women, who are at higher risk. We note that the growing number of female smokers is partly responsible for a recent narrowing of the gap in cancer mortality rates between men and women. Researchers do suggest, however, that if this trend continues, smoking-related deaths for women may soon equal those for men.

GENDER DIFFERENCES IN CANCER: IN PERSPECTIVE Cancer is an important illness, but it must be put in perspective. And because this is a critical issue, it bears repeating. Cancer is not the leading cause of death for either gender. Chapter 9, Cardiovascular Disease, revealed that heart disease is, in fact, the leading cause of death for men and women worldwide. Yet even today, when asked, many women believe that breast cancer claims more women's lives. In fact, many are surprised to learn that heart disease is the leading killer for women. This is literally a life-and-death issue, so it is important that we take a moment to review the statistics to clarify the mortality risks of cancer in comparison with other diseases.

Let's be clear: Mortality due to cancer is a significant health issue in all countries. Worldwide, however, cancer, specifically trachea, bronchus, and lung (TBL) cancers, account for only approximately 3.2% or just under 2 million deaths (WHO, 2023r). What is more, as of 2019, TBL cancers combined were the sixth leading cause of mortality worldwide (World Health Organization, 2023s). We will explore the issue of TBL cancers more thoroughly in the following section on smoking and cancer. For now, just note that current research shows that over a 10-year period, between 2010 to 2020, while the rates of TBL cancers have decreased for men globally, they have increased for women, specifically women in parts of Europe, Asia and Oceania, and among women over 50 years of age (Zhou et al., 2022). But, and this is an important point; only heart disease (all forms) surpassed cancer as the leading cause of death for males and females in developed and developing countries (World Health Organization, 2023r). Does this sound like we are repeating the statistics on heart disease? If so, it is true, but only because this is a life-and-death distinction.

Genetic Factors

GENETIC MARKERS FOR BREAST CANCER Over time, research discovers new information about genetic markers for specific diseases. This is the case with genetic markers for breast cancer.

Early Research Earlier research estimated that 5%–10% of breast cancer incidences were due to cancer-susceptible genes or other hereditary factors (Claus, Schildkraut, Thompson, & Risch, 1996; DeGreve, Sermijn, De Brakeleer, Ren, & Tengels, 2008). Medical researchers agree that in some racial and ethnic populations, two mutated genes, BRCA1 and BRCA2, have been linked to an increased risk for and incidences of early breast cancer (Brankovic-Magic, Dobricic, & Krivokuca, 2012). *Mutated genes* are defined here as genes that experience a change in their genetic material. The reason for the change is unclear but is usually attributed to a genetic error.

The link between BRCA1 and BRCA2 and breast cancer was identified in groups of British and Icelandic women (Anglican Breast Cancer Study Group, 2000; Tryggvadottir et al., 2001). Yet most studies suggest that the ethnic group showing the strongest association between BRCA1 and BRCA2 and breast cancer is Ashkenazi Jewish women. In several studies examining the mutated BRCA1 gene in women of various ethnic groups, Ashkenazi Jewish women accounted for between 12% and 20% of early incidences of the disease (Frey, Perez, Brewer, Fleischmann, & Silber, 2024; Warner et al., 1999).

The association was more pronounced in studies examining *lifetime risk* of breast cancer, meaning the likelihood of developing breast cancer over the course of one's lifetime. In these studies, Ashkenazi women with mutated BRCA1 or BRCA2 had an almost 70% chance of developing the disease (Frey et al., 2024). It is important to note that the risk of developing breast cancer increases with age. Therefore, statistics on lifetime risk must include the effects of age in addition to genetic factors.

Other studies show that a woman's chance of contracting breast cancer is influenced also by the number of female family members with prior early onsets of breast cancer (King, Marks, Mandell, & New York Breast Cancer Study Group, 2003), a phenomenon that occurs with other types of cancer as well.

Current Findings More recent developments in breast cancer research reveal that there are five additional cancer-susceptible genes linked to breast cancer: CDHI, PTEN, STK11, TP53, and PALB2 (Jones et al., 2021). But there is more. Researchers now believe that they may have missed other genetic signals. Studies by Jones et al. (2021) suggest that women, particularly minority women, may be at higher risk for breast cancer due to pathogenic or likely pathogenic cancer variants. What does this mean? We will discuss this more fully in the section on Race and Cancer. But for the moment, just note that the current research suggests that there are cancer-susceptible (*pathogenic*) or likely cancer-susceptible (*likely pathogenic*) genes that have not been fully identified that put these women at increased risk for breast cancer. Researchers now find that in order to identify women, specifically minority women, at potential risk for breast cancer, they must broaden their testing parameters, employing multigene testing panels to search for pathogenetic/likely pathogenic variants as well as variants of uncertain significance.

One additional point about breast cancer. Early studies that identified a genetic link for breast cancer also found a correlation between breast and *ovarian cancer*. In fact, many studies of breast cancer also include women with high risk factors or incidences of ovarian cancer. It appears that the mutated BRCA1, BRCA2, and other genes are risk factors for both types of cancers (Moslehi et al., 2000; Pietragalla, Arcieri, Marchetti, Scambia, & Fagotti, 2020), yielding a 35%–65% chance of cancer in the case of BRCA1 and a 5%–50% chance for BRCA2 (Rebbeck et al., 2018).

GENETIC MARKERS FOR COLON CANCER Gene mutation may also explain some forms of colon and rectal cancer, sometimes referred to as *colorectal cancer*. Some studies have linked a small percentage of colorectal cancers – approximately 3% – to Lynch syndrome, an inherited disease (Uhrhammer & Bignos, 2008; Win et al., 2017), whereas others note a higher risk of colon and rectal cancers among relatives (Tunio, Raf, & Hashmi, 2011).

As in the case of breast cancer, researchers have found a difference in outcomes between early versus later studies on colorectal cancers. Earlier studies of colorectal cancer among family members suggest that an individual's lifetime risk of the illness is increased when *first-degree relatives*, here meaning parents, siblings, or children, have been diagnosed with the disease (Fakheri, Bari, & Merat, 2011). Those studies noted that when a first-degree relative is diagnosed with colorectal cancer before age 55, an individual's own risk of contracting the disease is two to four times higher than someone without a familial risk factor (Fuches et al., 1994; St. John, McDermott, & Hopper, 1993). Such studies also concluded that the familial risk factor for colorectal cancer decreases when the affected person is a *second-degree* (grandparent, aunt, or uncle) or *third-degree* (cousin) relative (Safaee et al., 2010). Taken together, the studies strongly suggest a genetic component to colorectal cancer.

Later studies by Mangas-Sanjuan and Jover (2022) suggest that only people with one or more first-degree relatives who were diagnosed with colorectal cancer before 50 years of age, or two or more first-degree relatives with colorectal cancer – regardless of age of diagnosis (Mangas-Sanjuan & Jover, 2022) – should be categorized as people with familial risk of colorectal cancer. In essence, they suggest a tightening of this classification, suggesting that the former classification was overbroad.

However, of the few studies that examine genetic links for rectal cancers, work by Maul, Burt, and Cannon-Albright (2007) and Yu and Hemminki (2020) used extensive genealogical databases to examine familial associations. Maul et al. employed the Utah Population and Cancer Registry Database, one of three such databases worldwide linking cancer registry records to genealogy records. Yu and Hemminki used the Swedish Family-Cancer Database, the largest such database in the world, which includes all Swedish people born after 1931 and their biological parents (Yu & Hemminki, 2020). Both studies found a significant increase in the risk of rectal and colon cancers among the first-degree relatives of those diagnosed with the disease, here meaning the children of a diagnosed parent. The relative risks for colon or rectal cancer increased with an increase in the number of first-degree relatives with colon or rectal cancer (Yu & Hemminki, 2020). Maul and colleagues' and Yu and Hemminik's findings suggest a strong familial risk factor for rectal cancers and may challenge Mangas-Sanjuan and Jover's (2022) more restricted risk-categorization.

It is important to point out that much more research on colorectal cancers is needed. New statistics on colorectal cancer rates suggest why. New data show increases in cases of colorectal cancer, especially in higher-income countries, and especially among people less than 50 years of age (Feletto et al., 2019;

Stoffel & Murphy, 2020). Here, it appears that individual risk behaviors, particularly nutrition, diet, exercise, and colon cancer, could mitigate some of the proposed genetic determinants identified in current studies. We will explore the link between risk factors and colorectal cancers in more depth in the coming sections.

Race/Ethnicity and Cancer

The relationship between race/ethnicity and cancer can be examined from two perspectives: genetics and health outcomes. We mentioned that earlier studies suggest a higher likely occurrence of breast cancer among Ashkenazi Jewish women than among other ethnic/racial groups especially when examining the prevalence of BRCA1 and BRCA2 mutations. These studies also reported fewer incidences of breast cancer due to gene mutation in other ethnic groups. In those studies, African American and non-Jewish white American women with breast cancer reported only a 0%–3% chance of gene mutation. White women of Spanish descent showed only a 10% chance (de Sanjosé et al., 2003; Newman et al., 1998). Recent studies, however, present a different picture.

When using *multigene spectrum panels*, that is tests that look at mutations of multiple genes at once rather than just a single gene to test for breast cancer, studies suggest that minority women present with higher risks for breast cancer than suggested in previous studies. In a seven-year study (2010–2017) in New York City, Jones and colleagues (2021) found that African American women had the highest frequency of pathogenetic/likely pathogenetic cancer variants (18.6%), while Hispanic and Asian women had the highest frequency of variance of uncertain significance (19.0% and 21.9%, respectively).

But there is more. Rao and Shirts (2023) conducted a comprehensive review of the literature on the prevalence of genetic variance of BRCA1 and BRCA2. This review included 15 studies from North and South America, Europe, Asia, and Australia. Rao and Shirts (2023) found that an estimated 45%–88% of pathogenetic variances were missing. That is to say, these variants were present in the populations but not captured in the studies. What does this mean? Essentially, these findings tell us that these pathogenetic/likely pathogenetic variants and variance of uncertain significance may increase the likelihood of women at high risk for breast cancer who are undiagnosed. And it appears that minority women may be more likely to be impacted by this new discovery.

When we examine the mortality rates due to breast cancer, there emerges another and somewhat contradictory effect of race/ethnicity on cancer. Without a doubt, studies conducted in the U.S. show greater incidences of breast cancer – at least from known or readily identified factors – among white women than African American women or Latinas (Jacobellis & Cutter, 2002; Smith et al., 2008). Additionally, before the 1970s, death rates due to breast cancer was also higher among white women (1970: 32/100,000 deaths for non-Hispanic whites (NHW) versus 29/100,000 deaths for non-Hispanic blacks (NHB); Jutoi, Sung, & Jemal, 2022). But these trends in cancer survival rates reversed after the 1980s. Currently, African American women and Latinas have higher mortality rates from breast cancer than whites (Jutoi et al., 2022; Sighoko et al., 2018; Tian, Goovaertz, Zhan, & Wilson, 2010). The breast cancer death rates for NHWs decreased significantly by 2018 – now accounting for 20/100,000 deaths – while the breast cancer death rates for NHB is largely unchanged at 27/100,000. Furthermore, recent U.S. studies suggest that this trend persists. Cancer mortality rates for NHW are now consistently lower than that for NHB, regardless of the age category (see Figure 11.5; Sighoko et al., 2018).

How is it possible that some groups of women in the U.S. have a lower diagnosed incidence rate but a higher mortality rate attributed to the same disease? (See Figure 11.5.) There appear to be a number of possible explanations. Jutoi and colleagues (2022) suggests that the disparity in mortality rates for breast

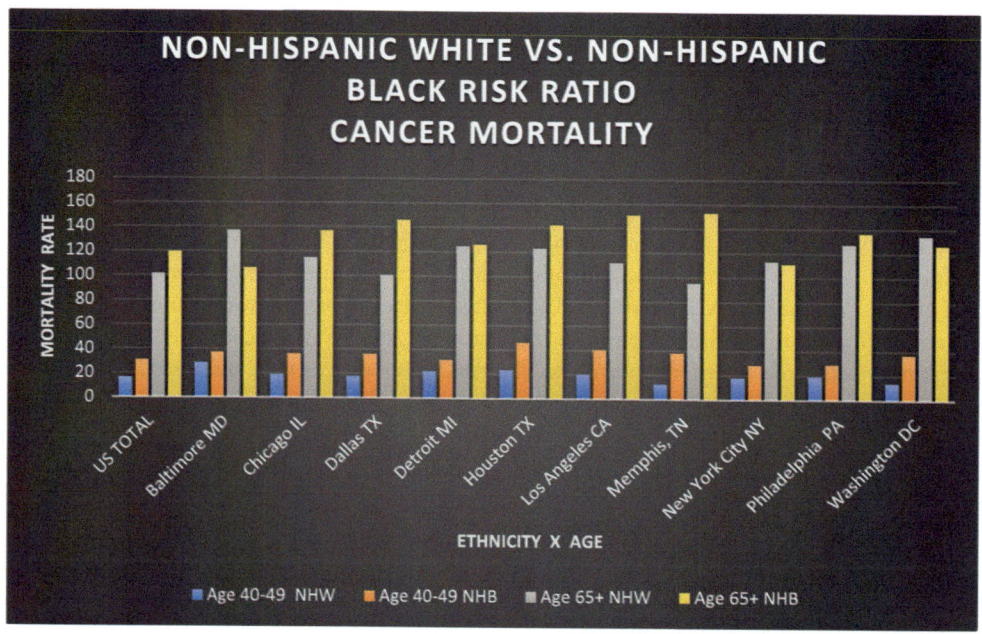

FIGURE 11.5 Cancer mortality risk ratios for non-Hispanic African American women are consistently higher than for non-Hispanic white women.

Source: Adapted from Sighoko et al. (2018).

cancer by race is a new phenomenon in the U.S., something that occurred after the 1980s. Specifically, they endorse the finding that the availability of new medical interventions, specifically *mammograms* for detection and *adjuvant endocrine therapy* for treatment, account for much of this disparity (: Is 3-D Mammography Worth The Extra Expense?: Shots – Health News: NPR, 2018). Research suggests that African American and Hispanic women are far less likely to undergo routine *mammograms*, a screening procedure to detect early stages of breast cancer. Mammograms have been shown to accurately identify 83%–95% of all early stage breast cancers. But one reason cited for the failure of African American and Hispanic women to obtain early testing is the lack of health insurance or of a regular medical provider who alerts the women to the need for such tests, or both (Jacobellis & Cutter, 2002; Orji, Kanu, Adelodun, & Brown, 2020).

Adjuvant endocrine therapy is a treatment for women and men with early stage, hormone receptor–positive breast cancer that reduces the risk of reoccurrence or death (Rao & Cobleigh, 2012). Women (and men) who lack either access to a medical care provider or who lack or have inadequate health insurance to cover the cost of these procedures and therapies will be unable to be screened or treated timely, thereby increasing the likelihood of mortality because of late-stage detection. There may be other reasons these women (and men) are unable to access these treatments, but whatever the reason, the result is that African American women and Latinas are less likely than whites to obtain the screening test that can help detect the disease in its earliest stages. As we noted earlier, one strategy proven effective in reducing mortality rates due to cancer or other diseases is early detection and treatment (Orji et al., 2020).

Some researchers note that socioeconomic class also explains, in part, the disparity in access to care and to potentially lifesaving tests like mammograms. Working-class and low-income women in the U.S. appear to experience greater delays between detection of breast abnormalities and treatment than do middle- and upper-middle-class women, in part due to the costs of such procedures and/or the lack of insurance to cover these costs (Mishra, DeForge, Barnet, Ntiri, & Grant, 2012; Smith et al., 2008). Because race/ethnicity is correlated highly with socioeconomic status in the U.S., African American women and Latinas – who are overrepresented in the lower socioeconomic groups – are more likely to experience delays in diagnosis and treatment than women in higher socioeconomic groups. Therefore, socioeconomic status may also contribute to the apparent racial/ethnic disparities in cancer diagnosis and treatment (Taplin, Ichikawa, & Yood, 2004).

It is important to note that the disparity in incidences and survival rates for cancer between ethnicities is true for all cancers, not just breast cancer. On average, African Americans (63%) are more likely to die five years or less after a diagnosis of cancer of any type than are white Americans (52%; Bach et al., 2002). In sum, although African Americans and Latinos report lower incidences of cancer than do white Americans, they have higher overall mortality rates, suggesting a disparity in access to timely and good-quality health care. And as we noted in previous chapters, access to health care is an individual, health systems, and health policy issue that will determine a person's health outcomes. In the case of cancer, it can also influence early mortality rates.

Environment and Cancer

Environmental factors (exposure to pesticides, air pollutants, and contaminants) and cultural or behavioral practices, specifically diet and exercise, are another determinant of the disparity in cancer survival rates for ethnic groups.

In Chapter 3, Theories and Models of Health Behavior Change, we identified hazardous waste sites as one of the environmental triggers for leukemia, lung, and breast cancers. Other environmental agents have also been identified as *carcinogens*. For example, research in Germany demonstrated significantly higher incidences of leukemia among children five years old or younger living near nuclear power plants (Kaatsch et al., 2008; see Leukemia, page 416). The list of possible environmental carcinogens is long. For that reason, we choose to focus on just two possible factors: cellular phones, an environmental and individual factor, and asbestos.

CELLULAR PHONES AND CANCER? Given the ubiquity of cell phones, the suggestion that cell phones might increase the risk of brain tumors or other cancers must be unwelcome news. One note of caution here. As we noted in Chapter 2, Research Methods, it is very important to maintain objectivity when reading about and interpreting study findings. Here is no exception. So, to maintain objectivity, please do put your cell phones away as you read this section!

Simply put, researchers are in a pitched battle over research exploring associations between cell phone use and cancer. Some scientists propose that radio waves from cellular phones contribute to the growth of tumors in the brain. One strong support for a link between mobile phones and tumors was reported in Sweden, where nearly 80% of the population own and use mobile phones (Lonn, Ahlbom, Hall, & Feychting, 2004). In a population-based study of all 20- to 69-year-olds in three Swedish geographical areas, Lonn and colleagues compared the relationship between long-term cell phone use and *acoustic neuroma*, a benign tumor. They report that individuals who reported heavy cell phone use were almost four times more likely to be diagnosed with an increased risk of acoustic neuroma than infrequent or non–cell phone users. Similar findings were reported by Hardell, Mild, and Carlberg (2003), who also studied cell phone use and incidences of cancer in a Swedish population. It is important to note that Hardell has conducted approximately ten studies on this topic.

In a meta-analysis of Hardell's work, Choi and colleagues (2020) found a marginally increased risk of tumors. They compare this to a series of studies – nine to be exact – by the INTERPHONE group also examining the association between cell phone use and tumor development. The meta-analysis of studies from the INTERPHONE group, conducted by Choi and colleagues (2020), yielded the opposite results. That is to say, cell phone use was associated with decreased tumor risk.

As if these two sets of contradictory findings are not confusing enough, there are other studies whose outcomes also differ, yielding no definitive answer. In the midst of these conflicting findings there are some important facts to consider. First, according to the International Agency for Research on Cancer (IARC), the radio-frequency radiation (RFR) emanating from cell phones and other wireless devices is a Group 2B human carcinogen. That means that it is considered a "possible" carcinogen by this very respected, expert panel (International Agency for Research on Cancer, 2013). Thus, there is reason for concern.

Second, most researchers, even some who contend that there is no statistically significant association between cell phones and tumors, acknowledge that duration of cell phone use could be a factor in tumor development. Essentially, researchers suggest that increased cumulative duration of cell phone use (Miller et al., 2019), that is using a cell phone for 10 or more years, significantly increases – some say doubles – the risk of brain tumors (Inskip et al., 2001; Khurana, Teo, Kundi, Hardell, & Carlberg, 2009).

Third, and this is critical, there is genuine concern about the effect of the RFR from cell phones on the developing brains of children. The skull's bone marrow of young children is considerably thinner than that of an adult with a fully formed brain. Consequently, children who use a cell phone will unwittingly expose their deeper brain structures to more radiation doses (Fernandez et al., 2018). To be clear, that is not a good outcome. To underscore that point, three large studies on the effects of the equivalent of lifetime, human exposures of RFR in rats revealed that rats developed malignant **gliomas** and damage to their DNA chromosomes (Falcioni et al., 2018; Lerchl et al., 2015).

Finally, a number of studies have shown that *ipsilateral* cell phone use, that is using the cell phone on the same side of the body, also increases the risk of tumor development. This finding is consistent with research suggesting that phones placed on the body – that is in back or breast pockets – also increase the risk of cancer.

One more point before moving on. We began this chapter emphasizing the importance of objectivity in reporting (remember the *Toronto Star* article). Therefore, it may be important to note that the research by the INTERPHONE group was partly funded by the mobile phone industry. Full disclosure is important.

As you have come to expect, there is research that contradicts the reports of an association or likely association between cell phones and cancers. There are, in fact, several such arguments. First, consider this: Muscat and colleagues (2000, 2002) conclude that their results do not support the association between mobile phones and cancer. But their findings show a trend in tumor development among cell phone users. Fully 63% of participants in their study developed cerebral tumors. Even more interesting, the tumors also occurred on the same side of the head participants used for their cell phones.

Second, as we mentioned a moment ago, the duration of use was another significant factor evaluated in the association between cell phone use and cancer. We know from earlier studies that short-term use, that is, less than 10 years, is considered a low-risk factor for tumor development. But 63% of participants in Muscat and colleagues' study developed tumors after just three years or less of continued cell phone use. It is possible that the trend toward cerebral tumors in Muscat and colleagues' study, even with such short use, suggests that even shorter cell phone exposure can increase the frequency and severity of tumor development in users.

Finally, several studies on cellular phone use, including those showing no association between cell phones and brain tumors, note that study participants report *subjective symptoms*, or symptoms that are self-identified, after increased use of the phones. The most frequently occurring subjective symptoms include fatigue, headaches, dizziness, and sensations of warmth or burning at the site where the phone is held (Chia, Chia, & Tan, 2000; Sandstrom, Wilen, Oftedal, & Hansson Mild, 2001). Such symptoms appear to pose no immediate health risks but do alert researchers that the radio signals may result in minor or short-term health symptoms at the same site of the brain at which tumors occur that may be related to cell use.

Putting all of this information together, it suggests that cellular phones suggest no danger of brain tumors from short-term use. But it is important to restate that studies examining the effects of digital cell phones have reported on short-term (less than 10 years) rather than long-term use as did earlier studies with analog phones. To fully examine the impact of the newer technology phone, more longitudinal research is needed. As we noted previously, the WHO is monitoring studies of the effects of electromagnetic fields on cancer, with a specific focus on brain cancers in children. For the moment, researchers must be content to follow the WHO's lead, monitoring and reporting if or when health risks occur.

And one more point, which should be obvious. Health psychologists can contribute here to preventive health behaviors by encouraging people to either limit their use of cell phones, or, failing that, to use earphones or the speaker function when talking on cell phones. This small change in health behaviors might reduce the risk of tumors.

ASBESTOS Another environmental agent classified as a carcinogen is *asbestos*. Asbestos is a bundle of fibers made of natural minerals. It was used commercially in the U.S. beginning in the 1800s, principally because of its natural properties as an insulator for heat and sound. As such, it was frequently used in buildings to insulate boilers, steam pipes, or hot-water pipes and for fireproofing because of its fire-retardant properties. But that is not all. According to the WHO, asbestos is found in a host of other products, including roofing shingles, water supply lines, and even in clutches and brake linings in automobiles (WHO, 2018).

The WHO estimates that even today, approximately 125 million people worldwide are exposed to asbestos at their places of work (WHO, 2018). But here is the problem. All forms of asbestos are carcinogenic for humans. Airborne asbestos can become trapped in lung tissues in the body, causing inflammation of the lungs and complicating breathing (Darton, McElvenny, & Hodgson, 2006; Frost, Hurdany Darnton, McElvenny, & Morgan, 2008). Exposure to asbestos has been linked to cancers of the lung, larynx, and ovaries. It is also a cause of *mesothelioma*, a cancer of the pleura, a thin layer of tissue that covers the lungs, and of the peritoneum, a tissue that lines the wall of the abdomen and covers most of the body's organs in the abdomen.

Given these health concerns, and in spite of its useful, natural properties, a health policy regulation issued by the U.S. Consumer Product Safety Commission banned the use of asbestos in 1970, especially in situations in which the fibers could be dislodged and released into the environment. Subsequently, in the late 1980s, the U.S. Environmental Protection Agency ordered the removal or encasement of all damaged asbestos insulation to prevent the release of the fibers into the air. Clearly the health risks of asbestos must have been considerable if two U.S. agencies issued health policies that banned its use and required its removal or containment (Agency for Toxic Substances and Disease Registry, 2001).

Similar actions to eliminate exposure to asbestos have been undertaken by the WHO. With the help of the World Health Assembly, the WHO has undertaken a global campaign to eliminate asbestos-related diseases (World Health Organization, 2018). It should be clear, however, that the best way of eliminating these diseases is to eliminate exposure to asbestos or use of asbestos.

Health Behaviors and Cancer

Up to this point, we have focused largely on nonbehavioral risk factors for cancer. We turn our attention now to the relationship between health-compromising behaviors and selected types of cancer. A report from a research group known as the Global Behavioral Diseases Cancer Risk Factors Collaborators, confirms that as of 2019, the leading risk factors contributing to global cancer burden were behavioral (GBD Cancer Risk Factors Collaborators, 2019). By now you should be thinking that addressing cancers caused by health behaviors is another role for health psychologists. If so, great! We will continue here to explore the behaviors linked to cancer and how health psychologists might help individuals or communities modify or change these behaviors.

Smoking and Cancer

Smoking causes cancer. We can make this causal statement because evidence from research supports such a strong declaration.

Studies over the past 30 years have demonstrated a causal link between cigarette smoke and lung tumors. As of 2019, the GBD Cancer Risk Factors Collaborators reported that smoking was the leading cause of cancer burden globally. In actual numbers, tobacco use (all forms, not just smoking) kills more than seven million people globally each year, accounting for more than 25% of all cancer deaths (World Health Organization, 2017, 2023t). In the U.S. over 80% of lung cancers are attributed to smoking (National Center for Chronic Disease Prevention and Health Promotion, 2014). Lower lung cancer rates attributed to cancer (61%) are reported in aggregate for 21 Asian countries (Zheng et al., 2014). As is shown in Table 11.4, the ten countries with the highest rates of lung cancer deaths are an eclectic mix. For males the top contenders include many low-income countries, whereas for females the majority of countries included in this list of the top ten countries for lung cancer mortalities are high-income countries.

Why is cigarette smoke so harmful? There are several reasons. First, consider this: Cigarettes introduce over 4,000 chemicals into the body. Researchers have not examined the health consequences of all 4,000 agents; however, information on three of the ingredients in cigarettes – tar, nicotine, and carbon monoxide – is sobering. Of these three elements, most attention had been focused on the damaging effects of tar. Most smokers report that they inhale and swallow the smoke emitted from cigarettes. As the inhaled smoke

TABLE 11.4 Global Trends in Lung Cancer Mortality by Gender: Top Ten Countries

Lung Cancer Mortality Rates – Males		Lung Cancer Mortality Rates – Females	
Armenia	65.6	Democratic Republic of Korea	30.7
Türkiye	57.5	Denmark	28.4
New Caledonia	55.6	Hungary	26.6
Kazakhstan	54.5	Canada	25.1
Democratic Republic of Korea	54.4	The Netherlands	24.5
French Polynesia	48.5	U.S.	23.4
China	48.3	French Polynesia	23.0
Uruguay	47.1	Iceland	22.9
Guam	42.7	Cuba	21.6
Cuba	39.6	U.K.	21.4

containing tar moves through the esophagus to the lungs, the smoke and tar damage the cells of the bronchial tubes. Over time, the damaged cells can form into tumors that spread from the bronchi to the lungs. From there, the cancerous tumors can metastasize to other parts of the body.

The effect of tar on the system is dangerous by itself, even without the other 3,999 elements. When added to addictive elements such as nicotine or to carbon monoxide, a poisonous substance when ingested in high quantities, it is no wonder that tobacco smoke is a deadly element.

Second, other studies provide additional evidence of the dangers of smoking. Individuals who smoke one or more packs of cigarettes a day are up to 22 times more likely to develop lung cancer than individuals who never smoked (World Health Organization, 2023t). And although cigar and pipe smokers also face an increased risk of cancer, the fact that cigar and pipe smoke is not swallowed appears to significantly decrease the risk of lung cancer among those groups.

Finally, cigarette smoke also presents health hazards for nonsmokers. The GBD study mentioned earlier showed that secondhand smoke was the tenth leading cause of cancer burden (GBD Cancer Risk Factors Collaborators, 2019). Why? An earlier study by the Harvard Medical School (2006) might help explain. It showed that approximately 3,000 people had been diagnosed with lung cancer who are not smokers themselves but have been exposed on a regular basis or at least frequently to secondhand smoke.

It may seem incredulous that a person can be harmed by someone else's health behavior, but it is exactly this information that motivated governments and public health officials to elevate cigarette smoking to a major public health risk in many city and regional public health departments globally. For example, in 1992, the U.S. Environmental Protection Agency classified environmental tobacco smoke, which includes secondhand smoke, as a Group A carcinogen, the most dangerous class of carcinogens (CDC, 2015). It is one reason why in the U.S., 28 states, in addition to Washington, D.C., the Navaho Nation, Puerto Rico, and the U.S. Virgin Islands, have adopted strict non-smoking regulations for workplaces, restaurants and bars. In addition, two states and the territory of Guam have no-smoking regulations in restaurants and bars (Campaign for Tobacco Free Kids, 2023).

For the global community, the WHO adopted health policies to assist countries in developing ways to limit the health-compromising behaviors of smokers in order to enhance the health status of both smokers and nonsmokers, with an emphasis on protecting the health of nonsmokers. Their regulations helped countries develop strategies to monitor the presence of secondhand smoke, promote smoke-free environments at home and in public spaces – including outdoor spaces, warn people about the dangers of smoking through mass media ads, require warnings on cigarette packages, and increase the monetary cost of smoking, in an effort to reduce smoking incidences (see Figure 11.6). As of 2017, more than 40% of the world's population has been exposed to warnings about the harmful effects of cigarette smoke through mass media or messages on packages (see again Figure 11.6).

Finally, if negative messages do not help health psychologists convince people not to smoke, consider the positive messages from Peto and colleagues (2000), Thun and colleagues (2013), and Jha (2020). Their work shows the benefits of not smoking. These researchers found that the life span of former smokers increases by 5 to 10 years after they stop smoking. Jha further illustrates that former smokers have a 25% decrease in the excess risk of death than do current smokers (Jha, 2020).

Smoking versus E-Cigarettes We introduced e-cigarettes and vaping in Chapter 5, Risky Health Behaviors, Part I, so we will not repeat that information here. Just remember that although e-cigarettes do not contain tobacco, they do contain a number of other elements, including nicotine, flavorings, and other chemicals that are converted into a mist that is then inhaled by the user.

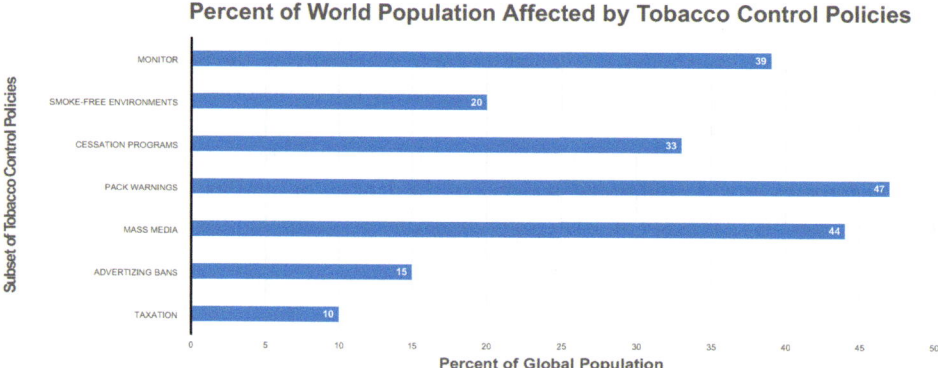

FIGURE 11.6 Impact of tobacco control policies worldwide. Worldwide, health warnings on cigarette packages occur most frequently.

Source: World Health Organization (2017).

Health professionals and e-cigarette manufacturers are debating the potential health effects of e-cigarettes. Some product manufacturers emphasize that e-cigarettes are good for tobacco harm reduction (Altria, 2023). Consistent with this argument, manufacturers claim that the "smoke-free" (also called non-combustible) element of e-cigarettes is a benefit since this would reduce nonsmoker's exposure to secondhand smoke (Altria Group, 2023; Juul, 2023). Additionally, they claim that it is the mix of other chemicals in cigarettes – not nicotine – that causes cancer. Finally, the majority of e-cigarette manufacturers believe that their product is intended for adult smokers only. They say they do not endorse the product for young smokers (Altria Group, 2023; Juul, 2023).

Needless to say, most health providers and many researchers take exception to all of these claims. There may be a debate about whether nicotine causes cancer. But it is generally agreed that nicotine is highly addictive, is considered dangerous to pregnant women and their fetuses, and can be harmful to the developing brain for young people if used before the mid-twenties (CDC, n.d.b). As for claims that e-cigarettes will help people to stop smoking, there is limited evidence to support this point (CDC, n.d.b; National Cancer Institute, n.d.).

Finally, as we saw earlier in Chapter 3, Theories and Models of Health Behavior Change, cigarette manufacturers may claim that their product is for adults, but interestingly, it is very attractive to a younger audience. In 2018 in the U.S., 40% of e-cigarette users between the ages of 18 and 24 had never been regular cigarette users. In contrast, in 2017, only 2.8% of adults were current e-cigarette users (CDC, n.d.b).

E-cigarette use is a popular activity globally as well. Globally, e-cigarettes are also widely popular among new and younger smokers, for example those ages 14–15 in New Zealand. In a 10-year, annual, cross-sectional survey of 14- and 15-year-old students, researchers found a significant increase in the proportion of students who ever tried e-cigarettes and a significant decrease in the proportion of students who ever smoked regular cigarettes (Walker et al., 2020). In this study, daily users of e-cigarettes or cigarettes were more likely to be Māori or Pacific Islander students, student from low socioeconomic backgrounds or gender diverse students (Walker et al., 2020). Finally, according to this study, while males were more likely to use e-cigarettes daily, female students were more likely to be daily cigarette smokers (Walker et al., 2020).

DIET AND EXERCISE Diet and exercise are other types of health-enhancing behaviors believed to minimize the risk of some forms of cancer. As you may remember, we discussed the effects of diet and exercise on other diseases, such as cardiovascular disease, chronic pain, and arthritis, in earlier chapters. Clearly, diet and exercise are general health-enhancing behaviors.

Researchers suggest a strong association between our consumption of foods that constitute the "Western diet," here meaning high consumption of red meat/processed meat, high-fat dairy, refined grains, sweet foods and drinks, and cancer (Baena & Salinas, 2015; Pischon et al., 2006). Instead, some researchers argue that a more aggressive dietary practice (e.g., large intake of fruits and vegetables, whole grains, fish, and white meats) is needed to reduce the risk of colorectal cancer (Baena & Salinas, 2015).

It should be reiterated, however, that high-fat foods, especially foods with trans-fatty acids and those that contain high levels of cholesterol, increase the risk for cardiovascular disease and are not considered best dietary practices. As we noted in Chapter 9, Cardiovascular Health, diets that include a recommended average of three to five cups of fruits and vegetables and foods high in fiber decrease cardiovascular risks. The point here is that the same guidelines that minimize the risk of heart disease also minimize risks of developing colon cancers.

With respect to exercise, researchers have found an inverse relationship between physical activity and cancer. In a European study of approximately 400,000 individuals, Friedenreich, Norat, and Steindor (2006) found that two hours of moderate physical activity or one hour of vigorous physical activity daily reduces the risk of colon cancer by 20%–25%, especially for premenopausal women. After menopause, however, the beneficial effect of lifelong physical activity appears to disappear.

SECTION III. CANCER TREATMENTS AND PREVENTION

By now it is clear that some forms of cancer are caused by genetic or other unknown factors whereas others are attributable to specific health-compromising behaviors, usually the same behaviors that increase risks for other types of chronic diseases. In some respects, therefore, prevention and treatment for cancers linked to lifestyle behaviors is similar to preventive strategies for other illnesses.

It is tempting to suggest that because the same health-enhancing behaviors minimize risks for cardiovascular disease, cancer, and other chronic illnesses, they would be readily adopted by many people. After all, this seems like a perfect example of a one-size-fits-all solution. But as we saw earlier when discussing motivation to change behaviors, sustaining changes in health behaviors can be difficult. Consider this: Many health promotion and healthy living programs report good initial behavior change and maintenance for the first six months but poor adherence thereafter. It is far more difficult to change unhealthy habits than to establish and maintain healthy behaviors, regardless of the health benefits. For this reason, health psychologists and other health professionals may want to emphasize programs that teach children to adopt healthy behaviors. Indeed, many schools, city and regional health departments, and health professionals are doing just that. Adopting healthy behaviors early in children's lives will reduce the struggle to learn these behaviors as adults. In the meantime, health professionals still need to attempt to change the poor health habits of adolescents and adults as well.

In the following section, we briefly review three types of health-behavior change programs designed to reduce risks or incidences of cancer: diet and exercise to minimize colon cancer; breast self-examination (BSE) for early detection and treatment of breast cancer; and immunization, the newest medical approach to prevent cervical cancer. Although the interventions address three distinct behaviors, they share one thing in common: All interventions were either initiated or strongly supported by health policy.

Preventive Health Behaviors

DIET, EXERCISE, AND COLON CANCER Consider this: When going to the movie theater, it is common for customers to purchase a snack to eat while watching the movie. The first problem with snacking at the movies is that consuming between-meal snacks while sitting passively for two or more hours adds fats, calories, and cholesterol – substances that increase fat deposits in the body and that contribute to weight gain. As if that were not enough, the types of snacks offered compound the problem. Popcorn saturated with artificial oils high in trans-fatty acids, sodium or sugars, candies, sodas (admittedly, diet sodas are available), and nacho chips with melted cheese are inconsistent with the food pyramid's recommended healthy eating behaviors. In recent years, movie theatres in the U.S. broadened their menus to include pretzel bites (dipped in salt or in cinnamon and sugar), pizzas, or hot dogs. These menu items are, like the other offerings, very high-fat and low-fiber items. Finally, consistent with the "supersize" Western diet culture, movie theaters, also in the U.S., often promote extra-large servings of their snacks for a nominal increase in cost. For the moviegoers' convenience, some even offer package deals: Get a large bag of popcorn, a box of candy, and a large soda for a special low price. Is it possible that high-fat, high-cholesterol snacks at the theater contribute to an increased risk of cancer, especially cancer of the colon?

The concession stand at movie theaters is just one example of the prevalent snack and fast-food culture, especially in industrialized nations. Fast-food chains that offer limited or no vegetables, fruits, or fiber-rich foods on their menus also promote poor nutrition and dietary habits that increase risks for colon cancer. Therefore, to answer the question, yes: The ready availability of very high-fat, high-cholesterol foods in movie theaters and at fast-food places increases cancer-related risks. Yet psychologists know that it is difficult to motivate individuals to give up the "good stuff" in favor of healthier dietary habits in part because of the heavily promoted junk-food culture in the U.S. and other countries. Challenges aside, health psychologists continue to promote and advocate for healthy alternatives.

We noted earlier that researchers have learned that eating habits are often developed early, usually during childhood. Therefore, health promotion programs must also begin early and may need to use health policy regulations to effect change. For example, new public health regulations that restrict the types of snacks and drinks sold in school vending machines in some U.S. cities are one example of a health policy initiative designed to shape healthy eating habits among children (see Chapter 5, Risky Health Behaviors). Instead of selling sodas and high-calorie juices, many school vending machines in, for example, New York City, Boston, and other cities now restrict beverages sold in schools to 2% white and chocolate milk and water. In addition, rather than filling vending machines with candies, cookies, and potato chips, schools in the same cities replace these snack items with fruits and sometimes granola or low-fat nuts. These changes are due to health policy initiatives proposed or adopted in over 16 states, including California, Connecticut, Mississippi, and Louisiana. These policies mandate changes in the marketing and selling of foods to adolescents in schools. Specifically, they aim to limit children's and adolescents' consumption of such snacks in an effort to reduce weight gain and decrease incidences of obesity among school children (National Conference of State Legislatures, 2006). The effects of the new policies, if enforced and maintained, could help lower rates of many chronic illnesses such as Type 2 diabetes (see Chapter 4, Global, Communicable, and Chronic Disease) and colon cancer for which diet and nutrition are contributing factors. Unfortunately, it may take several decades before the effects of the recently enacted health policies are realized.

BREAST SELF-EXAMINATION Prior to the introduction of *breast self-examinations (BSE)*, women relied on their physician or on diagnostic tests to detect possible cancerous tumors. But in the interval between annual physical exams, a small and undetected lump could grow to an appreciable size.

One solution was to teach women to use the same breast examination technique used by their physicians (see Box 11.3). Women could then perform the exams monthly rather than yearly. Increasing the frequency of breast exams would, theoretically, increase women's ability to detect irregularities and receive treatment well before the next physical exam.

VIDEO #54/60

Chapter 11: Cancer

- *Breast self-examination (BSE): Breast self-exams and what to look for*
- *Website: https://www.youtube.com/watch?v=fBC_umUbP7s www.mayoclinic.org/*
- *Mayo Clinic is publicly accessible since it provides medical-based information to the public at no cost (www.mayoclinic.org/)*

Unfortunately, the mass social-marketing campaign to promote BSE (see Chapter 3, Theories and Models of Health Behavior Change) was only partially successful. Some women were able to detect lumps before they became larger in size, but the early detection did not lead to a reduction in mortality rates due to breast cancer. Why?

In Chapter 3, we noted that one barrier to successful health behavior change is health maintenance. The easy part of health behavior change is initiation. Once an individual decides to change behaviors, the enthusiasm for beginning a new behavior and the expectation of improved or changed health status is a motivator in itself. Once the newness wears off, however, it is difficult for many individuals to maintain interest and to continue the behavior. Although some women did detect small lumps before they became problematic, the majority of women decreased the frequency of their BSE well before the development or detection of any lump small or large. As with other intervention programs that require long-term maintenance, many BSE programs reported a drop-off in self-examinations after six months. In the short term, the programs are successful. But if women are to be effective in performing early detection procedures, they must continue beyond the six-month period.

Box 11.3 Do Breast Self-Examinations (BSE) Prevent Deaths Due to Breast Cancer?

With the increased incidences of breast cancer and growing concern over the number of **mastectomies** – medical surgeries to remove breasts infected with malignant tumors – health care providers and researchers have searched for ways to detect breast tumors earlier and reduce the number of breast removal surgeries.

VIDEO #55/60

Chapter 11: Cancer

- *Mastectomy: 60 Seconds to Good Health: Breast Cancer Surgery*
- *Website: https://www.youtube.com/watch?v=Eyilkk3sxak*
- **The WakeMed Health and Hospitals website is publicly accessible and serves as a valuable resource for health-related information** *(Home | WakeMed)*

Mammograms, diagnostic tests that use X-rays or lasers to identify potential tumors in the breast, are effective in detecting precancerous and malignant tumors approximately 80% of the time (National Cancer Institute, 2023). Yet an 80% detection rate is considered low by most medical standards, with 90%–95% as the minimum accepted success rate. Women with "dense breasts," or breasts that have more supportive tissue than fatty tissue, are at higher risks for false negative test results, as are younger women. Newer techniques that involve the use of 3-D mammography, technically called **tomosynthesis**, that provide both 2-D and 3-D images of the breast have been proposed as more accurate in detecting breast cancers and reducing the rate of false positive results. Research from McDonald and colleagues (2017) suggests that fewer women received false positive results when tested using the 3-D technique than the 2-D technique. In addition, the 3-D technique reduced the numbers of women who were diagnosed with breast cancer between annual tests. Yet the debate about which method is preferred is ongoing. While some contend that the most accurate outcomes involve the use of both the 2-D and the 3-D tests, others point out that approach is not only costly, but it also exposes women to more radiation (National Public Radio, 2018).

So, what to do? Medical providers and health professionals realized that, to increase the probability of early breast cancer detection, they needed another tool. This time, however, the tool was not a sophisticated piece of equipment or even a highly trained specialist. The most effective tool, according to health specialists, was women – the same women who regularly schedule screening mammograms and annual visits to their gynecologists for preventive care, reproductive health visits (World Health Organization, 2006d).

The new strategy involved teaching women to perform the same breast examinations done in offices by their physicians. Researchers and health providers proposed that if women were taught to perform breast self-examinations (BSEs) every month, they would be better able to detect small growths or irregularities in their breasts between visits or diagnostic tests (Weiss, 2003). They may even identify some of the 20% of growths that are missed by mammograms. Two things to consider, however. First, the prevalence rates of breast cancer in women (all ages) are less than 10% in the U.S. And men – yes, men can get breast cancer, too – have a much smaller prevalence rate that never exceeds 0.1% at any age level (see Table 11.5).

TABLE 11.5 Prevalence Cases and Rates of Breast Cancer in the U.S.

Age	Females		Males	
	Prevalence (Cases)	Rates	Prevalence (Cases)	Rates
<15 years	26	<0.1%	0	<0.1%
15–39	46,961	0.1%	136	<0.1%
40–64	1,286,717	2.4%	5,140	<0.1%
65–74	1,156,166	7.0%	6,571	0.1%
75+	1,281,925	9.8%	9,311	0.1%

Source: National Cancer Institute (2019). Surveillance, Epidemiology & End Results Program

Disappointingly, however, this approach was jettisoned shortly after its introduction when large randomly controlled studies revealed that BSE had no clear impact on mortalities due to breast cancer. One reason was because of barriers to conducting BSE. These barriers included embarrassment, perceived

Psychotherapeutic Approaches

COGNITIVE-BEHAVIORAL THERAPIES In Chapter 10, Chronic Pain Management and Arthritis, we introduced three psychological intervention therapies used to treat arthritis pain and the resulting psychological problems: cognitive-behavioral therapies, biofeedback, and emotional disclosure. We noted that, with respect to arthritis pain, cognitive-behavioral therapies were the most widely used and consequently thought to be a more successful therapy in combination with medical or drug therapies. It should come as no surprise, therefore, that cognitive-behavioral therapies (CBT) are considered effective intervention techniques for coping with the discomforts and limitations of cancer and its medical treatments. For example, cognitive-behavioral therapy has been shown to reduce reports of depression or depressed moods for individuals at all stages of the disease (Sun et al., 2019). With cancer, CBT helps manage the discomfort of vomiting and pain, two frequently cited side effects of chemotherapy (Redd, Montgomery, & DuHamel, 2001; Tatrow & Montgomery, 2006).

Cognitive-behavioral therapies can also be employed to teach individuals about their illness and treatment as well as the psychological consequences (Moadei & Harris, 2008). The goal of the educational techniques in CBT is to inform the individual and prepare that person for potential problems and difficulties. In some respects, it takes the approach that "To be forewarned is to be forearmed." Educational intervention programs, such as the one developed and implemented by Fawzy and Fawzy (1994), that focus on health education, stress-management awareness, stress-management training, coping skills, and psychological support help to both reduce emotional distress and improve an individual's problem-focused coping skills (see Chapter 10, Chronic Pain Management and Arthritis).

EDUCATIONAL INTERVENTIONS There are two general types of educational therapy. One focuses on providing information about cancer and its treatments. Such support can be offered immediately, that is, as soon as the diagnosis has been shared, and can continue throughout the treatment and post-treatment phases. It can also serve as a useful means of support for patients when making decisions about their treatment options (Moadei & Harris, 2008).

The second type of intervention, psychoeducational intervention, focuses on the psychological aspects of cancer. The goal of this therapeutic approach is to help patients cope with the stress and emotional strain caused by the diagnosis. Here again, Fawzy and Fawzy's (1994) stress-management awareness, coping-skills training, and psychological support have been cited as effective psychotherapeutic techniques for cancer patients (Moadei & Harris, 2008).

COMPLEMENTARY AND ALTERNATIVE MEDICINES We introduced these concepts in Chapter 6, Emotional Health and Well-Being. Sometimes used interchangeably, the terms *complementary medicine* and *alternative medicine* refer to different concepts. *Complementary medicine* generally describes techniques, practices, or methods that are used alongside Western medical approaches. Yoga, acupuncture, meditation, and arts such as music or dance are now considered complementary forms of medicine (Moadei & Harris, 2008). Many researchers agree that these techniques help to address emotional or stressful situations, but there are few studies that suggest that these complementary medicines can retard disease progression or change the course of an illness.

The term *alternative medicine* refers to the use of traditional or herbal medicines in lieu of Western medicines. As we noted in Chapter 6, Emotional Health and Well-Being, herbal medicines have a long history. For example, Chinese traditional medicines and Native American medical practices have long employed plants and other natural elements to create herbal remedies to address chronic and acute illnesses.

In fact, proponents of traditional medicines prefer traditional or alternative medicines to Western medicines when addressing long-term or chronic illnesses.

Both forms of treatment may well be effective for certain illnesses. The paucity of research on complementary medicine (although the number of studies in this area is growing) limits our ability to assess its effectiveness compared with other medical approaches. On the other hand, although there is also limited research on the success of alternative medicines, centuries of history that documents the use of traditional medicines suggest that this field has met with considerable success in addressing health concerns.

COPING STRATEGIES For a refresher on the importance of social support systems and effective techniques when managing a life-threatening illness, return to Chapter 10, Chronic Pain Management and Arthritis, and Chapter 7, Stress and Coping. We will not repeat that information here, but instead highlight a few points.

Similar to the research in the field of stress and coping, research on coping and cancer suggests that individuals who employ a problem-centered approach to coping not only manage more effectively through the illness process, they also present healthier mental-health profiles after the crisis subsides.

Three studies serve as examples. In a study of 146 women with breast cancer, Ransom, Jacobson, Schmidt, and Andrykowski (2005) instructed women in an experimental group on problem-focused techniques they could use to address their diagnosis and treatment for breast cancer. They compared the women in the treatment group (problem-centered coping) with those in the control group (no special coping strategies) to assess women's perceived changes in quality of life after six months. These researchers found that the women in the control group reported focusing more on their cancer symptoms and reported a poorer physical and mental quality of life. Women in the experimental group, however, reported a better physical quality of life with less attention and focus on their symptoms. Interestingly, the experimental group's improved quality of life neither enhanced nor hindered their mental quality of life. The control group, however, reported setbacks in the quality of their mental health.

A second study examines coping strategies among women diagnosed with breast cancer. Hopko and colleagues (2011) found in their study of 80 women with breast cancer that individuals who relied on active, problem-solving coping style, and those who use behavioral activation treatment for depression (BATD) reported a better psychological adjustment to their illness and improved quality of life. Finally, when examining the strategies of adolescents and young adults with cancer, they, too, showed a stronger tendency to report problem-focused and appraisal-focused coping as helpful strategies in working through cancer. It should be noted, however, that in this group of 14 study participants, emotion-focused coping was also mentioned as an additional resource (Kyngas et al., 2001).

Coping through Spirituality We also introduced the use of spirituality to enhance overall well-being in Chapter 6, Emotional Health and Well-Being. Researchers studying the coping strategies of Jordanian adolescents (13–18 years of age) diagnosed with cancer found that adolescents employed four coping strategies, including "strengthening spiritual convictions," "being optimistic and rebuilding hope," "enhancing appearance," and "finding self again" to cope with their new diagnosis (Omari, Wynaden, Al-Omari, & Khatatbeh, 2016). Additionally, in a study of the role of religion and spirituality on women coping with cancer, Thune-Boyle and colleagues (2013) assessed after surgery 155 women newly diagnosed with breast cancer. Specifically, this study focused on aspects of religiousness/spirituality as it relates to anxiety and depression, including religiosity/spirituality, strength of faith, public and private practices, and perceived spiritual support, among others. The researchers concluded that religious and spiritual coping played an important role for the adjustment process for patients in the early stages of breast cancer.

Similar advances have been made in the treatment of the psychological and emotional health issues that often accompany the illness. These developments aside, it still may be a daunting task to assist a close friend or relative who is coping with cancer. The research we explored on coping strategies suggests that problem-focused coping is the most effective strategy for working with challenging and emotionally difficult issues. We agree; but remember the lessons learned in Chapter 6, Emotional Health and Well-Being. Caregivers or people who are called upon to assist people with chronic or debilitating diseases must remember to take good care of themselves as well. Caregivers must realize that the illness takes a toll on everyone, including them. Therefore, it is important that when assisting someone with such an illness, you take time to engage in activities that allow you to think, reflect, or enjoy a few moments free of the responsibilities you assumed. To that end, the coping strategies discussed here and in earlier chapters as well as other forms of relaxation, including music therapy, humor, and spirituality, all have been shown to be effective. But here is the key: Coping strategies are most effective with people who have prior exposure to and appreciation for those experiences. In other words, continue to make time to use those coping strategies that have been effective for you in other situations. Together, problem-focused (cognitive) coping, behavioral coping, and coping-support (social support) elements may be your most effective strategy.

Questions to Consider

1. Cell phones appear not to cause cancer, but they do appear to damage tissues. What might this suggest about the long-term impact of cell phones on our health?
2. What are the ethical considerations in the push to institute a health policy to vaccinate girls against the HPV virus?
3. Many countries have successfully found ways to integrate traditional medicines into their nations' health care systems. What barriers exist for doing the same in the U.S.? How might this impact the health of people who prefer these traditional approaches to health care?

True or False Questions

1. Leukemia is the most common form of cancer among children. True or False.
2. New discoveries in breast cancer show that there are many more variants than the BRCA1 and BRCA2 mutations. True or False.
3. Lymphomas are benign cancers that form in the lymphatic system. True or False.
4. Health psychologists are used in multitherapeutic treatment modalities to address the psychological comorbidities that often accompany cancer diagnosis and treatment. True or False.
5. Breast self-examination, a procedure that women can use themselves to detect new lumps in the breast, has been widely adopted worldwide. True or False.

Important Terms

Health Care Systems and Health Policy

Effects on Health Outcomes

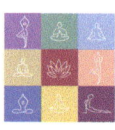

Source: 3xy/
Shutterstock.

Chapter Outline

Chapter Objectives

After studying this chapter, you will be able to:

1. List and describe the four major health care systems in the U.S.
2. Identify and describe three key features of the Affordable Care Act.
3. Identify three major barriers to access to health care.
4. Explain the relationship between consumer satisfaction and health outcomes.
5. Explain the importance of communication on health outcomes.
6. Identify three communication challenges for health care providers.
7. Describe single payer and multipayer health care systems.

DOI: 10.4324/9781003300670-13

OPENING STORY: MICHELLE'S DILEMMA

*Michelle often thought about changing her primary care physician. Dr. B., Michelle's doctor, was one of several physicians in her **health-maintenance organization** (HMO), a managed-care health insurance company in the U.S. that offers a variety of services by physicians, hospitals, and other health providers. Michelle chose Dr. B. because he had over 20 years of experience in medicine and because he was affiliated with one of the best teaching hospitals in Michelle's city. Given his background, she believed that Dr. B. could handle her routine health needs. But over the years, Michelle began to doubt her assumptions.*

Increasingly, Michelle felt that Dr. B. minimized her health complaints. For example, for several years she complained to Dr. B. about pain in her left ear and above her left eye. One time she remembered telling her doctor that if someone could just remove the left side of her face she would feel much better. Each time, after listening to Michelle's complaint, Dr. B. would do the same thing: look in her left ear, probe the sinus regions of her face, and say, "There is nothing wrong here."

On the advice of a friend, Michelle asked Dr. B. for a referral to a neurologist. She thought a specialist could help determine the cause of her headaches. Dr. B. referred Michelle to a neurologist at the same hospital, and she went the following week. After what was, in Michelle's opinion, a very basic exam, the neurologist told her that 50-year-old premenopausal women, like Michelle, often experience such discomforts. She was stunned and angry that a doctor would essentially dismiss her complaints, blaming her age and gender. When she asked the neurologist about specific tests that could confirm or rule out a reason for her pain, he indicated that there was no need for further tests. In addition, he doubted that her HMO would authorize tests based on Michelle's complaints.

One week later, Michelle had a bizarre accident that convinced her that both doctors were wrong. While at home, Michelle fainted and hit her head on a piece of furniture. The blow to her head caused several deep gashes on her face requiring emergency medical attention. Emergency department physicians repaired the wounds with 22 sutures. But after learning of Michelle's prior complaints of head and ear pain, the doctors suspected that neurological problems may have caused her loss of consciousness. They decided to admit Michelle to the hospital for two days to conduct neurological tests. You can imagine Michelle's surprise and feelings of relief when she learned that her complaints were finally being taken seriously. She was also thrilled to learn that her HMO approved all requested tests.

The two-day stay in the hospital gave Michelle plenty of time to think about the years she suffered with headaches, earaches, and facial pain. She also thought about her doctors' response – or lack thereof. If emergency department physicians could determine, in less than 12 hours, that she may be experiencing neurological problems and that additional tests were needed, she wondered why her own doctors could not have done the same. After 10 years with the same provider, Michelle decided that she had to change physicians to protect her health.

This time, instead of choosing a doctor from a list, Michelle asked her ophthalmologist for a recommendation. Michelle respected the ophthalmologist's professional judgment and knew that this doctor would choose someone who would listen carefully to her concerns.

Michelle's first appointment with the new physician confirmed that she had made a good choice. There was no doubt that her new doctor was competent, as was evident from the referral, a quick Internet search of her credentials, and the initial visit. The new doctor thoroughly reviewed the emergency department tests and identified the likely neurological cause for the loss of consciousness. Finally, Michelle had reason to hope that her bouts with headaches and other facial pain would soon come to an end. ■

It may seem strange to begin a chapter on health care systems and health policy with a story about choosing and changing *health care providers*, here meaning not just doctors, but nurses, nurse practitioners, physician assistants, and mental health professionals as well. But health care providers are often an individual's first or only point of contact with the large and sometimes daunting *health care system*. Health care providers serve as intermediaries between the individual and the system, helping to interpret the rules and regulations governing the types of services and treatments available to people from their health care system. As we will see, however, while serving as intermediaries, health providers can limit an individual's access to additional medical care on the belief that they are acting in ways consistent with the system's rules. Michelle's problems with her health care providers illustrate this point.

The opening story identified two additional problems: first, a consumer–provider communication problem between Michelle and both physicians; and second, an inability to access quality care. Michelle felt that neither Dr. B. nor the neurologist believed that her chronic pain was physiological. When they discounted her complaints, Michelle felt her doctors did not understand the effect of the pain on her overall well-being. In addition, she felt they were not sensitive to her continual discomfort.

The second problem involved an inability to obtain additional tests to identify or rule out possible causes for her illness. Specifically, after her experience in the emergency department, Michelle realized that the neurologist was restricting her access to additional medical services. But why would a doctor refuse to request a test that could help diagnose a problem?

We will explore both issues – consumer–provider communication and limited access to health services – and their effects on individual health outcomes more fully in the current chapter. For the moment it is important to note that the opening story also illustrates that often the health systems and individuals interact to shape health outcomes. Michelle's health system in the U.S. allows consumers to change health care providers when and if necessary. However, the decision to change is left to the individual. That is to say, a person must know that a change is possible and must take the initiative to obtain a new primary care provider according to the system's rules. Given Michelle's dissatisfaction, it seems logical that she would change physicians. But remember, it took her more than 10 years to come to that decision. Although some people would have changed physicians sooner, others never do, in spite of the fact that they are dissatisfied with their care. In essence, health care system rules and a knowledgeable and motivated individual can work jointly to improve that person's quality of care.

In the current chapter, we introduce common misconceptions about health care and the uninsured, focusing on the U.S., in Section I. We then continue by exploring how health care systems, health providers, and individual consumers contribute to an individual's health status.

In earlier chapters, we noted that one factor that enhances or impedes good health outcomes is access to timely and good quality care. Therefore, we begin Section II with an overview of the structure of health care systems in the U.S. because, as we will see, the system regulates access to care for many people, not just Michelle. We will also examine health care systems in other developed countries. We then briefly review the new Affordable Care Act, the health policy reforms that aim to make health care more accessible to the uninsured and underinsured in the U.S., and review this country's 100-plus-year attempts to reform its health care system.

We continue in Section III by examining frequently cited problems encountered by individuals when interacting with their health care system. Remember, by health system we mean the organization or structure that provides and regulates the type and frequency of services available to people in the health care group. We pay particular attention to the interaction between the individual, whom we refer to as the *consumer*, and the health care provider. As we mentioned before, in many cases the provider may be the consumer's first or only contact with the health system. We will review the research on *consumer–provider communication*, sometimes called patient–physician communication, and *consumer (patient) satisfaction* to explore their effects on individual health status.

In Section IV, we examine the health system from the perspective of the health care provider. Here, too, research on the interaction between the consumer and the provider suggests that the provider's response, independent of the consumer, can also affect an individual's health.

Finally, in Section V we review research that examines the impact of health care systems and health policies on an individual's health status. Recently, health psychologists have determined that both factors significantly affect the health status of individuals. Here we include a discussion of single payer, sometime called universal, health systems that have been shown to lead to the best, long-term, individual health outcomes in other industrialized nations. Interestingly, the only industrialized country that has not adopted universal health care for all of its citizens is the U.S.

SECTION I. ACCESS TO THE HEALTH CARE SYSTEM

Health Care: An Unnecessary Expense?

It may be difficult for 25-year-old recent college graduates, employed in their first "serious" or career-track job, to think about health insurance. At 25, most young adults feel great. Many believe they are in the best of health and may view health insurance as an unnecessary expense.

These perceptions are confirmed by many studies that show that in the U.S., young adults are the least likely age group to have health insurance. For example, in 2019 in the U.S., after the introduction of the Affordable Care Act, 15.6% of 19- to 34-year-olds were uninsured. This compares with an uninsured health rate of 11.3% for persons 35–64 years old and 5.7% of children 18 years of age or younger (Conway, 2020). We discuss the Affordable Care Act in detail later in the chapter. But briefly, this Act enabled U.S. citizens to obtain health care directly through health care exchanges without needing to rely on an employer or access restricted public health insurance programs. Nevertheless, young adults in good physiological health who have no immediate need for ongoing health care may consider health insurance unnecessary for their overall well-being.

What many young adults do not know is that individuals ages 21 through 29 have a higher incidence of emergency medical care and higher rates of automobile accidents, suicide, homicide, and tobacco and other substance abuse than adolescents (Lau, Adams, Boscardin, & Irwin, 2014). Given their high rates of unexpected medical problems or mishaps, they are, medically speaking, a high-risk group.

Being in a high-risk group for unanticipated medical care is one of the best reasons for purchasing health insurance in the U.S. In fact, the health insurance system is designed for just such people because they cannot accurately anticipate when or whether they will need medical attention. Rather than paying unexpected and expensive medical charges when an emergency occurs, health insurance allows individuals to pay a fixed rate, considerably less than what one would pay in emergency situations, for access to health care when needed. Consider this: When purchasing a car, U.S. car owners are required by many states to have motor vehicle insurance. Automobile insurance protects drivers from paying expensive repair or medical bills in the event of an accident. The same principle applies to health insurance. Although it is true that car owners are only required to carry liability insurance, defined as coverage to pay for the medical or material damage to other drivers, passengers, or vehicles, such monthly premiums are much less expensive than the cost of expensive and unanticipated repair bills or medical costs. In essence, health insurance protects people from large and unanticipated financial responsibilities due to medical emergencies.

Studies also show that without health insurance individuals are less likely to seek and obtain needed health care on a timely basis. Kotagal and colleagues' 2014 study demonstrates this point. Even after the introduction of the Affordable Care Act, people without health insurance were approximately 3.5 times *less* likely to see a doctor, four times *more* likely to indicate that they could not afford the price of prescription medications, and *less than half* as likely to get an annual physical examination (see Figure 12.1). Why would an individual neglect to obtain needed medical care? In the following sections, we identify several compelling reasons, one of which is the cost of care.

Health Care: An Unaffordable Expense?

Many young adults believe that health care is an unaffordable expense, perhaps even a luxury, especially when compared with other items thought to be essential for daily living, such as rent, car loan payments, or the cost of Internet and cell phone service. In fact, Kriss, Collins, Mahato, Gould, and Schoen (2008)

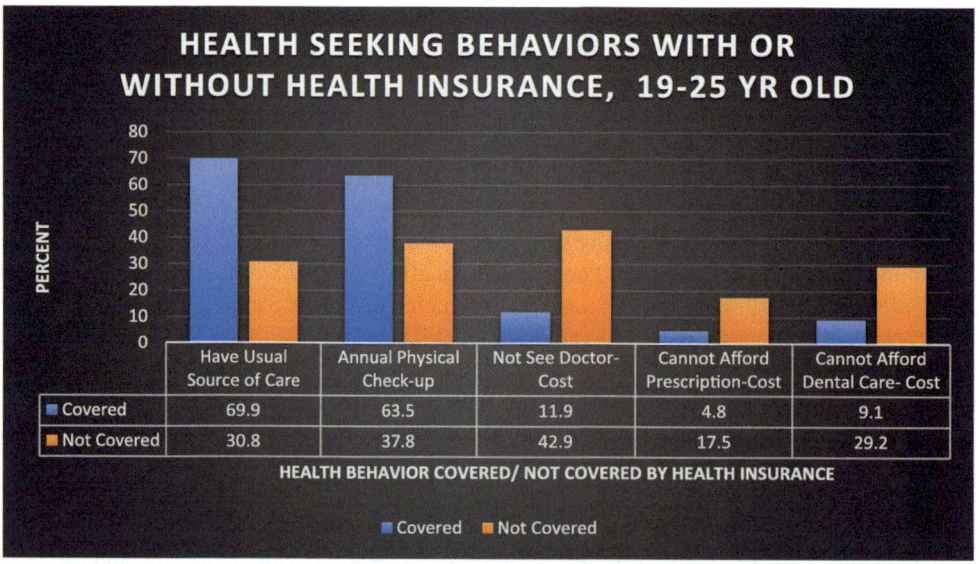

HEALTH SEEKING BEHAVIORS WITH OR WITHOUT HEALTH INSURANCE, 19-25 YR OLD

	Have Usual Source of Care	Annual Physical Check-up	Not See Doctor-Cost	Cannot Afford Prescription-Cost	Cannot Afford Dental Care- Cost
Covered	69.9	63.5	11.9	4.8	9.1
Not Covered	30.8	37.8	42.9	17.5	29.2

HEALTH BEHAVIOR COVERED/ NOT COVERED BY HEALTH INSURANCE

FIGURE 12.1 Health care behaviors of insured versus uninsured adults, ages 19 to 25. A bar chart compares the health-seeking behaviors of 19–25 year olds with and without health insurance. Those without insurance are less likely than insured 19–25 year olds to have a usual source of healthcare (30.8% vs. 69.6%), or to have annual physical checkups (37.8% vs. 63.5%), more likely NOT to see a doctor (42.9% vs. 11.9%), unable to afford prescription drugs (17.5% vs. 4.8%) or dental fees (29.2% vs. 9.1%).

Source: Kotagal, Carle, Kessler, & Flum (2014). Limited Impact on Health and Access to Care for 19- to 25-Year-Olds Following the Patient Protection and Affordable Care Act. *JAMA Pediatrics, 168, 11*, 1023–1029. https://doi.org/10.1001%2Fjamapediatrics.2014.1208

and Levine, McKnight, and Heep (2011) suggest that cost plays a key role in young adult's decisions not to obtain health insurance in the U.S. The high cost of the health care policies relative to young adult's unstable or part-time employment also contribute to the unaffordability of health insurance.

Unfortunately, the benefits of health insurance are often unappreciated until faced with a medical emergency. The out-of-pocket cost of emergency medical care is always greater for the uninsured than for insured individuals. We explain the payment arrangements of health insurance organizations in the U.S. later in the chapter. Briefly, however, the uninsured bear the full cost of all medical services at the time of treatment, whereas for insured individuals the monthly premiums they pay ensure that the full cost of care is subsidized by their insurance company.

One additional problem for uninsured individuals is the quality of care. When faced with a medical problem that requires immediate attention, there is no time to search for the best physician or the best medical care facility to address the need. Thus, uninsured individuals are a little like gamblers, taking a chance on whomever they are assigned much the same way a poker player takes a chance with the cards that are dealt. If lucky, the uninsured person will get a good hand: a skilled doctor or medical provider with experience treating the medical problem. An unlucky hand could result in an inexperienced or less skilled health provider and may result in an unsatisfactory medical repair, for example, an unsightly facial scar that could have been minimized or avoided. It could also result in a number of ongoing, long-term medical problems.

Up to this point, we have focused on young adults in the U.S. because, as statistics show, they are more likely to be uninsured than other age groups. However, uninsured young adults represent only one group that may underestimate the need for full-time and unlimited access to care. It is important to state that many individuals in all age groups prioritize other important – and sometimes not so important – issues over health care insurance. In the following sections, we will see that in the U.S., cost is only one of the many barriers to care for all age groups.

Let us return for the moment to our analogy of a car to emphasize the point that obtaining health care is as important as purchasing any other goods or services. Before buying a car, individuals usually consider their needs. For our purposes, we will assume that a car is necessary for transportation to and from work or school and for performing other basic daily activities. Exactly which type of car to purchase will depend on three main factors: the reliability and dependability of the car and its manufacturers, desired amenities, and, of course, cost. We contend that the same three main factors apply when choosing a health care plan. (We acknowledge that another minor factor – a nice-looking car that attracts attention – can influence one's choice. But few health plans are chosen on the basis of looks). In the following section, we examine the features of different health care systems in the U.S. and their impact on our health outcomes.

SECTION II. OVERVIEW OF HEALTH CARE SYSTEMS IN THE U.S.

In the Beginning

Prior to 1929, health insurance in the U.S. did not exist. When people became ill, they had two options. If financially able, they called a doctor who made house visits or went to the doctor's office to avoid the additional charge for a house call. Those who could not afford to pay a doctor's fee may have relied on traditional medicines or home remedies.

In 1929, *indemnity insurance*, the first form of health insurance, was introduced in the U.S. (Paharia, 2008a). *Indemnity* is a legal term that, when used in the context of health insurance, simply means that a person makes a contract with a company that allows the individual to be reimbursed all or part of the cost they incur as a result of their medical injury or need. With an indemnity insurance policy, an individual pays a fixed monthly or annual amount, called a *premium*, to the insuring company.

Think of it this way: a premium is like a membership fee. For the price of the premium, individuals gain access to the full range of health services available under the contract (see Box 12.1). When a person uses a health service in the contract, they pay the full cost of the service up front. The company then reimburses the individual for between 50% and 80% of the usual and customary medical charges associated with that health service. (We will return to this phrase "usual and customary" later in the chapter). In most instances, the monthly or annual premium for insurance is less than the actual cost of care.

Box 12.1 How Expensive Is Health Insurance?

Answering the question, "How expensive is health insurance?" could require a cost–benefit analysis. Monthly health insurance premiums that may range from $150 to $600 for a single person may seem unnecessary and expensive for a person who is currently healthy, who tries to "eat right," who exercises, and who neither drinks nor smokes. In fact, some would contend that the insurance premiums on a health plan could be put to better use paying housing costs, transportation expenses, and other necessities.

On the other hand, what would happen if the healthy person just described fell while bicycling and fractured his or her leg? Would the cost of health insurance premiums be more or less expensive than the cost of emergency health care? Consider this: The cost associated with doctors' fees, the use of the hospital's facilities, tests to determine the extent of the fracture, and medicines could exceed $70,000. Remember that this is the cost of treatment for just one day. Included in this figure would be approximately 12 hours in a hospital emergency department, X-ray tests to identify the fracture, consultations by orthopedic specialists, and the surgeon's time to repair the damaged leg. Yet this does not include the cost of perhaps a two-day stay in the hospital, follow-up care, or physical therapy to regain full use of the leg. Now we ask again, just how expensive is health insurance?

Blue Cross Blue Shield was the nation's earliest national private health insurance company, offering indemnity health insurance. It now insures approximately 115 million people nationwide (Blue Cross Blue Shield Association, 2024). Today, in addition to Blue Cross Blue Shield, there are a number of other private insurance companies as well as public or government-sponsored insurance programs available to eligible U.S. citizens or legal residents with more options now due to the Affordable Care Act. (More on that later in this section.) As we will see later in the chapter, public health systems are also quite common in many industrialized or developed countries.

Health Plans: Gatekeepers to Health Care

Health care systems in the U.S. today include many different private and public plans. Together, these private and public insurance programs provided access to health care for approximately 92.1% of U.S. citizens in 2022 or about 340 million people, a substantial increase from the 84% of the U.S. population insured in 2010. The remaining almost 8% (26 million) people are commonly referred to as the "uninsured" (U.S. Census Bureau, 2012b, 2023). We will explain the differences among these plans in just a moment. For now, it is important to know that most health care systems offer a number of different health plans, essentially a choice of insurance options that address the various health needs of individuals, couples, and families.

PRIVATE INSURANCE PLANS Private health insurance plans in the U.S. consist of either indemnity, commonly called *fee-for-service*, or *managed-care* plans. Collectively, the private plans insure approximately 67% of the U.S. population as of 2022 (Peter P. Peterson Foundation, 2023; U.S. Census Bureau, 2023; see Figure 12.2). As mentioned earlier, Blue Cross Blue Shield was the first national private indemnity plan. Partially for that reason it is referred to as *traditional indemnity health insurance*.

Traditional Indemnity Plans We explained earlier that individuals enrolled in traditional indemnity plans receive their health care from any provider they choose and are reimbursed 50%–80% of the usual and customary cost of the service. The term *usual (or reasonable) and customary* is critical to the plan and to understanding the cost of health care. Usual and customary means that the indemnity plan predetermines the cost for each medical service, including the provider's fee, tests, medicines, and other costs. Thus, reimbursement of 50%–80% of usual and customary costs does not mean reimbursement of 50%–80% of the actual billed costs, because reimbursement rates for the same procedure can vary depending on the fee charged by the provider or the institution. Consider this: A hospital in a major urban city may charge $130,000 for a knee replacement operation. The same operation at another hospital in the same city may cost $95,000. Traditional indemnity insurance may determine that the usual and customary cost for the procedure is $100,000 and reimburse 50%–80% of that cost, even if a patient paid $130,000 for the procedure.

Indemnity plans impose no restrictions on individuals when choosing a care provider and similarly impose no limits on the provider for the type or frequency of health services offered (CT.GOV, 2024). What does that mean? Consider, again, the case of Michelle in the opening story. If Michelle had been

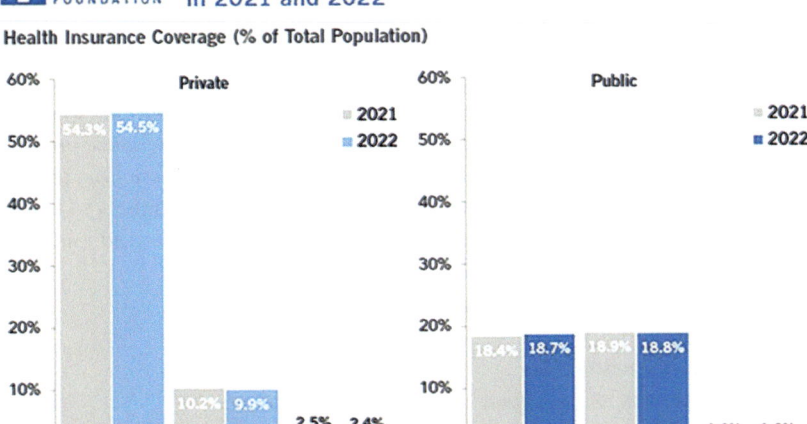

FIGURE 12.2 A bar chart compares the percentage of U.S. residents with private, public or no insurance coverage. Over half the population had private, employer-based health plans in 2021 (54.3%) and 2022 (54.5%). Public insurance through Medicare in 2021 (18.4%) and 2022 (18.7%) or Medicaid (18.9% in 2021; 18.8% in 2022) account for one-fifth of the population. Approximately 10% purchased insurance directly in 2021 (10.2% versus – 2022, 9.9%).

Source: Peter G. Peterson Foundation (2023). www.pgpf.org/blog/2023/11/the-share-of-americans-without-health-insurance-in-2022-matched-a-record-low#:~:text=The%20COVID%2D19%20Public%20Health,of%208.3%20percent%20in%202021

insured through a traditional indemnity plan rather than a managed-care plan, she would not have encountered resistance from her neurologist when asking for tests to diagnose her problem. Indemnity plans allow for unlimited access to and use of medical services – limited only by the consumer's willingness to pay.

A health system that offers an unlimited choice of health care providers and services would seem optimal. Yet traditional indemnity plans are the most expensive of all U.S. health plans and are prohibitively expensive for the average wage earner. For that reason, traditional indemnity plans in the U.S. are used by only a small percentage of the insured population.

Managed-Care Plans Private managed-care plans were first introduced in the 1970s by the Kaiser Corporation, which proposed the new system of health care for its employees. It was to be an alternative to the rising cost of health care under the traditional indemnity plans (Getzen, 2004). Unlike fee-for-service plans, managed care uses a system of tight controls to reduce the cost of health treatments. By reducing the cost of medical care, Kaiser passed the savings on to members enrolled in their managed-care plan. The low costs made managed care an appealing and affordable health insurance option. It also introduced apparent conflicts of interest that resulted in revisions to these plans in 2004.

Consider again Michelle in the opening story. The neurologist denied Michelle's request for additional tests. The restriction on services is, in part, consistent with a managed-care company's goal of limiting their own financial risks and reducing the cost of care (Paharia, 2008a). Yet there are times when medical services are necessary, albeit costly. In such instances, health plans require either preauthorization or preapproval from plan administrators for the specific service. The preapproval process allows the system to review the medical necessity of the requested procedure and thereby limit what it determines to be unnecessary expenses. It also leads to managed-care plans being called "gatekeepers," monitoring and controlling the delivery of services.

Following the lead by the Kaiser Corporation, many managed-care organizations were subsequently established. Today, private managed-care plans take the form of *health-maintenance organizations (HMOs), preferred-provider organizations (PPOs)*, or *point of service (POS;* see Box 12.2). All such plans use similar methods of financial incentives and controls to encourage their members to use the health care providers associated with the plans and to encourage health care providers to avoid unnecessary services.

VIDEO #56/60

Chapter 12: Health Care Systems and Health Policy

- HMO, PPO, and POS: *HMO, PPO, POS, EPO, and HDHP: What's the Difference – Aetna*
- *Website: https://www.aetna.com/health-guide/hmo-pos-ppo-hdhp-whats-the-difference.html?cid=smo-uhs-tw-gf----CP90258*
- *Aetna's corporate profile, health care initiatives, and information about their plans are publicly accessible on their official website.*

For example, consumers pay lower *copayments*, the part of the provider's fee paid directly by the individual to the provider, when using HMO or PPO providers or services. Managed-care plans also incentivize the provider. The incentives given to physicians are often unspecified, but in general, the plans encourage physicians to direct medical referrals to providers or services employed or owned by the HMO or PPO (Fang & Rizzo, 2008) and to limit the number of "unnecessary" medical procedures. As we saw in the opening story, however, the definition of "unnecessary" can be somewhat subjective.

Problems with Private Managed Care Encouraging or even requiring providers and customers to use managed care sponsored services is essential in this system to contain health care costs. So is denying medical procedures thought to be unnecessary. Yet research has shown that the practice of denying services introduces medical conflicts of interest between physicians and their consumers that causes problems for some managed-care systems and appears to jeopardize individual health outcomes.

Specifically, research suggests that such incentives encourage physicians to provide fewer medical services to the consumer even when such services are medically justified (Landon et al., 2009; Reschovsky, Rich, & Lake, 2015). These incentives cause two problems. First, a physician who knowingly refuses to authorize necessary medical services for a patient, perhaps in part to maximize the provider's own incentives from an HMO or PPO, is providing substandard or inadequate health care to the consumer: a violation of medical ethics. Second, if a consumer is denied needed health service, the physician's decision may contribute to that person's diminished health status and, over the longer term, a diminished quality of life.

Box 12.2 Sample of Managed–Health Care Systems in the U.S.

Name	Characteristics
Managed Care	Private or public organizations Individual consumers must be members Health care provided by medical and mental health providers Fixed or reduced fee for service Monthly or annual health insurance premiums
Private Managed-Care Organizations Health-maintenance organizations (HMO)	Health care providers employed by organization Hospitals, laboratories, and supplies owned or purchased by organization Individual consumers must be members Fixed or reduced fee when using HMO services Increased cost for non-HMO services Monthly or annual health insurance premium Additional services, tests, hospitalizations require preauthorization or preapproval
Preferred-provider organizations (PPO)	Subcontract with health care providers Providers negotiate reduced fee to be paid by organization Individual consumers must be members Fixed or reduced fee when using PPO providers Increased cost for non-PPO
Point of service (POS)	Hybrid HMO and PPO Allows members to use out-of-network providers Higher copayments apply
Public Managed-Care Organizations Medicaid	U.S. federal- and state-funded program Eligibility restrictions apply Membership based on income, disability, or related factors
Medicare	U.S.-sponsored program Care generally restricted to individuals 65 years or older with U.S. citizenship or permanent resident status – exceptions may be granted depending on the medical condition or type of care required

In Michelle's case, although we cannot claim that the neurologist refused additional tests because of incentives from the HMO, we can state that without such tests Michelle would have continued to suffer with chronic head and ear pain, undoubtedly leading to a poorer quality of life. Research by Pham, Landon, Reschovsky, Wu, and Schrag (2009) shows that a decrease in medical services negatively affects patients' perceived quality of care. It also lowers their overall satisfaction with their health care. As we will see shortly, decreased satisfaction also has a direct impact on an individual's overall well-being.

No one would disagree with managed-care's efforts to limit increases in health care costs, especially now when spending on health care is escalating in the U.S. The incentive system, however, puts health care providers in a difficult position: They could either request medical services for the consumer in spite of strong messages from the system to eliminate "unnecessary" medical services, or deny services in an effort to comply with the preferred practices of the system, and perhaps receive an incentive. Some research suggests, however, that changes to the managed-care systems that resulted in new procedures beginning in 2004 now show no difference in access to additional health services for individuals in managed care compared with those in fee-for-service plans (DeLaet, Shea, & Carrisquillo, 2002; Haas, Phillips, Sonneborn, McCulloch, & Liang, 2002).

PUBLIC (GOVERNMENT) HEALTH PLANS Public health insurance programs sponsored by the U.S. federal and state governments are also available. As of 2022, approximately 36% of the U.S. population was insured through a government-sponsored health insurance program, such as *Medicaid* for low-income and disabled individuals; *Medicare* for individuals over 65 years of age who also qualify; and health coverage for military personnel and veterans (again, see Box 12.2). The Affordable Care Act of 2010 is credited with increasing Medicaid coverage for eligible persons. We will review aspects of that act shortly.

VIDEO #57/60

Chapter 12: Health Care Systems and Health Policy

· **Medicare:** *How Medicare Plans to Pay to Support Family Caregivers*

· **Website:** *https://videos.aarp.org/detail/video/6344454237112/how-medicare-plans-to-pay-to-support-family-caregivers*

· **AARP is the American Association for Retired Persons and offers services and support for their members (www.aarp.org)**

How Medicare Plans to Pay to Support Family Caregivers – Top Videos and News Stories for the 50+ | AARP

Publicly sponsored and funded plans are also called single-payer plans because one payer, in this case, the U.S. and state governments, provides the sole financial support. For the moment, it is important to note that in *all* other developed countries, including Canada, England, France, Japan, and Sweden, a single-payer health care model is the norm for the majority of the populations (Crowley, Daniel, Cooney, & Engel, 2020). Although private insurers also offer health insurance in these countries, the vast majority of people in the industrialized countries mentioned previously and others rely on government-sponsored, single-payer plans for their primary source of care. We discuss the single-payer system in the section on health policy later in the chapter.

THE UNINSURED With access to either public or private health insurance plans in the U.S., it would seem inconceivable that anyone would be without health insurance. But as we noted, as of 2022, approximately 26 million people were not insured by either system (U.S. Census Bureau, 2023). This number may seem high, but it is actually an improvement from the year just prior to the Affordable Care

TABLE 12.1 (Continued)

Year	Organization	Proposal/Goal	Highlights of Plan	Outcome
1929	Baylor Hospital, Dallas Texas	Prepaid health plan for teachers	Prepaid health plan provides: • Guaranteed medical service, up to 21 days per year • Linked to single hospital	Spurred growth in prepaid health plans nationwide
1939	Wagner Bill—National Health Act of 1939	Furthered work of Tactical Committee on Medical Care of 1937 • Proposed National Health Act of 1937, a federally funded national health program	National health program • Federal government to provide grants to states • States administer program	Not adopted due to • Opposition in Congress • Impact of World War II • U.S. economic status
1943–1946	Wagner, Murray, & Dingle Bill (Continued under President Harry S. Truman)	National Health • Insurance • Add health insurance to Social Security	National Medical Care and Hospitalization • *Universal health care* • Available to all including self-employed and domestic workers • Comprehensive care • Unlimited doctor care, maximum 30 days hospitalization • Lab tests included • Insured choose physician from list of participating providers • Surgeon General of U.S. to establish standard of competence for specialists and hospitals	Bill proposed and defeated in Congress • Strong opposition from various groups • Bill reintroduced in Congress over 14 years
1944	Pres. Franklin D. Roosevelt	State of Union Speech	Proposed "economic bill of rights" that included adequate medical care and the opportunity to achieve and enjoy good health	Died shortly after beginning fourth term
1950	Pres. Harry S. Truman	Social Security Amendments • Amends FDR's SS system to include medical care	Federal funded program • Federal funds to states to administer • "Old-Age" assistance provides for medical care for poor older Americans • Foundation for Medicaid	Enacted in 1950

(Continued)

TABLE 12.1 (Continued)

Year	Organization	Proposal/Goal	Highlights of Plan	Outcome
1965	Pres. Lyndon B. Johnson	Medicare and Medicaid (Title XVIII and XIX of Social Security Act • National health insurance for elderly and poor	One of several single-payer health plans in the United States • Three-point plan • Comprehensive health insurance for poor and persons over 65 years (Part "A") • Medicaid: health services to those receiving welfare • Supplemental Medical Insurance (Part "B") voluntary program covering physician services	Signed into law 1965
1970	Pres. Richard M. Nixon	Two efforts under this administration • Expanded Medicare Eligibility • Proposed Comprehensive Health Insurance Plan	Under expanded Medicare • Social Security disability recipients now eligible for Medicare American Health Insurance Status Comprehensive Health Insurance Plan • *Mandated* employee health insurance plan • Employer pays 65% of premium years 1–3 & 75% thereafter • Annual deductible and out-of-pocket limits • No premiums for low-income families • Replace state run Medicaid programs • Cover all inpatient & outpatient physician costs, lab tests, x-rays, drugs, medical devices, ambulance services	Expanded Medicare enacted in 1972 American Health Insurance Status defeated by Congress
1993	Pres. William J. Clinton	Two proposals • Health Security Act • State Children's Health Insurance Plan	Proposed Health Security Act included: • Universal health care for all • Insurance from private insurers, not employers • Uniform benefit package	Stiff opposition to Health Security Act no bill proposed

(*Continued*)

TABLE 12.1 (Continued)

Year	Organization	Proposal/Goal	Highlights of Plan	Outcome
			• "Report card" on plans for consumers and doctors • Enforcement to prevent fraud, overcharging, bogus claims • Self-employed can deduct cost of plan from income tax Proposed State Children's Health Insurance Plan • Health insurance for children in families who exceed requirements for Medicaid but unable to purchase private health care	State Children's Health Insurance Plan passes Congress
2003	Pres. George W. Bush	Medicare Prescription, Drug, and Modernization Act (MMA)	Focus on changes to prescription drug benefits • Adds outpatient prescription drug benefit beginning 2006 • Adds prescription drug discount card valid 2003–2006 • New preventive benefits	MMA signed into law 2003
2010	Pres. Barack H. Obama	Affordable Care Act, or "ObamaCare"	Most comprehensive change to existing healthcare system, including: • "Health Insurance Marketplace" offering health coverage for U.S. citizens beginning 2014 • Children under 19 years cannot be denied coverage due to preexisting health conditions effective immediately upon passage • Preexisting Condition Insurance Plan for all U.S. citizens in participating states effective immediately upon passage	Signed into law in 2010

(*Continued*)

TABLE 12.1 (Continued)

Year	Organization	Proposal/Goal	Highlights of Plan	Outcome
			• Young adults (26 years or younger) eligible for health coverage under parent's plan effective immediately upon passage • End of lifetime limits on coverage for new health insurance plans effective 2014 • Prohibits lifetime dollar limit on benefits effective 2014 • Eligible for preventive services at no cost effective 2014	

Source: Based on Report of the Social Insurance Commission of the State of California. Sacramento, CA: California State Printing Office; Centers for Medicare & Medical Services (2013); Palmer (1999); Plaut & Arons (1994); Starr (1982); U.S. Department of Health & Human Services (2013); Zhou (2009).

The Affordable Care Act aims to assist people in acquiring health insurance through a number of options both public and private (see Box 12.4). But it is not a universal–health care or single-payer system similar to that in most other developed countries. That means that unlike other countries, the new health care system will make health care available to many thousands, but it will not insure everyone. The new health system under the Affordable Care Act is, however, the most significant health reform in the U.S. in over a century (see again Table 12.1 and Box 12.4).

Box 12.4 The Affordable Care Act of 2010: Also Known as "Obamacare"

More than a century after the U.S. first considered the concept of compulsory insurance for at least some segment of the population, the U.S. Congress adopted into law the Affordable Care Act of 2010.

The law, sometimes referred to as "Obamacare," a reference to the fact that it was passed under President Barack Obama's administration, aims to help millions of Americans obtain or retain health insurance coverage for themselves and their families. Some of the highlights of this plan are identified in Table 12.1. Included in this new legislation is the development of a "Health Insurance Marketplace" (sometimes called a health exchange), a place where any U.S. citizen who currently resides in the country and is not incarcerated can access information about health care plans and options and purchase health care for themselves and for their families. This option was developed to assist the approximately 49 million uninsured Americans obtain affordable and good-quality health care.

In addition to improving access, the law also prohibits insurance companies from denying coverage to children (19 years of age or younger) and to adults who have pre-existing health conditions with Pre-existing Coverage Insurance Plans. It stands to reason that a person with a health condition is most in need of health insurance. Without such protections, such a person may find their health care costs to be prohibitively expensive, forcing them to choose between obtaining necessary medical services or paying for food or housing. The law also allows for a portion of the least often insured group, young adults 26 years of age or younger, to remain on their parent's health insurance plan. As we saw earlier in the chapter, a segment of young adults in this age cohort has the highest uninsured rate of all age groups – an outcome that can be attributed to the need to accept employment with companies that do not offer health benefits or from their inability to find paid employment readily after completing school. Therefore, the new law offers a way to reduce substantially the number of medically uninsured Americans.

The good points notwithstanding, the law has its problems and its critics. One big concern is the cost of implementing and maintaining the new system. Although advocates for the system claim that it will help reduce the cost of health care, critics dispute that outcome. They point to the example of the Massachusetts health care policy enacted under then Governor Willard (Mitt) Romney. Health care costs in Massachusetts have increased as more people seek care, some for the first time. Additionally, researchers in Oregon have noted a similar outcome but with a twist. In 2008, Oregon, in an effort to offer health care to low-income individuals, instituted a lottery system. Anyone who met the qualifications would receive free health care. The problem was that Oregon could only accept 10,000 qualified applicants. Through a naturally occurring random-selection process, the first 10,000 Oregonians who called and were qualified received the free health care service. Finkelstein and colleagues (2012) saw Oregon's health lottery as an opportunity to compare the health outcomes of two matched groups of low-income Oregon state residents with similar demographics. The only difference between the groups was that one group won the right to obtain health insurance, whereas the other did not.

The results of Finkelstein and colleagues' two-year longitudinal study of low-income Oregonians with and without health insurance showed that the cost of providing health care to this new group of health care recipients did, indeed, increase. But they identified two surprising outcomes. First, they found that the newly insured group not only accessed care for the first time, but they stayed engaged. That is to say that they continued to seek health care services. Previously, these researchers suspected that this newly insured group would access care initially but not seek follow-up services.

What was most surprising to Finkelstein and her colleagues, however, was that the newly insured group also reported better emotional, psychological, and physical health than their counterparts. These outcomes suggest that the health care reforms instituted in Oregon, Massachusetts, and gradually throughout the U.S. should measure outcomes not just in terms of monetary cost, but also in terms of better overall health and well-being.

SECTION III. NEGOTIATING THE SYSTEM

Undoubtedly Michelle, the woman in the opening story, is pleased that she has a health care plan that gives her access to a network of health providers and health services, all under one system. But her story demonstrates that access to care does not automatically ensure quality care. In fact, at times it is necessary to negotiate with providers or others in the system to obtain the needed care. To improve her health outcomes, Michelle tried to negotiate two important changes. First, she asked for a referral and for neurological tests, and second, she requested a change of doctors. By requesting specific health services, Michelle became an active participant in her own health care rather than a passive recipient of services.

Later in this section, we will see that individuals who are active participants in their own care tend to have better health outcomes.

Michelle also negotiated to change her health care providers when it was apparent that her original providers were not responding to her as an active partner. By being an active participant, someone involved in the decision-making process, Michelle also improved her quality of care.

Transitioning from a passive to an active participant in one's care and changing one's care provider requires that an individual knows the rules of the system and can effectively negotiate the system to his or her advantage. Consider this analogy: After buying a car, the dealer or seller usually reminds the new owner to read the manual cover to cover. Few people actually do; many flip through the thick handbook to familiarize themselves with the features they will need and a few other interesting details. In the same way, individuals should at least flip through the health care system "handbook" to learn how to use the system effectively, particularly when encountering problems. Michelle may not have reviewed the health care manual for her HMO in its entirety before her dilemma, but no doubt she referred to the manual after her stay in the emergency department to determine how to change service providers.

By comparing our bodies to a car, we intend only to reinforce the point that we should give our body the same quality of care and attention that we give other things, such as the cars we rely on for our daily functioning. A poorly maintained car will not start reliably or when needed. Similarly, a body in poor repair will not allow us to function appropriately. We should take care to select, obtain, and maintain the services needed to function. As part of our self-servicing, we may need to negotiate for improved care.

All negotiations involve communication. Studies on consumer–provider communication show that two factors, the quality of the communication and consumer satisfaction, significantly influence health outcomes. We begin this section, therefore, with a review of the research on consumer satisfaction, followed by a discussion of the effect of consumer–provider communication on health outcomes.

We add one note before continuing. In health, many researchers and providers refer to "patient satisfaction" and "patient–provider communication." We substitute "consumer" for patient in this section to reinforce the concept of the individual as an active participant in his or her health process, someone who must be engaged and satisfied (D'Agostino et al., 2017). As we will see, engaging consumers in the care process increases their understanding of the problem and increases adherence to the recommended procedures, a process that should improve health results. But, as D'Agostino and colleagues notes, improved participation does not always result in improved health outcomes.

Consumer Satisfaction

DEFINING SATISFACTION Consumer satisfaction has been defined variably by health psychologists and medical researchers. For our discussion, we adopt Johannson, Oleni, and Fridlund's (2002) definition of consumer (patient) satisfaction as a comparison between a person's subjective assessment of his or her expectations regarding care and that person's perceptions of the actual care received. The actual care received is measured by the consumer's emotional and cognitive interaction with the provider.

Michelle expected to receive high-quality care from her first doctor given his years of experience, his affiliation with an excellent teaching hospital, and his 10 years serving as her primary care provider. As a result of poor consumer–provider communication with Dr. B. (discounting Michelle's complaints) and her dissatisfaction with the neurologist (unwillingness to authorize additional medical tests), it seems accurate to characterize Michelle as an unsatisfied consumer.

MEDICAL PROVIDER, EMOTIONAL INTELLIGENCE, PERSONALITY, AND DEMOGRAPHICS
Studies examining consumers' satisfaction with medical-care providers focus primarily on a person's

the consumer identify the health problem and agree on a course of action that will lead to better results. Health psychologists, with their combined knowledge of interpersonal interactions and health issues, are able to help providers and consumers build a good rapport for the purpose of advancing individual health outcomes. Health psychologists can also assist providers in developing the interpersonal skills that improve consumer–provider communication.

Studies on consumer–provider communication also identify psychosocial factors, similar to the consumer satisfaction variables we reviewed earlier, as critical to good communication. For example, in their study of Latinas and non-Latinas with abnormal mammogram test results (see Chapter 11, Cancer), Molina and colleagues (2014) found that while all 41 women in the study noted the importance of the provider's empathetic communication styles as important to them, Latinas further stressed the need for warm communication styles, whereas non-Latinas favored more information. They conclude that satisfaction with the provider's communication styles is associated with a positive view of follow-up treatment regimens.

Other studies examining consumer–provider communication in the context of medical decision-making find that here, too, psychosocial factors are important. For example, in a study examining the behaviors of physicians who help build a trusting relationship between consumer and provider, three factors were cited as critical for consumers to maximize their comfort and instill trust: effective communication, demonstrating care for their patient – including seeing them as a person, not just a patient, and a partner in the decision-making process – and demonstrating competence and knowledge about the medical issue(s) (Green & Ramos, 2021).

Remember Michelle, from the opening story? Researchers list active participation as yet another factor that is instrumental to establishing good consumer–provider communication and that also affects health outcomes. Studies show that patients who are less involved in the consultation process and who receive less information and support from their physicians tend to be less satisfied with their care, tend to understand less about their health and possible treatment options, and tend to be less likely to follow medical advice (Esch, Marion, Busato, & Heusser, 2008). We pause for a moment to underscore that less involvement in each of these areas means that a person is less likely to accept and use the medical advice given by the provider. It is not surprising that the combination of these factors leads to poorer health outcomes (Gordon, Street, Kelly, Souchek, & Wray, 2005; see Figure 12.4).

One final point: Although we are told many times to ask questions when we do not understand something, studies show that remarkably few consumers ask questions about their most pressing health concerns. Kirscht (1977), in reviewing the early literature on "patient"–provider communication, noted that consumers avoided asking questions either for fear of being seen as ignorant or due to concerns that they may delay a busy physician with their questions.

Other research on consumer–provider communication suggests that another reason individuals may not ask questions may be that they are not aware that they do not understand the information given. Sound incredible? Consider this: In a study of consumers' understanding of the discharge information and medical care instructions given after a visit to a hospital emergency department, researchers discovered that 78% of the persons discharged indicated that they did not understand the discharge care instructions. What is more, over 50% did not know that they did not understand the instructions (Health & Hospitals Network, 2008). A later study by Sheikh, Brezar, Dzwonek, Yau, and Calder (2018) revises these figures somewhat, but they reinforce the point. Sheikh and colleagues found that 24% of emergency department patients had a poor understanding of the discharge information they received upon leaving the emergency department, and perhaps worse, 42% did not receive complete discharge information, further compounding a lack of understanding.

Even when individuals are in less emotionally charged environments, receiving information about their health condition in nonemergency medical settings, researchers suggest that individuals still have a limited ability to process and recall negative news about their health (Lerner, Jehle, & Janicke, 2000).

It is important to state that communication is a two-way street, and misunderstandings concerning medical diagnosis and care instructions involve the physician also. We will address physician-related communication issues in the following section. For now, however, the main point is that consumers are subjected to a number of psychosocial factors that inhibit their ability to be fully conversant about and to understand aspects of their health condition. Whether consumers are self-conscious of their lack of medical knowledge, lack self-efficacy in becoming an active participant in their health, or are reacting to the personality characteristics or style of the provider, if they do not understand their condition or the medical advice given they are less likely to follow medical advice and therefore more likely to have poorer health outcomes. Improving communication, from both ends of the process, is essential to enhancing health (again, see Figure 12.4). Health psychologists are uniquely positioned to help consumers elicit specific information from their providers that helps them to better understand their health conditions.

We need to add one final point about consumer–provider communication. Many studies identify racial/ethnic background as a contributing or inhibiting factor in the communication process between consumer and provider (Ashton et al., 2003). In fact, a number of studies cite race/ethnicity as barriers to effective communication (Institute of Medicine, 2002b; LaVeist & Nuru-Jeter, 2002), whereas others suggest no significant effect (Lasser, Mintzer, Lambert, Cabral, & Bor, 2005; Stevens, Mistry, Zuckerman, & Halfon, 2005; Takeshita et al., 2020). Studies that cite race/ethnicity as a barrier also note specific differences in the communication patterns between consumers and providers of different races/ethnicities that interfere with the process. For example, Gordon and colleagues (2005) demonstrated that white physicians initiated less sharing of information with African American consumers, whereas African American consumers were less likely to initiate active participation in their own medical care than were white patients. A passive communication style both by physicians and consumers in cross-racial interactions will result in overall poorer health status due, in part, to the consumers' inability to understand their health problems and consequently their reluctance to adhere to the recommended health regimen not to mention poorer consumer satisfaction with their providers.

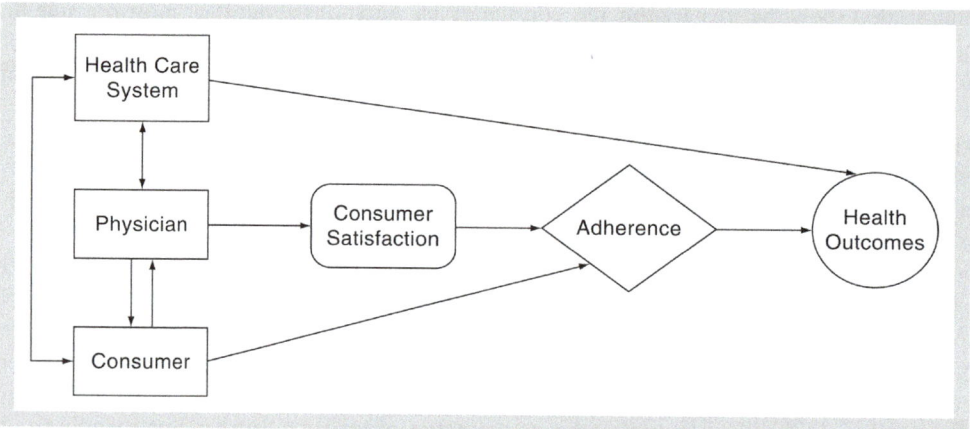

FIGURE 12.4 The flow chart illustrates how the health care system, a physician, and the consumer interact to impact consumer satisfaction, adherence to medical advice, and health outcomes. Both the consumer and the health care system also independently impact health outcomes.

Trust

An additional and important factor regarding race/ethnicity and consumer–physician relationships (including communication) is trust. Collins, Clark, Petersen, and Kressin (2002) stated that, before making decisions about their health care, African Americans in their study felt it essential to establish a level of trust with their health provider. When introducing that study, we did not mention that for many minorities, African Americans in particular, there is a long and deep-seated mistrust of the medical community and of medical providers (see Figure 12.5).

Much of the mistrust is rooted in a history of medical malpractice or questionable medical procedures conducted on African Americans. The Tuskegee experiment, explained in Chapter 2, Research Methods, is one of the worst examples of medical malpractice. Other and more recent examples continue to fuel the sense of mistrust of the health community by African Americans.

The Institute of Medicine's (2002b) report on the unequal treatment of minorities by the health professions in the U.S. has been reinforced by findings from the Commonwealth Fund showing that over 3,000 health care workers could identify specific instances of discrimination by other health care workers, against patients because of their ethnicity, race or language (Commonwealth Fund, 2024). These two findings from well-respected sources in the U.S. adequately documents the current experiences. Although there is no immediate remedy for the decades of medical mistrust, this psychological factor cannot be overlooked when addressing the health needs of African American consumers. For health psychologists, the challenge is to use our considerable knowledge of psychology and health to help both groups work together to improve communication and ultimately to improve the health outcomes of African Americans, and perhaps to begin rebuilding trust.

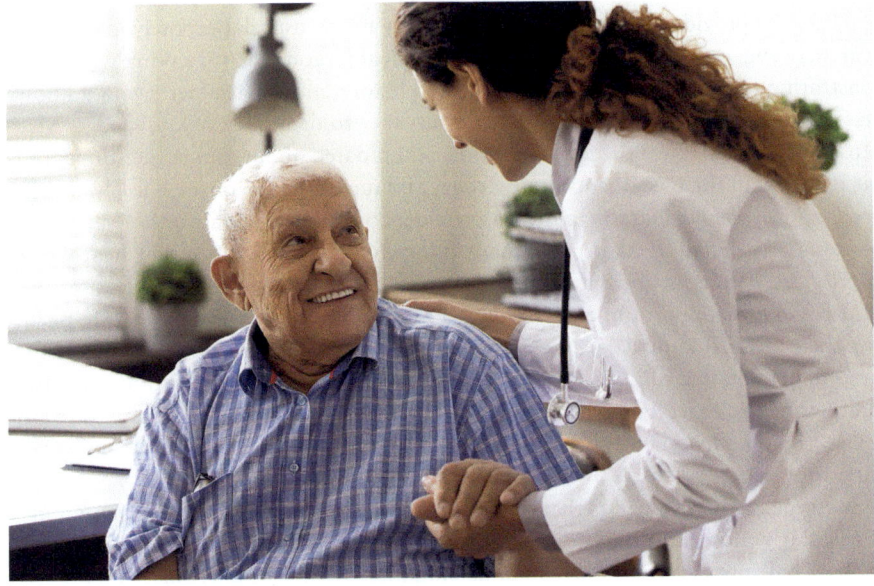

FIGURE 12.5 Consumer–provider relations. Two women, the healthcare provider in a white lab coat with stethoscope around her neck, consoles the patient, holding her hand while they talk.

Source: Getty #479243764.

SECTION IV. CHALLENGES FOR HEALTH CARE PROVIDERS

We have identified several consumer-related factors that may contribute to poor consumer– provider communication. Here we focus on the providers and their unique contributions that directly or indirectly affect outcomes. Although the focus is on the health provider in this section, it is important to remember that the physician is often the "face" of the health care system to the consumer. Therefore, the physician also represents the health system.

Physicians' Three "Fatal" Communication Errors

The "fatal" communication problems we address in this section rarely cause the death of a consumer. They may cause some health setbacks or delay the recovery process. At worst, they may end a consumer's relationship with their care provider, as in the case with Michelle and her primary-care physician in the opening story. In this section, we focus on three physician-related communication errors and their consequence not only for the consumer–provider relationship but also for the consumer's health outcomes. The errors addressed here are "medspeak," limited face time with consumers, and nonverbal communication miscues.

Medspeak

A term first coined by Christy (1979), describes health providers' use of medical terminology, sometimes called medical jargon, when speaking with consumers. Forsythe (2020) also used this term to characterize the need to use language that is clear and easy for patients to understand during the COVID-19 pandemic. It is important to point out that there is nothing problematic with medical providers using medspeak among themselves. It serves as an effective shorthand for communication among professionals. The problem occurs when medical providers use the same jargon when communicating with patients. Are medical providers oblivious to the knowledge gap between providers and consumers, or do they use medspeak purposely in those encounters?

Some researchers suggest that physicians may use medical jargon when speaking with consumers as a way of demonstrating their knowledge. As we indicated before, most consumers want a knowledgeable medical professional, but using medspeak is not the best way to demonstrate knowledge. Medspeak leaves patients confused about their own medical condition, intimidated about asking questions for fear they would appear ignorant in the face of such knowledge, and unwilling to converse freely with a provider. Although medspeak, or medical jargon, allows a provider to demonstrate his or her superior medical vocabulary – not a very difficult task because many patients are clueless when they hear words such as *angina* or *palpitations* (Thomas, Hariharan, Rana, Swain, & Andrew, 2014) – it increases the likelihood that the provider will miss opportunities to develop a rapport with his or her patient. In particular, when demonstrating their medical knowledge, the providers may be less inclined to demonstrate the emotional intelligence and understanding that contribute to individuals' feelings of satisfaction with their health providers and their health care. It also lessens the likelihood that patients will adhere to the medical regimen proposed by the physician. In sum, the negatives of medspeak outweigh any positives as a communication tool.

Interestingly, some research suggests that, in fact, the negative impact of medical jargon may benefit the doctor, particularly those with time constraints or those who would prefer not to explain an illness or procedure that challenges even the doctor's understanding. With consumers arriving for appointments throughout the day, providers compress the time spent with each person. Researchers suggest that providers in managed-care settings spend, on average, 15 minutes per person (Linzer et al., 2015). Think about it. Can you explain your medical problems, fears, and concerns adequately in 15 minutes? And how much time does that leave for the doctor to respond to your concerns? If pressed for time, some doctors may use medical jargon to quickly convey their observations and conclusions to the consumer. Having communicated the information, and with no questions from the confused but likely intimidated consumer, the provider can conclude the visit and move on to the next patient.

A more charitable explanation for the use of medspeak is that physicians overestimate consumers' knowledge. As we noted previously, consumers' medical vocabulary is usually limited. Rather than indicate they do not understand, consumers may remain silent, giving the impression that they grasp both the diagnosis and the medical care instructions (Fuhlbrigge et al., 2021). In such cases, medspeak may represent a misjudgment by the physician of the consumer's knowledge. Without questions from the consumer, physicians may be unaware that they are ineffectively communicating with the consumer. The lapse in communication may become apparent only later, when the individual does not comply with medical advice or delays returning for visits because of the lack of rapport with the physician. By now, you know the health consequences of such outcomes.

One final note here, caution against using medical or psychological jargon applies to health psychologists as well. We must take care to ensure that the consumer understands and has an opportunity to ask questions about anything they don't understand. Giving consumers permission to ask questions, using phrases such as "if I were you right now, I'd probably have lots of questions about things that sound strange to me, so don't be reluctant to ask," may give the consumer the opening they need to ask questions.

Physician Miscommunication or Patient Inattentiveness

Some consumers leave a doctor's office believing that they did not receive a diagnosis. Is it possible the doctor did not tell the consumer his or her medical problem? Did the consumer forget, or is this another example of medspeak?

According to several studies there is real disagreement between physicians and consumers over the issue of effective communication of diagnoses. Early studies by Ley and Spelman (1965) and Fried, Bradley, and O'Leary (2003) and later studies by Fuhlbrigge and colleagues (2021) suggest that consumers often do not remember or misremember, meaning that individuals make mistakes when recalling the information or their diagnosis. Tongue, Epps, and Forese (2005) conducted a national survey of surgeons and their patients in the U.S. to assess surgeons' communication clarity. They found that while 75% of surgeons believed they had communicated clearly with their patients, only 21% of patients agreed with this assessment. If 79% of consumers do not believe their surgeon communicates clearly, then how likely is it they will adhere to the surgeons' instructions? In such instances, the likelihood for improved health outcomes is slim.

Research by Fried and colleagues (2003) also suggests high error rates in individuals' recall. But even more telling, these researchers found that providers and consumers disagreed over whether a discussion about diagnosis ever took place. When comparing the consumer's and provider's recall concerning a poor health diagnosis, Fried and colleagues found that, in 46% of the cases, clinicians reported telling the individual about his or her poor prognosis, but the same individuals claimed not to recall the discussion.

Realizing that it may be difficult to hear distressing news about oneself, the researchers also tested the agreement in recall between providers and caregivers for the patient. The outcomes were marginally worse, with only 38% of clinicians and caregivers agreeing that such discussions took place.

What does all this mean? The lack of agreement about whether discussions occurred, the content of those discussions, and the difficulty communicating about health issues and concerns suggest that consumer–provider communication is a complicated process that becomes more difficult when dealing with personal and perhaps emotional issues like one's health (see Box 12.5). In such instances, good communication skills are essential. This, then, is yet another role for health psychologists as an aid or facilitator in communications between provider and consumer.

The recent attention to interpersonal skills in medicine is due largely to a break from the more traditional, paternalistic approach of medicine in the U.S. (Driever, Tolhuizen, Duvivier, Stigglebout, & Brand, 2022; Driever, Stiggelbout, & Brand, 2020). In that model, the physician was considered the knowledgeable entity, and consumers were expected to comply with all medical directives without question. But as we indicated earlier in the chapter, modern medical practices have evolved to view individuals as consumers of services and therefore as participants in their own health care. The new approach requires continued training of health providers on interpersonal skills, including listening, and all communication skills. Included in this new approach is a focus on nonverbal communication.

Nonverbal Communication Cues

More than 30 years ago, psychologists established that communication involves more than just the spoken or written word. Nonverbal signals, such as facial expressions, a touch, a gaze, or even a tone of voice, also communicate information to the listener. In classic, early research on *nonverbal communication* by the late psychologist Robert Rosenthal, Hall, DiMatteo, Rogers, and Archer (1979), they demonstrated that, in psychotherapy settings, counselors who were more sensitive to their own bodies' nonverbal communication were more effective with their clients than were counselors who were unaware of their nonverbal communication. According to this study, facial, body, and voice cues all conveyed information to the clients that was interpreted along with the counselor's verbal message.

Box 12.5 Introducing Difficult Topics

We indicated that communication is a two-way street. But who is responsible for introducing difficult or unanticipated topics, such as risky health behaviors or illicit behaviors that also affect an individual's health? For example, who should raise the subject of illicit drug use, dependence on sleeping pills, or unprotected sexual behaviors? Additionally, should the physician or the consumer raise concerns about an intimate relationship that is causing emotional distress?

Topics such as these tend to be avoided by many physicians. They are sensitive and can be embarrassing to both the consumer and the provider, not to mention simply being awkward to discuss. As we have discussed, however, health is more than one's physiological state. Emotional health, psychological health, and risky health behaviors all affect physiological functioning.

Research on adolescent health reveals that among that age group, physicians rarely asked about teens' exposure to or experience with risky health behaviors. Fewer than half of physicians who treat adolescent-initiated discussions or sought to counsel teens about risky sexual or substance-use activities even though, as we saw in Chapter 5, Risky Health Behaviors, experimentation begins early in the adolescent years. Studies by Klein, Wilson, and McNulty (1999) and Ziv, Boulet, and Slap (1999) suggest that less than 3% of adolescents report ever being asked about STDs or HIV/AIDS, and less than one-quarter of adolescent boys or girls were asked or counseled about pregnancy prevention. More surprisingly, less than one-third of adolescents discussed mental health issues at their last physical health visit, a disturbing finding given our current understanding of the role of mental and emotional health issues on adolescents' overall well-being.

In truth, few would expect adolescents to initiate such discussions with an adult, especially if the adult is an authority figure or a virtual stranger. After all, adolescents are reluctant to admit to behaviors that are viewed negatively by society or that are illegal. Therefore, physicians or other health care providers need to broach the topic to signal to adolescents that health settings are the appropriate place to talk about *any* behaviors that influence health.

Research by Mulvihill and colleagues (2005) suggests that adolescents who are given regular access to a health care provider trained to address such topics report a significant increase in discussions on risky and mental health behaviors. In their study on the SCHIP program, these researchers reported a 50% increase in discussions about mental health and even greater gains in discussions about STDs, HIV/AIDS, and other health-risk behaviors. If the goal of health care providers is to reduce health-compromising behaviors and to increase the likelihood of health-enhancing behaviors, they should raise such topics even in the absence of physical or psychological symptoms. Raising the question indicates to adolescents that the provider not only expects to discuss such topics, but that such topics are appropriate in the context of a health care visit and that the provider is prepared to provide information and guidance on these issues in a confidential setting.

Applying this research to medicine, researchers have concluded that nonverbal cues may also affect a physician's ability to establish a rapport with consumers. For example, a provider's body language can suggest impatience or an intention to leave imminently, which can be interpreted as a physician's lack of interest in talking with the consumer. Other body language, such as fully facing the consumer when talking, using facilitative nodding, and looking at the consumer while both speaking and listening, are nonverbal body language cues that individuals attend to when rating a physician's interest in them and their health issues (Ishikawa, Hashimoto, Kinoshita, & Fujimori, 2008).

Training medical students and other health professionals about the importance of interpersonal communication style, including nonverbal communication, is one way health psychologists can contribute to more effective consumer–provider communication, a first step on the road to enhancing consumer-health outcomes.

In sum, consumer–provider communication is a complex process with many factors and many possibilities for error. Research by social and health psychologists suggests that provider characteristics and demographics (age and experience), consumer characteristics (active participant versus passive recipient), consumer demographics (ethnicity and gender), and the health care setting can contribute to miscommunication. A good rapport and good communication with one's health provider will improve a consumer's level of satisfaction with their health care. More important, it will increase trust and the likelihood that the consumer will adhere to the medical advice given – all of which ultimately affects health outcomes.

SECTION V. HEALTH POLICY

The term *health policy* can describe the system of rules and regulations that apply to managed-care organizations. In this section, however, we define *health policy* as the regulations on health behavior and health services designed to improve an individual's or community's health status. Government agencies, including regional and federal agencies, rather than health systems are responsible for establishing and enforcing such policies. The Affordable Care Act discussed in earlier sections is a recent example of health policy.

In earlier chapters, we identified a number of health policy initiatives by international, regional and local entities. For example, the decision by the WHO to put forth the Framework Convention on Tobacco Control (see Chapter 5, Risky Health Behaviors, Part I) is an example of a global health policy regulation to limit exposure to secondhand smoke, a known carcinogen. Additionally, the implementation of the policy to end electronic nicotine delivery systems (ENDS), also put forth by the WHO and adopted by 32 countries, is a health policy initiative that also educates individuals about the hidden risk of this newest smoking product.

In this section, we focus on local and federal health policy that could affect health care delivery rather than health behaviors. Specifically, we examine two policy initiatives that, if adopted in the U.S., could help improve access to and quality of care: preventive care–focused health plans and single-payer health care systems.

Preventive Care

As we noted in Chapter 6, Emotional Health and Well-Being, Western medicine is based on the biomedical model, a reactive approach to health and illness. The model responds to illnesses or dysfunctions after they have occurred but does not address, nor is it designed to address, ways of preventing illness or dysfunction.

Admittedly, many illnesses are unanticipated or unforeseen, and we will always need a system for responding to the unexpected. But as we have seen in earlier chapters, other illnesses, especially chronic illnesses, are wholly preventable. Currently there are many things that individuals can do to prevent illnesses such as obesity (see Chapter 5, Risky Health Behaviors, Part II) or specific forms of cancer (see Chapter 11, Cancer). It is the case, however, that many individuals are unaware of the behaviors that put them at risk for chronic illnesses. Others may not understand that their self-initiated preventive behaviors are insufficient to avoid the onset of illnesses.

Take smoking, for example. Many smokers were unaware of the dangers of secondhand smoke until public-health advertisements appeared in print media and on radio and television. When realizing the potential harm to family members who were nonsmokers, many smokers tried to make adjustments in their smoking habits. For example, when smoking in a car, the smoker would take pains to lower the window even in the coldest of weather. Although admirable, their self-initiated efforts to reduce risks would have minimal effects. Educating consumers about the benefits and limitations of individually initiated preventive health behaviors is one way to achieve health-behavior change.

It is important to note that some managed-care plans provide continuing education to their members as part of a preventive-care campaign. Pamphlets and informational brochures sent to managed-care plan members provide information about general health-enhancing behaviors as well as information about specific behaviors to improve knowledge. In addition, some managed-care plans now offer *wellness visits*, annual physical exams to review the health status of an individual and to identify problems or potential problems in their early stages before they become severe.

The operative word here is *some*. Preventive-care programs and wellness visits have not been implemented by all health systems. Without a health policy mandate that requires preventive-care services, it is unlikely that all health care systems will adopt such a strategy. In addition, changing from the reactive health model (biomedical model) most prevalent in the U.S. to a preventive model requires more than voluntary change on the part of a few willing systems. Such a change requires concerted effort by government and private businesses.

Single-Payer Health Care System

One difference between the single-payer health care system found in many developed countries and the multipayer system in the U.S. is the conceptual difference in the concept of health care. A *single-payer system* fits a preventive approach to health care, whereas, as we noted previously, *multipayer systems* are rooted more closely in a reactive approach to health and wellness.

We mentioned earlier that Canada, the U.K., and France, along with most other developed countries, use single-payer health care systems that serve the health needs of the majority of their populations. They offer universal and comprehensive care without impeding access (Munn & Woznick, 2007). A critical goal is to offer services at a low cost, all the while maximizing productivity of health care workers in the system. But the system is implemented somewhat differently in each country.

In England, the National Health Service (NHS), a government-run entity, is responsible for administering the universal system. The NHS owns the health care facilities and employs the doctors who work in the system. The delivery of care is managed by physicians clustered in primary-care groups. The groups are organized according to geographic region and are located throughout the U.K. Therefore, the process of deciding and delivering medical care is made at the local level by physicians (Klein, 2001).

Even though the majority of the population in the U.K. is registered with the NHS, there are also private physicians for individuals who prefer to receive their medical care from health care providers not affiliated with the national system. It is important to note, however, that regardless whether one uses a private or an NHS physician, all consumers use the same hospital and laboratory facilities for their care needs.

By comparison, in the Canadian system, control of both the administrative and medical portions of the service are managed by local agencies: in other words, the territories and provinces in Canada. Each territory is able to establish its own set of procedures as long as they are consistent with the Canada Health Act, the national governing document that sets the general guidelines for the system (Munn & Woznick, 2007). In Canada, although approximately 95% of the physicians are in private practice, about the same proportion of the health care facilities – such as hospitals – are publicly owned.

The point here is that there are many different models of universal care. Each country developed the system that fits best with its larger government and culture. When examining the benefits of a universal, or single-payer, system, one fact is quite clear: Preventive health care as a concept appears more consistent with single-payer rather than multipayer systems.

Consider this: Multipayer systems of care, like the many managed-care organizations in the U.S., assume that individuals will change health care systems several times over a 10- to 20-year period. For this reason, they are less vested in establishing and promoting wellness and preventive-care programs because they assume some level of turnover in their membership (Hussey, 2005). Put another way, they focus on the short-term health needs of their members. As a result, few resources are spent to prevent or identify and treat health problems at their earlier stages because the consumer is expected to change to another health system or carrier in short order.

On the other hand, single-payer systems show less turnover in membership during the same period of time. Once enrolled in a single-payer system, members tend to stay for 20 or more years. It is important to note that the lack of turnover may be due, in part, to the lack of other good or affordable options. Whatever the reason, the absence of turnover encourages such single-payer systems to introduce and promote preventive-care services because they will serve a relatively stable population of clients for several decades. By focusing on preventive care, the single-payer system is more expensive in the short term but more cost effective in the long term as it avoids more expensive medical treatments for health ailments that have been ignored or overlooked.

When considering the two options it appears that single-payer systems have two strong advantages. First, they provide unfettered access to care for all eligible individuals. Those truly in need of care, with urgent or emergency medical needs, are covered. It is true, however, that in some systems, such as England's, individuals may be placed on a waiting list for some services. Usually, however, these waiting lists are maintained for nonessential or elective care such as elective surgeries. Second, because individuals in universal health care systems remain for several decades on average, the system strongly promotes preventive health care as a concept and offers preventive-care services as a regular feature of the system. And, in the long run this focus on preventive care results in cost savings for the payer.

Does the system work? In an earlier chapter, we cited a study by Banks et al. (2006) comparing the health status of individuals in the U.S. versus those in England. The researchers were surprised to learn that English residents were reported to be in better overall health relative to Americans. Specifically, the study found that even the wealthiest Americans in the study had poorer health profiles than the average working-class English person. Although there are many possible explanations, one conclusion proposed by the researchers was that the national health system in England, which provides individuals with unfettered access to care, gives even those of limited socioeconomic status better and more consistent health care and better health outcomes than comparable or even higher-income Americans. It would appear from this study that there may be some benefits to a universal health care system.

To be sure, the single-payer system has some disadvantages. We noted that consumers may be placed on a waiting list for some procedures deemed nonurgent or elective. Remember, however, that nonurgent can be a subjective judgment. Recall the research on knee replacement surgery in Chapter 6, Emotional Health and Well-Being. Researchers Toye et al. (2006) found that participants' decision to have knee replacement surgery was based primarily on their discomfort with being dependent on others and with their limited mobility. This is not to negate the psychological- and emotional-health consequences of the loss of one's independence. (We addressed these issues as critical to overall health in previous chapters). In single-payer systems, these issues of psychological or emotional discomfort may not elevate the physical-health problem to a level of urgent or necessary treatment. In countries with single-payer systems, it may be difficult to convince some individuals that their psychological or emotional health does not result in a higher placement on the waiting list.

Personal Postscript

HOW IS THIS CHAPTER RELEVANT TO COLLEGE AND UNIVERSITY STUDENTS?

If you are attending college or university, you may have thought that this chapter is not relevant to you at the moment. Many students are required to enroll in their university's health care plan, so you may feel that you are covered, at least for now. But what does "covered" mean? You may know where to go if you are feeling ill, but do you know what services are offered and whether any require a copayment from you? You may want to take a few moments to review your school's health manual to acquaint yourself with the provisions of the health care service at your university. Pay specific attention to the answers to the following questions:

Hours of Operation

What are the working hours of the health service?
Do you need an appointment for service, or can you be a walk-in?
Are there emergency hours?

Medical Staff

What medical specialties are represented at the health service?
Are referrals possible if you have a medical condition not covered by the university's health service?
Are referrals to non-university physicians covered by your insurance?
Is dental and optical care available through the health service?
Can you choose one physician as your primary-care provider while at the university, or are you randomly assigned to whomever is available?
Are mental health care visits included in the plan?

Payment for Services

Is there a copayment for services?
Can the copayment be billed to your term bill?
If you need a prescription, does the health service have a preferred pharmacist who fills prescriptions for students covered under the university's health plan?

Health Care Services During Vacation

Is the health service open during vacations and semester breaks?
If you are away from campus but need medical care, are you still covered under the university's health policy?

This is not an exhaustive list of questions, but it will help you to begin the process of understanding the rules and regulations of your current health plan. Chances are you will have very few occasions to use your university's health services. When you do, however, you will be better prepared if you know the answers to these basic questions.

Questions to Consider

1. Some people in countries with universal health care complain about the wait-times to receive elective care surgeries under their system. They believe such services are more readily available in the U.S. for all who request them. Do you agree? Who or why not?
2. What additional challenges will the increased access to care occasioned by the Affordable Care Act pose for health care providers, including health psychologists?
3. Communication between a consumer and provider is important to ensuring good health outcomes. How might this also pertain to health psychologists? What challenges do health psychologists encounter when communicating with a consumer about necessary changes in their health behaviors?

True or False Questions

1. Medspeak is a medical term for a specific type of emotional distress. True or False.

2. The Affordable Care Act is the U.S. equivalent of universal health care and is comparable to the universal care plans of other developed countries. True or False.
3. Young people between the ages of 21 and 30 have more emergency medical incidences than any other age group. True or False.
4. Until the Affordable Care Act, many in the U.S. obtained their health insurance from either their employer or the U.S. government. True or False.
5. Studies show that more than 80% of patients report they fully understood their health provider's diagnosis and treatment plan for them. True or False.

Important Terms

CHAPTER 13

The Health Psychologist's Role

Research, Application, and Advocacy

Chapter Outline

Opening Story: John and Ahmed: Aspiring Health Psychologists

Section I. Working with Individuals

Section II. Working with Communities

Section III. Working with Health Care Systems

Section IV. Working in Health Policy

Personal Postscript

Questions to Consider

True or False Questions

Important Terms

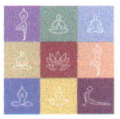

Source: 3xy/
Shutterstock.

Chapter Objectives

After studying this chapter, you will be able to:

1. Describe the health psychologist's likely role in developing four education strategies used with individuals.

2. Identify and define six self-advocacy behaviors to monitor health.

3. Define and explain the health psychologist's role in developing program evaluations.

4. Define euthanasia.

5. Explain the ethical arguments supporting and countering euthanasia.

6. Define and explain community-based participatory research and programs.

7. Define the role of community advocates in improving health outcomes.

8. Explain why health policy is a form of self-advocacy.

9. Identify and describe two health policies influenced by research on health and health behaviors.

10. Describe how health psychologists contribute to healthy workplace environments.

11. Identify two ways in which health psychologists can be health advocates.

DOI: 10.4324/9781003300670-14

OPENING STORY: JOHN AND AHMED: ASPIRING HEALTH PSYCHOLOGISTS

John and Ahmed share a common goal: Both want to pursue a career in health psychology. But while talking about the field they realized they had very different concepts of what health psychologists do. For example, John understood that health psychologists work directly with people, offering education and health-intervention programs to improve an individual's health status. John is particularly interested in cardiovascular disease. He would like to work in a hospital outpatient clinic or community-based center, providing health information and guidance to individuals with heart disease.

For Ahmed, health psychology means health policy. His views on the field were influenced by his father, a public health advocate who worked closely with researchers to change their city's policy on free school lunches for high school students. Roughly 50% of the high school students in Ahmed's small town qualified for free lunches because their families' household incomes were below the poverty level. Yet on average, less than 10% of students took school lunch daily.

A change in the city's policy made school lunches available to all students. School officials reported that since the change, 80% of students consumed a school lunch daily. Health researchers suggested that by removing the eligibility restrictions on school lunches, they unknowingly removed another barrier: the perceived stigma based on socioeconomic class associated with school lunches.

Ahmed is fascinated by the complex interaction of human motivation and human behavior, particularly when it involves health. The response to the change in the school-lunch policy is an example of just such an interaction. His ideal job would be working in a department of health to develop policies that improve the health status of communities.

Are John and Ahmed thinking about the same profession?   ■

Although John and Ahmed seem to have different concepts of what health psychologists do, they are both correct. As John observed, some health psychologists work with individuals and small groups to improve health outcomes or to help people manage their health problems. John's concept is consistent with the work performed by health psychologists in the early years of the profession when the field focused primarily on individual and community health issues. They addressed the relationship between diseases and the *psychosocial*, here meaning psychological and sociological, needs of individuals.

Recently, however, the field has expanded. As we explained in Chapter 1, An Interdisciplinary View of Health, psychologists now also examine the effects of external factors such as the environment, health policies, and health systems on health outcomes. Currently, many health psychologists take an *ecological* view of health, consistent with the belief that an individual's health cannot be evaluated independent of his or her environment. In addition, emerging research in the field of psychoneuroimmunology adds a new dimension to health psychology: the complex interaction between psychology, neurology, and immunology.

You have heard the term *ecological* before. In Chapters 1 (An Interdisciplinary View of Health) and 6 (Emotional Health and Well-Being), we explained that the ecological model examines the social, systemic, and environmental factors that contribute to health (Eriksson et al., 2018; Stokols, 1996). An ecological perspective also requires an interdisciplinary approach to the study and practice of health, drawing on work from economics, epidemiology, medicine, psychology, public health, and sociology (McLeroy, Bibeau, Steckler, & Glanz, 1988).

The American Psychological Association's Society for Health Psychology has also adopted a view of health psychology that approximates the ecological perspective. In 2002, the Society for Health Psychology revised their mission statement to reflect the changed perspective. They now note that psychology serves as a "means for promoting health, education, and human welfare" (American Psychological Association, 2004, Article I). In this context, "human welfare" refers to the cultural, economic, and organizational influences that contribute to an individual's health status (Smith & Suls, 2004).

Why is this relevant for individuals interested in health psychology? The expanded field has created more professional opportunities. As we will see in the current chapter, health psychologists now work in a variety of capacities, including working directly with patients with medical conditions, working with research teams designing health-intervention programs or evaluating such programs, and working with health policy professionals. This range of options is available to people who are trained as clinicians as well as researchers. For example, as part of their work on health policy, psychologists – clinicians as well as researchers – may advocate for the health needs of specific communities. Both types of training can be used also as preparation for careers in more specialized health or *allied health professions*, including physical or occupational therapy, social work, or even medicine.

With regard to psychoneuroimmunology, as we saw in Chapter 8, Psychoneuroimmunology, researchers are integrating environmental factors in their study of the effects of the environment on psychological and immunologic functions, and vice versa. Health psychologists interested in research opportunities that examine the interaction between physiological, emotional, and environmental factors will find ample opportunities in this growing research field.

In the current chapter, we examine health psychologists' roles in four domains: individual, community, health care systems, and health policy. Through specific examples of the type of work health psychologists do in each of the major areas, we describe the breadth of the field and perhaps help you identify your area of interest in health psychology.

SECTION I. WORKING WITH INDIVIDUALS

Consider this example: a 45-year-old woman suddenly experiences extreme fatigue, excessive weight loss, and blurry vision. She makes an appointment with her physician to determine the cause of the symptoms. She learns she has Type 2 diabetes (see Chapter 4, Global, Communicable, and Chronic Disease). She is instructed by her physician to change her diet. She also must check her blood sugar levels regularly and begin taking insulin (see Chapter 4). The woman's doctor starts her on a regimen of oral medication but warns that if it is not effective in reducing her blood sugar levels, she may need to receive daily injections of insulin. In effect, the woman is told to make major changes in her daily health habits immediately.

This is a large undertaking. As is often the case, her physician is not able to devote the time needed to guide her through the health-behavior changes, challenges, and questions she will inevitable encounter. Will the woman be able to significantly change years of health behaviors by herself to control the progression of Type 2 diabetes?

Change is possible; however, effective change, one that slows disease progression or reverses the adverse effects, is almost impossible without the help of knowledgeable and trained professionals. In this case, the woman could seek assistance from an allied health professional, such as a therapist or nutritionist who works with patients to change their diet (Association of Schools of the Allied Health Professions, 2009). But health psychologists who also focus on nutrition and diet may be another resource for the woman. Health psychologists would use their knowledge about nutrition and diet along with their understanding of the psychosocial issues that influence health behavior change to assist the woman in setting and maintaining her required new behaviors. Both health psychologists and allied health professionals would be sure to devote time to educating the woman about her new condition.

Education

Working with an *interdisciplinary* team of health professionals, here meaning individuals from other fields, health psychologists often design education, training, and support programs to help individuals make and sustain changes to their health behaviors. There are, however, many types of education, training, and support programs. For example, education programs can be conducted through mass-media advertisements; formal education programs in schools, clinics, or health seminars; or informal information sessions. It should come as no surprise that health psychologists can and do contribute to the development of all forms of health-education programs.

MASS-MEDIA ADVERTISEMENTS Mass-media advertisements help raise awareness about a specific disease among large groups of potentially at-risk individuals. In fact, raising awareness is one of the principal goals of mass advertisements.

Remember social marketing, introduced in Chapter 3, Theories and Models of Health Behavior Change? Social marketing campaigns often begin with mass-media advertisements. Consider, for example, a media campaign to increase awareness of diabetes. In such campaigns, brochures and posters may be used to identify the problem and the behaviors that control or prevent diabetes. The advertising campaign helps to provide basic information about the illness – such as symptoms, risk factors, or behavior modification – to large numbers of people in specific target groups who may be at risk for the identified health problem.

What role do health psychologists play in developing such materials? First, it is important to state that psychologists often work on all types of advertising campaigns. Using their knowledge of human motivation, they contribute to advertising campaigns that motivate individuals to purchase a product, perhaps a piece of clothing, or engage in a specific activity, such as taking a trip. You encounter examples of advertisements that are intended to influence your behaviors every day.

Similarly, health psychologists involved in advertising campaigns to improve health outcomes integrate their knowledge of human motivation and health behaviors to design ads that motivate the targeted group to change behaviors or to purchase healthy products. Many health-promotion ads are found in print media and television commercials. The number of promotional ads has increased in the past three decades due, in part, to a growing emphasis on health-enhancing behaviors.

FORMAL EDUCATION PROGRAMS Health education is also delivered in small group presentations in schools, clinics, or seminars (see Figure 13.1). The programs usually provide in-depth information about the disease and an individual's risk of contracting the disease, details not usually offered in advertisements.

Formal educational programs may be designed as a one-time event or may include multiple presentations spanning weeks or months. Recall that Walter and colleagues (1992, 1993) designed and implemented an eight-week educational program to teach HIV/AIDS prevention to adolescents in a high school health class (see Chapter 5, Risky Health Behaviors, Part I). The goal of the program was to educate adolescents about HIV/AIDS and the risky health behaviors that transmit the virus. Included in the eight-week program were role-playing exercises to help adolescents develop skills to abstain from sexual behavior or to negotiate safer sexual practices.

Educational programs that impart skills usually require more than a single session. It is not surprising, therefore, that Walter and colleagues (1992, 1993) chose to deliver their program over several weeks. And because the goal of the intervention study was to educate and to impart skills, it is also not surprising that the research team who developed the program included health psychologists, adolescent-medicine physicians, cognitive psychologists, health educators, psychiatrists, and biostatisticians (see Box 13.1).

INFORMAL EDUCATIONAL PROGRAMS Educational programs may also take place in informal settings. Remember Kelly and colleagues' (1991) traffic light logo to create opportunities to talk about HIV/AIDS and HIV prevention? Kelly chose to conduct the educational campaign in a neighborhood bar patronized largely by gay men (see Chapter 3, Theories and Models of Health Behavior Change). A more recent example of informal educational programs is the barbershop-based health-promotion programs in the U.S., specifically in California, Texas, Georgia, Florida, New York, and Pennsylvania (Wippold, Frary, Garcia, & Wilson, 2023). Thirteen programs reviewed by Wippold and colleagues evaluated the success of these informal programs in recruiting and retaining a sample of African American men, and documenting changes in their knowledge and health behaviors with respect to prostate cancer, hypertension, and, in one case, violence prevention. We need to point out that most of the programs reported significant health changes and benefits, as reported by the participants.

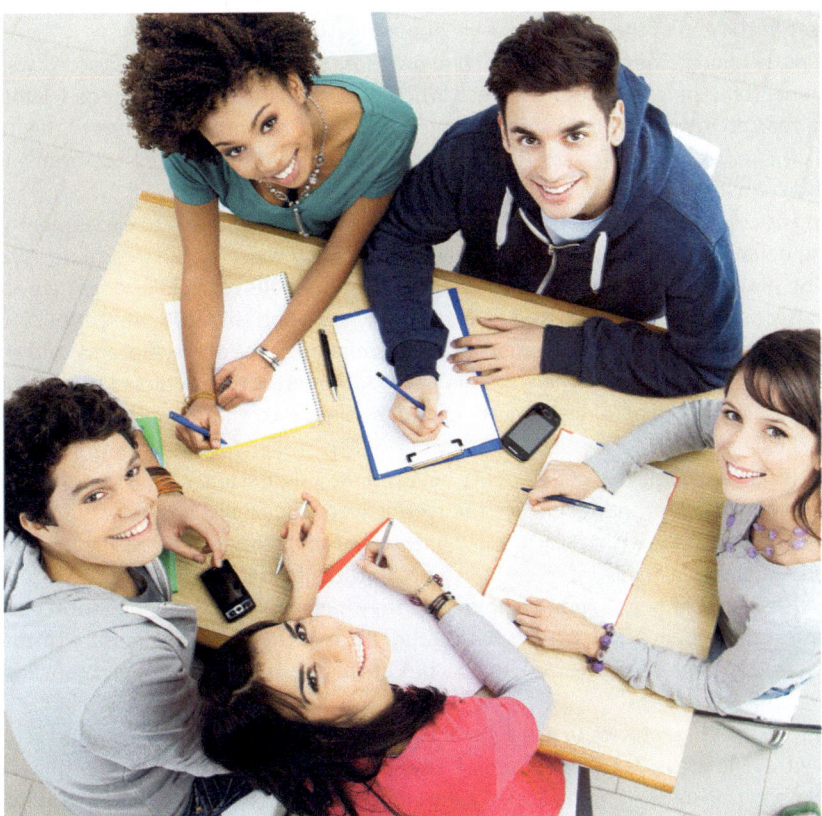

FIGURE 13.1 A diverse group of five students (two boys, three girls) around a table with pads and pens, smiling up at the camera.

Source: Shutterstock# 133717982.

The point here is that there are many ways to educate people about health, including mass-media advertisements, formal group instruction in schools or other settings, informal instruction like the conversations conducted in Kelly's study, or the informal programs conducted in African American barbershops. Regardless of the educational approach or setting, health psychologists are often involved in developing health education, health research, or health programs. Their research-method skills (see Chapter 2, Research Methods) together with their knowledge of human behaviors and health are valuable when planning, implementing, and evaluating such programs.

Box 13.1 The Art of Negotiation

Consider the following scenario: Two adolescent boys, James and Eric, are at a party at a friend's house. They managed to join the party even though it was restricted to varsity sports team members and their guests. Because no one questioned them when they arrived, they decided to stay and look as if they fit in.

In one corner, a group of adolescents was chugging beer, another group nearby was playing video games, and a third group was outside smoking. James decided to watch and possibly play a video game. He did not drink and was not interested in smoking. Eric preferred to go outside. Before separating, they agreed to meet at the end of the party and drive home together.

When the party ended, Eric found James sitting on a sofa staring blankly into space. It was clear that James was drunk, something Eric did not expect. When he asked James what happened, James told him about feeling coerced to participate in a drinking game because two of the captains of the football team told him he had to drink if he wanted to stay at the party. Eric faced similar pressure from another group who teased him about not smoking, but he was not persuaded to smoke.

Do adolescents succumb easily to pressure from friends or acquaintances to experiment with health-compromising behaviors? Apparently so, according to studies by Walter and colleagues (1992, 1993). In an intervention project designed to teach students negotiating skills to avoid or negotiate safer sexual behaviors, Walter and colleagues delivered an eight-week course on HIV/AIDS prevention. Students received information about HIV/AIDS, its modes of transmission, signs and symptoms, and skills training to negotiate safer sexual behaviors. The students watched vignettes that depicted successful and failed negotiation scenarios on video. They also participated in role-play scenarios in the class to practice their negotiation skills.

At the conclusion of the class, most students believed they significantly improved their negotiation skills and were confident that they could use them effectively. They believed they would be able either to withstand pressure to engage in risky sexual behaviors or to negotiate safer sexual behaviors – with one exception. Responding in postintervention surveys, students indicated that they would not be able to effectively use their new negotiation techniques if they had consumed alcohol or other substances prior to the attempted negotiation. What is more, students reported that the pressure to engage in risky sexual behaviors was greatest when attending parties at which drinking alcohol and consuming other substances was the norm.

Is it realistic to tell students not to use substances at a party? Perhaps as realistic as assuming that James could withstand pressure to drink from varsity sports team captains, a group with whom he wanted to fit in. Walter and colleagues' findings clearly showed a willingness on the part of students to practice health-enhancing behaviors. It also identified real barriers that effectively limit students' ability to perform the safer behaviors.

SUPPORT GROUPS Support groups are another type of educational program in which the groups provide much of the health information. Consider this: Weight Watchers, a well-known international organization that now goes by the name WW, guides and advises individuals striving to lose weight using both formal and informal group sessions. They contend that supportive networks are an important feature of any behavior-change program because the groups contribute to the long-term success of the intended outcome.

Weight Watchers (WW) even makes use of Web-based networks to help people attain their goals. For example, a person can attend in-person weekly Weight Watchers meetings or participate in an online support service. Using the computer, people can still weigh in by reporting their weight online (note that this is a self-report versus monitored and observed reporting) and receive immediate feedback of congratulations, encouragement, or helpful hints for doing better. In addition, online participants have access to a wealth of recipes and helpful suggestions from other members who also use the Web to share their experiences. And, adapting to the new research on weight loss, WW even supports its members' use of new GLP-1s, the weight loss medications that appear to help people lose and keep off excess weight (see Chapter 5, Risky Health Behaviors, Part II).

If this concept sounds familiar, it may be because in earlier chapters we reviewed research that explained the relationship between support groups and health-behavior change (see, for example Chapter 10, Chronic Pain Management and Arthritis). Specifically, we explained that individuals who must adopt new health behaviors – such as increased exercise regimens to control joint stiffness due to arthritis – usually are more successful in initiating and maintaining such behaviors when they have supportive networks. Research suggests that the psychological support from the groups enhances the chances of success in changing and maintaining the targeted behavior (Turk et al., 2008).

WW's support networks may be premised on such research. Through monthly meetings or online exchanges using the program's Web page, Weight Watchers provides its members with supportive social networks as well as other resources.

A reasonable question at this point might be: How are health psychologists involved in educational programs that involve social support? They contribute in two ways. First, they may help design and facilitate formal or informal support groups, such as the Weight Watchers group meetings. Second and equally as important, some of the research we identified earlier concerning the contributions of support networks was conducted by health psychologists. The research may be used by organizations that include support networks as part of their program's plan to achieve behavior change.

Evaluation of Interventions

We noted that health psychologists contribute to the design and implementation phase of health programs. Yet programs must be evaluated to determine their effectiveness in changing health outcomes. Here, too, we may find health psychologists working as members of a research-evaluation team. For example, to determine whether 30 minutes of an aerobic exercise program will help individuals achieve weight loss, researchers would design an evaluation of the intervention that measures the program's stated goals (weight loss), the exercise techniques employed to reach the goals (aerobic exercise), individuals' adherence to the goals, and individual outcomes at the conclusion of the program. As trained researchers, health psychologists can use their research design and analysis skills to assess an intervention program's effectiveness in achieving its goals. This is particularly important for commercial programs that purport to be effective in realizing specific health-enhancing outcomes.

Most effective health intervention programs develop the evaluation plan at the outset. What is more, it is common to find that health psychologists who conduct evaluations are involved in the initial design of the program as well as the evaluation and planning process. When health psychologists design intervention programs, they pay close attention to the variables needed to measure change and to assess the program's success.

Consider the following example: Bayne-Smith and colleagues (2004) tested the effectiveness of the PATH Program, a new cardiovascular health program developed for adolescent girls in New York City. Their program consisted of vigorous aerobic and strength-building exercises, health and nutrition education, and lessons in physiology that emphasized the cardiovascular system. The goal of the study was to determine whether education, exercise, and dietary changes would result in improved cardiovascular health for the adolescents.

Bayne-Smith and colleagues (2004) measured the adolescents' weight, body mass index (the percentage of body fat to height; see Chapter 5, Risky Health Behaviors, Part II), blood pressure, and cholesterol level two weeks prior to and two weeks after the 12-week program. Their results showed improvements in cholesterol levels, dietary habits, blood pressure, cardiovascular knowledge, and percentage of body fat, all essential factors for improving cardiovascular health. The variables included as part of the program design are the same factors used to demonstrate the program's effectiveness in reaching its goal. Program evaluation is a task well suited to health psychologists.

Promoting Individual Self-Advocacy

Health psychologists also work with individuals on ways to monitor and enhance their own outcomes independently. The ability to effectively address one's own health needs is the first step in health advocacy. In this section, we explore simple self-advocacy health techniques.

To be an effective health advocate for ourselves, we must know our health history. Here we mean not just our own history, but the illness and disease histories of our first-degree (father, mother, and siblings) and second-degree (grandparents, aunts, and uncles) relatives.

Does this sound easy? It really is not. For example, perhaps someone told you that your maternal grandmother had heart problems. But does that mean that she had coronary artery disease (see Chapter 9, Cardiovascular Disease) or a birth defect of the heart? If your paternal grandfather had a weight problem, was it caused by obesity, a thyroid disorder, or a problem that current GLP-1s might address by working to circumvent the brain's reward circuitry? The medical histories of family members may be incomplete. The origins of the problems can be misidentified. In some instances, health histories may be unknown. This is especially so in the case of someone who is adopted. Finally, in some families, medical histories are considered personal information and therefore not to be shared.

Although family members have the right to privacy concerning their health, information about common or recurring family health problems may help others in the family understand their health outcomes or anticipate potential problems. Consider this example: A 33-year-old woman experiences irregular bowel symptoms. She consults her physician, who refers her to a colon specialist. The specialist performs a *colonoscopy*, an examination of the large colon using a fiber-optic camera. The exam reveals several small *polyps*, small growths on the lining of the colon. The doctor removes the polyps and examines them to determine whether they are cancerous (see Chapter 11, Cancer). The polyps are benign, meaning noncancerous, but the doctor advises the woman to return in five years for a follow-up colonoscopy.

When relaying her experiences to her mother, the woman learns that her father, who died when she was a young child, had colon cancer. After telling her doctor about her father's illness, the doctor shortened the interval for colonoscopies to every three years from every five. Is there a connection between the health outcomes of the woman and her father's illness that led the doctor to change health care plans? Remember our discussion of colon cancer in Chapter 10, Chronic Pain Management and Arthritis? If so, you know that the answer may be yes. A child has a higher risk of colon cancer if their father (a first-degree relative) had colon cancer. In the absence of a family history of cancer, her risk levels would be lower. What is important here is that the father's disease and the woman's new symptoms signal a need for regularly scheduled colonoscopies at more frequent intervals. Therefore, family histories can inform the type or frequency of health care other family members should receive.

Box 13.2 Modified Family Health History Form

Do you know your family's health history? See how many of the following questions you can answer about your family members.

Health Condition	Mother	Father	Maternal Grandmother	Maternal Grandfather	Paternal Grandmother	Paternal Grandfather
Medical health conditions						
Alzheimer's disease						
Allergic rhinitis (hay fever)						
Anemia						
Anesthesia problems						
Arthritis (rheumatoid)						
Arthritis (osteoarthritis)						
Asthma						
Birth defects						
Bleeding problems						
Cancer (breast)						
Cancer (lung)						
Cancer (melanoma)						
Cancer (prostate)						
Cancer (skin, other than melanoma)						
Cancer (ovarian)						
Cancer (other)						
Depression						
Diabetes, Type 1						
Diabetes, Type 2						
Epilepsy						
Eye condition						
Glaucoma						
Heart problems						
Heart disease						

(Continued)

(Continued)

Health Condition	Mother	Father	Maternal Grandmother	Maternal Grandfather	Paternal Grandmother	Paternal Grandfather
High cholesterol						
High blood pressure						
Kidney disease						
Lungs						
Mental retardation						
Migraine headaches						
Miscarriages						
Stroke						
Thyroid disorder						
Tuberculosis						
Ulcer						
Other						
Behavioral health conditions						
Alcoholism						
Drug use						
Obesity						
Smoking						

SELF-MONITORING Family health history is one type of health-advocacy activity. Another activity of involves self-monitoring, meaning a systematic process of checking health indicators such as weight, blood pressure, cholesterol, and other measures that could signal impending health problems. We discussed many of the risky behaviors that could create negative health outcomes in Chapter 5, Risky Health Behaviors. Here, we focus on simple and easy-to-obtain measures that allow individuals to monitor their own health status.

Weight Scales In earlier chapters, we discussed body weight management as one health-enhancing behavior. Weight management helps reduce the likelihood of obesity, diabetes, cardiovascular disease, and even some forms of cancer. Because weight management is an important health-enhancing activity, we might assume that many people would weigh themselves regularly. In fact, they do not. In an international study of scale obsessions, fast-food addictions, and obesity, researchers examined the self-weighing behaviors of individuals in 13 countries: Australia, Brazil, Canada, the Czech Republic, France, Hong Kong, Malaysia, Romania, Saudi Arabia, Singapore, the United Arab Emirates, the U.K., and the U.S. The results revealed that very few study participants reported frequent weight monitoring. Although approximately 50% of American and French participants reported weighing themselves on average once per week, more than 37% of Singaporeans reported *never* weighing themselves (Amerinfo, 2008).

Because research suggests that frequent weighing is associated with better weight loss and improved weight management (O'Neil & Brown, 2005), infrequent monitoring poses at least two disadvantages. In the short term, it results in less weight loss. In the long term, it leads to a higher likelihood of chronic disease.

Exercise The 13-country international study also noted that when asked about weight-loss strategies, most individuals (for example, approximately 57% of Americans) chose controlling food intake as their preferred weight-loss strategy. Indeed, limiting the intake of foods high in fats and calories will contribute to weight loss. Yet studies also stress the role of exercise in sustained weight loss. A 2005 study by Carels and colleagues revealed that individuals who monitored their exercise frequency reported increased and sustained weight loss.

The beneficial effects of exercise can be seen also in chronic diseases such as arthritis. Exercise minimizes the discomfort and stiffness associated with arthritis. It also increases mobility. Aquatic exercises and other water sports are particularly helpful for arthritis sufferers because they facilitate joint movement while minimizing discomfort. Although some avid exercisers boast "No pain, no gain," for people with arthritis, water-based exercises take away the pain and ensure gain.

Self-Examinations We discussed the benefits of breast self-examinations as a form of early detection for breast cancer in Chapter 11, Cancer. What we did not mention at the time, however, was the benefits of self-examination to monitor other forms of illnesses or diseases. Take, for example, skin cancer. Many individuals who enjoy sunbathing may not notice sudden discolorations or moles on their face or other parts of the body as they perform their regular hygiene. However, periodic self-examinations for skin irregularities could help detect early symptoms of skin cancer should they appear.

We learned that although there will be an estimated 1 million cases of skin cancer in the U.S., fewer than 100 cases will result in death (see Chapter 11, Cancer). Yet with early detection, some of those 100 incidences might be prevented. In other words, self-examination for irregularities of any form is recommended to detect early warning signs of health problems. Self-examination, therefore, is another form of health self-advocacy.

Third Party Review Assume for the moment that you have carefully gathered information about your family's health history. You try to monitor your weight and make an effort to exercise regularly. You are reasonably observant of your health status, taking note of things that may signal a health problem. What else can you do?

Consider having an independent assessment of your health. An annual physical examination to confirm your opinion of your health or to explore any unusual findings is another form of individual health advocacy. An annual physical exam, or *wellness examination*, may help prevent unexpected health problems or detect and treat new problems as early as possible. Annual exams are checkups: checking to ensure that all is well or making it possible to address new problems quickly.

There is one additional benefit of annual checkups: the opportunity to learn new strategies for improving one's current health. If asked, physicians will share information about new medical findings or recommendations that may help maintain or improve one's health status. For example, some individuals who exercise regularly may not see a change in their stamina or endurance within four to six weeks, as suggested by many exercise experts. Therefore, in the annual exam, an individual might ask the physician for recommendations for new or different exercises to achieve their goal.

Annual checkups also allow patients to learn about the risk of contracting illnesses or diseases common to family members. If learning that two relatives, a first cousin and an aunt, both contracted breast cancer, the annual exam could be an opportunity for the individual to determine, in consultation with her health provider, whether the changed health status of relatives increases her own risks of contracting breast cancer. In essence, the annual checkup should be viewed as an opportunity to do two things: check on one's current health status and improve one's knowledge about health-enhancing behaviors and health risks.

We need to make one additional point. In Chapter 12, Health Care Systems and Health Policy, we noted that some individuals are reluctant to ask questions of their health care providers. They may be concerned about appearing medically uninformed or taking too much of the busy provider's time. Questions are a necessary part of learning about one's health. No health care provider should be too busy to respond to questions. But if a provider is truly too overwhelmed on a given day to respond to specific questions at that time, an individual should ask for a time when the provider would be available to have a fuller discussion, perhaps by phone. Physicians know that timely medical advice is also a form of health advocacy.

We pause here to ask, again, how can health psychologists be helpful in the self-assessment process? One way would be to partner with primary care physicians to develop a limited set of questions they can ask their consumers at each annual or biannual visit. Consumers may not respond as fully as physicians may like the first several times the questions are posed. But, just by asking the questions, consumers will begin to understand that they, too, can play a vital role in monitoring and maintaining good health outcomes. They will also come to expect such questions and be prepared to respond more fully in subsequent visits.

Box 13.3 Superman to the Rescue

Christopher Reeve may be best known for his Hollywood portrayal of the fictional character Superman (see Figure 13.2). In real life, however, his advocacy work on behalf of individuals with spinal cord injuries made him a true Superman for many with the same disorder.

An avid equestrian, Reeve was performing in a sporting competition in May of 1995 when he fell from his horse. Reeve broke two vertebrae, which appeared at first to result in permanent paralysis, a loss of sensation and voluntary movement of his body below his neck (Christopher & Dana Reeve Foundation, 2009). Consistent with spinal cord injuries that originate at the neck region, Reeve was unable to move his legs or arms. Such conditions also compromise breathing functions. Therefore Reeve also relied on a ventilator to breathe (Mayo Clinic, 2009).

Many feared that Reeve would be dependent on a ventilator for the duration of his life. Many also predicted a poor overall quality of life for Reeve. It seemed, however, that Superman had other ideas. Having honed his skill as an advocate for many other causes, Reeve seemed determined this time to use his advocacy skills to improve health outcomes for him and others similarly afflicted.

After six months, Reeve was able to breathe for 15 minutes at a time without the respirator. But according to reports, even before these signs of notable improvements, Reeve was beginning to advocate for research on spinal cord injuries.

From 1995 to his death in 2004, Christopher Reeve became the public face of advocates for spinal cord research. Specifically, Reeve and others pushed for increased funding for stem cell research, which appeared to be a vital link to understanding and repairing spinal cord injuries.

While spearheading the charge for research on stem cells, Reeve also championed causes to accommodate the needs of people with disabilities. For example, he worked with TEAM Sport to create athletic competitions that challenged athletes like him who became disabled as a result of an accident. And he lobbied U.S. senators to enable people with disabilities to continue receiving disability benefits after returning to work.

Almost 10 years after his accident, Reeve died of heart failure, one of several complications he developed in the aftermath of his fall. But his legacy of promoting research with potentially lifesaving and life-enhancing benefits continues.

Reeve will remain a superhero in the hearts and minds of millions who benefited from his advocacy.

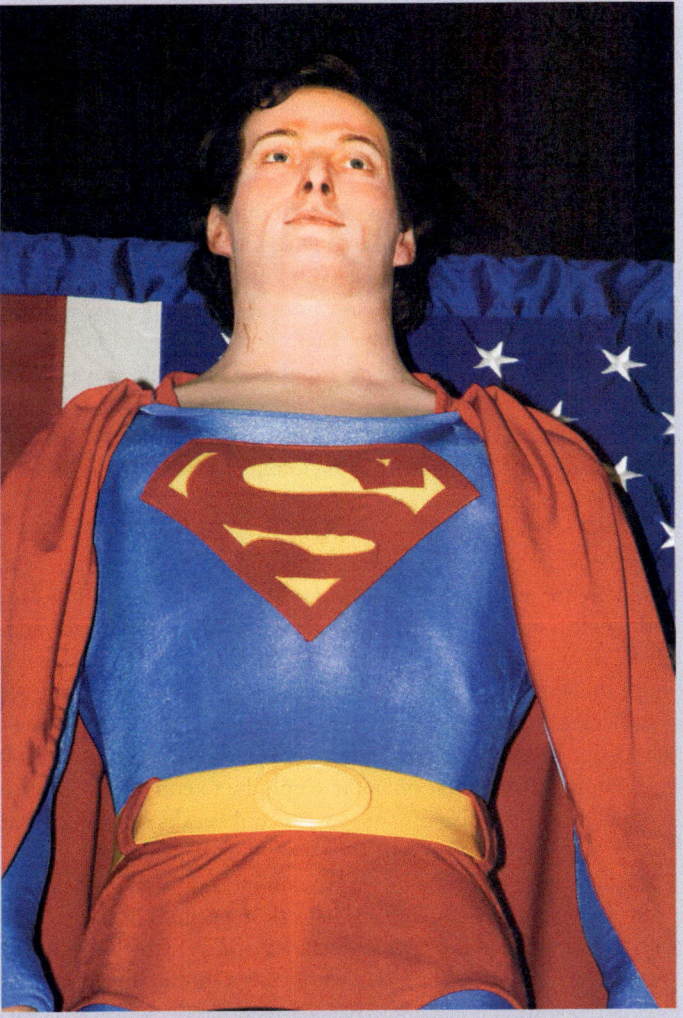

FIGURE 13.2 A full-body photo of Christopher Reeve in the Superman suit with cape, standing on top of a building.

Source: Getty Images78982015.

FINAL SELF-ADVOCACY Irrespective of health habits and behaviors, there may be times when individuals experience debilitating physical health problems. For some, the problem occurs suddenly and without warning. Others may have experienced a gradual deterioration of their health over weeks or months.

Each person's response to debilitating illnesses or accidents will differ according to the person, her lifestyle, and her coping styles. Some may explore new studies about their illnesses, hoping that new treatments may better control or cure them. For such individuals, one strategy for coping with terminal or debilitating illnesses is to advocate for continued research on their specific illnesses. One well-known health advocate for a debilitating disease is Christopher Reeve (see Box 13.3).

Some know Christopher Reeve best for his role as Superman. Whatever name is used, it is a fact that Reeve became an active and effective advocate for stem cell research, a new and controversial research technique believed to be a vital tool for repairing spinal cord injuries. Reeve not only advocated for stem cell research, but he also established a foundation to help people who, like him, were disabled due to an injury to the spinal cord that resulted in paralysis.

other advocates for ending life with dignity Consider the following scenario:

Every morning Emily awakes to the same thought: "I did not expect my life to end this way."

Emily used to be an active, energetic, 67-year-old grandmother of two. She fondly described herself as "healthy as a horse." She was rarely sick, traveled frequently, and enjoyed regular outings to the pool and to the tennis courts. All that changed, however, when Emily was in a near-fatal car accident.

Emily remembers little about the accident. She recalls driving home alone from an evening out with friends. It began to rain. At one point, it was raining so hard that it was difficult to see the road. But Emily's biggest problem that night was neither the roads nor the rain: It was another driver. An oncoming car swerved suddenly as if to avoid an object in the road. As a result of the shift in direction, the car headed straight for her. There was no time to react. Emily remembers the head-on collision, but everything else is a blur.

Now, six weeks after the accident, Emily is paralyzed from the neck down. She is unable to move her arms or legs. She spends her days either in bed or in a wheelchair and depends on her home health care assistants, who are with her 24 hours a day, to help her with all basic and bodily needs. Because speaking is difficult, Emily often prefers to communicate with a slight nod of the head. Most of the time she is silent.

Nighttime is perhaps the worse for Emily. Alone and lonely, she thinks about the active life she once led: the social gatherings, the tennis teams, and the summer parties. Her family visits regularly, but their visits are short due to Emily's limited communication ability. This is not the life Emily envisioned for herself. Emily feels the best outcome would be to end her life, but she is unable to communicate her strong desire because she cannot write and speaks only with great difficulty.

Like many others suffering from debilitating or terminal illnesses, Emily is having difficulty coping with her current existence (few who experience such paralysis call it a "life"). It appears that Emily is thinking about *euthanasia*, a word adopted from the Greek word *euthanatos*, which means "the good death." Euthanasia has been called "mercy killing" by some who see it as a dignified end to life. For others it is "another form of murder." To be sure, it is a controversial issue.

Dr. Jack Kevorkian is perhaps one of the better known advocates for euthanasia. And he, too, is controversial. Nicknamed "Dr. Death," Dr. Kevorkian pioneered a process that enabled patients suffering from an interminable illness or pain to end their life with the assistance of a physician. The procedure became known as *physician-assisted suicide*. He also developed a method that allowed patients to participate in the act without the assistance of others, known as *active euthanasia*. Kevorkian is credited for (or accused of, depending on your point of view) assisting or enabling more than 45 patients to end their lives. Many question Kevorkian's motives, and others support his belief that individuals should have the right to end their life in dignity. Emily's condition and her strong desire to end her suffering may be similar to that of many other patients who sought Dr. Kevorkian's help.

Euthanasia may seem like an unusual topic for a section on health advocacy. Most discussions of health advocacy focus on ways to improve one's state of health by, for example, improving access to good-quality health care or improving environmental conditions in communities, such as air or water quality. Advocates such as Dr. Kevorkian suggest that an individual's ability to choose a dignified end to life is inherent in the definition of quality of life. He and others who hold similar beliefs support the right of individuals to choose not to endure years of pain, clinical depression, or other psychological problems that contribute to a poor quality of life.

The principal question concerning euthanasia appears to be whether it is ethical to require a person to live life in constant pain or suffering or whether it is ethical to permit that person to painlessly end his or her life. Consider this: In the majority of euthanasia cases, an individual is either terminally ill or, like Emily, suffers from a debilitating injury for which there are few, if any, life-enhancing treatments. According to advocates of euthanasia, the physical suffering together with the mental and emotional "pain" that accompanies the illness are sufficient reasons to allow individuals to choose a dignified end. Others contend that individuals can be helped to overcome the pain, discomfort, and depression by learning and using appropriate coping techniques.

It is impossible to determine which group has the more compelling claim. For the moment we make the following two points. First, the right of individuals to die with dignity or for individuals to cope and live with challenging physical- and mental-health problems are two examples of health advocacy at work.

Second, health psychologists can contribute to the research and debate on euthanasia. Many psychologists would agree that anyone considering an early termination to his or her life, even those with terminal or painful illnesses, should first seek psychological and emotional support and counseling. Health psychologists working with such individuals can introduce coping techniques that may marginally improve a person's overall well-being. But they can also address the holistic health needs of a person considering euthanasia.

Advocates for euthanasia are aware that the act is illegal in most U.S. states. In fact, physician-assisted suicide is legal on only ten states in the U.S. Only Oregon has enacted a "death with dignity" law that allows a person to end their own life with physician-prescribed medication. In this case the physician can prescribe, but not administer, a lethal dose of medication for the patient. The patient must be shown to be mentally competent to make the request (Oregon.gov, n.d.). Worldwide, only 11 countries permit euthanasia.

Some see Oregon's law as precedent setting, potentially influencing other states to consider a similar law. Oregon's law is an example also of advocacy using public policy. We will discuss other uses of public policy to advocate for health later in the chapter.

EUTHANASIA AND MEDICAL ETHICS The issue of euthanasia also raises concerns about medical ethics. Specifically, some wonder whether it is ethical for physicians to participate in such acts given their Hippocratic oath, an oath taken by many physicians in which they essentially promise to "first do no harm" to any individual or patient. It also raises questions about who is better equipped to make such judgments: the afflicted individual or someone with medical training.

Research on the ending of life suggests that, if needing to consider such requests, both laypersons and medical professionals prefer to hear the request from the individual with the illness, not the medical doctor (Guedi et al., 2005). What is more, research on physicians who respond to requests for end-of-life assistance indicate that they were significantly more likely to respond with assistance when the patient himself or herself made the request and when the requests were made repeatedly (Meier, Emmons, Litke, Wallenstein, & Morrison, 2003).

Finally, both laypersons and medical professionals are more inclined to accept such requests when the reason for euthanasia is to end *intractable physical suffering* (Guedi et al., 2005), here meaning severe pain, seizures, delirium, or other painful or disorienting symptoms.

It is important to note that other research also shows that the most commonly cited reasons for euthanasia in fact are not related to intractable physical suffering. Instead, patients most often cite loss of autonomy, loss of ability to control bodily functions, loss of enjoyment of life, and a preference to control their manner of death when terminally ill (American Psychological Association, 2024). Does this mean that individuals who request euthanasia due largely to severe psychological or emotional distress are considered less credible than those in clear physical pain? Perhaps not. The research suggests that when making difficult decisions that involve ethical judgments, it may be easier for medical persons to accept a request for euthanasia when they can readily see and understand the extent of someone's pain and discomfort. We must add, however, that the mental and psychological distress associated with illnesses, something that may be less apparent to another individual, must be considered also because such factors influence overall well-being. Once again, health psychologists can contribute to the important decisions pertaining to euthanasia by examining both the physical and emotional health of a person to assess well-being.

Can an individual considering euthanasia also be an advocate for himself or herself? The answer appears to be "sometimes." But this, too, is highly controversial. Remember that we noted that in Oregon physicians can assist only someone who is mentally competent to make such a request. Some health care providers believe that patients suffering from terminally ill or debilitating conditions can be lucid and are able to distinguish between momentary discomfort and intractable discomfort that shows no hope of abating. Others contend that the pain and suffering can be so intense that the wish to die is more likely an intense desire to remove the immediate pain or discomfort and to regain part of the quality of life the individual enjoyed previously.

This highly controversial topic will continue to engage health professionals. Questions about the ethics of living with unremitting pain versus the right to choose to end such suffering will not be resolved easily. An embedded issue in this debate is whether individuals can advocate for and win the right to choose to end a painful existence.

SECTION II. WORKING WITH COMMUNITIES

We described the ways in which health psychologists help design health programs and research to change individual health behaviors. They use some of the same techniques when working in community settings. Each of the educational approaches explained earlier – mass-media ad campaigns, formal and informal educational programs, and support groups – can be used, with some modifications, when working with communities. One important difference is the need to involve the community in the planning and implementation process of the health program.

Community Needs Assessment

When working in communities, many health care workers understand that the community, not the individual, is the focus. But like individuals, a community will be more responsive to new behavior-change programs if the members of the community believe the program addresses their perceived health needs.

Recall that in Chapter 3, Theories and Models of Health Behavior Change, some Western health professionals in southern Africa labeled the growing HIV/AIDS epidemic the most important health issue in the region. Yet many of the residents in southern Africa did not agree. They understood the potential long-term impact of such a disease. Many villagers and government health officials, however, were more concerned about other health problems that they believed posed a greater and more immediate risk to the community. For example, in South Africa incidence rates of HIV were increasing rapidly for several years. Yet the health department (or ministry as it is called there) was struggling to address the need to expand a health care system, which provided easy access to care for white South Africans, into a system that provided health services to more than 24 million black, coloured, and Indian South Africans who were denied basic care under the apartheid regime (Schneider & Stein, 2001). In this case, the health department's first concern was providing immediate, basic health services to 24 million neglected individuals. It took precedence over treating the rapid escalation of HIV/AIDS.

Similar problems were encountered by health workers in other countries in which the need to focus on basic survival, including food, shelter, or attention to other diseases such as cholera or malaria that result in death in the short term, were determined to be more immediate and more critical to improving the health status of the community (Loewenson, 2007).

Conflicting views on the most important health concerns often pit health researchers against the community. Such problems have been noted in the U.S. as well and have led to similar "turf wars" when attempting to identify a community's most pressing health need (American Hospitals Association Community Health Improvement, 2024).

How do health psychologists introduce and implement a specific education and intervention program in a community when the community is focused on other pressing concerns? As public health workers know, health psychologists will be more effective in identifying and developing successful health programs if they first assess the needs of the community from the community's perspective. Most important, psychologists must include community residents, especially the community's own health professionals, in the assessment. The first job of health psychologists when working in communities is to assist the community members in conducting their own needs assessment.

Many health care workers understand that when working in communities, individuals and their behaviors must be evaluated in their *social milieu*, or social context (Merzel & D'Afflitti, 2003). By social context we mean the community values, norms, and behaviors that shape the attitudes that help shape the behaviors. You may recall that in Chapter 3, Theories and Models of Health Behavior Change, several theories proposed that a society's norms and values influence an individual's behavior. Similarly, any effort to change health outcomes at the community level must consider the community norms, here meaning behavioral practices and beliefs, in addition to the social environment.

Let us put this in perspective. Earlier we recalled the intervention program by Walter and colleagues (1992, 1993) designed to teach adolescents techniques for negotiating safer sexual behaviors to prevent the risk of HIV infection. Unfortunately, these researchers did not anticipate the social context that gives rise to high-risk sexual behaviors. In a posttest analysis, Walter and colleagues (1993) noted that the adolescents felt able to use the training and negotiation skills learned in the intervention program to negotiate safer sexual behaviors, but they also noted that they would be less able to use the newly acquired skills after drinking or using drugs.

Why is this relevant? In most instances, adolescents report a higher risk of engaging in sexually risky behaviors after consuming alcohol or other substances. In essence, they identify substance use as an important context in which the risky behavior occurs, a context that was not tested by Walter and colleagues (1993). Their intervention program did not consider the social context of adolescents. Community-based participatory research offers one method for overcoming similar obstacles.

Program Implementation

There is currently an emphasis on *community-based participatory research* or *programs*, here meaning research or programs that involve the community from inception through to the conclusion. Community-based participatory programs usually include community members as part of the planning team. Their knowledge of the community's values and belief systems, together with their interest in the health problem, facilitates the researcher's or practitioner's introduction into the community as well as the effective delivery of the program. Examples of successful community-based programs or studies exist for a range of health issues throughout the world. They include a program to increase women's physical activity and cardiovascular health in the Persian Gulf (Pazoki, Nabipour, Seyednezami, & Imami, 2007), and programs to promote weight loss among Turkish and Moroccan women to promote healthy lifestyles (Wagemakers et al., 2008).

The common factor in all of the studies is a partnership between the community and the health practitioner or health researcher in designing, conducting, and evaluating the program's effectiveness. Such programs are based on the assumption that individuals are inextricable from their context and that a supportive context will reinforce and sustain the behavior. Community-based participatory programs may use as their foundation theories of health behavior that include social context as one factor that shapes behavior.

In sum, the current work of community-based health intervention programs recognizes that an individual is linked to his or her context. Efforts to improve a community's – and therefore an individual's – health will be more successful if health professionals carefully study the community and its perceived needs, take account of the community's values and attitudes in the proposed health behavior, and include the community as a partner in the project. Health psychologists often work on such community-based participatory programs.

We must make one final observation. Some researchers suggest that when working in communities, health psychologists need to change the community's social norms or attitudes to obtain the targeted behavior change. We caution that changing social norms and values is a process that occurs slowly, if at all. Programs that require substantial changes to norms and attitudes may be successful only for the duration of the program. Once the program ends or the health professionals leave, it is unlikely that the health behaviors will be self-sustaining. In essence, a community-based health behavior change must be a community-led initiative if it is to be effective and enduring.

Selecting Populations within Communities

An effective strategy for changing a community health behavior involves selecting a specific (or target) population and a health problem or behavior prevalent in that population. As we noted in Chapter 3, Theories and Models of Health Behavior Change, social-marketing programs demonstrate that effective behavior change programs focus on one target group, even though the behavior may be evident in other groups in the community.

Targeting one group to receive a health intervention is troublesome to some in the health field. It means that others with similar health behaviors may not benefit from the intervention program. In point of fact, health professionals and researchers regularly segment populations to develop and deliver effective health-intervention programs. Consider this: What advertising message would you use to inform all audiences, including adolescents, about the dangers of smoking? Would a warning about the dangers of cigarette smoke to pregnant women and their fetuses be equally as effective with adolescents as with women contemplating pregnancy? We contend that it would not. Rather, a campaign that derides smoking as "uncool" among popular students or that suggests that smoker's breath is a turnoff when speaking up close with someone attractive may have more impact for teens than messages about the dangers of smoking for the unborn child. Health psychologists, like marketers, must select the most impactful message and program for a specific group and work with that group to increase the likelihood of effective message communication and successful behavior change.

Promoting Community Advocates

After participating in the community needs assessment and assisting with program development to address the health needs of the community, health psychologists may also advocate for the change on behalf of the community. Health issues of interest to *community health advocates* include ensuring access to nutritious and fresh produce, access to clean water, environments that are free of toxic waste sites, and violence reduction in neighborhoods. As we indicated in earlier chapters, each of these issues affects the health of the community as well as the individual.

Research by nursing students from a university in southern Georgia provides an example of community advocacy by health researchers and community members. The university students chose to work in a community adjacent to their university that also included family members and friends of some of the students. No doubt the students' familiarity with the community and their existing social networks increased the community's receptivity to the health advocates and their proposed health programs.

The students and the community conducted a community needs assessment and identified five health problems, one of which was lack of fluoridation in the water (Wold, Brown, Chastain, Griffis, & Wingate, 2008). Fluoride in water helps to prevent dental cavities, especially in small children (Adain et al., 2001; Truman et al., 2002). Together, the community and students developed programs to address the individual and community dental-health needs of the children. They then developed a teaching plan on preventive dental care that was adopted by and implemented at a local elementary school. The educational program was geared to elementary school children because they are the most susceptible to tooth decay when fluoride is in short supply.

The resulting program provided a benefit to the individual children and the community. Each child received immediate dental health care and learned dental hygiene habits that could help to arrest future tooth decay. In addition, the community gained a dental health program that could be incorporated into the school's health program and used annually to educate future elementary school students. It will provide ongoing dental health benefits for children in the community.

SECTION III. WORKING WITH HEALTH CARE SYSTEMS

When health psychologists work with health care systems (see Chapter 12, Health Care Systems and Health Policy), most often they are engaged in research to explain patterns of health care–seeking behaviors or barriers to using the health care systems. Yet studies of health care behaviors must also consider the effects of the regulations and restrictions of the health care system on individual health behaviors.

As we noted in Chapter 12, Health Care Systems and Health Policy, health care systems offer a prescribed set of services and specify the frequency of services to be provided to individuals who subscribe to the plan. A system that regulates access to care by defining when, what, and how frequently health services can be provided will certainly affect an individual's health outcomes.

Assessing Access to Health Care

What is more likely to influence a person's decision to obtain needed health care: the individuals, their families/communities, or the health care system – including physicians – from which they usually obtain medical care? There is broad agreement that all three factors – individuals, family and community, and health care systems – influence individuals' decisions to seek care. Yet there is little agreement about the relative contribution of each of the factors. Simply stated, we do not know which factor is more instrumental in affecting an individual's health or health-seeking behaviors. Consider this example: An individual with a chronic cough but no other cold symptoms decides not to obtain medical advice. If the cough evolves into bronchitis, it would be fair to assume that the individual's own inattention to his or her health contributed to the poorer health status.

Now assume that the same individual with the same cough condition calls his or her physician for an appointment but is told that the next available appointment is in three weeks. While the consumer is waiting three weeks, the cough worsens and progresses to bronchitis. In this instance, the worsening health condition can be attributed to a delay in medical care. This time, however, the delay is caused by the physician, not the individual.

Finally, assume that the same individual with the same cough condition calls and receives an appointment with the physician within 48 hours. The doctor determines that a chest X-ray is needed to check for possible pneumonia. Unfortunately, the individual's managed-care plan (see Chapter 12, Health Care Systems and Health Policy) denies authorization for the X-ray, and the individual cannot afford to pay for the test out of pocket. Once again, the cough evolves into bronchitis. In this instance, it is clear that the delay in diagnosis and treatment is the fault of the health care system, not the health care provider or the individual.

The examples cited are simplistic and clearly link the cause of the worsening health condition to a specific factor. In most instances the causes of poor health outcomes are not so easily determined. What is more, there are a number of characteristics imbedded in each of the three factors (individual, provider, or health system) that also influence health outcomes.

Early studies suggested that individual factors largely explained why individuals delayed obtaining health care. For example, some studies report that people in lower socioeconomic classes, males, and less educated individuals tend to delay care (Baker, Stevens, & Brook, 1994; Wilson & Klein, 2000; Zuckerman & Shen, 2004). Yet a study by Lowe and colleagues (2005) suggests that the type of health services and the structure of the services provided by primary care physicians also contribute to an individual's decision to delay medical care.

Lowe and colleagues (2005) examined patients' decisions to obtain medical care in a hospital emergency department rather than from their primary-care physician for nonemergency medical needs. Results of their study showed that three factors influenced an individual's likelihood of seeking care from someone other than his or her primary-care physician: patient volume, here meaning the number of patients in a doctor's private or group practice, a factor that affects the amount of time patients have to wait to be examined; availability of evening appointments; and the range of medical services available in office. These researchers found that physicians with a large number of patients; physicians who allocated fewer than 12 hours per week for evening appointments; physicians who reported no support services available through their office, such as nurse practitioners; and those who reported no special equipment available for special needs, such as asthma, were more likely to have patients who sought medical care from hospital emergency departments than were physicians who reported some or all of the aforementioned services (see Table 13.1).

Why is Lowe's research important to health psychology? His research suggests that the quality of services provided by the doctor is not the most significant factor when explaining patients' decisions to postpone or find alternative sources of medical care. Rather, they found that the packet of services, such as hours of operation or volume of patients – in other words, psychosocial factors – is critical to explaining the health care–seeking behaviors of individuals. Lowe's research suggests additional reasons that individuals may choose alternative care options even when they have a relationship with one physician. Their findings affirm the role of psychosocial factors on seeking timely care. The study may also help explain decisions to refrain from seeking care altogether.

Promoting Access to Health Care through Advocacy

Many providers have changed their office practices by taking the psychosocial factors identified by Lowe and colleagues into account. The most common change has been adding evening appointments and expanding staff to include other health providers who may address a variety of special needs. Lowe and colleagues' research (2005) and that of other psychologists offer one way to advocate for changes to the health care system to improve access to care (Goin, Hays, Landeman, & Hobbs, 2009; Prentice & Pizer, 2007).

DeVoe (2009) offers another approach for advocating greater access to health care by offering an interesting glimpse into the problems of access to health care in the U.S. DeVoe developed a hypothetical scenario in which access to education was regulated in the same manner as access to health care. His example, which refers specifically to publicly funded health care (such as Medicaid or Medicare), illustrates the unexpected and, for many, unacceptable consequences of such a system.

In DeVoe's (2009) scenario, access to education for children would require insurance, as does health care. Children without insurance would be denied access to a school and consequently to daily instruction. Proof of insurance would be required before admission is granted. Once in the educational arena, parents and children might find that their access to various educational experiences is limited by restrictions imposed by their education insurance carrier. For example, some education insurance companies may restrict access to foreign-language instruction or art or music, holding those as special services available only to parents enrolled in enhanced education programs. These enhanced programs are more expensive

TABLE 13.1 Influences on Health Status: Individual, Provider, and Health-Service Characteristics

Individual	Provider	Health Services
Age	Hours of operation	Number of providers in network
Gender	Evening hours	Out-of-network option
Ethnicity	Weekend hours	Covered medical test
Socioeconomic status	Telephone advice	Referrals available
Level of education	Returns patient calls	Preauthorization needed for tests and referrals
Inner city versus rural	Urgent appointments	Limits on additional services
Health insurance	Practice type (office, hospital, clinic)	
Medicaid eligibility	Hospital inpatient care	
Prior medical condition	Availability of special equipment	
Current health status		

options. Furthermore, they may also find that many teachers refuse to accept the children's educational insurance (called educaid by DeVoe), making it difficult to find a teacher who will enroll the child in his or her class.

Educational insurance would be linked to employment. Parents who are employed and who work for an employer that offers insurance would be able to acquire educational insurance for their child. In the event of parental job loss, the child's educational insurance would be terminated as well. What is more, should the parent find employment that would allow him or her to restart the educational insurance, children may find educators doubtful that they could bridge the months or years of missed educational experience.

Sound incredible? Perhaps so. But DeVoe's (2009) hypothetical story helps to illustrate the problems with access to health care in the U.S. Few parents would willingly accept the limitations to access to education for their children posed by DeVoe's scenario. Yet these very restrictions to access to health care exist for both children and adults. DeVoe's approach of analogizing education insurance to health insurance clarifies the need for changes in the health care system in the U.S.

SECTION IV. WORKING IN HEALTH POLICY

It may seem unlikely, at first, that health psychologists would have much involvement with health policy. But think back to the opening story. Ahmed's father, a public health professional, worked with health researchers, some of whom could be health psychologists, to change policies that directly affect health. Such a pairing is indeed quite common. Some health psychologists work directly with policy makers, whereas others conduct research that helps inform the development of new regulations that also shape or, in some cases, restrict behaviors that affect health. Examples of health policies influenced by research include smoking restrictions in public places, workplace safety regulations, and healthy workplace rules.

Smoking Bans as Health Policy

The ban on smoking on all U.S. domestic airline flights (GPO Access, 2008) and the ban on smoking in public places, including bars, restaurants, and bowling alleys, are two examples of health policy regulations initiated to reduce the incidences of a health-compromising behavior, smoking, and its health implications for individuals. Similar bans enacted worldwide with the support of WHO reinforced the importance of banning cigarette smoking as a public health initiative.

We have discussed the association between smoking and respiratory illnesses and cancer in Chapter 11, Cancer, so we will not review it here. The fact that cigarette smoke harms the smoker has long been accepted in the research community. What is new, however, is that nonsmokers face some of the same health hazards from *secondhand smoke*, or smoke from another individual's cigarette. Overwhelming evidence of the dangers of secondhand smoke was the basis for the ban on smoking in many public places, including workplaces, by 27 states, as well as the federal ban on smoking in airplanes.

We now add to this research on the dangers of cigarette smoking and secondhand smoke, and as of yet, inconclusive research on the dangers of vaping. As we noted in Chapter 5, Risky Health Behaviors, Part I, preliminary findings suggest that adolescents who vape frequently are at increased risk of damage to their lungs, heart, and other vital organs. Part of the problem stems from the thousands of ingredients in vape products and their unknown effects on the body. Unfortunately, while these studies progress, many, many more youth will be exploring this newest product (Figure 13.3).

Health psychologists can and must contribute to this research effort.

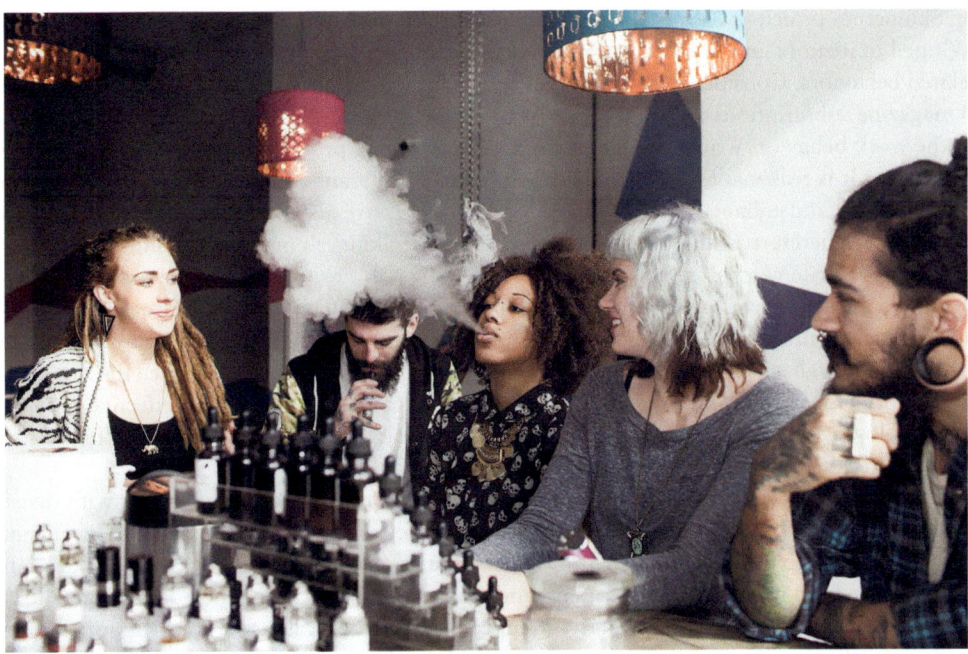

FIGURE 13.3 Above a horizontal cloud of smoke the photo asks: "What's in a vape cloud?" Six answers, written in the cloud, are "nicotine," "tobacco-specific nitrosamines," "formaldehyde," "carcinogens," "benzene," and "acetaldehyde."

Workplace Safety

Another health policy influenced by researchers is workplace safety. The concept of workplace safety in the U.S., specifically the employer's role in creating a safe work environment, is relatively new. It began with the concept of behavioral safety introduced by Herbert Heinrich in the 1930s. Heinrich's research examining the causes of workplace injuries and accidents suggested that the actions of the workers, not the work environment, were responsible for the majority of injuries on the job (Heinrich, Petersen, & Roos, 1980; Wirth & Sigurdsson, 2008). In other words, Heinrich suggested that individual, not environmental, determinants contributed to workplace injury. Recent studies on workplace safety, however, criticize Heinrich's assessment that the worker bore the greatest responsibility for workplace accidents and injuries (Cooper, 2003). Instead, later studies determined that workplace hazards caused by the environment and by poor safety guidelines contributed significantly to injuries and accidents at work sites.

Can psychologists contribute to the research on workplace safety? Absolutely! In fact, B.F. Skinner, the famous behavioral psychologist, demonstrated that psychologists could contribute to efforts to improve employees' safe behavior in the workplace.

Skinner, as you may recall, was the psychologist who developed the principle of *operant conditioning*, a process by which individuals and animals could learn to perform a specific behavior by gradual shaping of their behavior. Skinner demonstrated that, through operant conditioning, individuals can learn to adopt and maintain behaviors such as safety behaviors. Key to Skinner's theory is the principle of reinforcement or reward. When individuals are appropriately rewarded, Skinner showed that they not only will perform but will retain the desired behavior.

Using Skinnerian principles, industrial/organizational (I/O) psychology, a new discipline in psychology, was developed to identify and test strategies that would motivate employees to adopt and maintain desired work-related behaviors. Consider this: Employees at a magazine company may be told that if they sell at least 20 magazine subscriptions they will receive a bonus. The bonus is the incentive or reward offered to shape the work behavior. Would the same operant-conditioning process work to shape workplace safety behaviors? It is reasonable to conclude that if Skinner's operant-conditioning principles can shape workplace behavior and enhance productivity, they can be effective also in shaping and reinforcing safe workplace habits. Therefore health psychologists can also use Skinner's operant-conditioning theory to shape and reinforce safe workplace behaviors.

For example, health psychologists can work with employees to identify workplace safety behaviors unique to their environments. Together with the employees, health psychologists can introduce safety plans and procedures through small group presentations or seminars, use posters to reinforce the message (a Skinnerian principle again) and to remind workers of the goal. Some of the most effective posters reminding employees of workplace safety behaviors are cartoons. Humorous posters can attract attention and are easy to recall while reminding workers of the safety goals.

Currently, the U.S. Occupational Safety and Health Administration (OSHA), together with divisions of workplace safety administered by state agencies, conducts evaluations of workplace sites to identify potential and specific job hazards (OSHA, 1989). U.S. regulations mandate that state workplace safety plans must include both management leadership and employee participation when developing and maintaining a safe and hazard-free workplace. It appears that the federal regulations support the view that the environment, the management company (policy), and the worker all contribute to establishing and maintaining a safe workplace environment.

In spite of the regulations, U.S. workplaces still report accidents in the millions. In 2006, the U.S. Bureau of Labor Statistics reported more than 3.9 million nonfatal workplace injuries and approximately 5,700 fatalities (Wirth & Sigurdsson, 2008). The injuries and fatalities included in the statistics represent a mix of all three causal factors: individual, company policy, and environment. As the statistics suggest, much more work is needed to establish and ensure a safe work environment for employees.

A Healthy Workplace

Some work environments have few physical hazards or hazardous jobs. For example, the average office worker or employee in educational institutions is not required to work with dangerous chemicals or heavy machinery. Yet even in office or educational settings, many employers are establishing healthy workplace rules.

Work environments that promote a healthy workplace do so for two reasons. First, they consider the productivity loss when one person is ill. If an employee is absent from work due to illness, that worker's work production may be lost for the duration of the illness. His or her lost productivity can result in lost earnings for both the employer and the employee. Second, employers consider the potential impact on other workers. Consider the effect on work productivity when several employees are absent due to illness. The potential loss of revenue when several employees are absent could financially strain some employers.

Programs that promote healthy workplace environments offer potential benefits to both the workers and to the employer. For the worker, less absenteeism may mean less lost income or, equally as important, overall good health. We already noted the benefits to the employer of no loss of productivity and therefore no loss of potential revenue due to illness.

For those reasons, healthy workplace programs, sometimes called worksite health-promotion programs, are being implemented in many businesses. Studies that evaluate the effect of healthy workplace programs on worker absenteeism and worker productivity demonstrate the dual benefit of these programs. Kuoppala, Lamminpaa, and Husman (2008) showed that workplace health-promotion programs were credited with decreasing absenteeism, increasing the mental well-being of the workers, and increasing the productivity of the workers. Similarly, Mills, Kessler, Cooper, and Sullivan (2007) studied the effects of a workplace health intervention program in the U.K. office of a multinational company, a company with major operations in more than one country. They compared workers' responses to questionnaires before the program and 12 months after the program. Mills and coauthors' (2007) results showed that workers reported a decrease in health-risk factors and an increase in productivity as a result of the healthy workplace program.

Clearly a healthy workplace benefits workers by increasing the likelihood that they will remain in good physical health with less exposure to and risk of physical illness. However, as these studies suggest, they also improve employees' mental health and overall well-being. It appears, therefore, that some healthy workplace programs address the holistic health of individuals.

Advocating for New Health Policies

Can health policy be a form of health advocacy? In the current and prior chapters we provided examples of health policy developed and implemented for the purpose of improving the health status of individuals, communities, special populations, and workplace environments. And according to our definition of health advocacy stated in the beginning of the chapter, a principal goal of health advocacy is to promote behavior and practices that improve an individual's or a community's state of health.

Consistent with the definition, therefore, health policy can be a form of health advocacy. Consider this: A state mandate that requires all passengers and drivers to wear seat belts when riding in automobiles is a health policy. Most would agree that the policy is also a form of health advocacy that promotes automobile safety. Similarly, state regulations that ban the use of handheld cell phones while driving is a health policy intended to reduce accident rates due to cell phone use.

In most cases, health policies are developed and implemented to improve health or at least remove health hazards. There are times, however, when health policies appear to jeopardize, rather than enhance, the health outcomes of individuals. Consider the case of childhood immunizations. In Chapter 4, Global, Communicable, and Chronic Disease, we described the benefits of vaccines that, when given to children by age five, help to reduce incidences of serious illnesses and death primarily of children. Recently, however, parental concern about the measles, mumps, and rubella (MMR) vaccine routinely given to children in most developed and many developing countries has raised questions about the safety of the vaccine. We will not revisit the work on vaccine hesitance or vaccine refusal here, but it is important to identify the origins of this debate, and we do here.

Parents raised concerns about the likelihood that the MMR vaccine increases the risk of autism in young children. Results from a study in 1998, in addition to increased levels of *ethyl mercury* in the vaccine between 1987 and 1995, led some researchers, but mostly parents, to see a causal link between the higher levels of ethyl mercury and alarmingly higher rates of autism in children within the past 10 to 15 years (Fombonne, Zakanan, Bemuth, Meny, & McLean-Heywood, 2006; Wakefield et al., 1998). More important, parents who participated in the original study with Wakefield and colleagues and who learned of the increased level of ethyl mercury also believed that the MMR vaccine resulted in developmental delays associated with autism (see Box 13.4).

Numerous studies that attempted to replicate Wakefield and colleagues' (1998) claim of an increase in autism rates linked to the MMR vaccine found no such link (Dales, Hammer, & Smith, 2001; Fombonne & Chakvabarti, 2001; Smith, Ellenberg, Bill, & Ruben, 2008). They argue for the maintenance of the health policy that requires children to receive the MMR vaccine by the time they enter elementary school.

Unfortunately, public opinion on the issue appears to favor the proposed link. As a result, a growing number of parents in the U.S. and in England are choosing to refuse the MMR vaccine for their children (Jansen et al., 2003). The effect of even a small number of parents refusing to vaccinate their children caused a spike in the incidence rates of measles in England in 2001 and 2002 (Jansen et al., 2003). Some researchers and health workers fear that, should parents continue to refuse the vaccine for their children, new cases of measles will result in a significant increase in serious illness and even death of children. And remember, as we noted in Chapter 4, Global, Communicable, and Chronic Disease, measles is one of the deadliest diseases for children under five years of age worldwide.

Box 13.4 Does the Measles, Mumps, and Rubella (MMR) Vaccine Cause Autism?

According to approximately 40 parents and some researchers, the MMR vaccine is the cause of a new variant of autism that involves severe gastrointestinal symptoms.

Claims of the new variant of autism took many researchers by surprise. The reports of a new strain of autism were first published by Wakefield and colleagues in 1998. They noted that, in their initial study of 12 children, parents reported that the children's severe gastrointestinal symptoms and progressive developmental disorders began within days of their children receiving an MMR vaccine. The symptoms included abdominal pain, diarrhea, bloating, and food intolerance. Wakefield and colleagues determined that because previous studies showed that children with autism also reported intestinal disorders, it was possible and perhaps likely that the gastrointestinal problems and other behavioral disorders evidenced in 12 children could be related to autism (Reichert et al., 1993; Shattock, Kennedy, Powell, & Berney, 1991). Some earlier studies even suggested a link between gastrointestinal disorders and disruption of normal brain development. Wakefield and colleagues believed that their study had indeed identified a link between the vaccine and autism when an additional 27 children were identified whose parents reported the same symptoms shortly after their children were administered an MMR vaccine. With a total of 39 cases, these researchers believed they identified a health policy problem: The MMR vaccine appeared to cause a new variant of autism.

This claim by Wakefield and colleagues (1998) puzzled health psychologists. Up to this point, most researchers believed autism to be a largely genetic and neurological disorder, a defect that occurred in embryonic development. Few were able to understand how a vaccine given after the first year of life could be responsible for a disorder that up to now was thought to occur in utero (DeStefano & Chen, 2008). Even more puzzling to some were the statistics on the increased rates of autism in California used to support the association between MMR vaccines and autism.

It is true that between 1980 and 1994 California saw its rates of diagnosed cases of autism increase by over 373%. In 1980, incidence rates of autism were 44 per 100,000 children. By 1994, however, the incidence rates had increased to 208 per 100,000 children. But at the same time, the rates of MMR vaccine only increased 14%, far too little to explain the dramatic increase of over 300% in autism (Dales et al., 2001).

In the face of numerous studies that refuted the association between autism and MMR vaccines and earlier research demonstrating that autism was a neurological disorder that occurred in utero, how could researchers explain the dramatic increase in rates?

For many researchers, the answer lay with improvements in medical knowledge. DeStefano and Chen (2008) and Fombonne and colleagues (2006) suggest that the most likely reason for the dramatic rise in autism rates is broader diagnostic criteria used to identify the illness and better detection of early indicators of autism. Broader diagnostic criteria allowed health professionals to classify children as autistic who, in the past, would not have been identified as such. In addition, physicians and other medical providers are now better able to detect early signs of the disease, leading to earlier diagnosis. Together, both may account for some, though not all, of the dramatic increase in cases of autism.

One thing appears to be clear, however. The fear that a childhood immunization may cause autism in one's child is sufficient to deter many parents from an otherwise safe and effective vaccine. It will no doubt take time for the public to review the evidence showing no clear link between the MMR vaccine and autism and to lose their fear of the vaccine. In the meantime, however, unvaccinated children are at increased risk of contracting measles, a potentially fatal and wholly preventable childhood illness.

Are researchers' fears exaggerated? Clearly not, from what we have illustrated in Chapter 4, Global, Communicable, and Chronic Disease. Consider again the escalating rates of measles and now mumps, especially in developed countries. These illnesses were all but eradicated 10 years ago. Researchers and health care providers worry that this escalation may continue and risk a return of pre-vaccine levels if more parents refuse the vaccine for their children.

Health Psychologists as Health Advocates

We explained how individuals can become their own advocates for health. We also explained how nursing students with a connection to a community can become community advocates. But how can health psychologists serve as health advocates and inspire change?

By addressing euthanasia, we saw how health psychologists may demonstrate their ability to serve as advocates for terminally ill or debilitated patients for one of two outcomes: ending life with dignity or coping with debilitating illnesses or injuries. In addition, throughout the book and indeed throughout this chapter we identified ways in which social determinants affect health outcomes. Some of the effects of social determinants on health are known due to the research of health psychologists. And through that same research, health psychologists can integrate their expertise in research design, their knowledge of health and the health problems of a community, and their understanding of social determinants of health to present a carefully designed and carefully executed study that can advocate for health change.

Some health psychologists will use their research or that of others to work closely with policy professionals to implement the changes recommended by the research. When implementing policy, health psychologists will evaluate the effects of the policy in much the same way they evaluate the impact of an intervention program designed to change behaviors.

Finally, some health psychologists may be particularly intrigued by the new research that delves into the physiological and emotional connection to health and well-being. For those health psychologists, more coursework and training in biology and close collaboration with biologists and medical researchers will be essential if they want to play a pivotal role in this line of research.

These are only a sample of the ways in which health psychologists may use their own work or that of others to advocate for improved health outcomes for individuals and communities.

Personal Postscript

WHAT ARE YOUR CAREER PLANS?

Are you considering a career as a health psychologist? If so, after reading this chapter you may see that there are a number of options available to you.

Before deciding on one approach, or "domain," as identified in the chapter, we suggest a few things to help you learn more about the field in general and to help you make an informed choice.

First, consider volunteering in areas in which health psychologists work. For example, health psychologists can be found in many hospital outpatient clinics that provide support programs for individuals with chronic health issues. Teaching hospitals, particularly those affiliated with major universities, are more likely to employ health psychologists in such settings.

Second, health psychologists also work as researchers in major teaching hospitals. Research directors are often willing to have volunteers work on their research teams. By volunteering, you will gain valuable experience to help you determine whether you enjoy working as part of a research team with other health psychologists. In addition, you may have an opportunity to identify a health issue of interest to you.

Third, explore the role of health psychologists in public health settings, such as departments of health or community health settings, in your city or town. In such settings, health psychologists could be involved in either research or policy making or in designing or administering public-health programs.

Finally, consider the work of health psychologists in community-based intervention projects. Community-based participatory research is fast becoming the preferred method of conducting community-health research or intervention programs. Volunteering with a community-based participatory project may provide opportunities to test both the research and the direct-service side of health psychology.

Questions to Consider

1. How can a health psychologist contribute to the development of new policy regulations to improve the safety conditions in the workplace?
2. Community-based participatory research requires that the targeted community be involved in the project from its inception. What challenges does that present for investigators who have a strong interest in a specific health topic?
3. What ethical issues must health psychologists consider when counseling patients about euthanasia?

Alyahya, M. S., Al-Sheyab, N., Alqudah, J., Younis, O. B., & Khader, Y. S. (2021). Effect of multimedia messaging service on exercise self-efficacy in diabetic patients. *American Journal of Health Behavior*, *45*(5), 902–915. doi: 10.5993/AJHB.45.5.10

Alzahrani, A. Y. (2020). Teenage cigarette smoking and the situation in Saudi Arabia in terms of prevalence, predicting and preventing factors: A narrative review. *European Journal of Medical & Health Sciences*, 2(3).

American Cancer Society. (2006). *Cancer facts and figures 2006*. Atlanta, GA: Author.

American Cancer Society. (2008). *Cancer facts & figures, 2008*. Retrieved from www.cancer.org

American Cancer Society. (2022). *What is melanoma skin cancer?* Retrieved February 2, 2023, from www.cancer.org/content/dam/CRC/PDF/Public/8823.00.pdf

American Diabetes Association. (2013). *Diabetes basics*. Retrieved October 24, 2013, from www.diabetes.org/diabetes-basics/?loc=GlobalNavDB

American Heart Association. (2004). *Automated external defibrillation funding fact sheet*. Retrieved from www.americanheart.org

American Heart Association. (2013). *Atherosclerosis*. Retrieved October 25, 2013, from www.heart.org/HEARTORG/Conditions/Conditions_UCM_001087_SubHomePage.jsp#f2

American Heart Association. (2024). Smoking and heart disease in women. *Go Red for Women*. Retrieved February 12, 2024.

American Lung Association. (n.d.). *COPD trends brief: Mortality*. Retrieved November 30, 2023.

American Non-Smoker's Rights Foundation. (2013). *State, commonwealth & municipalities with 100% smokefree laws in workplace, restaurants & bars*. Retrieved from www.no-smoke.org/goingsmokefree.php?id=519

American Pain Foundation. (2009). *Pain facts & figures*. Retrieved September 4, 2009, from http://www.painfoundation.org/newsroom/reporter-resources/pain-facts-figures.html

American Pain Society. (2002). *Guidelines for the management of pain in osteoarthritis, rheumatoid arthritis and juvenile chronic arthritis*. Glenview, IL: Author.

American Psychological Association. (1992). Ethical principles of psychologists and code of conduct. *American Psychologist*, *47*, 1597–1611.

American Psychological Association. (2004). *Bylaws of the American Psychological Association, Article I, 1*. Retrieved from www.apa.org/about/governance/bylaws/index.aspx

American Psychological Association. (2024). *Biofeedback and applied psychophysiology*. Retrieved March 1, 2024, from apa.org

American Hospital Association Community Health Improvement. (2024). *Community health assessment toolkit*. Retrieved May 20, 2024, from https://www.healthycommunities.org/resources/community-health-assessment-toolkit

American Rhetoric. (2001). *Press conference announcing HIV infection and retirement*. Retrieved November 1, 2008, from www.americanrhetoric.com/speeches/magicjohnsonhivretirement.htm

Amerinfo.com. (2008). *Global weight survey look at scale obsession, fast food addiction, and obesity*. Retrieved October 24, 2013, from www.bi-me.com/main.php?id=16148&t=1&c=36&cg=4&mset=

AMFAR. (2006). *Statistics worldwide*. Retrieved from www.amfar.org/abouthiv/article.aspx?id=3592&terms=latin+america

Amnesty International. (2010). *Commissioning justice truth commissions and criminal justice*. London: Author.

An, Y., Zhang, Y., Wang, L., Chen, C., & Fan, X. (2022). The relationship between uncertainty in illness and quality of life in patients with heart failure: Multiple mediating effects of perceived stress and coping strategies. *The Journal of Cardiovascular Nursing*, *37*(3), 257–265. doi: 10.1097/JCN.0000000000000799

Anderson, B. L., Kiecolt-Glaser, J. K., & Glaser, R. (1994). A biobehavioral model of cancer stress and disease course. *American Psychologist*, *49*, 389–404.

Anderson, G. F., & Chu, E. (2007). Expanding priorities: Confronting chronic diseases in countries with low income. *The New England Journal of Medicine*, *356*(3), 209–211.

Anderson, K. M., Odell, P. M., Wilson, P. W., & Kannel, W. B. (1991). Cardiovascular disease risk profiles. *American Heart Journal*, *121*, 293–298.

Anderson, K. O., Bradley, L. A., Young, L. D., McDaniel, L. K., & Wise, C. M. (1985). Rheumatoid arthritis: Review of psychological factors related to etiology, effects and treatment. *Psychological Bulletin*, *98*, 358–387.

Anderson, N. W., Gustafsson, L. N., Okkels, N., Taha, F., Cole, S. W., Munk-Jorgensen, P., & Goodwin, R. D. (2015). Depression and the risk of autoimmune disease: A nationally representative, prospective longitudinal study. *Psychological Medicine*, *45*(16), 3559–3569. doi: 10.1017/S0033291715001488

Anderson, R. N., Kochanek, K. D., & Murphy, S. L. (1995). Report on final mortality statistics. *Monthly Vital Statistics Report*, *45*(suppl. 2), 23–33.

Andreasen, A. R. (1995). *Marketing social change: Changing behavior to promote health, social development, and the environment*. San Francisco: Jossey-Bass Publishers.

Andrews, J. A., Tildesley, E., Hops, H., & Li, F. (2002). The influence of peers on young adult substance use. *Health Psychology*, *21*(4), 349–357.

Angelino, A. C., Evans, Y., Moore, K., & Bell, S. (2023). Ending the erasure of American Indian and Alaska native adolescents and young adults in research in the United States. *Journal of Adolescent Health*, *73*(1), P15–P16. doi: 10.1016/j.jadohealth.2023.03.015

Anglican Breast Cancer Study Group. (2000). Prevalence and penetration of BRCA1 and BRCA2 mutations in a population-based series of breast cancer cases. *British Journal of Cancer*, *83*, 1301–1308.

Annals of Internal Medicine. (2008). Health consequences. *Annals of Internal Medicine*, *149*(7), 14.2–14.3.

Annemans, L., Spaepen, E., Gaskin, M., Bonnemaire, M., Malier, V., Gilbert, T., & Nuki, G. (2008). Gout in the UK & Germany: Prevalence, comorbidities & management in general practice 2000–2005. *Annals of Rheumatoid Disease*, *67*, 960–966. doi: 10.1136/ard.2007.076232

Antczak, E., & Miszczyńska, K. M. (2021). Causes of sickness absenteeism in Europe – Analysis from an intercountry and gender perspective. *International Journal of Environmental Research and Public Health*, *18*(22), 11823. doi: 10.3390/ijerph182211823

Anteghini, M., Fonseca, H., Ireland, M., & Blum, R. W. (2001). Health risk behaviors and associated risk and protective factors among Brazilian adolescents in Santos, Brazil. *Journal of Adolescent Health*, *28*(4), 295–302.

Appelman, Y., van Rijn, B. B., Ten Haaf, M. E., Boersma, E., & Peters, S. A. E. (2015). Sex differences in cardiovascular risk factors and disease prevention. *Atherosclerosis*, *241*(1), 211–218. doi: 10.1016/j.atherosclerosis.2015.01.027

Arabi-Mianrood, H., Hamzehgardeshi, Z., Khoori, E., Moosazadeh, M., & Shahhosseini, Z. (2021). Influencing factors on high-risk sexual behaviors in young people: An ecological perspective. *International Journal of Adolescent Medicine and Health*. doi: 10.1515/ijamh-2016-0162

Arce, J. S. S., Warren, S. S., Meriggi, N. F., Scacco, A., McMurry, N., Voors, M., . . . Omer, S. B. (2021). COVID-19 vaccine acceptance and hesitancy in low- and middle-income countries. *Nature Medicine*, *27*, 1385–1394.

Arena, J. G., & Blanchard, E. B. (2001). Biofeedback training for chronic pain disorders: A primer. In J. Loeser, D. Turk, R. Chapman, & S. Butler (Eds.), *Bonica's management of pain* (3rd ed., pp. 1755–1763). Baltimore: Williams and Wilkins.

Arévalo Avalos, M. R., Ayers, S. L., Patrick, D. L., Jager, J., González Castro, F., Konopken, Y. P., . . . Shaibi, G. Q. (2020). Familism, self-esteem, and weight-specific quality of life among Latinx adolescents with obesity. *Journal of Pediatric Psychology*, *45*(8), 848–857. doi: 10.1093/jpepsy/jsaa047

Aridi, Y. S., Walker, J. L., Roura, E., & Wright, O. R. L. (2020). Adherence to the Mediterranean diet and chronic disease in Australia: National Nutrition and Physical Activity Survey analysis. *Nutrients*, *12*(5), 1251. doi: 10.3390/nu12051251

Armstead, C. A., Lawler, K. A., Gorden, G., Cross, J., & Gibbons, J. (1989). Relationship of racial stressors to blood pressure responses and anger expression in black college students. *Health Psychology*, *8*, 541–556.

Armstrong, D. (2002). Theoretical tensions in biopsychosocial medicine. In D. Marks (Ed.), *The health psychology reader*. London: Sage Publications.

Arrogante, O., González-Romero, G. M., Carrión-García, L., & Polo, A. (2021). Reversible causes of cardiac arrest: Nursing competency acquisition and clinical simulation satisfaction in undergraduate nursing students. *International Emergency Nursing*, *54*. doi: 10.1016/j.ienj.2020.100938

Arroyo, C., Hu, F. B., Ryan, L. M., Kawachi, I., Colditz, G. A., Speizer, F. E., & Manson, J. (2004). Depressive symptoms and risk of type 2 diabetes in women. *Diabetes Care*, *27*, 129–133.

Arruda, L. K., Vailes, L. D., Ferriani, V. P., Santos, A. B., Pomes, A., & Chapman, M. D. (2001). Cockroach allergens and asthma. *Journal of Allergy & Clinical Immunology*, *107*(3), 419–428.

Arthritis Foundation. (2008). *Osteoarthritis*. Retrieved from www.arthritis.org

Arthritis Foundation. (2013). *Arthritis fact sheet*. Retrieved October 25, 2013, from www.arthritis.org/presscenter/arthritis-statistics/

Arthritis Foundation. (n.d.-a). *Juvenile arthritis patient education & resources*. Retrieved March 1, 2024.

Arthritis Foundation. (n.d.-b). *Osteoarthritis: Symptoms, diagnosis, and treatment*. Retrieved March 1, 2024.

Aryan, L., Younessi, D., Zargari, M., Banerjee, S., Agopian, J., Rahman, S., . . . Eghbali, M. (2020). The role of estrogen receptors in cardiovascular disease. *International Journal of Molecular Sciences*, *21*(12), 4314. doi: 10.3390/ijms21124314

Asano, Y. (1996). Varicella vaccine: The Japanese experience. *Infectious Diseases*, *174*(Suppl. 3), S310–S313. doi: 10.1093/infdis/174.supplement_3.s310

Aschengrau, A., Weinberg, J. M., Janulewicz, P. A., Romano, M. E., Gallagher, L. G., Winter, M. R., . . . Ozonoff, D. M. (2012). Occurrence of mental illness following prenatal and early childhood exposure to tetrachloroethylene (PCE)-contaminated drinking water: A retrospective cohort study. *Environmental Health*, *11*, 2.

Ashley, C. D., Smith, J. F., Robinson, J. B., & Richardson, M. T. (1996). Disordered eating in female collegiate athletes and collegiate females in an advanced program of study: A preliminary investigation. *International Journal of Sport Nutrition*, *6*, 391–401.

Ashton, C. M., Haidet, P., Paterniti, D. A., Collins, T. C., Gordon, H. S., O'Malley, K., . . . Street, R. L., Jr. (2003). Racial & ethnic disparities in the use of health services. *Journal of General Internal Medicine*, *18*, 146–152.

Aspinwall, L. G., & Staudinger, U. M. (2003). A psychology of human strengths: Some critical issues of an emerging field. In L. G. Aspinwall & U. M. Staudinger (Eds.), *A psychology of human strengths: Fundamental questions & future directions for a positive psychology* (pp. 9–22). Washington, DC: American Psychological Association.

Association of Schools of the Allied Health Professions. (2009). *Allied health professions*. Retrieved from www.explorehealthcareers.org/en/Field.1aspx

Astle, S., McAllister, P., Emanuel, S., Rogers, J., Toews, M., & Yazedjian, A. (2021). College students' suggestions for improving sex education in schools beyond 'blah blah blah condoms and STDs'. *Sex Education*, *21*(1), 91–105. doi: 10.1080/14681811.2020.1749044

Atkinson, J. H., Grant, I., & Kennedy, C. J. (1988). Prevalence of psychiatric disorders among men infected with human immunodeficiency virus. *Archives of General Psychiatry*, *45*, 859–864.

Aubel, J., Touré, I., & Diagne, M. (2004). Senegalese grandmothers promote improved maternal and child nutrition practices: The guardians of tradition are not averse to change. *Social Science & Medicine*, *59*, 945–959.

Aufiero, M., Stankewicz, H., Quazi, S., Jacoby, J., & Stoltzfus, J. (2017). Pain perception in Latino vs. Caucasian and male vs. female patients: Is there really a difference? *Western Journal of Emergency Medicine*, *18*(4), 737–742. doi: 10.5811/westjem.2017.1.32723

Australian Institute of Health & Welfare. (2002). *Australia's health*. AIWA: Cat. No. AUS 25. Canberra: Author.

Avdic, D., & Johansson, P. (2013). *Gender differences in preferences for health-related absences from work*. IZA Discussion Paper No. 7480. doi: 10.2139/ssrn.2293297. Retrieved February 1, 2024, from https://ssrn.com/abstract=2293297

Avery, C. (1991). Native American medicine: Traditional healing. *Journal of American Medical Association*, *265*(17), 2271–2273.

Avery, L., Hutchinson, D., & Whitaker, K. (2002). Domestic violence & intergenerational rates of child sexual abuse: A case record analysis. *Child Adolescent Social Work*, *19*, 77–90.

Ayouba, A. J., Nerrienet, A., Menu, E., Lobe, M., Thonnon, J., & Leke, R. (2003). Mother-to-child transmission of human immunodeficiency virus type 1 in relation to the season in Yaounde, Cameroon. *American Journal of Tropical Medicine and Hygiene*, *69*(4), 447–449.

Babic, M. J., Smith, J. J., Morgan, P. J., Eather, N., Plotnikoff, R. C., & Lubans, D. R. (2017). Longitudinal associations between changes in screen-time and mental health outcomes in adolescents. *Mental Health and Physical Activity*, *12*, 124–131. doi: 10.1016/j.mhpa.2017.04.001

Bach, P. B., Schrag, D., Brawley, O. W., Galaznik, A., Yakren, S., & Begg, C. B. (2002). Survival of blacks and whites after a cancer diagnosis. *JAMA*, *287*, 2106–2113.

Baena, R., & Salinas, P. (2015). Diet and colorectal cancer. *Maturitas*, *80*, 258–264.

Bagley, C., & Mallick, K. (2000). Prediction of sexual, emotional, and physical maltreatment and mental health outcomes in a longitudinal cohort of 290 adolescent women. *Child Maltreatment*, *5*, 218–226.

Bahl, S., Hampton, L. M., Bhatnagar, P., Rao, G. S., Haldar, P., Sangal, L., . . . Nalavade, U. P. (2017). Notes from the field: Detection of Sabin-like type 2 poliovirus from sewage after global cessation of trivalent oral poliovirus vaccine – Hyderabad and Ahmedabad, India, August–September 2016. *Morbidity and Mortality Weekly Report*, *65*(52), 1493–1494. Retrieved from www.cdc.gov/mmwr/index.html

Baker, D. W., Stevens, C. D., & Brook, R. H. (1994). Regular source of ambulatory care and medical care utilization by patients presenting to a public hospital emergency department. *Journal of the American Medical Association*, *271*, 1909–1912.

Baker, K. R., Nelson, M. E., Felson, D. T., Layne, J. E., Sarno, R., & Roubenoff, R. (2001). The efficacy of home based progressive strength training in older adults with knee osteoarthritis: A randomized controlled trial. *Journal of Rheumatology*, *18*, 1655–1665.

Balasooriya-Smeekens, C., Walter, F. M., & Scott, S. (2015). The role of emotions in time to presentation for symptoms suggestive of cancer: A systematic literature review of quantitative studies. *Psychooncology*, *24*(12), 1594–1604. doi: 10.1002/pon.3833

Balsa, A. I., Homer, J. F., French, M. T., & Norton, E. C. (2011). Alcohol use & popularity: Social payoffs from conforming to peers' behaviors. *Journal of Research on Adolescents, 21,* 559–568.

Bandura, A. (1977). Self-efficacy: Towards a unifying theory of behavioral change. *Psychological Review, 84*(2), 191–215.

Bandura, A. (1982). Self-efficacy mechanism in human agency. *American Psychologist, 37*(2), 122–147.

Bandura, A. (1986). *Social foundations of thought & action: A social cognitive theory.* Englewood Cliffs, NJ: Prentice-Hall.

Banerjee, B. (2015). Background, controversies, and misuse of post traumatic stress disorder diagnostic criteria: A review. *Indian Journal of Health and Wellbeing, 6*(4), 400–406.

Banks, J., Marmot, M., Oldfield, Z., & Smith, J. P. (2006). Disease and disadvantage in the United States and in England. *Journal of the American Medical Association, 295*(17), 2037–2045.

Banks, S. M., & Kerns, R. D. (1996). Explaining high rates of depression in chronic pain: A diathesis–stress framework. *Psychological Bulletin, 119,* 95–110.

Bao, W., Srinivasan, S. R., Valdez, R., Greenlund, K. J., Wattigney, W. A., & Berenson, G. S. (1997). Longitudinal changes in cardiovascular risk from childhood to young adulthood in offspring of parents with coronary artery disease. *JAMA, 278,* 1749–1754.

Barbieri, R., Drancourt, M., & Raoult, D. (2021). The role of louse-transmitted diseases in historical plague pandemics. *The Lancet: Infectious Diseases, 21*(2), e17–e25. doi: 10.1016/S1473–3099(20)30487–4

Barbiero, V. K. (2020). Ebola: A hyperinflated emergency. *Global Health: Science and Practice, 8*(2), 178–182. doi: 10.9745/GHSP-D-19-00422

Barksdale, D. J., Farrug, E. R., & Harkness, K. (2009). Racial discrimination & blood pressure: Perceptions, emotions, and behaviors of black American adults. *Issues of Mental Health Nursing, 30*(2), 104–111.

Barlow, J. H., Cullen, L. A., & Rowe, I. F. (2002). Education preferences, psychological well-being and self-efficacy among people with rheumatoid arthritis. *Patient Education and Counseling, 46,* 11–19.

Barnett, J. C., & Vornovitsky, M. (2015). *Health insurance coverage in the United States: 2015* (U.S. current population reports). U.S. Census Bureau.

Baron, R., Binder, A., & Wasner, G. (2010). Neuropathic pain: Diagnosis, pathophysiological mechanisms & treatment. *Lancet Neurology, 9*(8), 807–819.

Barrett, B., Shadick, K., Schilling, R., Spencer, L., del Rosario, S., Moua, K., & Vang, M. (1998). Hmong/medicine interactions: Improving cross-cultural health care. *Family Medicine, 30*(3), 179–184.

Barrett-Connor, E., & Stuenkele, C. (1999). Hormones & heart disease in women's health and estrogen/progesterone replacement studies in perspective. *Journal of Clinical Endocrinology & Medicine, 84*(6), 1848–1853.

Barry, E. (2023, August 10). U.S. watchdog halts studies at N.Y. Psychiatric Center after a subject's suicide. *The New York Times.* Retrieved September 10, 2023, from nytimes.com.

Bar-Shalita, T., & Cermak, S. A. (2020). Multi-sensory responsiveness and personality traits predict daily pain sensitivity. *Frontiers in Integrative Neuroscience, 13.* doi: 10.3389/fnint.2019.00077

Bashir, A., Doreswamy, S., Narra, L. R., Patel, P., Guarecuco, J. E., Baig, A., . . . Heindl, S. E. (2020). Childhood obesity as a predictor of coronary artery disease in adults: A literature review. *Cureus, 12*(11), e11473. doi: 10.7759/cureus.11473

Bashour, H., & Mamaree, F. (2003). Gender differences and tuberculosis in the Syrian Arab republic: Patients' attitudes, compliance and outcomes. *East Mediterranean Health, 9*(4), 757–768.

Basic Documents. (2006). *Constitution of the World Health Organization* (45th ed.). Retrieved October 4, 2013, from www.who.int/governance/eb/who_constitution_en.pdf

Batbaatar, E., Dorjdagva, J., Luvsannyam, A., Savino, M. M., & Amenta, P. (2017). Determinants of patient satisfaction: A systematic review. *Perspectives in Public Health*, *137*(2), 89–101. doi: 10.1177/1757913916634136

Baum, A., & Posluszny, D. M. (1999). Health psychology: Mapping biobehavioral contributions to health & illness. *Annual Review of Psychology*, *50*, 137–163.

Bayne-Smith, M., Farder, P. S., Azzollini, A., Magel, S., Schmitz, K. H., & Agin, D. (2004). Improvements in heart health behaviors, reduction in coronary artery disease risk factors in urban teenage girls through a school-based intervention. *American Journal of Public Health*, *94*(9), 1538–1543.

Beaglehole, R., Ebrahim, S., Reedy, S., Voute, J., Leeder, S., & Chronic Disease Action Group. (2007). Prevention of chronic diseases: A call to action. *The Lancet*, *370*(9605), 2152–2157.

Beavis, A., Krakow, M., Levinson, K., & Rositch, A. F. (2018). Reasons for lack of HPV vaccine initiation in NIS-teen over time: Shifting the focus from gender and sexuality to necessity and safety. *Journal of Adolescent Health*, *63*(5), 652–656. doi: 10.1016/j.jadohealth.2018.06.024

Beck, L. F., Dellinger, A. M., & O'Neil, M. E. (2007). Motor vehicle crash injury rates by modes of travel, United States: Using exposure-based methods to quantify differences. *American Journal of Epidemiology*, *166*(2), 212–218.

Becker, L. B. (1996). The epidemiology of sudden death. In N. A. Paradis, H. R. Halperin, & R. M. Nowak (Eds.), *Cardiac arrests: The science and practice of resuscitation medicine* (pp. 28–47). Baltimore: Williams & Wilkins.

Beenstock, M., & Rahav, G. (2002). Testing gateway theory: Do cigarette prices affect illicit drug use? *Journal of Health Economics*, *21*(4), 679–698.

Behbehani, A. M. (1983). The smallpox story: Life and death of an old disease. *Microbiological Reviews*, *47*(4), 455–509.

Belknap, R. A., & Cruz, N. (2007). When I was in my home I suffered a lot: Mexican women's description of abuse in family of origin. *Health Care for Women International*, *28*(5), 506–522.

Bell, D., Ragin, D. F., & Cohall, A. (1999). Cross-cultural issues in prevention, health promotion, and risk reduction in adolescence. *Adolescent Medicine: Prevention Issues in Adolescent Health Care. State of the Art Reviews*, *10*(1), 57–70.

Belluz, J. (2015, February 21). How the Toronto Star massively botched a story about the HPV vaccine- and corrected the record. *Vox Media*. Retrieved January 14, 2023, from www.vox.com/2015/2/10/8009973/toronto-star-hpv-vaccine

Benjamin, E. J., Muntner, P., Alonso, A., Bittencourt, M. S., Callaway, C. W., Carson, A. P., . . . Virani, S. S. (2019). Heart disease and stroke statistics – 2019 update: A report from the American Heart Association. *Circulation*, *139*(10).

Benkel, I., Arnby, M., & Molander, U. (2020). Living with a chronic disease: A quantitative study of the views of patients with a chronic disease on the change in their life situation. *SAGE Open Medicine*, *8*. doi: 10.1177/2050312120910350

Bennington, D., Tetsch, N., Kunzendorf, S., & Jantschek, G. (2007). Body image in patients with eating disorders and their mothers' and the role of family functioning. *Comprehensive Psychiatry*, *48*, 118–123.

Benoit, D. (2018). iPhones and children are a toxic pair, say two big Apple investors. *Wall Street Journal*.

Bentacourt, J. R. (2006). Eliminating racial and ethnic disparities in health care: What is the role of academic medicine? *Academic Medicine*, *81*(9), 788–794.

Bentley, M. (1988). The household management of childhood diarrhea in rural north India. *Social Science & Medicine*, *27*, 75–85.

Berenson, G. S., Srinivasan, S. R., Bao, W., Newman, W. P., Tracy, R. E., & Wattigney, W. A. (1998). Association between multiple cardiovascular risk factors and atherosclerosis in children and young adults. *New England Journal of Medicine, 338*, 1650–1656.

Bermejo, P. M., Sánchez Valdés, L., Somarriba López, L., Valdivia Onega, N. C., Vidal Ledo, M. J., & Alfonso Sánchez, I. (2021). Equity and the Cuban National Health System's response to COVID-19. *Revista Panamericana de Salud Pública, 45*. doi: 10.26633/RPSP.2021.80

Berna, C., Leknes, S., Holmes, E. A., Edwards, R. R., Goodwin, G. M., & Tracey, I. (2010). Induction of depressed moods disrupts emotion regulation neurocircuitry and enhances pain unpleasantness. *Biological Psychiatry, 67*, 1083–1090.

Bersani, F. S., Wolkowitz, O. M., Milush, J. M., Sinclair, E., Eppling, L., Aschbacher, K., . . . Mellon, S. H. (2016). A population of atypical CD56-CD16 natural killer cells is expanded in PTSD and is associated with symptom severity. *Brain, Behavior & Immunity, 56*, 264–270.

Bertram, M. Y., Sweeny, K., Lauer, J. A., Chisholm, D., Sheehan, P., Rasmussen, B., . . . Deane, S. (2018). Investing in non-communicable diseases: An estimation of the return on investment for prevention and treatment services. *The Lancet Taskforce on NCDS and Economics, 391*(10134), 2071–2078.

Bethel, J. W., & Schneker, M. B. (2005). Acculturation and smoking patterns among Hispanics: A review. *American Journal of Preventive Medicine, 29*(2), 143–148.

Beveridge, W. I. (1991). The chronicle of influenza epidemics. *History and Philosophy of the Life Sciences, 13*, 223–235.

Bielak, L. F., Yu, P., Ryan, K. A., Rumberger, J. A., Sheedy, P. F., II., Turner, S. T., . . . Peyser, P. A. (2007). Differences in prevalence and severity of coronary artery calcification between two non Hispanic white populations with diverse lifestyles. *Atherosclerosis, 196*(2), 888–895.

Bieliauskas, L. A. (2019). *Stress and its relationship to health and illness.* New York, NY: Routledge.

Biglan, A., Metzler, C. W., & Wirt, R. (1990). Social and behavioral factors associated with high-risk sexual behaviors among adolescents. *Journal of Behavioral Medicine, 13*, 245–261.

Bingham, S. A. (2000). Diet and colorectal cancer prevention. *Biochemical Social Transmission, 28*, 12–16.

Binkin, N. J., Vernon, A. A., Simone, P. M., McCray, E., Miller, B. I., & Schieffelbein, C. W. (1999). Tuberculosis prevention and control activities in the US: An overview of the organization of TB screening. *International Journal of Tuberculosis Lung Disease, 3*(8), 663–674.

Bin Zarah, A., Enriquez-Marulanda, J., & Andrade, J. (2020). Relationship between dietary habits, food attitudes and food security status among adults living within the United States three months post-mandated quarantine: A cross-sectional study. *Nutrients, 12*(11). doi: 10.3390/nu12113468

Bjorck, J. P., Hopp, D. P., & Jones, L. W. (1999). Prostate cancer and emotional functioning: Effects on mental adjustment, optimism and appraisal. *Journal of Psychosocial Oncology, 17*(1), 71–85.

Bjordal, J. M., Klovning, A., Ljunggren, A. E., & Slordal, L. (2007). Short-term efficacy of pharmapsychotherapeutic interventions in osteoarthritic knee pain: A meta-analysis of randomized placebo-controlled trials. *European Journal of Pain, 11*, 125–138.

Blackadar, C. B. (2016). Historical review of causes of cancer. *World Journal of Clinical Oncology, 7*(1), 54–86.

Blake, L. V. (1992, July 19). *Hemophilia and HIV – A hidden majority.* Paper presented at the International Conference on AIDS.

Bledsoe, G. H., Schexnayder, S. M., Carey, M. J., Dobbins, W. N., Gibson, W. D., Hindman, J. W., . . . Ferrer, T. J. (2002). The negative impact of the repeal of the Arkansas motor cycle helmet law. *Journal of Trauma, 53*(6), 1078–1086.

Bleiker, E. M., Hendricks, J. T., Otten, J. D., Verbeck, A. L., & van der Ploeg, H. M. (2008). Personality factor and breast cancer risk: A 13-year follow-up. *Journal of the National Cancer Institute*, *100*, 213–218.

Blount, B. C., Karwowski, M. P., Shields, P. G., Morel-Espinosa, M., Valentin-Blasini, L., Gardner, M., . . . Pirkle, J. L. (2020). Vitamin E acetate in bronchoalveolar-lavage fluid associated with EVALI. *The New England Journal of Medicine*, *382*(8), 697–705.

Blue Cross Blue Shield Association. (2024). *The Blue Cross Blue Shield system*. Retrieved February 29, 2024, from bcbs.com

Blum, R. W., Beuhring, T., Shew, M. L., Beavinger, L. H., Sieving, R. E., & Resnick, M. D. (2000). The effects of race/ethnicity, income and family structure on adolescent risk behaviors. *American Journal of Public Health*, *90*(12), 1879–1884.

Boddington, P. (2009). Theoretical & practical issues in the definition of health: Insight from Aboriginal Australia. *Journal of Medicine and Philosophy*, *34*(1), 49–67.

Boehmer, T. K., Lovegreen, S. L., Haire-Joshu, D., & Brownson, R. C. (2006). What constitutes an obesogenic environment in rural communities? *American Journal of Health Promotion*, *20*(6), 411–421.

Boets, S., Meunier, J-C., & Kluppels, L. (2016). Implementing graduated driving license in Europe: Literature review on practices and effects, and recommendation of an ideal model. *Recherche Transports Sécurité*, *2016*(1–2), 81–96.

Bojuwoye, O., & Moletsane-Kekae, M. (2018). African indigenous knowledge systems and healing traditions. In S. Fernando & R. Moodley (Eds.), *Global psychologies*. London: Palgrave Macmillan.

Bolen, J., Sniezek, T., Theis, K., Helmich, C., Hootman, J., Brady, T., & Langmaid, G. (2005). Racial/ethnic differences in the prevalence and impact of doctor-diagnosed arthritis: United States, 2002. *Morbidity & Mortality Weekly Report*, *54*, 119–123.

Bolger, N., Foster, M., Vinoker, A. D., & Ng, R. (1996). Close relationships & adjustments to a life crisis: The case of breast cancer. *Journal of Personal & Social Psychology*, *70*, 283–294.

Bolland, J. M. (2003). Hopelessness and risk behavior among adolescents living in high-poverty inner-city neighborhoods. *Journal of Adolescence*, *26*, 145–158.

Boney, F. H. (1967). Doctor Thomas Hamilton: Two views of a gentleman of the old South. *Phylon*, *28*, 288–292.

Bor, J., Herbst, A. J., Newell, M. L., & Barnighausen, T. (2013). Increase in adult life expectancy in rural South Africa: Valuing the scale-up of HIV treatment. *Science*, *339*, 961–965.

Borders, A. (2004). Predicting problem behaviors with multiple expectancies: Expanding expectancy-value theory. *Adolescence*, *39*(155), 539–550.

Borod, M. (2006). SMILES – Toward a better laughter life: A model for introducing humor in the palliative care setting. *Journal of Cancer Education*, *21*, 30–34.

Borrell, B. (2023). Flawed protocol for levodopa clinical trial brings retractions. *The Transmitter*. Retrieved November 11, 2023.

Borstelmann, N. A., Rosenberg, S. M., Ruddy, K. J., Tamimi, R. M., Gelber, S., Schapira, L., & Come, S. (2015). Partner support and anxiety in young women with breast cancer. *Psychooncology*, *24*(12), 1679–1685.

Boscarino, J. (2004). Posttraumatic stress disorder & physical illness: Results from clinical and epidemiological studies. *Annals of New York Academy of Science*, *1032*, 141–153.

Bosswell, G. H., Kahana, E., & Dilworth-Anderson, P. (2006). Spirituality and healthy lifestyle behaviors: Stress counter-balancing effects on the wellbeing of older adults. *Journal of Religion and Health*, *45*(4), 587–602.

Bourgeois, A. P. (1980). Kakungu among the Yaku and Suku. *African Arts*, *14*(1), 42–46.

Bourguignon, D., Teixeira, C. P., Koc, Y., Outten, H. R., Faniko, K., & Schmitt, M. T. (2020). On the protective role of identification with a stigmatized identity: Promoting engagement and discouraging disengagement coping strategies. *European Journal of Social Psychology*, *50*(6), 1125–1142. doi: 10.1002/ejsp.2703

Bourne, P. A. (2009). Health inequalities in Jamaica, 1988–2007. *Australian Journal of Basic and Applied Science*, *3*(3), 3040–3052.

Bowen-Reid, T. L., & Harrell, J. P. (2002). Racist experiences and health outcomes: An examination of spirituality as a buffer. *Journal of Black Psychology*, *28*, 18–36.

Bowie, J. V., Sydnor, K. D., Granot, M., & Pargament, K. J. (2004). Spirituality and coping among survivors of prostate cancer. *Journal of Psychosocial Oncology*, *22*(2), 41–56.

Boyd, B., & Wandersman, A. (1991). Predicting undergraduate condom use with the Fishbein and Azjen and the Triandis attitude-behavior models: Implications for public health intervention. *Journal of Applied Social Psychology*, *21*, 1810–1830.

Boylston, A. (2012). The origins of inoculation. *Journal of the Royal Society of Medicine*, *105*(7), 309–313. doi: 10.1258/jrsm.2012.12k044

Brady, S. S., Dolcini, M. M., Harper, G. W., & Pollack, L. M. (2009). Supportive friendships moderate the association between stressful life events and sexual risk taking among African American adolescents. *Health Psychology*, *28*(2), 238–248.

Brady, S. S., & Donenberg, G. R. (2006). Mechanisms linking violence exposure to health risk behavior in adolescence: Motivation to cope and sensation-seeking personality. *Journal of the American Academy of Child and Adolescent Psychiatry*, *45*, 673–680.

Brankovic-Magic, M., Dobricic, J., & Krivokuca, A. (2012). Genetics of breast cancer: Contribution of BRCA1/2 genes alterations to hereditary predisposition. *Vojnosanitetski Pregled: Military Medical & Pharmaceutical Journal of Serbia & Montenegro*, *69*, 700–706.

Bratberg, E., Dahl, S. A., & Risa, A. E. (2002). The double burden: Do combinations of career and family obligations increase sickness absence among women? *European Sociological Review*, *18*(2), 233–249.

Braun, S., Mejia, R., Ling, P. M., & Perez-Stable, E. J. (2008). Tobacco industry target youth in Argentina. *Tobacco Control*, *17*(2), 111–117.

Breitbart, W. (1995). Identifying patients at risk for a treatment of major psychiatric complications of cancer. *Supportive Cancer Care*, *3*, 45–60.

Breitbart, W., McDonald, M. V., Rosenfeld, B., Passik, S. D., Hewitt, D., Thaler, H., & Portenoy, R. K. (1996). Pain in ambulatory AIDS patients I: Pain characteristics and medical correlates. *Pain*, *68*, 315–321.

Breman, J. G., Heymann, D. L., Lloyd, G., McCormick, J. B., Miatudila, M., Murphy, F. A., . . . Johnson, K. M. (2016). Discovery and description of Ebola Zaire virus in 1976 and relevance to the West African epidemic during 2013–2016. *Journal of Infectious Diseases*, *214*(Suppl. 3), S93–S101. doi: 10.1093%2Finfdis%2Fjiw207

Bremner, D., Wittbrodt, M. T., Gurel, N. Z., Shandhi, M. H, Gazi, A. H., Jiao, Y., . . . Inan, O. T. (2021). Transcutaneous cervical vagal nerve stimulation in patients with posttraumatic stress disorder (PTSD): A pilot study of effects on PTSD symptoms and interleukin-6 response to stress. *Journal of Affective Disorders Reports*, *6*. doi: 10.1016/j.jadr.2021.100190

Brender, N. D., & Collins, J. L. (1998). Co-occurrence of health-risk behaviors among adolescents in the United States. *Journal of Adolescent Health*, *22*, 209–213.

Brendgen, M., & Vitaro, F. (2008). Peer rejection and physical health problems in early adolescence. *Journal of Developmental and Behavioral Pediatrics*, *29*(3), 183–190.

Brendgen, M., Vitaro, F., Bukowski, W. M., Doyle, A. B., & Markiewicz, D. (2001). Developmental profiles of peer social preference over the course of elementary school: Associations with trajectories of externalizing and internalizing behaviors. *Developmental Psychology*, 37, 308–320.

Brennan, F. (2015). The US congressional "Decade on pain control and research" 2001–2011: A review. *Journal of Pain & Palliative Care Pharmacotherapy*, 29(3), 212–227. doi: 10.3109/15360288.2015.1047553

Brennan, M., Singer, S., Maki, R., & O'Sullivan, B. (2004). Sarcomas of the soft tissue and bone. In V. T. DeVita, S. Hellman, & S. A. Rosenberg (Eds.), *Cancer: Principle & practice of oncology* (Vol. 2, 7th ed.). Philadelphia: Lippincott, Williams & Wilkins.

Brentlinger, P. E., Behrens, C. B., & Kublin, J. G. (2007). Challenges in the prevention, diagnosis & treatment of malaria in human immunodeficiency virus infected adults in sub-Saharan Africa. *Archives of Internal Medicine*, 167(17), 1827–1836.

Bright, K., Mills, A., Bradford, J. P., & Stewart, D. J. (2023). RAPID framework for improved access to precision oncology for lethal disease: Results from a modified multi-round Delphi study. *Frontiers in Health Service*, 3, 1015621. doi: 10.3389/frhs.2023.1015621

British Heart Foundation. (2021). *How your heart works*. Retrieved February 12, 2024.

Britto, M. T., Klostermann, B. K., Bonny, A. E., Altum, S. A., & Hornung, R. W. (2001). Impact of a school-based intervention on access to healthcare for underserved youth. *Journal of Adolescent Health*, 29, 116–124.

Broadhead, W. E., Kaplan, B. H., James, S. A., Wagner, E. H., Schoenbach, V. J., Grimson, R., . . . Gehlbach, S. H. (1983). The epidemiologic evidence for a relationship between social support and health. *American Journal of Epidemiology*, 117, 521–537.

Brod, S., Rattazzi, L., Piras, G., & D'Acquisto, F. (2014). 'As above, so below' examining the interplay between emotion and the immune system. *Immunology*, 143(3), 311–318. doi: 10.1111/imm.12341

Brondolo, E., Rieppi, R., Kelly, K. P., & Gerin, W. (2003). Perceived racism and blood pressure: A review of the literature and conceptual and methodological critique. *Annals of Behavioral Medicine*, 25, 55–66.

Bronfenbrenner, U. (1977). Toward an experimental ecology of human development. *American Psychologist*, 32(7), 513.

Bronfenbrenner, U. (1986). Ecology of the family as a context for human development: Research perspectives. *Developmental Psychology*, 22(6), 723–742.

Broome, B., & Broome, R. (2007). Native Americans: Traditional healing. *Urologic Nursing*, 27(2), 161–173.

Brosseau, L., Pelland, L., Wells, G., Macleay, L., Lamothe, C., Michaud, G., . . . Tugwell, P. (2004). Efficacy of aerobic exercises for osteoarthritis (Part II): A meta-analysis. *Physical Therapy Review*, 9, 125–145.

Brown, L. K., & DiClemente, R. J. (1992). Predictors of condom use in sexually active adolescents. *Journal of Adolescent Health*, 13(8), 651–657.

Bruce, A., Bray, D., Lewis, J., Raff, M., Roberts, K., & Watson, J. D. (2002). *The molecular biology of the cell*. Retrieved February 26, 2010, from www.ncbi.nlm.nih.gov/books/NBK20684/

Bruce, K. R., & Steiger, H. (2005). Treatment implications of Axis-II comorbidity in eating disorders. *Eating Disorders*, 13, 93–108.

Brunchmann, A., Thomsen, M., & Fink-Jensen, A. (2019). The effect of glucagon-like peptide-1 (GLP-1) receptor agonists on substance use disorder (SUD)-related behavioural effects of drugs and alcohol: A systematic review. *Physiology & Behavior*, 206(1), 232–242. doi: 10.1016/j.physbeh.2019.03.029

Bruni, L., Albero, G., Serrano, B., Mena, M., Collado, J. J., Gómez, D., Muñoz, J., Bosch, F. X., & de Sanjosé, S. (2021, October 22). *Human papillomavirus and related diseases in the world*. Summary

Report. ICO/IARC Information Centre on HPV and cancer (HPV Information Centre). Retrieved August 18, 2022.

Bryant, R.A. (2022). Controversies in posttraumatic stress disorder. In C.L. Cobb, S.J. Lynn, & W. O'Donohue (Eds.), *Toward a science of clinical psychology*. Cham: Springer. doi: 10.1007/978-3-031-14332-8_18

Bucko, R.A., & Cloud, S.I. (2008). Lakota health and healing. *Southern Medical Journal, 101*(6), 596–598.

Bullman, D.C., & Svarsted, B.L. (2000). Effects of physician communication style on client medication beliefs and adherence with antidepressant treatment. *Patient Education and Counseling, 40*(2), 173–185.

Bunin, G.R. (2004). Nongenetic causes of childhood cancers: Evidence from international variation, time trends & risk factor studies. *Toxicology & Applied Pharmacology, 199*, 91–103.

Burke, A.P., Farb, A., Malcom, G.T., Liang, Y., Smialek, J.E., & Virmani, R. (1999). Plaque rupture and sudden death related to exertion in men with coronary artery disease. *JAMA, 281*(10), 921–926.

Burnam, A.M., Telles, C.A., Karno, M., & Hough, R.I. (1987). Measurement of acculturation in a community of Mexican Americans. *Hispanic Journal of Behavioral Science, 9*, 105–130.

Burt, W., & Overpeck, M.D. (2001). Emergency visits for sports-related injuries. *Annals of Emergency Medicine, 37*(3), 301–308.

Burton, L.E., Smith, H.H., & Nichols, A.W. (1980). *Public health and community medicine* (3rd ed.). Baltimore: Williams & Wilkins.

Caban, A.J., Lee, D.J., Fleming, L.E., Gomez-Martin, O., Leblanc, W., & Pitman, T. (2005). Obesity in U.S. workers: The national health interview survey 1986–2002. *American Journal of Public Health, 95*(9), 1614–1622.

Cafferky, B.M., Mendez, M., Anderson, J.R., & Stith, S.M. (2018). Substance use and intimate partner violence: A meta-analytic review. *Psychology of Violence, 81*, 110–131.

Calcagni, E., & Elenkov, I. (2006). Stress system activity, innate & T helper cytokines & susceptibility to immune-related diseases. *Annals of the New York Academy of Science, 1069*, 62–76.

Callan, M.J., Kim, H., & Matthews, W.J. (2015). Predicting self-rated mental and physical health: The contributions of subjective socioeconomic status and personal relative deprivation. *Frontiers in Psychology, 6*, 1415. Retrieved July 22, 2023, from www.frontiersin.org/articles/10.3389/fpsyg.2015.01415/full

Calogero, R., Boroughs, M., & Thompson, J. (2007). The impact of Western beauty ideals on the lives of women: A sociocultural perspective. In V. Swami & A. Furnham (Eds.), *The body beautiful* (pp. 259–298). Palgrave Macmillan.

Caminero Luna, J.A. (2003). *Guia de la tuberculosis para medicos especialistas*. Paris: International Union Against Tuberculosis and Respiratory Disease.

Campaign for Tobacco Free Kids. (2023). *Smoke-free states in the United States*. Retrieved March 28, 2023, from tobaccofreekids.org

Campaign for Tobacco-Free Kids. (2024). *Smoke-free states in the United States*. Retrieved February 8, 2024, from 0332.pdf (tobaccofreekids.org)

Campbell, L.C., Keefe, F.J., Scipio, C., McKee, D.C., Edwards, C.L., & Herman, S.H. (2006). Facilitating research participation & improving quality of life for African American prostate cancer survivors & their intimate partners. *Cancer, 109*(suppl. 2), 414–424.

Campsmith, M.L., Rhodes, P.H., Hall, H.I., & Green, T.A. (2010). Undiagnosed HIV prevalence among adults & adolescents in the US at the end of 2006. *Journal of Acquired Immune Deficiency Syndrome, 53*(3), 619–624.

Cancer Australia. (2022). *Sarcoma*. Retrieved February 10, 2023.

Cannon, W. B. (1929). *Body changes in pain, hunger, fear & rage*. New York: Appleton.

Cantor, D. (2000). The diseased body. In R. Cooter & J. E. Pickstone (Eds.), *Medicine in the 20th century*. London: Harwood Press.

Cao, W., Fang, Z., Hou, G., Han, M., Xu, X., Dong, J., & Zheng, J. (2020). The psychological impact of the COVID-19 epidemic on college students in China. *Psychiatry Research, 287*. doi: 10.1016/j.psychres.2020.112934

Capaldi, D. M., & Clark, S. (1998). Prospective family prediction of aggression towards female partner for at-risk young men. *Developmental Psychology, 34*, 1175–1188.

Carels, R. A., Darby, L. A., Ryder, S., Douglas, O. M., Cacciapaglia, H. M., & O'Brien, N. H. (2005). The relationship between self-monitoring, outcome expectations, difficulty with eating and exercise and physical activity and weight loss treatment outcome. *Annals of Behavioral Medicine, 30*(3), 182–190.

Carreira, H., Williams, R., Dempsey, H., Stanway, S., Smeeth, L., & Bhaskaran, K. (2021). Quality of life and mental health in breast cancer survivors compared with non-cancer controls: A study of patient-reported outcomes in the United Kingdom. *Journal of Cancer Survivorship, 15*, 564–575.

Carroll, D., Smith, G. D., & Bennett, P. (2002). Some observations on health and socio-economic status. In D. F. Marks (Ed.), *The health psychology reader*. London: Sage Publications.

Carstensen, L. I., & Charles, S. T. (2003). Human aging: Why is even good news taken as bad? In L. G. Aspinwall & U. M. Staudinger (Eds.), *A psychology of human strengths* (pp. 75–86). Washington, DC: American Psychological Association.

Cartwright, M., Wardle, J., Steggles, N., Simon, A. E., Croker, J. E., & Jarvis, M. J. (2003). Stress and dietary practices in adolescents. *Health Psychology, 22*, 362–369.

Case, A., Lubotsky, D., & Paxson, C. (2002). Economic states and health in childhood: The origins of the gradient. *American Economic Review, 92*, 1308–1334.

Cassels, A. K. (2007). Vaccination against human papillomavirus. *Canadian Medical Association Journal, 177*, 1526.

Caswell-Jin, S. L. (2018). Racial/ethnic differences in multiple-gene sequencing results for hereditary cancer risk. *Genetic Medicine, 20*(2), 234–239.

Cavanagh, S. E. (2007). Peers, drinking, and the assimilation of Mexican American youth. *Sociological Perspectives, 50*(3), 393–416.

Cavender, A. P., & Albin, M. (2009). The use of magical plants by curanderos in the Ecuador highlands. *Journal of Ethnobiology & Ethnomedicine, 5*, 3.

Centers for Disease Control. (1992). *1993 revised classification system for HIV infection and expansion of surveillance case definition for AIDS among adolescents and adults* (Mortality and Morbidity Weekly reports, Dec.18, 41(RR-17)).

Centers for Disease Control. (1999). *National center for health statistics*. National Vital Statistics.

Centers for Disease Control. (2000). *Boy's growth chart: Weight vs. height*. CDC: National Center for Health Statistics. Retrieved February 24, 2009, from www.cdc.gov/growthcharts/data/set1clinical/cj41c025.pdf

Centers for Disease Control. (2001). *Sexually transmitted disease surveillance, 2000*. Atlanta, GA: U.S. Department of Health and Human Services.

Centers for Disease Control. (2004a). *Dracunculiasis, parasites and health*. Retrieved May 12, 2007, from www.dpd.cdc.gov.dpdx/HTML/Frames/A-F/Dracunculiasis/body

Centers for Disease Control. (2004b). *Excite: An introduction to epidemiology*. Retrieved March 23, 2009, from www.cdc.gov/excite/classroom/intro-epi.htm

Centers for Disease Control. (2004c). *National program of cancer registry: United States cancer statistics.* Retrieved July 15, 2009, from http://apps.nccd.cdc.gov/uscs/toptencancers.aspxh

Centers for Disease Control. (2004d). *Tobacco use in the US.* Washington, DC: National Centers for Disease Control and Prevention and Health Promotion, Tobacco Information & Promotion Source.

Centers for Disease Control. (2004e). *West Nile virus background: Virus history and distribution.* Retrieved May 15, 2007, from www.cdc.gov/ncidod/dvbid/westnile/background/html

Centers for Disease Control. (2004f). *National Center for occupational safety & health.* Worker's Health Chartbook.

Centers for Disease Control. (2004g). Alcohol-attributable deaths & years of potential life lost United States, 2001. *MMWR: Morbidity and Mortality Weekly Report, 53*(37), 866–870.

Centers for Disease Control. (2005a). Surveillance for illnesses and injury after Hurricane Katrina – New Orleans, Louisiana, September 8–25. *MMWR: Morbidity and Mortality Weekly Report, 54*(40), 1018–1021.

Centers for Disease Control. (2005b). Annual smoking-attributable mortality, years of potential life lost & productivity losses – U.S. 1997–2001. *MMWR: Morbidity and Mortality Weekly Report, 54*(25), 625–628.

Centers for Disease Control. (2005c). *Avian influenza A virus infection of humans.* Retrieved October 25, 2013, from www.cdc.gov/flu/avian/gen-info/avian-flu-humans.htm

Centers for Disease Control. (2005d). *Web-based injury statistics querie and reporting system.* WISQARS 2005. National Center for Injury Prevention and Control, CDC. Retrieved from www.cdc.gov/injury/wisqars/pdf/WISQARS-FactSheet20120425-a.pdf

Centers for Disease Control. (2006a). *Avian influenza infections of humans.* Retrieved May 30, 2008, from www.cdc.gov/flu/avian/gen-info/avian-flu-humans.htm

Centers for Disease Control. (2006b). Racial/ethnic disparities in diagnoses of HIV/AIDS. *Morbidity and Mortality Weekly Report, 55*, 121–125.

Centers for Disease Control. (2006c). *Multi-state outbreak of E-coli 0157 infections. November–December, 2006.* Foodborne & Diarrheal Disease Branch. Retrieved May 23, 2007, from www.cdc.gov/ecoli/2006/december/121406.htm

Centers for Disease Control. (2007a). *Prevention of specific infectious diseases.* Retrieved September 26, 2007, from www.cdc.gov/travel/yellowBookCh4-TB.aspx

Centers for Disease Control. (2007b). *Tuberculosis factsheet.* Division of Tuberculosis and Elimination. Retrieved February 10, 2010, from www.cdc.gov/tb/publications/factsheets/statistics/TBTrends.htm

Centers for Disease Control. (2007c). *HIV/AIDS basics.* Retrieved October 25, 2013, from http://www.cdc.gov/actagainstaids/basics/

Centers for Disease Control. (2008a). *Arthritis types – Overview: Childhood arthritis.* Retrieved from www.cdc.gov/arthritis/arthritis/childhood.htm

Centers for Disease Control. (2008b, November 14). Smoking-attributable mortality, years of potential life loss & productivity losses, U.S., 2000–2004. *Morbidity & Mortality Weekly Report, 57*(45), 1226–1228.

Centers for Disease Control. (2008c). *Alcohol.* Retrieved May 22, 2009, from www.cdc.gov/alcohol

Centers for Disease Control. (2008d). *Alcohol & public health.* Retrieved May 23, 2009, from www.cdc.gov/alcohol/

Centers for Disease Control. (2008e). *Fact sheets: Alcohol use and health.* Retrieved October 25, 2013, from www.cdc.gov/alcohol/fact-sheets/alcohol-use.htm

Centers for Disease Control. (2008f). *Surveillance summaries, 57, No. SS12, 1–60.* Retrieved July 12, 2010, from www.cdc.gov/mmwr/pdf/ss/ss5712.pdf

Centers for Disease Control. (2009a). *HIV mortality (through 2006)*. Retrieved February 26, 2010, from www.cdc.gov/hiv/topics/surveillance/resources/slides/mortality/index.htm

Centers for Disease Control. (2009b). *HIV, statistics and surveillance: Basic statistics*. Retrieved from www.cdc.gov/hiv/topics/surveillance/basic.htm#hivaidsexposure

Centers for Disease Control. (2009c). *Overweight and obesity*. CDC: National Center for Health Statistics. Prevalence of Overweight Children and Adolescents US 2003-2004. Retrieved February 24, 2010, from www.cdc.gov/nchs/data/hestat/overweight/overweight_child_03.htm

Centers for Disease Control. (2009d). *Travelers' yellowbook*. Retrieved February 19, 2010, from http://www.cdc.gov/travel/yellowbook/2010/Chapter-5/tuberculosis.aspx#1315

Centers for Disease Control. (2010). *FluView: A weekly influenza surveillance report*. Prepared by Influenza Division, Week ending January 8, 2010. Retrieved June 2, 2010, from www.cdc.gov/h1n1flu/updates/us/011510.htm

Centers for Disease Control. (2011, June 3). HIV surveillance – United States, 1981–2008. *Morbidity and Mortality Weekly Report*, 60(21), 689–693.

Centers for Disease Control. (2012a). Youth risk behavior surveillance, United States 2011. Surveillance summary Vol. 61, No. 4. *Morbidity & Mortality Weekly Report*. Atlanta, GA: U.S. Department of Health & Human Services.

Centers for Disease Control. (2012b). *Alcohol & public health frequently asked questions*. Retrieved January 5, 2013, from www.cdc.gov/alcohol/faqs.htm#moderateDrinking

Centers for Disease Control. (2012c). *Behavioral risk factor surveillance survey data*. Atlanta, GA: U.S. Department of Health and Human Services, CDC.

Centers for Disease Control. (2012d, September 14). *Surveillance for violent deaths*. National violent death reporting system, 16 states 2009. Surveillance summary 61, No. 6. *Morbidity &Mortality Weekly Report*. Atlanta, GA: U.S. Department of Health & Human Services.

Centers for Disease Control. (2012e). Vital signs, testing & risk behaviors among youth U.S. *Morbidity and Mortality Weekly Report*, 61(47), 971–976.

Centers for Disease Control. (2012f). *Lesson 1: Introduction to epidemiology*. Retrieved June 14, 2023, from www.cdc.gov/csels/dsepd/ss1978/lesson1/section1.html

Centers for Disease Control. (2015). *2000 Surgeon General's report highlights: Tobacco timeline*. Retrieved March 28, 2023.

Centers for Disease Control. (2017). *Opioids*. Retrieved May 30, 2023.

Centers for Disease Control. (2019). *Influenza (flu). 2009 H1N1 Pandemic (H1N1pdm09 virus)*. Retrieved April 8, 2023.

Centers for Disease Control. (2020a). *Ten leading causes of death and injury*. Retrieved May 12, 2023, from www.cdc.gov/injury/wisqars/LeadingCauses.html

Centers for Disease Control. (2020b). *WISQARS. Leading causes of death visualization tool*. Retrieved May 17, 2023, from cdc.gov

Centers for Disease Control. (2021). *HPV infections*. Retrieved June 18, 2022.

Centers for Disease Control. (2022a). *Cancers associated with human papillomavirus, United States, 2015–2019*. United States Cancer Statistics Data Briefs, No. 31.

Centers for Disease Control. (2022b). *Symptoms of COVID-19*. Retrieved April 12, 2023.

Centers for Disease Control. (2022c). *Chickenpox (varicella): Chickenpox vaccine saves lives and prevents serious illness infographic*. Retrieved April 12, 2023.

Centers for Disease Control. (2022d). *How many cancers are linked to HPV each year?* Retrieved January 26, 2023.

Centers for Disease Control. (2022e). *Smoking and tobacco use: Youth and tobacco use.* Retrieved May 8, 2023.

Centers for Disease Control. (2022f). *Fast facts: Preventing intimate partner violence.*

Centers for Disease Control. (2022g). *Violence prevention.* Retrieved May 22, 2023.

Centers for Disease Control. (2022h). *Cancer treatments.* Retrieved March 30, 2023.

Centers for Disease Control. (2022i). *Drug overdose.* Retrieved May 30, 2023, from www.cdc.gov/drugoverdose/data/od-death-data.html

Centers for Disease Control. (2022j). *Distracted driving.* Retrieved from https://cdctransportation.org/www.cdc.gov/transportationsafety/Distracted_Driving/index.html

Centers for Disease Control. (2023a). *CDC Museum COVID-19 timeline.* David J. Sencer CDC Museum: In Association with the Smithsonian Museum. Retrieved April 1, 2023.

Centers for Disease Control. (2023b). *COVID-19. People with certain medical conditions.* Retrieved March 31, 2023.

Centers for Disease Control. (2023c). *Physical activity helps prevent chronic diseases.* Retrieved February 2, 2024.

Centers for Disease Control. (2023d). *What is diabetes?.* Retrieved November 25, 2023, from www.cdc.gov/diabetes/basics/diabetes.html#:~:text=With%20diabetes%2C%20your%20body%20doesn,vision%20loss%2C%20and

Centers for Disease Control. (2023e). *Current cigarette smoking among adults in the United States.* Retrieved May 18, 2023.

Centers for Disease Control. (2023f). *WISQARS.* Retrieved June 11, 2023, from cdc.gov

Centers for Disease Control. (2023g). *Fast facts: Preventing teen dating violence.* Retrieved January 2, 2024.

Centers for Disease Control. (2023h). *Dating matters toolkit.* Retrieved January 2, 2024, from cdc.gov

Centers for Disease Control. (2023i). *Childhood arthritis.* Retrieved March 1, 2024, from www.cdc.gov/arthritis/types/childhood.htm

Centers for Disease Control. (2023j). *Leading causes of death.* Retrieved May 5, 2023, from https://wisqars.cdc.gov/lcd/?o=LCD&y1=2022&y2=2022&ct=10&cc=ALL&g=00&s=0&r=0&ry=2&e=0&ar=lcd1age&at=groups&ag=lcd1age&a1=0&a2=199

Centers for Disease Control. (n.d.-a). *E-cigarettes, or vaping, products visual dictionary.* Retrieved May 22, 2023, from cdc.gov

Centers for Disease Control. (n.d.-b). *Electronic cigarettes: What's the bottom line?* Retrieved March 29, 2023, from cdc.gov

Centers for Disease Control & Prevention. (2011). *Vital signs, prescription painkiller overdoses in the U.S.* Retrieved November 9, 2016, from www.cdc.gov/vitalsigns/PainkillerOverdoses/index.html

Centers for Disease Control & Prevention. (2013a). Vital signs: Binge drinking among women & high school girls, United States, 2011. *Morbidity & Mortality Weekly Report, 62*(1), 9–13.

Centers for Disease Control & Prevention. (2013b). Suicide among adults aged 35–64 years. United States 1999–2010. *Morbidity & Mortality Weekly Report, 62*(17), 321–325.

Centers for Disease Control & Prevention. (2015a). Tuberculosis. *Traveler's Yellowbook.* Retrieved October 23, 2016, from http://wwwnc.cdc.gov/travel/yellowbook/2016/infectious-diseases-related-to-travel/tuberculosis#4718

Centers for Disease Control & Prevention. (2015b). Trends in tuberculosis. *Fact Sheet*. Retrieved October 23, 2016, from www.cdc.gov/tb/publications/factsheets/statistics/TBTrends.htm

Centers for Disease Control & Prevention. (2016a). *Ten leading causes of death & injury*. Injury Prevention & Control Data & Statistics (WISQARS). Retrieved April 15, 2016, from www.cdc.gov/injury/wisqars/leadingcauses.html

Centers for Disease Control & Prevention. (2016b). *Suicide: Facts at a glance*. Retrieved October 30, 2016, from www.cdc.gov/ViolencePrevention/pdf/Suicide-DataSheet-a.pdf

Centers for Disease Control & Prevention. (2016c). *Heroin overdose data: Injury prevention & control opioid overdose*. Retrieved November 9, 2016, from www.cdc.gov/drugoverdose/data/heroin.html

Centers for Medicare & Medical Services. (2013). *Presidential milestones*. Tracing the History of CMS Programs: From President Theodore Roosevelt to President George W. Bush. Retrieved June 30, 2013, from www.cms.gov/About-CMS/Agency-Information/History/downloads/presidentcmsmilestones.pdf

CERD Working Group on Health & Environmental Health. (2008). *Unequal health outcomes in the United States: Racial & ethnic disparities in health care treatment & access, the role of social & environmental determinants of health & the responsibilities of the state* (A report to the U.N. Committee on the Elimination of Racial Discrimination). Retrieved September 22, 2009, from www.prrac.org/pdf/CERDhealthEnvironmentReport.pdf

Cha, M. Y., & Hong, H. S. (2015). Effect and path analysis of laughter therapy on serotonin, depression and quality of life in middle-aged women. *Journal of Korean Academy of Nursing, 45*(2), 221–230. doi: 10.4040/jkan.2015.45.2.221

Chadwick, S. E. (1842). *Report from the Poor Law Commission on an inquiry into the sanitation conditions of the labouring population of Great Britain*. United Kingdom: Craig Thornber Publisher.

Chafin, S., Roy, M., Gerin, W., & Christenfeld, N. (2004). Music can facilitate blood pressure recovery from stress. *British Journal of Health Psychology, 9*(3), 393–403.

Chambers, D. W. (2001). A brief history of conflicting ideals in health care. *Journal of the American College of Dentists, 68*(3), 48–51.

Chamorro, R., & Florez-Ortiz, Y. (2000). Acculturation and disordered eating patterns among Mexican American women. *International Journal of Eating Disorders, 28*, 125–129.

Chan, C. H., Ting, T. T., Chen, Y. T., Chen, C.-Y., & Chen, W. J. (2015). Sexual initiation and emotional/behavioral problems in Taiwanese adolescents: A multivariate response profile analysis. *Archives of Sexual Behavior, 44*, 717–727. doi: 10.1007/s10508-014-0265-7

Chan, C. L., Tso, I. F., Ho, R. T., Ng, S. M., Chan, C. H., Chan, J. C., . . . Evans, P. D. (2006). The effect of a one-hour Eastern stress management session on salivary cortisol. *Stress Health, 22*, 45–49.

Chandrashekara, S. (2021). Research methodology and psychoneuroimmunology. In D. F. Ragin & J. P. Keenan (Eds.), *Handbook of research methods in health psychology*. New York, NY: Routledge/Taylor & Francis Group.

Chandrashekara, S., Jayashree, K., Veeranna, H. B., Vadiraj, H. S., Ramesh, M. N., Shobha, A., . . . Vikram, Y. K. (2007). Effects of anxiety on TNF-α levels during psychological stress. *Journal of Psychosomatic Research, 63*(1), 65–69.

Chang, W. L., Liu, H. T., Lin, T. A., & Wen, Y. S. (2008). Influence of family communication structure & vanity trait on consumption behavior: A case study of adolescent students in Taiwan. *Adolescent, 43*(170), 417–435.

Chang, Y.-H., Fu, C.-H., Hsu, M.-H., Okoli, C., & Guo, S.-E. (2024). The effectiveness of a transtheoretical model-based smoking cessation intervention for rural smokers: A quasi-experimental longitudinal study. *Patient Education and Counseling, 122*, 108136. doi: 10.1016/j.pec.2024.108136

Chang, Y.-P., Schneider, J. K., & Sessanna, L. (2011). Decisional conflict among Chinese family caregivers regarding nursing home placement of older adults with dementia. *Journal of Aging Studies, 25*(4), 436–444.

Chapman, W. P., & Jones, C. M. (1944). Variations in cutaneous & visceral pain sensitivity in normal subjects. *Journal of Clinical Investigations, 23*, 81.

Chapple, A., Ziebland, S., & McPherson, A. (2004). Qualitative study of men's perceptions of why treatment delays occur in the UK for those with testicular cancer. *British Journal of General Practice, 54*, 25–32.

Chaves, E., Lunes, D. H., Moura, C., Carvalho, L. C., Silva, A. M., & Carvalho, E. C. (2015). Ansiedade e espiritualidade em estudantes universitários: um estudo transversal. *Revista Brasileria de Enfermagem (Brazilian Journal of Nursing), 68*(3). doi: 10.1590/0034-7167.2015680318i

Chaves, S. S., Gargiullo, P., Zhang, J. X., Civen, R., Guris, D., Mascola, L., & Seward, J. F. (2007). Loss of vaccine-induced immunity to varicella over time. *The New England Journal of Medicine, 356*, 1121–1129.

Chávez-Rodríguez, A. (2021). La "Brujería" en Tonalá: Reconceptualización de la medicina tradicional, la alternativa y el curanderismo. *Psicología Unemi, 5*(9), 85–97. doi: 10.29076/issn.2602-8379vol5iss9.2021pp85-97p

Checkland, K., Harrison, S., McDonald, R., Grant, S., Campbell, S., & Guthrie, B. (2008). Biomedical, holism & general medical practice: Responses to the 2004 general practitioner contract. *Sociology of Health & Wellness, 30*(5), 788–803.

Chee, V. A. (1991). Medicine men. *Journal of the American Medical Association, 265*(17), 2276.

Chen, Y., & VanderWeele, T. J. (2018). Associations of religious upbringing with subsequent health and well-being from adolescence to young adulthood: An outcome-wide analysis. *American Journal of Epidemiology, 187*(11), 2355–2364. doi: 10.1093/aje/kwy142

Cheney, M. K., & Mansker, J. (2014). African American young adult smoking initiation: Identifying intervention points and prevention opportunities. *American Journal of Health Education, 45*(2), 86–96. doi: 10.1080/19325037.2013.875959

Chesney, M. A., Darber, L. A., Hoerster, K., Taylor, J. M., Chambers, D. B., & Anderson, D. E. (2005). Positive emotions: Explaining the other hemisphere in behavioral medicine. *International Journal of Behavioral Medicine, 12*(2), 50–58.

Chia, S. E., Chia, H. P., & Tan, J. S. (2000). Prevalence of headache among handheld cellular telephone users in Singapore: A community study. *Environmental Health Perspective, 108*, 1059–1062.

Chida, Y., Hamer, M., Wardle, J., & Steptoe, A. (2008). Do stress-related psychosocial factors contribute to cancer incidence and survival? *National Clinical Practice Oncology, 5*, 466–475.

Chida, Y., & Steptoe, A. (2008). Positive psychological wellbeing and mortality: A qualitative review of prospective observational studies. *Psychosomatic Medicine, 70*, 741–756.

Chida, Y., & Vedhara, K. (2009). Adverse psychosocial factors predict poorer prognosis in HIV disease: A meta-analytic review of prospective investigations. *Brain, Behavior, and Immunity, 23*, 434–445.

Child Trends Data Bank. (n.d.). *Teen births*. Retrieved February 2, 2009, from www.childtrends.org/news/news-releases/teen-birth-rates-continue-their-dramatic-decline/

Chipperfield, J. G., Hamm, J. M., Perry, R. P., Parker, P. C., Ruthing, J. C., & Lang, F. R. (2019). A healthy dose of realism: The role of optimistic and pessimistic expectations when facing a downward spiral in health. *Social Science & Medicine, 232*, 444–452.

Chisuwa, N., & O'Dea, J. A. (2010). Body image and eating disorders amongst Japanese adolescents: A review of the literature. *Appetite, 54*(1), 5–15.

Choi, H., Yorgason, J. B., & Johnson, D. R. (2016). Marital quality and health in middle and later adulthood: Dyadic associations. *The Journals of Gerontology: Series B, 71*(1), 154–164. doi: 10.1093/geronb/gbu222

Choi, H. K., Atkinson, K., Karlson, L. W., Willett, W., & Curhan, G. (2004a). Alcohol intake & risk of incident of gout in men: A prospective study. *Lancet, 363*, 1277–1281.

Choi, H. K., Atkinson, K., Karlson, L. W., Willett, W., & Curhan, G. (2004b). Purine-rich foods, dairy & protein intake & the risk of gout in men. *New England Journal of Medicine, 350*, 1093–1103.

Choi, Y.-J., Moskowitz, J. M., Myung, S.-K., Lee, Y.-R., & Hong, Y.-C. (2020). Cellular phone use and risk of tumors: Systematic review and meta-analysis. *International Journal of Environmental Research and Public Health, 17*(8079), 1–20. doi: 10.3390/ijerph17218079

Christaki, C., Orovou, O., Dagla, D., Sarantaki, S., Moriati, M., Kirkou, K., & Antoniou, A. (2023). Domestic violence during women's life in developing countries. *Materia Sociomedica, 35*(1), 58–64. doi: 10.5455%2Fmsm.2023.35.58-64

Christenfeld, N., Glynn, L. M., & Gerin, W. (2000). On the reliable assessment of cardiovascular recovery: An application of curve-fitting techniques. *Psychophysiology, 37*, 543–550.

Christensen, H. C., Schuz, J., Kosteljanetz, M., Poulsen, H. S., Thomsen, J., & Johansen, C. (2004). Cellular telephone use and risk of acoustic neuroma. *American Journal of Epidemiology, 159*, 277–283.

Christensen, P. (2003). "In these perilous times": Plagues and plague policies in early modern Denmark. *Medical History, 47*(4), 413–450.

Christopher and Dana Reeve Foundation. (2009). *The history of the Reeve foundation.* Retrieved November 27, 2009, from www.christopherreeve.org/site/c.ddJFKRNoFiG/b.4506337/apps/s/content.asp?ct=5856133

Chua, J. L., Touyz, S., & Hill, A. J. (2004). Negative mood-induced overeating in obese binge eaters: An experimental study. *International Journal of Obese Related Metabolism Disorders, 28*, 606–610.

Chung, V. C. H., Ma, P. H. X., Lau, C. H., Wong, S. Y. S., Yeoh, E. K., & Griffiths, S. M. (2014). Views on traditional Chinese medicine amongst Chinese population: A systematic review of qualitative and quantitative studies. *Health Expectation, 17*(5), 622–636. doi: 10.1111/j.1369-7625.2012.00794.x

Cintron, A., & Morrison, R. S. (2006). Pain & ethnicity in US: A systematic review. *Journal of Palliative Medicine, 9*(6), 1454–1473.

Clark, J. D., & Winterowd, C. (2012). Correlates and predictors of binge eating among Native American women. *Journal of Multicultural Counseling and Development, 40*(2), 117–127. doi: 10.1002/j.2161-1912.2012.00011.x

Clark, R. (2006). Perceived racism and vascular reactivity in black college women: Moderating effects of seeking social support. *Health Psychology, 25*(1), 20–25.

Claudpierre, P. (2005). Spa therapy for ankylosing spondylitis: Still useful? *Joint, Bone Spine, 72*, 283–285.

Claus, E. B., Schildkraut, J. M., Thompson, W. D., & Risch, N. J. (1996). The genetic attributable risk of breast and ovarian cancer. *Cancer, 77*, 2318–2324.

Clauss-Ehlers, C. C. C. (2003). Promoting ecological health resilience for minority youth: Enhancing health care access through the school health center. *Psychology in the Schools, 40*(3), 265–278.

Clay, R. (1977, December). *Prevention is theme of the '98 presidential year* (The American Psychological Association Monitor, p. 35). Washington, DC: The American Psychological Association.

Clearing House for Military Family Readiness. (2023). *What parents need to know about vaping and JUULing.* Retrieved December 20, 2023, from psu.edu

Cleeland, C. S., & Ryan, K. M. (1994). Pain assessment: Global use of the brief pain inventory. *Annals of Academic Medicine of Singapore, 23*, 129–138.

Clennett, B., & Yiu, K. (2022). China orders 51 million into lockdown as COVID surges. *ABC News.* Retrieved December 1, 2023, from go.com.

Cleveland Clinic. (2024a). *Atherosclerosis: Symptoms, causes & treatment*. Retrieved February 20, 2024, from clevelandclinic.org

Cleveland Clinic. (2024b). *Dopamine agonists: What it is, uses, side effects & risks*. Retrieved January 4, 2024, from clevelandclinic.org

Cleveland Clinic. (2024c). *Bone marrow: What it is & why it is important*. Retrieved March 1, 2024, from clevelandclinic.org

Cleveland Clinic. (2024d). *Sudden cardiac arrest: Causes & symptoms*. Retrieved February 20, 2024, from clevelandclinic.org

CNN. (2023). TB is still here – New CDC data show U.S. cases increased again in 2022. Retrieved November 11, 2023, from www.cnn.com/2023/03/23/health/tuberculosis-2022-cdc-report/index.html

Coburn, D. (2004). Beyond the income inequality hypothesis: Class, neo-liberalism, and health inequalities. *Social Science & Medicine, 58*, 41–56.

Cockerham, W. C. (2001). *Medical sociology*. Upper Saddle River, NJ: Prentice Hall.

Cohen, D. A., Farley, T. A., Bedimo-Etame, J. R., Scribner, R., Ward, W., Kendall, C., & Rice, J. (1999). Implementation of condom social marketing in Louisiana. *American Journal of Public Health, 89*, 204–208.

Cohen, J. B., & Reed, D. (1985). Type-A behavior & coronary heart disease among Japanese men in Hawaii. *Journal of Behavioral Medicine, 8*, 343–352.

Cohen, K. (2003). *Honoring the medicine: The essential guide to Native American healing*. New York: Random House.

Cohen, M. (2006). Jim Crow's drug war: Race, Coca Cola and the southern origins of the drug prohibition. *Southern Cultures, 12*(3), 55–79.

Cohen, S. (2004). Connecting social relationships and health. *Monitor on Psychology, 35*, 14–15.

Cohen, S. (2005). Keynote presentation at the Eighth International Congress of Behavioral Medicine: The Pittsburgh common cold studies: Psychosocial predictors of susceptibility to respiratory infectious illness. *International Journal of Behavioral Medicine, 12*(3), 123–131.

Cohen, S., Doyle, W. J., Skoner, D. P., Fireman, P., Gwaltney, J. M., & Newsom, J. T. (1995). State and trait negative affect as predictors of objective and subjective symptoms of respiratory viral infections. *Journal of Personality and Social Psychology, 68*, 159–169.

Cohen, S., Kaplan, G. A., & Salonen, J. T. (1999). The role of psychological characteristics in the relations between socioeconomic status and perceived health. *Journal of Applied Social Psychology, 29*, 445–468.

Cohen, S., & McKay, G. (1984). Social support, stress & the buffering hypothesis: A theoretical analysis. In A. Baum, J. E. Singer, & S. E. Taylor (Eds.), *Handbook of psychology and health* (Vol. 4, pp. 253–267). Hillsdale, NJ: Erlbaum.

Cohen, S., Murphy, M. L. M., & Prather, A. A. (2019). Ten surprising facts about stressful life events and disease risk. *Annual Review of Psychology, 70*, 577–597. doi: 10.1146/annurev-psych-010418-102857

Cohen, S., Tyrrell, D. A. J., & Smith, A. P. (1991). Psychological stress and susceptibility to the common cold. *New England Journal of Medicine, 325*, 606–612.

Cohen, S., Tyrrell, D. A. J., & Smith, A. P. (1993). Life events, perceived stress, negative affect and susceptibility to the common cold. *Journal of Personality and Social Psychology, 64*, 131–140.

Cohen, S., & Williamson, G. M. (1991). Stress & infectious diseases in humans. *Psychological Bulletin, 109*, 5–24.

Cohen, S., & Wills, T. A. (1985). Stress, social support & the buffering hypothesis. *Psychological Bulletin, 98*(2), 310–357.

Cold, J., Petruckevitch, A., Feder, G., Chung, W., Richardson, J., & Moorey, S. (2001). Relation between childhood sexual and physical abuse and risk of revictimization in women: A cross-sectional survey. *Lancet, 258,* 450–454.

Coll, C. V. N., Ewerling, F., Garcia-Moreno, C., Hellwig, F., & Barros, A. J. D. (2020). Intimate partner violence in 46 low-income and middle-income countries: An appraisal of the most vulnerable groups of women using national health surveys. *BMJ Global Health, 5,* e002208. doi: 10.1136/bmjgh-2019-002208

Collins, T. C., Clark, J. A., Petersen, L. A., & Kressin, N. R. (2002). Racial differences in how physicians communication regarding cardiac testing. *Medical Care, 40*(suppl. 1), 127–134.

Committee on Ethical Standards of Psychologists. (1958). Standards of ethical behavior for psychologists. Report of the committee on ethical standards of psychologists. *American Psychologists, 13,* 266–271.

Committee on Injury, Violence, and Poison Prevention and Committee on Adolescence. (2006). The teen driver. *Pediatrics, 118,* 2570–2581.

Commonwealth Fund. (2024). *Revealing disparities: Health care workers' observations of discrimination against patients.* Retrieved February 26, 2024, from

Compas, B. E., Connor-Smith, J. K., Saltzman, H., Thomsen, A. H., & Wadsworth, M. E. (2001). Coping with stress during childhood & adolescence: Problems, progress & potential in theory & research. *Psychological Bulletin, 127,* 87–127.

Compston, A. (2000). The genetics of multiple sclerosis. *Journal of Neurovirology* (suppl. 2), S5–S9.

Compton, W. M., Jones, C. M., & Baldwin, G. T. (2016). Relationship between nonmedical prescription opioid use and heroin use. *The New England Journal of Medicine, 374,* 154–163.

Conde Nast Traveller. (2022). *These are the countries where marijuana is legal.* Retrieved May 22, 2023, from cntraveller.in

Connolly, M. A., Gayer, M., Ryan, M. J., Salama, P., Spiegel, P., & Heymann, D. L. (2004). Communicable diseases in complex emergencies: Impact and challenges. *Lancet, 364,* 1974–1983.

Conway, D. (2020). *Health insurance coverage among young adults aged 19 to 34: 2018 and 2019.* Retrieved February 20, 2024, from census.gov

Conway, J. (2023). Top countries in terms of annual cannabis use in 2020. *Statista.* Retrieved January 4, 2024.

Cooke, B., & Ernst, E. (2000). Aromatherapy: A systematic review. *British Journal of General Practice, 50,* 493–496.

Cooke, M., Holzhauser, K., Jones, M., Davis, C., & Finucan, J. (2007). The effect of aromatherapy massage with music on stress & anxiety levels of emergency nurses: Comparison between summer and winter. *Journal of Clinical Nursing, 16*(9), 1695–1703.

Cooper, D. C., Mills, P. J., Bardwell, N. A., Ziegler, M. G., & Dimsdale, J. E. (2009). The effect of ethnic discrimination and socioeconomic status on etidothelin-1 among blacks and whites. *American Journal of Hypertension, 22*(7), 698–704.

Cooper, M. D. (2003). Behavior based safety still a viable strategy. *Safety and Health, 167,* 46–48.

Cooper-Patrick, L., Gallo, J. J., Gonzales, J. J., Vu, H. T., Powe, N. R., Nelson, C., & Ford, D. E. (1999). Race, gender and partnership in the patient–physician relationship. *Journal of the American Medical Association, 282*(6), 583–589.

Coovadia, H. M., Rollins, N. C., Bland, R. M., Little, K., Coutsoudis, A., Bennish, M. L., & Newell, M. L. (2007). Mother-to-child-transmission of HIV-1 infection during exclusive breastfeeding in the first 6 months of life: An intervention cohort study. *Lancet, 369,* 1107–1116.

Corcoran, J. L., Li, P., Davies, S. L., Knight, C. C., Lanzi, R. G., & Landores, S. L. (2021). Adolescent chlamydia rates by region, race, and sex: Trends from 2013 to 2017. *Journal of Pediatric Health Care*, *35*, 172–179. doi: 10.1016/j.pedhc.2020.09.004

Corso, P. S., Mercy, J. A., Simon, T. R., Finkelstein, E. A., & Miller, T. R. (2007). Medical costs and productivity losses due to interpersonal and self-directed violence in the United States. *American Journal of Preventive Medicine*, *32*(6), 474–482.

Corter, C. M., & Flemming, A. S. (1995). Psychobiology of maternal behavior in human beings. In M. H. Bornstein (Ed.), *Handbook of parenting Vol. 2: Biology & ecology of parenting* (pp. 87–116). Mahwah, NJ: Erlbaum.

Cosdon, N. (2022). Today's Google Doodle honors Dr. Michiaki Takahashi, Inventor of the chickenpox vaccine. *HCP Live Network: Contagion Live, Infectious Diseases Today*. Retrieved April 1, 2023, from contagionlive.com.

Coursen, C. C. (2009). Inequalities affecting access to healthcare: A philosophical reflection. *International Journal for Human Caring*, *13*(1), 7–15.

Crandall, C. S., Priesler, J. J., & Aussprung, J. (1992). Measuring life event stress in the lives of college students: The undergraduate stress questionnaire. *Journal of Behavioral Medicine*, *15*, 627–662.

Creamer, P., Lethbridge-Cejku, M., & Hochberg, M. C. (1999). Determinants of pain severity & knee osteoarthritis: Effects of demographic & psychosocial variables using 3 pain measures. *The Journal of Rheumatology*, *26*, 1785–1792.

Cressey, T. R., & Lallemant, M. (2007). Pharmacogenetics of antiretroviral drugs for the treatment of HIV-infected patients: An update. *Infection, Genetics and Evolution*, *7*, 333–342.

Crombez, G., Eccleston, C., Van Hamme, G., & De Vlieger, P. (2008). Attempting to solve the problem of pain: A questionnaire study in acute and chronic pain patients. *Pain*, *137*(3), 556–563.

Crosby, A. W. (1989). *America's forgotten pandemic: The influenza of 1918*. Cambridge: Cambridge University Press.

Crowley, R., Daniel, H., Cooney, T. G., & Engel, L. S. (2020). Envisioning a better U.S. health care system for all: Coverage and cost of care. *Annals of Internal Medicine*, *172*(2 Suppl.), S7–S32. doi: 10.7326/M19-2415

Croy, I., Springborn, M., Lotsch, J., Johnston, A. N. B., & Hummel, T. (2011). Agreeable smellers & sensory neurotics – Correlates among personality traits & sensory thresholds. *PLoS One*, *6*(4), e18701.

Cruces, J., Venero, C., Pereda-Perez, I., & Fuentes, M. D. (2014). A higher anxiety state in old rats after social isolation is associated to an impairment of the immune response. *Journal of Neuroimmunology*, *277*(1–2), 18–25.

Cruz, M. L., Christie, S., Allen, E., Meza, E., Nápoles, A. M., & Mehta, K. M. (2022). Traditional healers as health care providers for the Latine community in the United States, a systematic review. *Health Equity*, *6*(1), 412–426. doi: 10.1089/heq.2021.0099

Cruz-Coke, R. M. (2007). Peregrinaciones a las Fuentes de la medicina clasica. *Revista Medica De Chile*, *135*(8), 1076–1081.

CT.GOV. (2024). *How indemnity plans work*. Retrieved February 28, 2024, from ct.gov

Cummings, J. R., Ackerman, J. M., Wolfson, J. A., & Gearhardt, A. N. (2021). COVID-19 stress and eating and drinking behaviors in the United States during the early stages of pandemic. *Appetite*, *162*(1). doi: 10.1016/j.appet.2021.105163

Cummings, K. M., Hyland, A., Giovino, G. A., Hastrup, J. L., Bauer, J. E., & Bansal, M. A. (2004). Are smokers adequately informed about the health risks of smoking and medicinal nicotine? *Nicotine Tobacco Research*, *6*(suppl. 3), S333–S340.

Cuthbertson, C. A., Newkirk, C., Ilardo, J., Loveridge, S., & Skidmore, M. (2016). Angry, scared, and unsure: Mental health consequences of contaminated water in Flint, Michigan. *Journal of Urban Health*, *93*(6), 899–908.

Cutts, F. T., Franceschi, S., Golden, S., Castellasque, X., de San Jose, G., & Garnet, G. (2007). Human papillomavirus and HPV vaccines: A review. *Bulletin of the World Health Organization*, *85*(9), 719–726.

DA. (2007). *Drugs, brains, and behavior: The science of addiction* (NIDA report).

D'Acquisto, F. (2016). Editorial overview: Immunomodulation: Exploiting the circle between emotions and immunity: Impact on pharmacological treatments. *Current Opinion in Pharmacology*, *29*, viii–xii. doi: 10.1016/j.coph.2016.07.008

D'Acquisto, F. (2017). Affective immunology: Where emotions and the immune response converge. *Dialogues in Clinical Neuroscience*, *19*(1), 9–19. doi: 10.31887/DCNS.2017.19.1/fdacquisto

D'Agostino, T. A., Atkinson, T. M., Latella, L. E., Rogers, M., Morrissey, D., DeRosa, A. P., & Parker, P. A. (2017). Promoting patient participation in healthcare interactions through communication skills training: A systematic review. *Patient Education and Counseling*, *100*(7), 1247–1257. doi: 10.1016/j.pec.2017.02.016

D'Alberto, A. (2006, September). The withering of yin: A mid-life crisis? *Positive Health*, 18.

Dabelea, D. (2007). The predisposition to obesity and diabetes in offspring of diabetic mothers. *Diabetes Care*, *30*(suppl. 2), 169–174.

Dageid, W., & Duckert, F. (2008). Balancing between normality and social death: Black, rural, South African women coping with HIV/AIDS. *Quantitative Health Research*, *18*(2), 182–195.

Dahl, A. A. (2010). Link between personality and cancer. *Future Oncology*, *6*(5), 691–707.

Dai, K., Gakidou, E., & Lopez, A. D. (2022). Evolution of the global smoking epidemic over the past half century: Strengthening the evidence base for policy action. *Tobacco Control*, *31*(2), 129–137. doi: 10.1136/tobaccocontrol-2021-056535

Dai, W.-S., Huang, S.-T., Xu, N., Chen, Q., & Cao, H. (2020). The effect of music therapy on pain, anxiety and depression in patients after coronary artery bypass grafting. *Journal of Cardiothoracic Surgery*, *15*, 81. doi: 10.1186/s13019-020-01141-y

Dales, L., Hammer, S. J., & Smith, N. J. (2001). Time trends in autism and in MMR immunization coverage in California. *Journal of the American Medical Association*, *285*, 1183–1185.

Daniel, T. M. (2006). The history of tuberculosis. *Respiratory Medicine*, *100*(11), 1862–1870.

Dariotis, J. K., Sonenstein, F. L., Gates, G. J., Astone, N. M., Pleck, J. H., Sifakis, F., & Zeger, S. (2008). Changes in sexual risk behaviors as young men transition into adulthood. *Perspectives on Sexual and Reproductive Health*, *40*(4), 218–225.

Darton, A. J., McElvenny, D. M., & Hodgson, J. T. (2006). Estimating the number of asbestos related lung cancer deaths in GB from 1980–2000. *Annals of Occupational Hygiene*, *50*(1), 29–38.

Das, S. (2019). The relationship between healthcare and economy. *HATI International*. Retrieved December 10, 2023, from hatiintl.com.

Dashti-Khavidaki, S., Saidi, R., & Lu, H. (2021). Current status of glucocorticoid usage in solid organ transplantation. *World Journal of Transplantation*, *11*(11), 443–465. doi: 10.5500/wjt.v11.i11.443

Dassow, P. (2005). Setting educational priorities for women's preventive health: Measuring beliefs about screening across disease states. *Journal of Women's Health*, *14*(4), 324–330.

Daughtery, J. D., & Houry, D. E. (2008). Intimate partner violence screening in the emergency department. *Journal of Postgraduate Medicine*, *54*(4), 301–305.

Davis, A., & Robson, J. (2016). The dangers of NSAIDs: Look both ways. *British Journal of General Practice*, *66*(645), 172–173. doi: 10.3399/bjgp16X684433

Davis, A. L. (1996). History of the sanatorium movement. In W. N. Rom & S. M. Garay (Eds.), *Tuberculosis*. Boston, MA: Little Brown.

Davis, J. M., & Liang, C. T. H. (2015). A test of the mediating role of gender role conflict: Latino masculinities and help-seeking attitudes. *Psychology of Men & Masculinity, 16*(1), 23–32. https://psycnet.apa.org/doi/10.1037/a0035320

Davis, K., Dickman, E. D., Ferris, D., & Dias, J. K. (2004). Human papillomavirus among parents of 10–15 year old adolescents. *Journal of Lower Genital Track Disease, 8*(3), 188–194.

Dawber, T. R., & Kannel, W. B. (1966). The Framingham study: An epidemiological approach to coronary heart disease. *Circulation, 34*(4), 553–555.

de Barros, B. V., da Costa Proenca, R. P., Kliemann, N., Hilleshein, D., de Souza, A. A., Cembranel, F., . . . Fernanades, A. C. (2022). Trans-fat labeling in packaged foods sold in Brazil before and after changes in regulatory criteria for trans-fat-free claims on food labels. *Frontiers in Nutrition, 9*. doi: 10.3389/fnut.2022.868341

De Figueiredo, A., Simas, C., Karafillakis, E., Paterson, P., & Larson, H. J. (2020). Mapping global trends in vaccine confidence and investigating barriers to vaccine uptake: A large-scale retrospective temporal modelling study. *The Lancet, 396*(10255), 898–908.

DeFilippis, E. M., & Van Spall, H. G. C. (2021). Is it time for sex-specific guidelines for cardiovascular disease. *Journal of the American College of Cardiology, 78*(2), 189–192. doi: 10.1016/j.jacc.2021.05.012

de Freitas, P. P., de Menezes, M. C., dos Santos, L. C., Pimenta, A. M., Ferreira, A. V. M., & Lopes, A. C. S. (2020). The transtheoretical model is an effective weight management intervention: A randomized controlled trial. *BMC Public Health, 20*, 652. doi: 10.1186/s12889-020-08796-1

Degenhardt, L., Dierker, L., Chiud, W. T., Medina-Mora, M. E., Neumark, Y., Sampsond, N., & Alonso, J. (2010). Evaluating the drug use "gateway" theory using cross-national data: Consistency and associations of the order of initiation of drug use among participants in The WHO World Mental Health Surveys. *Drug and Alcohol Dependence, 108*, 84–97.

DeGreve, J., Sermijn, E., De Brakeleer, S., Ren, Z., & Tengels, E. (2008). Heredity breast cancer: From bench to bedside. *Current Opinions in Oncology, 20*(6), 605–613.

Dehelean, L., Papava, I., Musat, M. I., Bondrescu, M., Bratosu, F., & Buscatos, B. O. (2021). Coping strategies and stress related disorders in patients with COVID-19. *Brain Sciences, 11*(10). doi: 10.3390/brainsci11101287

Dehlin, M., Jacobsson, L., & Roddy, E. (2020). Global epidemiology of gout: Prevalence, incidence, treatment patterns and risk factors. *Nature Reviews Rheumatology, 16*(7), 380–390. doi: 10.1038/s41584-020-0441-1

de Jager Meezenbroek, E., Garssen, B., van den Berg, M., van Dierendonck, D., Visser, A., & Schaufeli, W. B. (2012). Measuring spirituality as a universal human experience: A review of spirituality questionnaires. *Journal of Religion and Health, 51*, 336–354. doi: 10.1007/s10943-010-9376-1

deKloet, C. S., Vermetten, E., Bekker, A., Meulam, A., Geuze, E., & Kavelaars, A. (2007). Leukocyte glucocorticoid receptor expression and immunoregulation in veterans with and without post-traumatic stress disorder. *Molecular Psychiatry, 125*, 443–453.

DeLaet, D. E., Shea, S., & Carrisquillo, O. (2002). Receipt of preventive services among privately insured minorities in managed care versus fee-for-service insurance plans. *Journal of General Internal Medicine, 17*(6), 451–457.

DelBocca, F. K., Darkes, J., Goldman, M. S., & Smith, G. T. (2002). Advancing the expectancy concept via the interplay between research and theory. *Alcoholism: Clinical and Experimental Research, 26*, 926–935.

Del Castillo, F. A. (2021). Health, spirituality and Covid-19: Themes and insights. *Journal of Public Health*, 43(2), e254–e255. doi: 10.1093/pubmed/fdaa185

Del Castillo, R., Fernandez, I. T., & Luna, L. L. (2020). Traditional healing practices in curanderismo. In L. Grayshield & R. Del Castillo (Eds.), *Indigenous ways of knowing in counseling*. International and Cultural Psychology. Cham: Springer. doi: 10.1007/978-3-030-33178-8_6

Delgado, D. J., Lin, W. Y., & Coffey, M. (1995). The role of Hispanic race/ethnicity and poverty in breast cancer survival. *Puerto Rican Health Science Journal*, 14, 103–116.

Delgado, M. K., Wanner, K. J., & McDonald, C. (2016). Adolescent cellphone use while driving: An overview of the literature and promising future directions for prevention. *Media and Communication*, 4(3), 79–89. doi: 10.17645%2Fmac.v4i3.536

Delucchi, K. L., Matzger, H., & Weisner, C. (2008). Alcohol in emerging adulthood: 7-Year study of problem and dependent drinkers. *Addictive Behaviors*, 33(1), 134–142.

Dembroski, J. M., MacDougall, J. M., Williams, R. B., Haney, T. L., & Blumenthal, J. A. (1985). Components of type-A, hostility & anger in relationship to angiographic findings. *Psychosomatic Medicine*, 47, 219–233.

Denning, P., & DiNenno, E. (2011). *Communities in crisis: Is there a generalized HIV epidemic in impoverished urban areas in the United States?* Atlanta, GA: Centers for Disease Control and Prevention. Retrieved February 1, 2013, from www.cdc.gov/hiv/pdf/statistics_poverty_poster.pdf

Denollet, J., Pedersen, S. S., Vrints, C. J., & Conraads, V. M. (2006). Usefulness of Type D personality in predicting five-year cardiac events above and beyond concurrent symptoms of stress in patients with coronary heart disease. *American Journal of Cardiology*, 97, 970–973.

De Oliveira, B. I. R., Smith, A. J., O'Sullivan, P. P. B., Haebich, S., Fick, D., Khan, R., & Bunzli, S. (2020). 'My hip is damaged': A qualitative investigation of people seeking care for persistent hip pain. *British Journal of Sports Medicine*, 54, 858–865.

de Ridder, D., Kroese, F., Evers, C., Adriaanse, M., & Gillebaart, M. (2017). Healthy diet: Health impact, prevalence, correlates, and interventions. *Psychology & Health*, 32(8), 907–941. doi: 10.1080/08870446.2017.1316849

Derlega, V. J., Winstead, B. A., Oldfield, E. C., & Barbee, A. P. (2003). Close relationships and social support in coping with HIV: A test of sensitive interaction systems. *AIDS Behavior*, 7, 119–129.

Derry, H. M., Fagundes, C. P., Andridge, R., Glaser, R., Malarkey, W. B., & Kiecolt-Glaser, J. K. (2013). Lower subjective social status exaggerates interleukin-6 responses to a laboratory stressor. *Psychoneuroendocrinology*, 38(11), 2676–2685. doi: 10.1016/j.psyneuen.2013.06.026

de Sanjosé, S., Leone, M., Berez, V., Izquierdo, A., Font, R., Brunet, J. M., . . . Sinilnikova, O. M. (2003). Prevalence of BRCA1 and BRCA2 germline mutations in young breast cancer patients: A population-based study. *International Journal of Cancer*, 106, 588–593.

De Smet, P. A. G. M. (1998). Traditional pharmacology and medicine in Africa: Ethnopharmacological themes in sub-Saharan art objects and utensils. *Journal of Ethnopharmacology*, 63, 1–175.

de Souza, R. J., Mente, A., Maroleanu, A., Cozma, A. I., Ha, V., Kishibe, T., . . . Anand, S. S. (2015). Intake of saturated and trans unsaturated fatty acids and risk of all cause mortality, cardiovascular disease, and type 2 diabetes: Systematic review and meta-analysis of observational studies. *BMJ*, 351, h3978. doi: 10.1136/bmj.h3978

DeStefano, F., & Chen, R. T. (2008). Autism and measles-mumps-rubella vaccination: Controversy laid to rest? *CNS Drugs*, 15(11), 831–837.

DeVoe, J. E. (2009). Educaid: What if the US systems of education and healthcare were more alike? *Family Medicine*, 41(9), 652–655.

Dewi, T. K., & Zein, R. A. (2017). Predicting intention perform breast self-examination: Application of the theory of reasoned action. *Asian Pacific Journal of Cancer Prevention, 8*(11), 2945–2952. doi: 10.22034/APJCP.2017.18.11.2945

Deyle, G. D., Henderson, N. E., Matekel, R. L., Ryder, M. G., Garber, M. B., & Allison, S. C. (2000). Effectiveness of manual physical therapy & exercise in osteoarthritis of the knee: A randomized control trial. *Annals of Internal Medicine, 132*, 173–181.

Dhabhar, F. S. (2014). Effects of stress on immune function: The good, the bad, and the beautiful. *Immunologic Research, 58*, 193–210. doi: 10.1007/s12026-014-8517-0

Dhabhar, F. S. (2018). The short-term stress response – Mother nature's mechanism for enhancing protection and performance under conditions of threat, challenge, and opportunity. *Frontiers in Neuroendocrinology, 49*, 175–192. doi: 10.1016/j.yfrne.2018.03.004

Dhabhar, F. S., & McEwen, B. C. (2001). Bidirectional effects of stress & glucocorticoid hormones on immune function: Possible explanations for paradoxical observations. In R. Ader, D. I. Felten, & N. Cohen (Eds.), *Psychoneuroimmunology* (3rd ed., pp. 301–338). San Diego: Academic Press.

Dhabhar, F. S., Saul, A. N., Daughtery, C., Holmes, T. H., Bouley, D. M., & Oberyszyn, T. M. (2010). Short-term stress enhances cellular immunity and increases early resistance to squamous cell carcinoma. *Brain, Behavior, and Immunity, 2*(1), 127–137. doi: 10.1016/j.bbi.2009.09.004

Dharod, J. M., Drewette-Card, R., & Crawford, D. (2011). Development of the Oxford Hills healthy moms project using a social marketing process: A community-based physical activity & nutrition intervention for low socioeconomic-status mothers in a rural area in Maine. *Health Promotion Practice, 12*, 312–321.

Diaz, D. P. (1993). Foundations for spirituality: Establishing the variables of spirituality within the disciplines. *Journal of Health Education, 24*(6), 24–326.

DiClemente, R. J., Lodico, M., Grinstead, O. A., Harper, G., Rickman, R. L., Evans, P. E., & Coates, T. J. (1996). African American adolescents residing in high-risk urban environments do use condoms: Correlates and predictors of condom use among adolescents in public housing developments. *Pediatrics, 98*, 269–278.

Diener, E. (2000). Subjective well-being: The science of happiness and a proposal for a national index. *American Psychologist, 55*, 34–43.

Diener, E., & Chan, M. (2011). Happy people live longer: Subjective well-being contributes to health and longevity. *Applied Psychology: Health and Well-Being, 3*, 1–43.

Diener, E., & Suh, E. M. (2000). *Culture & subjective wellbeing.* Cambridge, MA: MIT Press.

Diener, E., Pressman, S., Hunter, J., & Delgadillo-Chase, D. (2017). If, why, and when subjective well-being influences health, and future needed research. *Applied Psychology: Health and Well-Being, 9*, 133–167.

Dienlin, T., Masur, P. K., & Trepte, S. (2017). Reinforcement or displacement? The reciprocity of FtF, IM, and SNS communication and their effects on loneliness and life satisfaction. *Journal of Computer-Mediated Communication, 22*(2), 71–87. doi: 10.1111/jcc4.12183

Diesfled, K. (2008). Interpersonal issues between pin physicians and patient: Strategies to reduce conflict. *Pain Medicine, 9*(8), 1118–1124.

DiFranza, J. R., Richards, J. W., Paulman, P. M., Wolf-Gillespie, N., Fletcher, C., Jaffe, R. D., & Murray, D. (1991). RJR Nabisco's cartoon panel promotes camel cigarettes. *JAMA, 266*(22), 3149–3153.

Dinh, N. M. H., & Groleau, D. (2008). Traumatic amputation: A case of Laotian indignation and injustice. *Culture, Medicine & Psychiatry, 32*, 440–457.

DISA. (2023). *Marijuana legality by states.* Retrieved May 23, 2023.

DiSpezio, M. (1997). *The science of HIV.* A National Science Teachers' Association Publication. USA: Automated Graphic Systems.

Distefan, J. M., Pierce, J. P., & Gilpin, E. A. (2004). Do favorite movie stars influence adolescent smoking initiation? *American Journal of Public Health*, *94*(7), 1239–1244.

Dixon, B. N., Ugwoaba, U. A., Brockmann, A. N., & Ross, K. M. (2020). Associations between the built environment and dietary intake, physical activity, and obesity: A scoping review of reviews. *Obesity Reviews*, *22*(4), e13171. doi: 10.1111/obr.13171

Dixon, K. E., Keefe, F. J., Scipio, C. D., Perri, L. M., & Abernethy, A. P. (2007). Psychological interventions for arthritis pain management in adults: A meta-analysis. *Health Psychology*, *26*(3), 241–250.

Doctors Without Borders. (2006). *Malnutrition*. Retrieved January 7, 2008, from www. doctorswithoutborders.org/news/malnutrition/background.cfm

Dodds, C. (2006). HIV-related stigma in England: Experiences of gay men & heterosexual African immigrants living with HIV. *Journal of Community & Applied Social Psychology*, *16*(6), 472–480.

Dodgen, C. E. (2005). *Nicotine dependence: Understanding and applying the most effective treatment interventions*. Washington, DC: American Psychological Association.

Doherty, M. (2009). New insights into the epidemiology of gout. *Rheumatology*, *48*(suppl. 2), ii1–ii8.

Dominguez, A., EchoHawk, A., & Liu, K. (2019). Indigenous epidemiology: Identifying health disparities and health priorities. *Journal of Public Health Information*, *11*(1), e350. doi: 10.5210%2Fojphi. v11i1.9797

Donatuto, J., Campbell, L., & Gregory, R. (2016). Developing responsive indicators of indigenous community health. *International Journal of Environmental Research and Public Health*, *13*(9), 899. doi: 10.3390/ijerph13090899

Dong, T., Guo, M., Zhang, P., Sun, G., & Chen, B. (2020). The effects of low-carbohydrate diets on cardiovascular risk factors: A meta-analysis. *PLoS One*, *15*(1), e0225348. doi: 10.1371/journal. pone.0225348

Donoghue, H. D., Lee, O. Y.-C., Minnikin, D. E., Besra, G. S., Taylor, J. H., & Spigelman, M. (2009). Tuberculosis in Dr Granville's mummy: A molecular re-examination of the earliest known Egyptian mummy to be scientifically examined and given a medical diagnosis. *Proceedings of the Royal Society B: Biological Sciences*, *277*, 51–56. doi: 10.1098/rspb.2009.1484

Dorn, T., Yzermans, C. J., Guiju, H., & Zee, J. (2007). Disaster-related stress as a prospective risk factor for hypertension in parents of adolescent fire victims. *American Journal of Epidemiology*, *165*, 410–417.

Doucleff, M. (2023). Diabetes drug Ozempic and weight-loss drug Wegovy seem to curb other cravings. *National Public Radio*. Retrieved December 20, 2023.

Downing, R. G., Otten, R. A., Marem, E., Biryahwaho, B., Alwano-Edyegu, M. G., & Sempala, S. D. (1998). Optimizing the delivery of HIV counseling and testing services: The Ugandan experience using rapid HIV antibody test algorithms. *Journal of Acquired Immune Deficiency Syndromes and Human Retrovirology*, *18*(4), 384–388.

Driever, E. M., Stiggelbout, A. M., & Brand, P. L. P. (2020). Shared decision making: Physicians' preferred role, usual role and their perception of its key components. *Patient Education and Counseling*, *103*(1), 77–82. doi: 10.1016/j.pec.2019.08.004

Driever, E. M., Tolhuizen, I. M., Duvivier, R. J., Stigglebout, A. M., & Brand, P. L. P. (2022). Why do medical residents prefer paternalistic decision making? An interview study. *BMC Medical Education*, *22*, 155. doi: 10.1186/s12909-022-03203-2

Duberstein, P., Meldren, S, Fiscella, K., Shields, C. G., & Epstein, R. M. (2007). Influences on a patient's ratings of physicians: Physician demographics & personalities. *Patient Education & Counseling*, *65*, 270–274.

Dunbar, H. F. (1943). *Psychosomatic diagnosis.* New York: Hoeber Press.

Duncan, C. J., & Scott, S. (2005). What caused the Black Death? *Postgraduate Medical Journal, 81,* 315–320.

Duncan, M. S., Freiberg, M. S., Greevy, R. A., Kundu, S., Vasan, R. S., & Tindle, H. A. (2019). Association of smoking cessation with subsequent risk of cardiovascular disease. *JAMA, 322*(7), 642–650. doi: 10.1001/jama.2019.10298

Dunlop, S. M., & Romer, D. (2010). Relation between newspaper coverage of 'light' cigarette litigation and beliefs about 'lights' among American adolescents and young adults: The impact on risk perceptions and quitting intentions. *Tobacco Control, 19,* 267–273. doi: 10.1136/tc.2009.032029

Dusek, J. A., & Benson, H. (2009). Mind–body medium: A model of the comparative clinical impact of the acute stress & relaxation response. *Minnesota Medicine, 92*(5), 47–50.

Dushoff, J., Plotkin, J. B., Viboud, C., Earn, D. J. D., & Simonsen, L. (2006). Mortality due to influenza in the US: An annualized regression approach using multiple cause mortality data. *American Journal of Epidemiology, 163*(2), 181–187.

Duterte, E. E., Bonomi, A. E., Kernic, M. A., Schiff, M. A., Thompson, R. S., & Rivara, F. P. (2008). Correlates of medical and legal help-seeking among women reporting intimate partner violence. *Journal of Women's Health, 17*(1), 85–95.

Dworkin, R. H., O'Connor, A. B., Audette, J., Baron, R., Gourlay, G. K., Haanpää, M. L., . . . Wells, C. D. (2010). Recommendations for the pharmacological management of neuropathic pain: An overview & literature update. *Mayo Clinic Proceedings, 85*(suppl. 3), S3–S14.

Dyer, M. L., Easey, K. E., Heron, J., Hickman, H., & Munafo, M. R. (2019). Associations of child and adolescent anxiety with later alcohol use and disorders: A systematic review and meta-analysis of prospective cohort studies. *Addiction, 114*(6), 968–982. doi: 10.1111/add.14575

East, K., McNeill, A., Thrasher, J. F., & Hitchman, S. C. (2021). Social norms as a predictor of smoking uptake among youth: A systematic review, meta-analysis and meta-regression of prospective cohort studies. *Addiction, 116*(11), 2953–2967. doi: 10.1111/add.15427

Easton, D., Iverson, E., Cribbin, M., Wilson, E., Weiss, G., & The Community Intervention Trial for Youth Group. (2007). Space: The new frontier in HIV prevention for young men who have sex with men. *AIDS Education & Prevention, 19*(6), 465–478.

Ebrahim, A. H., & Atrash, H. (2006). Managing persistent preventable threats to safer pregnancies and infant health in the United States: Beyond silos and into integration, early, intervention, and prevention. *Journal of Women's Health, 15*(9), 1090–1092.

Eby, C. H., & Evjen, H. D. (1962). The plague at Athens: A new oar in muddied waters. *Journal of the History of Medicine,* 258–263.

Eckerling, A., Ricon-Becker, I., Sorski, L., Sandbank, E., & Ben-Eliyahu, S. (2021). Stress and cancer: Mechanisms, significance and future directions. *Nature Reviews Cancer, 21,* 767–785. doi: 10.1038/s41568-021-00395-5

Edberg, M. C., Cleary, S. D., Andrade, E. L., Evans, W. D., Quinteros-Grady, L., Alvayero, R. D., & Gonzalez, A. (2022). The Adelante project: Realities, challenges and successes in addressing health disparities among Central American immigrant youth. *Cultural Diversity and Ethnic Minority Psychology, 28*(3), 402–412. doi: 10.1037/cdp0000368

Education Week. (2023, January 6). *School shootings this year: How many and where.* Retrieved June 19, 2023, from edweek.org

Edwards, C. L., Fillingim, R. B., & Keefe, F. (2001). Race, ethnicity & pain. *Pain, 94,* 133–137.

Edwards, R. R., Moric, M., Husfeldt, B., Buvanendran, A., & Ivankovich, O. (2005). Ethnic similarities & differences in the chronic pain experience: A comparison of African American, Hispanic & White patients. *Pain Medicine, 6,* 88–98.

Eggleston, P. A. (1999). The environment and asthma in US inner cities. *Environmental Health Perspectives, 107*(3), 439–450.

Eisenberg, M. S. (1995). The problem of sudden cardiac death. In M. S. Eisenberg, L. Bergner, & A. P. Hallstrom (Eds.), *Sudden cardiac death in the community* (pp. 1–16). New York: Praeger.

Eisler, R., & Levine, D. S. (2002). Nurture, nature, and caring: We are not prisoners of our genes. *Brain and Mind, 3,* 9–52. doi: 10.1023/A:1016553723748

Eisner, M. D., Klein, J., Hammond, S. K., Koren, G., Lactao, G., & Iribarren, C. (2005). Directly measured second hand smoke exposure and asthma health outcomes. *Thorax, 60,* 814–821.

El Boghdady, M., & Ewalds-Kvist, B. M. (2020). The influence of music on the surgical task performance: A systematic review. *International Journal of Surgery, 70,* 101–112. doi: 10.1016/j.ijsu.2019.11.012

Eley, J. W., Hill, H. A., Chen, V. W., Austin, D. F., Wesley, M. N., Muss, H. B., . . . Edwards, B. K. (1994). Racial differences in survival from breast cancer: Results of the National Cancer Institute Black/White Cancer Survival Study. *JAMA, 272*(12), 947–954.

Eligon, J., & Moyo, J. (2024, February 13). Deadliest cholera outbreak in past decade hits southern Africa. *The New York Times.* Retrieved February 13, 2024, from nytimes.com.

Elkington, K. S., Bauermeister, J. A., & Zimmerman, M. A. (2011). Do parents and peers matter? A prospective socio-ecological examination of substance use and sexual risk among African American youth. *Journal of Adolescence, 34*(5), 1035–1047. doi: 10.1016/j.adolescence.2010.11.004

Elliot, G. R., & Eisdorfer, C. (1982). *Stress and human health: An analysis and implications of research.* A Study by the Institute of Medicine, National Academy of Sciences. New York: Springer Publishing.

El-Sadig, M., Alam, M. S., Carter, A. O., Fares, K., Al-Taneuiji, H. O. S., Romilly, P., . . . Lloyd, O. (2004). Evaluation of effectiveness of safety seatbelt legislation in the United Arab Emirates. *Accident Annals Prevention, 36*(3), 399–404.

Elsaid, N., Saied, A., Kandil, H., Soliman, A., Taher, F., Hadi, M., . . . El-Baz, A. (2021). Impact of stress and hypertension on the cerebrovasculature. *Frontiers in Bioscience, 26*(12), 1643–1652. doi: 10.52586/5057

El Sayed, S. M., Abdelrahman, A. A., Ozbak, H. A., Hemeg, H. A., Kheyami, A. M., Rezk, N., . . . Fathy, Y. M. (2016). Updates in diagnosis and management of Ebola hemorrhagic fever. *Journal of Research in Medical Science, 21,* 84. doi: 10.4103/1735-1995.192500

Emadi, M., Delavari, S., & Bayati, M. (2021). Global socioeconomic inequality in the burden of communicable and non-communicable diseases and injuries: An analysis on global burden of disease study 2019. *BMC Public Health, 21,* 1771. doi: 10.1186/s12889-021-11793-7

Engel, G. L. (1977). The need for a new medical model: A challenge for biomedicine. *Science, 196,* 129–136.

Engel, G. L. (2002). The need for a new medical model: A challenge for biomedicine. In D. L. Marks (Ed.), *The health psychology reader.* London: Sage Publications.

Enos, W. F., Holmes, R. H., & Beyer, J. (1953). Coronary disease among United States soldiers killed in action in Korea; preliminary report. *JAMA, 152*(12), 1090–1093.

Environmental Health Information Services. (2000). *Ninth report on carcinogens.* Washington, DC: U.S. Department of Health and Human Services, Public Health Service, National Toxicology Program.

Environmental Protection Agency. (2007a). *Clean Air Act 42 U.S.C. s/s 7401 et seq. (1970).* Retrieved July 15, 2007, from www.epa.gov/region5/defs/html/caa/htm

Environmental Protection Agency. (2007b). *Climate change basic information.* Retrieved July 15, 2007, from www.epa.gov/climatechange/basicinfo.html

Epel, E., Lapidus, R., McEwen, B., & Brownell, K. (2001). Stress may add bite to appetite in women: A laboratory study of stress-induced cortisol & eating behaviors. *Psychoneuroendocrinology, 26*(1), 37–49.

Epel, E. A., Crosswell, A. D., Mayer, S. E., Prather, A. A., Slavich, G. M., Puterman, E., & Mendes, W. B. (2018). More than a feeling: A unified view of stress measurement for population science. *Frontiers in Neuroendocrinology, 49*, 146–169.

Erdine, S., & Ari, O. (2006). ESH-ESC guidelines for the management of hypertension. *Herz, 31*, 331–338.

Eriksson, M., Ghazinour, M., & Hammarström, A. (2018). Different uses of Bronfenbrenner's ecological theory in public mental health research: What is their value for guiding public mental health policy and practice? *Social Theory & Health, 16*, 414–433. doi: 10.1057/s41285-018-0065-6

Erlbich, J., Boubjerg, D. H., & Valdimarsdottir, R. B. (2000). Psychosocial distress, health and beliefs and frequency of breast self-examination. *Journal of Behavioral Medicine, 23*, 277–292.

Escalante, A., del Rincon, I., & Mulrow, C. D. (2000). Symptoms of depression and psychological distress among Hispanics with rheumatoid arthritis. *Arthritis Care and Research, 13*(3), 156–167.

Esch, B. M., Marion, F., Busato, A., & Heusser, P. (2008). Patient satisfaction with primary care: An observational study comparing anthroposophic and conventional care. *Health Quality Life Outcomes, 30*(6), 74.

Eskandarieh, S., Sahraiain, M. A., Molazadeh, N., & Moghadasi, A. N. (2019). Pediatric multiple sclerosis and its familial recurrence: A population based study (1999–2017). *Multiple Sclerosis and Related Disorders, 36.* doi: 10.1016/j.msard.2019.101377

Eskenazi, B., Bradman, A., & Castorina, R. (1999). Exposures of children to organophosphate pesticides and their potential adverse health effects. *Environmental Health Perspectives, 107*(S3), 409–414.

Esler, M., Eikelis, N., Schlaich, M., Lambert, G., Alvarenga, M., & Dawood, T. (2008). Chronic mental stress is a cause of essential hypertension: Presence of biological markers of stress. *Clinical and Experimental Pharmacology and Physiology, 35*(4), 498–502. doi: 10.1111/j.1440-1681.2008.04904.x

Essajee, S. M. (1999). Immunologic and virologic responses to HAART in severely immunocompromised HIV-1 infected children. *AIDS, 13*, 2523–2532.

Euesden, J., Danese, A., Lewis, C. M., & Maughan, B. (2017). A bidirectional relationship between depression and the autoimmune disorders: New perspectives from the National Child Development Study. *PLoS One, 12*(3). doi: 10.1371/journal.pone.0173015

Evans, J. J. (1997). Oxytocin in the humans – Regulation of derivations & destinations. *European Journal of Endocrinology/European Federation of Endocrine Societies, 137*, 559–571.

Evers, A. W. M., Kraaimaat, F. W., Geenen, R., Jacobs, J. W. G., & Bijlsma, J. W. J. (2003). Pain coping and social support as predictors of long-term functional disability and pain in early rheumatoid arthritis. *Behavioral Research and Therapy, 41*, 1295–1310.

Ezzati, M., Vander-Hoorn, S., & Lowes, C. M. M. (2005). Re-thinking the disease of affluence paradigm: Global patterns of nutritional risks in relation to economic development. *Public Library of Science and Medicine, 2*(5), e133.

Faerstein, E., Chor, D., Loureiro Werneck, G., de Souza Lopes, C., & Kaplan, C. (2014). Race and perceived racism, education, and hypertension among Brazilian civil servants: The Pró-Saúde Study. *Revista Brasileira de Epidemiologia, 17*(Suppl. 2), 81–87. doi: 10.1590/1809-4503201400060007

Fakheri, H., Bari, Z., & Merat, S. (2011). Familial aspects of colorectal cancers in Southern Littoral of Caspian Sea. *Archives of Indian Medicine, 14*, 175–178.

Falagas, M., Vardakas, K., & Paschalis, V. (2007). Underdiagnosis of common chronic disease prevalence and impact on human health. *International Journal of Clinical Practice*, *61*, 1569–1579.

Falagas, M. E., Zarkadoulia, E. A., & Samonis, G. (2006). Arab science in the golden age (750–1258 CE) and today. *The FASEB Journal: Official Publication of the Federation of American Society for Experimental Biology*, *20*(10), 1581–1586.

Falcioni, L., Bua, L., Tibaldi, E., Lauriola, M., De Angelis, L., Gnudi, F., . . . Belpoggi, F. (2018). Report of final results regarding brain and heart tumors in Sprague-Dawley rats exposed from prenatal life to natural death to mobile phone radiofrequency field representative of a 1.8 GHz GSM base station environmental emission. *Environmental Research*, *165*, 496–503. doi: 10.1016/j.envres.2018.01.037

Famularo, R., Kinscherff, R., & Fenton, T. (1992). Parental abuse and the nature of child maltreatment. *Child Abuse and Neglect*, *16*, 475–483.

Fang, C. Y., & Myers, H. F. (2001). The effects of racial stressors and hostility on cardiovascular reactivity in African American and Caucasian men. *Health Psychology*, *20*, 64–70.

Fang, H., & Rizzo, J. A. (2008). The changing effect of managed care on physicians. *American Journal of Managed Care*, *14*, 653–660.

Farahmand, M., Tehrani, F. R., Amiri, P., & Aziz, F. (2012). Barriers to healthy nutrition, perceptions & experiences of Iranian culture. *BMC Public Health*, *12*, 1064–1070.

Fardin, M. A. (2020). COVID-19 epidemic and spirituality: A review of the benefits of religion in times of crisis. *Journal of Chronic Disease Care*, *9*(2). doi: 10.5812/jjcdc.104260

Faria, N. R., Rambaut, A., Suchard, M. A., Baele, G., Bedford, T., Ward, M. J., . . . Lemey, P. (2014). The early spread and epidemic region of HIV-1 in human populations. *Science*, *346*(6205), 56–61.

Farmer, P. (2020). *Fever, feuds, and diamonds: Ebola and the ravages of history*. New York, NY: Farrar, Straus & Giroux.

Faucett, J., Gordon, N., & Levine, J. (1994). Differences in postoperative pain severity among four ethnic groups. *Journal of Pain Symptom Management*, *9*, 383–389.

Fawzy, F. L., & Fawzy, N. W. (1994). A structured psycho-educational intervention for cancer patients. *General Hospital Psychiatry*, *60*, 100–103.

Fekete, E. M., Antoni, M. H., Duran, R., Stoelb, B. L., Kumar, M., & Schneiderman, N. (2009a). Disclosing HIV serostatus to family members: Effects on psychological and physiological health in minority women living with HIV. *International Journal of Behavioral Medicine*, *16*(4), 367–376.

Fekete, E. M., Antoni, M. H., Lopez, C. R., Durán, R. E., Penedo, F. J., Bandiera, F. C., . . . Schneiderman, N. (2009b). Men's serostatus disclosure to parents: Associations among social support, ethnicity & disease status in men living with HIV. *Brain, Behavior, and Immunity*, *23*(5), 693–699.

Feldscher, K. (2023). *Botswana lab known for identifying Omicron variant receives new recognition*. The Harvard T. H. Chan School of Public Health. Retrieved November 11, 2023.

Feletto, E., Yu, X. Q., Lew, J.-B., St. John, J. B., Jenkins, M. A., Macrae, F. A., . . . Canfell, K. (2019). Trends in colon and rectal cancers incidence in Australia from 1982 to 2014: Analysis of data on over 375,000 cases. *Cancer Epidemiology, Biomarkers & Prevention*, *28*(1), 83–90. doi: 10.1158/1055-9965.EPI-18-0523

Fergus, K. D., & Gray, R. E. (2009). Relationship vulnerabilities during breast cancer: Patient & partner perspectives. *Psycho-Oncology*, *18*, 1311–1322.

Ferlay, J., Bray, F., Pisani, P., & Parkin, D. M. (2004). International Agency for Research on Cancer (IARC). *GLOBOCAN 2002: Cancer incidences and prevalence worldwide* (Cancer Base, No. 5, Version 2.0). Lyon: IARC Press.

Fernandez, C., de Salles, A. A., Sears, M. E., Morris, R. D., & Davis, D. L. (2018). Absorption of wireless radiation in the child versus adult brain and eye from cell phone conversation or virtual reality. *Environmental Research*, *167*, 694–699.

Ferreira-Valente, A., Sharma, S., Torres, S., Smothers, Z., Pais-Ribeiro, J., Abbott, J.H., & Jensen, M.P. (2022). Does religiosity/spirituality play a role in function, pain-related beliefs, and coping in patients with chronic pain? A systematic review. *Journal of Religion and Health*, *61*, 2331–2385. doi: 10.1007/s10943-019-00914-7

Fiala, C., & Pasic, M.D. (2020). Aspirin: Bitter pill or miracle drug? *Clinical Biochemistry*, *85*, 1–4. doi: 10.1016/j.clinbiochem.2020.07.003

Fields, T.R. (2024). Gout: Risk factors, diagnosis and treatment. *HSS*. Retrieved February 28, 2024.

Filardo, T.D., Feng, P., Pratt, R.H., Price, S.F., & Self, J.L. (2022). Tuberculosis – United States, 2021. *Morbidity and Mortality Weekly Report*, *71*, 441–446. doi: 10.15585/mmwr.mm7112a1

Finch, E.A., Linde, J.A., Jeffery, R.W., Rothman, A, J., King, C.M., & Levy, R.L. (2005). The effects of outcome expectations and satisfaction on weight loss and maintenance: Correlational and experimental analyses – A randomized trial. *Health Psychology*, *24*, 608–616.

Finer, L.B., Darroch, J.E., & Singh, S. (1999). Sexual partnership patterns as a behavioral risk factor for sexually transmitted diseases. *Family Planning Perspective*, *31*(3), 228–236.

Finkelstein, A.M., Taubman, S., Wright, B., Bernstein, M., Gruber, J., Newhouse, J.P., . . . Oregon Health Study Group. (2012). The Oregon health insurance experiment: Evidence from the first year. *The Quarterly Journal of Economics*, *127*(3), 1057–1107.

Finn, R. (1993, February 8). Arthur Ashe, tennis star is dead at 49. *The New York Times Obituary*. Retrieved October 25, 2013. www.nytimes.com/learning/general/onthisday/bday/0710.html

Fischer, C. (2008). *The corpus: The Hippocratic writings (Kaplan classics of medicine)*. New York: Kaplan.

Fischer, P.M., Schwartz, M.P., Richards, J.W., Goldstein, A.O., & Rojas, T.H. (1991). Brand logo recognition by children aged 3 to 6 years. Mickey Mouse and Old Joe the Camel. *Journal of the American Medical Association*, *266*(22), 3185–3186.

Fishbein, M., & Ajzen, I. (1975). *Beliefs, attitudes, intentions and behaviour: An introduction to theory and research*. Reading, MA: Addison-Wesley.

Fitzgerald, M.P., Donovan, K.R., Kees, J., & Kozup, J. (2019). How confusion impacts product labeling perceptions. *Journal of Consumer Marketing*, *36*(2), 306–316. doi: 10.1108/JCM-08-2017-2307

Flaherty, M.R., Kim, A.M., Salt, M.D., & Lee, L.K. (2020). Distracted driving laws and motor vehicle crash fatalities. *Pediatrics*, *145*(6), e20193621. doi: 10.1542/peds.2019-3621

Flake, J. K., Barron, K. E., Hulleman, C., McCoach, B. D., & Welsh, M. E. (2015). Measuring cost: The forgotten component of expectancy-value theory. *Contemporary Educational Psychology*, *41*, 232–244. www.sciencedirect.com/science/article/abs/pii/S0361476X15000089

Fleury, M.-J., Imboua, A., Aube, D., & Farand, L. (2012). Collaboration between general practitioners (GP) and mental health care professionals within the context of reforms in Quebec. *Mental Health in Family Medicine*, *9*(2), 77–90.

Flood, D.M., Weiss, N.S., Cook, L.S., Emerson, J.C., Schwartz, S.M., & Potter, J.D. (2000). Colorectal cancer incidences in Asian immigrants to the US and their descendants. *Cancer Cause and Control*, *11*, 403–411.

Flores, G., & Vega, L. (1998). Barriers to health care access for Latino children: A review. *Family Medicine*, *30*(3), 196–205.

Folkman, S., & Greer, S. (2002). Promoting psychological well-being in the face of serious illness: When theory, research and practice inform each other. *Psychooncology*, *9*, 11–19.

Folkman, S., & Moskowitz, J. T. (2000). Positive affect and the other side of coping. *American Psychologist*, *55*(6), 647–654.

Fombonne, E., & Chakvabarti, S. (2001). No evidence for a new variant of measles-mumps rubella-induced autism. *Pediatrics*, *108*(11), e58.

Fombonne, E., Zakanan, R., Bemuth, A., Meny, L., & McLean-Heywood, D. (2006). Pervasive developmental disorders in Montreal, Quebec, Canada: Prevalence and links with immunization. *Pediatrics*, *118*(1), e139–e150.

Ford, D., Easton, D. F., Stratton, M., Nurod, S., Goldgar, D., & Devilee, P. (1998). Genetic heterogeneity and penetrance analysis of the BRCA1 and BRCA2 genes in breast cancer families. *American Journal of Human Genetics*, *62*, 676–689.

Forde, A. T., Lewis, T. T., Kershaw, K. N., Bellamy, S. L., & Diez Roux, A. V. (2021). Perceived discrimination and hypertension risk among participants in the multi-ethnic study of atherosclerosis. *JAMA*, *10*(5). doi: 10.1161/JAHA.120.019541

Forsythe, R. A. (2020). Considerations of low health literacy during the COVID-19 pandemic. *International Journal of Nursing Didactics*, *10*(11), 1–6.

Foundation for a Smoke-Free World. (2022). *State of smoking in the United Kingdom*. Retrieved May 18, 2023, from smokefreeworld.org

France, C. R., Keefe, F. J., Emery, C. F., Affleck, G., France, J. L., Waters, S., . . . Edwards, C. (2004). Laboratory pain perception & clinical pain in post-menopausal women & age-matched men with osteoarthritis: Relationship to pain coping & hormonal status. *Pain*, *112*(3), 274–281.

Franco, D. A., & Williams, C. E. (2000). "Airs, waters, places" and other Hippocratic writings: Inferences for control of foodborne and waterborne diseases. *The Journal of Environmental Health*, *62*, 9–12.

Franco-Paredes, C., Tellez, I., & del Rio, C. (2006). Rapid HIV testing: A review of the literature and implications for the clinician. *Current HIV/AIDS Report*, *3*(4), 169–175.

Fregoso, G., Wang, A., Tseng, K., & Wang, J. (2019). Transition from acute to chronic pain: Evaluating risk for chronic postsurgical pain. *Pain Physician*, *22*, 479–88.

Frey, M. K., Perez, L. R., Brewer, J. T., Fleischmann, A. K., & Silber, E. (2024). Breast cancer in the Ashkenazi Jewish population. *Current Breast Cancer Reports*, *16*, 98–105. doi: 10.1007/s12609-024-00528-3

Freynhagen, R., Parada, H. A., Calderon-Ospina, C. A., Chen, J., Rakhmawati Emril, D., Fernández-Villacorta, F. J., . . . de Andrade, D. C. (2019). Current understanding of the mixed pain concept: A brief narrative review. *Current Medical Research and Opinion*, *35*(6), 1011–1018. doi: 10.1080/03007995.2018.1552042

Fried, T. R., Bradley, E. H., & O'Leary, J. (2003). Prognosis communication in serious illnesses: Perceptions of older patients, caregivers & clinicians. *Journal of the American Geriatrics Society*, *51*, 1398–1403.

Friedenreich, C., Norat, T., & Steindor, F. K. (2006). Physical activity and risk of colon and rectal cancer: The European prospective investigation into cancer. *Cancer Epidemiology Biomarkers Prevention*, *15*, 2398–2407.

Friedman, E. H. (1991). Role of Type A behavior pattern (TABP) in the pathogenesis of coronary heart disease (CHD). *Social Science and Medicine*, *32*(11), 1317–1318.

Friedman, H., Newton, C., & Klein, T. W. (2003). Microbial infections, immunomodulation and drugs of abuse. *Clinical Microbiology Review*, *16*(2), 209–219.

Friedman, M. (1989). Type A behavior, its diagnosis, cardiovascular relation and the effects of its modification on occurrences of coronary artery disease. *American Journal of Cardiology*, *64*(6), C12–C19.

Friedman, M., & Rosenman, R. H. (1959). Association of specific over behavior pattern with blood and cardiovascular findings. *Journal of the American Medical Association*, *169*, 1286–1296.

of age in the United States: Third National Health and Nutrition Examination study, 1988 to 1994. *Pediatrics, 101*(2), E8.

Getzen, T. E. (2004). *Health economics: Fundamentals and flows of funds* (2nd ed.). Danvers, MA: Wiley & Sons.

Ghaed, S. G., & Gallo, L. C. (2007). Subjective social status, objective socioeconomic status, and cardiovascular risk in women. *Health Psychology, 26*(6), 668. https://psycnet.apa.org/doi/10.1037/0278-6133.26.6.668

Ghazisaeidi, S., Muley, M. M., & Salter, M. W. (2023). Neuropathic pain: Mechanisms, sex differences, and potential therapies for a global problem. *Annual Review of Pharmacology and Toxicology, 63*(1), 565–583. doi: 10.1146/annurev-pharmtox-051421-112259

Ghebreyesus, T. A. (2023, August 17). *WHO Director-General's opening remarks at WHO Traditional Medicine Global Summit – Gandhinagar, India.* Retrieved September 7, 2023.

Giancane, G., Consolaro, A., Lanni, S., Davì, S., Schiappapietra, B., & Ravelli, A. (2016). Juvenile idiopathic arthritis: Diagnosis and treatment. *Rheumatology and Therapy, 3*, 187–207. doi: 10.1007/s40744-016-0040-4

Gibbons, C. (2022). Understanding the role of stress, personality and coping on learning motivation and mental health in university students during a pandemic. *BMC Psychology, 10*(1), 261. doi: 10.1186/s40359-022-00971-w

Gibbons, C. (2023). Untangling the role of optimism, pessimism and coping influences on student mood, motivation and satisfaction. *Innovations in Education and Teaching International.* doi: 10.1080/14703297.2023.2260780

Gili, M., Roca, M., Ferrer, V., Obrador, A., & Cabeza, E. (2006). Psychosocial factors associated with the adherence to a colorectal cancer screening program. *Cancer Detection & Prevention, 30*(4), 354–360.

Gilkey, M. B., & McRee, A.-L. (2016). Provider communication about HPV vaccination: A systematic review. *Human Vaccine & Immunotherapeutics, 12*(6), 1454–1468. doi: 10.1080/21645515.2015.1129090

Gillum, R. F., Folsom, A., Luepker, R. V., Jacobs, D. R., Kottle, T. E., & Gomez-Martin, O. (1983). Sudden death and acute myocardial infarction in a metropolitan area, 1970–1980. The Minnesota Heart Survey. *New England Journal of Medicine, 309*(22), 1353–1358.

Ginzler, J. A., Cochran, B. N., Domenech-Rodriguez, M., Cauce, A. M., & Whitbeck, L. B. (2003). Sequential progression of substance use among homeless youth: An empirical investigation of gateway theory. *Substance Use and Misuse, 38*(1–6), 725–758.

Gioscia-Ryan, R. A., Clayton, Z. S., Zigler, M. C., Richey, J. J., Cuevas, L. M., Rossman, M. J., . . . Seals, D. R. (2021). Lifelong voluntary aerobic exercises prevents age- and Western-diet induced vascular dysfunction, mitochondrial oxidative stress and inflammation in mice. *Journal of Physiology, 599*(3), 911–925. doi: 10.1113/JP280929

Glantz, S. A., & Parmley, W. W. (1991). Passive smoking and heart disease: Epidemiology, physiology and biochemistry. *Circulation, 83*, 1–12.

Glassman, A. H., & Shapiro, P. A. (1998). Depression and the course of coronary artery disease. *American Journal of Psychiatry, 155*, 4–11.

Gobodo-Madikizela, P. (2002). *A human being died that night: A South African story of forgiveness.* New York: Houghton Mifflin.

Gobodo-Madikizela, P. (2003). Remorse, forgiveness & rehumanization: Stories from South Africa. *Journal of Humanistic Psychology, 42*(1), 7–32.

Godfrey, J. R., & Felson, D. T. (2008). Toward optimal health: Managing arthritis in women. *Journal of Women's Health, 17*(5), 729–734.

Goebels, M. U., Mills, P. J., Irwin, M. R., & Zeigler, M. G. (2000). Interleukin-6 and tumor factor-α production after acute psychological stress, exercise, and infused isoproterenol: Differential effects and pathways. *Psychosomatic Medicine, 62,* 591–598.

Goin, R. T., Hays, J. C., Landeman, D. R., & Hobbs, G. (2009). Access to healthcare and self-rated health among community-dwelling older adults. *Journal of Applied Gerontology, 20*(3), 307–321.

Gok, M. S., & Sezen, B. (2013). Analyzing the ambiguous relationship between efficiency, quality and patient satisfaction in healthcare services: The case of public hospitals in Turkey. *Health Policy, 111*(3), 290–300. doi: 10.1016/j.healthpol.2013.05.010

Gola, H., Engler, H., Sommershof, A., Adenauer, H., Kolassa, S., Schedlowski, M., . . . Kolassa, I. T. (2013). Posttraumatic stress disorder is associated with and enhanced spontaneous production of pro-inflammatory cytokines by peripheral blood mononuclear cells. *BMC Psychiatry, 13,* 1.

Gold, M. R., Hurley, R., Lake, T., Ensor, T., & Berenson, R. (1995). A national survey of the arrangements managed care plans make with physicians. *New England Journal of Medicine, 333*(25), 1678–1683.

Goldbach-Mansky, R., Lee, J., McCoy, A., Hoxworth, J., Yarboro, C., Smolen, J. S., . . . El-Gabalawy, H. S. (2002). Rheumatoid arthritis associated auto antibodies in patients with synovitis of recent onset. *Arthritis Research, 3,* 236–243.

Goldring, M. B. (2006). Update on the biology of the chondrocyte & new approaches to treating cartilage disease. *Best Practices & Research in Clinical Rheumatology, 20*(5), 1003–1025.

Goldsby, R. A., Kindt, T. J., Osborne, B. A., & Kuby, J. (2003). *Immunology.* New York: W. H. Freeman and Co.

Goldsmith, S. K., Pellmar, T. C., Kleinman, A. M., & Bunney, W. E. (2002). *Reducing suicide: A national imperative.* Washington, DC: National Academy Press.

Gollurtzer, P. W. (1993). Goal achievement: The role of intentions. In W. Strobe & M. Hewstone (Eds.), *European review of social psychology* (Vol. 4, pp. 141–188). Chichester, UK: Wiley & Sons.

Gong, G., Phillips, S. G., Hudson, C., Curti, D., & Phillips, B. U. (2019). Higher US rural mortality rates linked to socioeconomic status, physician shortages, and lack of health insurance. *Health Affairs, 38*(12), 2003–2010. doi: 10.1377/hlthaff.2019.00722

Goodman, R. M., Wandersman, A., Chinman, M., Imm, P., & Morrissey, E. (1996). An ecological assessment of community-based interventions for prevention and health promotion: Approaches to measuring community coalitions. *American Journal of Community Psychology, 24*(1), 33–61.

Goodnough, A. (2003, June 25). Schools cut down on fat and sweets in menus. *The New York Times.*

Goodwin, A. H., Wells, J. K., Foss, R. D., & Williams, A. F. (2006). Encouraging compliance with graduated driver licensing restrictions. *Journal of Safety Research, 37,* 343–351.

Goodyear, I. M., Herbert, J., Tamplin, A., & Altham, P. M. (2000). First-episode major depression in adolescents: Affective, cognitive and endocrine characteristics of risk status and predictors of onset. *British Journal of Psychiatry, 176,* 142–149.

Gordon, H. S., Street, R. L., Kelly, P. A., Souchek, J., & Wray, N. P. (2005). Physician-patient communication following invasive procedures: An analysis of post-angiogram consultations. *Social Science & Medicine, 61*(5), 1015–1025.

Gorelick, D. A. (2023). Cannabis-related disorders and toxic effects. *The New England Journal of Medicine, 389,* 2267–2275. doi: 10.1056/NEJMra2212152

Gorman, J. M., & Kertzner, R. (1990). Psychoneuroimmunology and HIV infection. *Neurosciences, 2,* 241–252.

Gorodeski, G. (2002). Update on cardiovascular disease in post-menopausal women. *Best Practice & Research Clinical Obstetrics and Gynecology, 16*(3), 329–355.

Gottschalk, A., & Flocke, S. A. (2005). Time spent in face-to-face patient care and work outside the examination room. *Annals of Family Medicine, 3*(6), 488–493.

Gouin, J. P., Kiecolt-Glaser, J. K., Malarkey, W. B., & Glaser, R. (2008). The influence of anger expression on wound healing. *Brain, Behavior, and Immunity, 22,* 699–708.

Gowland, R. L., & Chamberlain, A. T. (2005). Detecting plague: Palaeodemographic characterisation of a catastrophic death assemblage. *Antiquity, 79,* 146–157.

GPO Access. (2008). *Electronic code of federal regulations.* Title 14: Aeronautics & Space. National Archives & Records Administration. Retrieved October 2, 2009, from www.gpo.gov/fdsys/pkg/CFR-2004-title14-vol1/content-detail.html

Graff, R. E., Moller, S., Passarelli, M. N., Witte, J. S., Skytthe, A., Christensen, K., . . . Hjelmborg, J. B. (2017). Familial risk and heritability of colorectal cancer in the Nordic Twin Study of Cancer. *Clinical Gastroenterology & Hepatology, 15*(8), 1256–1264.

Grann, V., Troxel, A. B., Zojwalla, N., Hershman, D., Glied, S. A., & Jacobsen, J. S. (2006). Regional & racial disparities in breast cancer-specific mortality. *Social Science & Medicine, 62,* 337–347.

Grant, I., Atkinson, J. H., & Hesselink, J. R. (1987). Evidence for early central nervous system involvement in the acquired immunodeficiency syndrome (AIDS) and other human immunodeficiency virus (HIV) infections: Studies with neuropsychological testing and magnetic resonance imaging. *Annals of Internal Medicine, 107,* 828–836.

Green, A. C., Fong, G. T., Borland, R., Quah, A. C. K., Seo, H. G., Kim, Y., & Elton-Marshall, T. (2015). The importance of the belief that "light" cigarettes are smoother in misperceptions of the harmfulness of "light" cigarettes in the Republic of Korea: A nationally representative cohort study. *BMC Public Health, 15,* 1108. doi: 10.1186/s12889-015-2472-0

Green, C. R., Anderson, K. O., Baker, T. A., Campbell, L. C., Decker, S., Fillingim, R. B., . . . Vallerand, A. H. (2003). The unequal burden of pain: Confronting racial and ethnic disparities in pain. *Pain Medicine, 4*(3), 277–294.

Green, J., & Ramos, C. (2021). A mixed methods examination of health care provider behaviors that build patients' trust. *Patient Education and Counseling, 104*(5), 1222–1228. doi: 10.1016/j.pec.2020.09.003

Greenberg, D. R., & LaPorte, D. J. (1996). Racial differences in body type preferences of men for women. *International Journal of Eating Disorders, 19,* 275–278.

Greenblatt, R. M., & Hessol, N. A. (2001). Epidemiology and natural history of HIV infection in women. In R. J. Anderson (Ed.), *A guide to the clinical care of women with HIV* (pp. 1–32). Washington, DC: U.S. Department of Health and Human Services, Health Resources and Services Administration.

Greene, C. A., Haisley, L., Wallace, C., & Ford, J. D. (2020). Intergenerational effects of childhood maltreatment: A systematic review of the parenting practices of adult survivors of childhood abuse, neglect, and violence. *Clinical Psychology Review, 80.* doi: 10.1016/j.cpr.2020.101891

Greenlund, K. J., Johnson, C. C., Webber, L. S., & Berenson, G. S. (1997). Cigarette smoking attitudes and first use among third-through sixth-grade students: The Bogalusa heart study. *American Journal of Public Health, 87*(8), 1345–1348.

Greeno, C. G., & Wing, R. R. (1994). Stress-induced eating. *Psychological Bulletin, 115,* 444–464.

Greenwald, J. L., Burstein, G. R., Pincus, J., & Branson, B. (2006). A rapid review of rapid antibody tests. *Current Infections Disease Reports, 8,* 125–131.

Gregus, A. M., Levine, I. S., Eddinger, K. A., Yaksh, T. L., & Buczynski, M. W. (2021). Sex differences in neuroimmune and glial mechanisms of pain. *Pain*, *162*(8), 2186–2200. doi: 10.1097/j. pain.0000000000002215

Greydanus, D. E., & Merrick, J. (2020). Liver and gallbladder: A historical perspective. *International Journal of Child Health and Human Development*, *13*(3), 229–261.

Griep, R. H., Nobre, A. A., Alves, M. G. M., Fonseca, M. J. M., Cardoso, L. O., Giatti, L., . . . Chor, D. (2015). Job strain and unhealthy lifestyle: Results from the baseline cohort study, Brazilian Longitudinal Study of Adult Health (ELSA-Brasil). *BMC Public Health*, *15*, 309. doi: 10.1186/s12889-015-1626-4

Grillo, C. M., Crosby, R. D., & Machado, P. P. P. (2019). Examining the distinctiveness of body image concerns in patients with anorexia nervosa and bulimia nervosa. *International Journal of Eating Disorders*, *52*(11), 1229–1236. doi: 10.1002/eat.23161

Grond, S., Zech, D., Lynch, J., Schug, S., & Lehmann, K. A. (1992). Tramadol – A weak opioid for relief of cancer pain. *Pain Clinic*, *5*, 241–247.

Grosse, L., Hoogenboezem, T., Ambrée, O., Bellingrath, S., Jörgens, S., de Wit, H. J., . . . Drexhage, H. A. (2016). Inflammatory monocyte activation is associated with natural T regulatory cell deficiencies and co-occurs with cellular immune defects in major depressive disorder. *Neurology, Psychiatry and Brain Research*, *22*(1), 12.

Grunbaum, J. A., Kann, L., Kinchen, S. A., Williams, B., Ross, J. G., Lowry, R., & Kolbe, L. (2002). Youth risk behavior survey: Surveillance summaries. *Morbidity and Mortality Weekly Report*, *51*(SS04), 1–64.

Guay, L. A., Muskoe, P., Fleming, T., Bagenda, D., Allen, M., & Nakabiito, C. (1999). Intrapartum and neonatal single-dose nevirapine compared with zidovudine for prevention of mother-to-child transmission of HIV-1 in Kampala, Uganda. *Lancet*, *354*, 795–802.

Guedi, M., Gilbert, M., Maudet, A., Munoz-Sastre, M. T., Mullet, E., & Sorun, P. C. (2005). The acceptability of ending of patient's life. *Journal of Medical Ethics*, *31*, 311–317.

Guiliani, N. R., McRae, K., & Gross, J. J. (2008). The up- and down-regulation of amusement: Experimental, behavioral & autonomic consequences. *Emotion*, *8*, 714–719.

Gutmann, F. D., Gardner, J. W., Potter, R. N., & Kark, J. A. (2002). Nontraumatic exercise related deaths in the U.S. military, 1996–1999. *Military Medicine*, *167*(12), 964–970.

Guyll, M., Matthews, K. A., & Bromberger, J. T. (2001). Discrimination and unfair treatment: Relationship to cardiovascular reactivity among African American and European American women. *Health Psychology*, *20*, 315–325.

Gyurcsik, N. C., Cary, M. A., Sessford, J. D., Flora, P. K., & Brawley, L. R. (2014). Pain, anxiety, and negative outcome expectations for activity: Do negative psychological profiles differ between the inactive and active? *Arthritis Care & Research*, *67*(1), 58–64. doi: 10.1002/acr.22421

Haas, C. (2006). The Antonine plague. *Bulletin de L'Académie Nationale de Médecine*, *190*(4–5), 1093–1098.

Haas, J. S., Phillips, A. S., Sonneborn, D., McCulloch, C. E., & Liang, S. Y. (2002). Effects of managed care insurance on the use of preventive care for specific ethnic groups in the U.S. *Medical Care*, *40*(9), 743–751.

Haas, S. A., & Schaefer, D. F. (2014). With a little help from my friends? Asymmetrical social influence on adolescent smoking initiation & cessation. *Journal of Health & Social Behavior*, *55*(2), 126–143.

Haddock, C. K., Jahnke, S. A., Poston, W. S. C., & Williams, L. N. (2013). Cigarette prices in military retail: A review and proposal for advancing military health policy. *Military Medicine*, *178*(5), 563–569. doi: 10.7205/MILMED-D-12-00517

Hadley, J., & Holahan, J. (2004, May). The cost of care for the uninsured: What do we spend, who pays and what would full coverage add to medical spending? *KCMU Issue Update*. Kaiser Commission on Medicaid and the Uninsured, Henry J. Kaiser Family Foundation.

Hadlow, J., & Pitts, M. (1992). The understanding of common health terms by doctors, nurses and patients. *Social Science and Medicine*, *32*, 193–196.

Hafeez, A., Ahmad, S., Ali Siddqui, S., Ahmad, M., & Mishra, S. (2020). A review of COVID-19 (coronavirus disease-2019) diagnosis, treatments and prevention. *Eurasian Journal of Medicine and Oncology*, *4*(2), 116–125. doi: 10.14744/ejmo.2020.90853

Haidt, J., & Rausch, Z. (2023). Kids who get smartphones earlier become adults with worse mental health. *After Babel*. Retrieved December 3, 2023, from afterbabel.com

Hajat, A., MacLehose, R. F., Rosofsky, A., Walker, K. D., & Clougherty, J. E. (2021). Confounding by socioeconomic status in epidemiological studies of air pollution and health: Challenges and opportunities. *Environmental Health Perspectives*, *129*(6). doi: 10.1289/EHP7980

Haj-Yahia, M. M., Sokar, S., Hassan-Abbas, N., & Malka, M. (2019). The relationship between exposure to family violence in childhood and post-traumatic stress symptoms in young adulthood: The mediating role of social support. *Child Abuse & Neglect*, *92*, 126–138. doi: 10.1016/j.chiabu.2019.03.02

Hale, H. I., Song, R., Rhodes, P., Prejean, J., An, Q., & Lee, L. M. (2008). Estimates of HIV incidences in the US. *Journal of the American Medical Association*, *300*(5), 520–529.

Hales, C. M., Fryar, C. D., Carroll, M. D., Freedman, D. S., & Ogden, C. L. (2018). Trends in obesity and severe obesity prevalence in US youth and adults by sex and age, 2007–2008 to 2015–2016. *JAMA*, *319*(16), 1723–1725. doi: 10.1001/jama.2018.3060

Hall, J. A., & Valente, T. W. (2007). Adolescent smoking networks: The effects of influence & selection on future smoking. *Addictive Behavior*, *32*(12), 3054–3059.

Halpern-Felsher, B. L., Biehl, M. A., Kropp, R. Y., & Rubenstein, M. D. (2004). Perceived risks and benefits of smoking: Differences among adolescents with different smoking experiences and intentions. *Preventive Medicine*, *39*(3), 559–567.

Halpern-Felsher, B. L., & Rubinstein, M. D. (2004). Clear the air: Adolescents' perceptions of the risks associated with secondhand smoke. *Preventive Medicine*, *41*(1), 16–22.

Hamadeh, N., van Rompaey, C., Metreau, E., & Eapen, S. G. (2022). *New World Bank country classifications by income level: 2022–2023*. Retrieved on November 11, 2023, from https://blogs. worldbank.org/opendata/new-world-bank-country-classifications-income-level-2022–2023

Hamilton, B. E., Martin, J. A., & Ventura, S. J. (2007). Births: Preliminary data for 2006. *National Vital Statistics Reports*, *56*(7), 1–23. U.S. Department of Health and Human Services, Centers for Disease Control and Prevention.

Hamilton-West, K. E., & Quine, L. (2007). Effects of written emotional disclosure on health outcomes in patients with ankylosing spondylitis. *Psychology and Health*, *22*(6), 637–757.

Hamlin, C., & Sheard, S. (1998). Revolutions in public health: 1848–1998. *British Medical Journal*, *317*, 587–591.

Hammen, C. (2006). Stress generation in depression: Reflections on origins, research, and future directions. *Journal of Clinical Psychology*, *62*(9), 1065–1082.

Hammonds, E. M. (1994). Your silence will not protect you: Nurse Eunice Rivers and the Tuskegee Syphilis study. In E. C. White (Ed.), *The Black woman's health book: Speaking for ourselves* (pp. 323–331). Seattle, WA: Seal Press.

Hampl, S. E., Hassink, S. G., Skinner, A. C., Armstrong, S. C., Barlow, S. E., Bolling, C. F., . . . Okechukwu, K. (2023). Clinical practice guideline for the evaluation and treatment of children and adolescents with obesity. *Pediatrics*, *151*(2), e2022060640. doi: 10.1542/peds.2022-060640

Hancox, R. J., Poulton, R., Ely, M., Welch, D., Taylor, D. R., McLachlan, C. R., . . . Sears, M. R. (2010). Effects of cannabis on lung function: A population-based cohort study. *European Respiratory Journal*, *35*(1), 42–47. doi: 10.1183/09031936.00065009

Handel, A. E., Handrennetthi, L., Giovannoni, G., Ebers, G. C., & Ramagopalan, S. V. (2010). Genetic & environmental factors & the distribution of multiple sclerosis in Europe. *European Journal of Neurology*, *17*, 1210–1214.

Haney, C., Banks, W., & Zimbardo, P. (1973). Interpersonal dynamics in a simulated prison. *International Journal of Criminology and Penology*, *1*, 69–97.

Haney, C., & Zimbardo, P. (1998). The past and future of U.S. prison policy: Twenty-five years after the Stanford prison experiment. *American Psychologist*, *53*(7), 709–727.

Hanna, L. R., Avila, P. F., Meteer, J. D., Nicholas, D. R., & Kaminsky, L. A. (2008). The effects of a comprehensive exercise program on physical function, fatigue and mood in patients with various types of cancer. *Oncology Nursing Forum*, *35*(3), 461–469.

Hansen, J., Hanewinkel, R., & Morgenstern, M. (2020). Electronic cigarette advertising and teen smoking initiation. *Addictive Behaviors*, *103*. doi: 10.1016/j.addbeh.2019.106243

Hardell, L., Mild, K. H., & Carlberg, M. (2002). Case-control study on the use of cellular and cordless phones and the risk for malignant brain tumors. *International Journal of Radiation Biology*, *78*, 931–935.

Hardell, L., Mild, K. H., & Carlberg, M. (2003). Further aspects on cellular and cordless telephones and brain tumors. *International Journal of Oncology*, *22*, 339–407.

Hardt, J., Jacobsen, C. Goldberg, J., Nickel, R., & Buchwald, D. (2008). Prevalence of chronic pain in a representative sample in the United States. *Pain Medicine*, *9*, 803–812.

Hargreaves, M. K., Schundt, D. G., Buchowaki, M. S., Hardy, R. E., Rossi, S. R., & Rossi, J. S. (1999). Stages of change and the intake of dietary fat in African-American women: Improving stage assignment using the eating styles questionnaire. *Journal of the American Dietetic Association*, *99*(11), 1392–1399.

Harlow, L. L., Prochaska, J. O., Redding, C. A., Rossi, J. S., Velicer, W. F., Snow, M. G., . . . Rhodes, F. (1999). Stages of condom use in a high HIV-risk sample. *Psychology & Health*, *14*, 143–157.

Harrell, Z. A. T., & Karim, N. M. (2008). Is gender relevant only for problem alcohol behaviors? An examination of correlates of alcohol use among college students. *Addictive Behaviors*, *33*(2), 359–365.

Harris, P. G., & Siplon, P. (2001). International obligation and human health: Evolving policy responses to HIV/AIDS. *Ethics & International Affairs*, *15*(2), 29–52.

Hartung, T. J., Brahler, E., Faller, H., Harter, M., Hinz, A., Johansen, C., . . . Mehnert, A. (2017). The risk of being depressed is significantly higher in cancer patients than in the general population: Prevalence and severity of depressive symptoms across major cancer types. *European Journal of Cancer*, *72*, 46–53.

Harvard Health. (2004). *Rheumatoid arthritis?* Retrieved August 20, 2008, from www.health.harvard.edu/joint/Diseases_RA.htm

Harvard Medical School. (2006). *Lung cancer: Not just for smokers*. Healthbeat: Harvard Medical School Family Health Guide. Retrieved October 20, 2013, from www.health.harvard.edu/fhg/updates/Lung-cancernot-just-for-smokers.shtml

Harvard Medical School. (2024). *Arthritis*. Retrieved March 1, 2024, from

Harvard School of Public Health. (2008). *The nutrition source: Carbohydrates: Good carbs guide the way*. Retrieved from www.hsph.harvard.edu/nutritionsource/carbohydrates/

Ibrahim, S. A., Whittle, J., Mayberry, B., Kelley, M. E., Good, C., & Conigliaro, J. (2003). Racial/ethnic variation in physician recommendations for cardiac revascularization. *American Journal of Public Health*, *93*(10), 1689–1693.

Ibrahim, W. H. (2007). Recent advances and controversies in adult cardiopulmonary resuscitation. *Postgraduate Medical Journal*, *83*(984), 649–654. doi: 10.1136%2Fpgmj.2007.057133

Icahn School of Medicine at Mount Sinai. (2023). *Atypical pneumonia information*. Retrieved April 6, 2023.

ICNIRP, Ahlbom, A., Green, A., Kheifets, L., Savitz, D., & Swerdlow, A. (2004). Epidemiology of health effects of radiofrequency exposure. *Environmental Medicine*, *112*, 1741–1754.

IFRC. (2023). *Homepage*. Retrieved December 9, 2023.

Ilic, M., & Ilic, I. (2022). Worldwide suicide mortality trends (2000–2019): A joinpoint regression analysis. *World Journal of Psychiatry*, *12*(8), 1044–1060. doi: 10.5498/wjp.v12.i8.1044

Inskip, P. D., Tarone, R. E., Hatch, E. E., Wilcosky, T. C., Shapiro, W. R., Selker, R. G., . . . Linet, M. S. (2001). Cellular-telephone use and brain tumors. *New England Journal of Medicine*, *344*, 79–86.

Institute for Health Metrics and Evaluation. (2023a). *Podcast: Chronic respiratory disease*. Retrieved November 30, 2023, from healthdata.org

Institute for Health Metrics and Evaluation. (2023b). *The Lancet: New study reveals the most common form of arthritis, osteoarthritis, affects 15% of the global population over the age of 30*. Retrieved February 29, 2024, from healthdata.org

Institute for Justice. (2013). *Bone marrow statistics*. Retrieved January 23, 2013, from www.ij.org/bonemarrow-statistics

Institute of Medicine. (2000). *American's health care safety net: Intact but endangered*. Washington, DC: National Academy Press.

Institute of Medicine. (2002a). *Reducing suicides: A national imperative*. Committee on Pathophysiology & Prevention of Adolescent & Adult Suicide, board on Neuroscience & Behavioral Health. Washington, DC: National Academies Press.

Institute of Medicine. (2002b). *Unequal treatment: Confronting racial & ethnic disparities in health care*. Washington, DC: National Academy Press.

International Agency for Research on Cancer. (2004). *Tobacco smoke and involuntary smoking*. IARC Monograph on the Evaluations of Carcinogenic Risks to Humans (83). Lyon, France: Author.

International Agency for Research on Cancer. (2013). *Non-ionizing radiation. Part 2: Radiofrequency electromagnetic fields*. Monographs on the Evaluation of Carcinogenic Risks to Humans. Lyon: International Agency for Research on Cancer.

International Agency for Research on Cancer. (2014). *World cancer report 2014*. Lyon: Author.

International Agency for Research on Cancer. (2022). *Global cancer observatory*. Retrieved February 10, 2023, from iarc.fr

International on Line. (2004). *SA approves law to recognize sangomas*. Retrieved June 30, 2008, from www.int.iol.co.za

Ironson, G., & Hayward, H. (2008). Do positive psychosocial factors predict disease progression in HIV-1? A review of the evidence. *Psychosomatic Medicine*, *70*(5), 546–554.

Ironson, G., O'Cleirigh, C., Fletcher, M. A., Laurenceau, J. P., Balbin, E., Klimas, N., . . . Solomon, G. (2005). Psychosocial factors predict CD4 and viral load change in men and women with human immunodeficiency virus in the era of highly active antiretroviral treatment. *Psychosomatic Medicine*, *67*, 1013–1021.

Ironson, G., Stuetzle, R., & Fletcher, M. A. (2006). An increase in religiousness/spirituality occurs after HIV diagnosis & predicts slower disease progression over four years in people with HIV. *Journal of General Internal Medicine*, 21(suppl. 5), S62–S68.

Irving, M., & Schweiger, A. (1991). Individual and family characteristics of middle class adolescents hospitalized for alcohol & other drug abuses. *British Journal of Addictions*, 86(11), 1435–1447.

Irwin, M. R. (2008). Human psychoneuroimmunology: 20 Years of discover. *Brain, Behavior & Immunity*, 22(2), 129–139.

Irwin, M. R., Cole, S., Olmstead, R., Breen, E. C., Cho, J. J., Moieni, M., & Eisenberger, N. I. (2019). Moderators for depressed mood and systemic and transcriptional inflammatory responses: A randomized controlled trial of endotoxin. *Neuropsychopharmacology*, 44, 635–641. doi: 10.1038/s41386-018-0259-6

Ishikawa, H., Hashimoto, H., Kinoshita, M., & Fujimori, S. (2008). Evaluating medical students' non-verbal communication during the objective structured clinical examination. *Medical Education*, 40(12), 1180–1187.

Islami, F., Torre, L. A., & Jemal, A. (2015). Global trends of lung cancer mortality and smoking prevalence. *Translational Lung Cancer Research*, 4(4), 327–338. doi: 10.3978/j.issn.2218-6751.2015.08.04

Iversen, M. D., Frits, M., von Heideken, J., Cui, J., Weinblatt, M., & Shadick, N. A. (2016). Physical activity and correlates of physical activity participation over three years in adults with rheumatoid arthritis. *Arthritis Care & Research*, 69(10), 1535–1545. doi: 10.1002/acr.23156

Jackson, T., Thomas, S., Stabile, V., Shotwell, M., Han, X., & McQueen, K. (2016). A systematic review and meta-analysis of the global burden of chronic pain without clear etiology in low-and middle-income countries: Trends in heterogeneous data and a proposal for new assessment methods. *Anesthesia & Analgesia*, 123(3), 739–748.

Jacobellis, J., & Cutter, G. (2002). Mammography screening and differences in stage of disease by race/ethnicity. *American Journal of Public Health*, 92(7), 1144–1150.

Jacobs, B. M., Noyce, A. J., Bestwick, J., Belete, D., Giovannoni, G., & Dobson, R. (2021). Gene-environment interactions in multiple sclerosis: A UK biobank study. *Neurology Neuroimmunology & Neuroinflammation*, 8(4), e1007. doi: 10.1212/NXI.0000000000001007

Jacobs, G. D. (2001). The physiology of mind–body interactions: The stress response and the relaxation response. *Journal of Alternative & Complementary Medicine*, 7, S83–S92.

Jacobus, J., Squeglia, L. M., Meruelo, A. D., Castro, N., Brumback, T., Giedd, J. N., & Tapert, S. F. (2015). Cortical thickness in adolescent marijuana and alcohol users: A three-year prospective study from adolescence to young adulthood. *Developmental Cognitive Neuroscience*, 16, 101–109.

Jacoby, J., Chestnut, R. W., & Silberman, W. (1977). Consumer use and comprehension of nutritional information. *Journal of Consumer Research*, 4, 119–128.

Jaiswal, Y., Liang, Z., & Zhao, Z. (2016). Botanical drugs in ayurveda and traditional Chinese medicine. *Journal of Ethnopharmacology*, 194, 245–259. doi: 10.1016/j.jep.2016.06.052

Jamal, A., Agaku, I. T., O'Connor, E., King, B. A., Kenemer, J. B., & Neff, L. (2015). Current cigarette smoking among adults – United States 2005–2014. *Morbidity and Mortality Weekly Report*, 64(44), 1233–1240.

James, R. D., West, K. M., Claw, K. G., EchoHawk, A., Dodge, L., Dominguez, A., . . . Burke, W. (2018). Responsible research with urban American Indians and Alaska Natives. *American Journal of Public Health*, 108(12), 1613–1616. doi: 10.2105/AJPH.2018.304708

James, S. A., LaCroix, A. Z., Kleinbaum, D. G., & Strogatz, D. S. (1984). John Henryism & blood pressure differences among black men: II. The role of occupational stressors. *Journal of Behavioral Medicine*, 7, 259–275.

James, W. (1961). *The varieties of religious experiences: A study in human nature*. Cambridge, MA: Harvard University Press.

Jamieson, J. P., Nock, M. K., & Mendes, W. B. (2012). Mind over matter: Reappraising arousal improves cardiovascular and cognitive responses to stress. *Journal of Experimental Psychology: General*, *141*(3), 417–422. doi: 10.1037/a0025719

Janeway, C. A., Travers, P., Jr., & Walport, M. (2001). *The immune system in health and disease* (5th ed.). New York: Garland Science.

Jansen, C. E., Miaskowski, C., Dodd, M., Dowling, G., & Kramer, J. (2005). A meta-analysis of studies of the effects of cancer chemotherapy on various domains of cognitive functions. *Cancer*, *104*(10), 2222–2233.

Jansen, V. A. A., Stollenwerk, N., Jensen, H. J., Ramsay, M. E., Edmunds, W. J., & Rhodes, C. J. (2003). Measles outbreak in a population with declining vaccine uptakes. *Science Magazine*, p. 804.

Janz, N. K., & Becker, M. H. (1984). The health belief model: A decade later. *Health Education Quarterly*, *11*, 1–47.

Jaremka, L. M., Fagundes, C. P., Peng, J., Bennett, J. M., Glaser, R., Malarkey, W. B., & Kiecolt-Glaser, J. K. (2013). Loneliness promotes inflammation during acute stress. *Psychological Science*, *24*(7), 1089–1097.

Javier, S. J., & Belgrave, F. Z. (2019). "I'm not White, I have to be pretty and skinny": A qualitative exploration of body image and eating disorders among Asian American women. *Asian American Journal of Psychology*, *10*(2), 141–153. doi: 10.1037/aap0000133

Jayedi, A., Soltani, S., Abdolshahi, A., & Shab-Bidar, S. (2020). Healthy and unhealthy dietary patterns and the risk of chronic disease: An umbrella review of meta-analyses of prospective cohort studies. *British Journal of Nutrition*, *124*(11), 1133–1144. doi: 10.1017/S0007114520002330

Jelenchick, L. A., Eickhoff, J. C., & Moreno, M. A. (2013). Facebook depression? Social network site use and depression in older adolescents. *The Journal of Adolescent Health*, *52*, 128–130.

Jessor, R., Donovan, J. E., & Costa, F. M. (1991). *Beyond adolescence: Problem behavior and young adult development*. Cambridge, UK: Cambridge University Press.

Jha, P. (2020). The hazards of smoking and the benefits of cessation: A critical summation of the epidemiological evidence in high-income countries. *eLife*, *9*, e49979. doi: 10.7554/eLife.49979

Jiao, J., Shi, L., Chen, H., Wang, X., Yang, M., Yang, J., . . . Sun, G. (2022). Containment strategy during the COVID-19 pandemic among three Asian low and middle-income countries. *Journal of Global Health*, *12*, 05016. doi: 10.7189%2Fjogh.12.05016

Johannson, P., Oleni, M., & Fridlund, B. (2002). Patient satisfaction with nursing care in the context of health care: A literature study. *Scandinavian Journal of Caring Science*, *16*(4), 337–344.

Johansen, C., Boice, J. D., McLaughlin, J. K., & Olsen, J. H. (2002). Cellular telephone and cancer: A nationwide cohort study in Denmark. *Journal of the National Cancer Institute*, *93*, 203–207.

Johns Hopkins University. (2001). *Report of internal investigation into the death of a volunteer research subject*. Retrieved January 15, 2007, from www.hopkinsmedicine.org/press/2001/july/report_of_internal_ investigation.htm

Johnsen, K., Espnes, G. A., & Gillard, S. (1998). Associations between type A/B behavioral dimensions & type 2/4 personality patterns. *Journal of Personality & Individual Differences*, *25*, 937–945.

Johnson, G. (2006). *Successful folk healing course returning for 5th summer at University of New Mexico*. Retrieved March 30, 2009, from www.unm.edu/news/06JunNewsRelease/06-05-folkhealing.htm

Johnson, J. L., Sher, K. J., & Rolf, J. E. (1991). Models of vulnerability to psychopathology in children of alcoholics: An overview. *Alcoholic Health & Research World*, *15*(1), 32.

Johnson, S. S., Paiva, A. L., Cummins, C. O., Johnson, J. L., Dyment, S. J., Wright, J. A., . . . Sherman, K. (2008). Transtheoretical model-based multiple behavior intervention for weight management: Effectiveness on a population basis. *Preventive Medicine, 2*, 238–246. doi: 10.1016/j.ypmed.2007.09.010

Johnston, K. L., White, K. M., & Norman, P. (2004). An examination of the individual-difference approach to the role of norms in the theory of reasoned action. *Journal of Applied Social Psychology, 34*(12), 2524–2549.

Joint Commission on Accreditation of Healthcare Organizations. (1999). *Report of the Joint Commission on Accreditation of Healthcare Organizations.* Washington, DC: Author.

Jones, J. (1981). *Bad blood: The Tuskegee syphilis experiment: A tragedy of race and medicine.* New York: The Free Press.

Jones, T., Trivedi, M. S., Jiang, X., Silverman, T., Underhill, M., Chung, W. K., . . . Crew, K. D. (2021). Racial and ethnic differences in BRCA1/2 multigene panel testing among young breast cancer patients. *Journal of Cancer Education, 36*, 463–469.

Jordan, M. S., Lumly, M. A., & Leisen, J. C. (1998). The relationship of cognitive coping & pain control beliefs to pain & adjustment among African American & Caucasian women with rheumatoid arthritis. *Arthritis Care Research, 11*, 80–88.

Joseph, A. M., Muggli, M., & Pearson, K. C. (2005). Cigarette manufacturers' efforts to promote tobacco in the U.S. military. *Military Medicine, 10*, 874–880.

Journal of the American College of Cardiology. (2024). *Global Burden of Cardiovascular Diseases and Risks Collaboration 1990–2021.* Retrieved February 12, 2024, from jacc.org

Joy, J. E., Penhoet, E. E., & Petitti, D. B. (2004). *Saving women's lives: Strategies for improving breast cancer detection and diagnosis.* Washington, DC: National Academic Press.

Jukkala, T., Makinen, I. H., Kislitsyna, O., Ferlander, S., & Vagero, D. (2008). Economic strain, social relations, gender and binge drinking in Moscow. *Social Science and Medicine, 66*(3), 663–674.

Jung, C.-H., Son, J. W., Kang, S., Kim, W. J., Kim, H.-U., Kim, H. S., . . . Yoon, K. H. (2021). Diabetes fact sheets in Korea, 2020: An appraisal of current status. *Diabetes & Metabolism Journal, 45*(1), 1–10. doi: 10.4093/dmj.2020.0254

Jutoi, I., Sung, H., & Jemal, A. (2022). The emergence of the racial disparity in US breast-cancer mortality. *The New England Journal of Medicine, 386*(25), 2349–2352.

Juul Labs Inc. (2023). *Juul.* Retrieved March 29, 2023.

Kaatsch, P., & Mergenthaler, A. (2008). Incidence, time trends & regional variations in childhood leukaemia in Germany and Europe. *Radiation Protection Dosimetry, 132*(2), 107–113.

Kaatsch, P., Spix, C., Schulze-Rath, R., Schmiedel, S., & Blettner, M. (2008). Leukaemia in young children living in the vicinity of German nuclear power plants. *International Journal of Cancer, 122*, 721–726.

Kagee, A., & van der Merwe, M. (2006). Predicting treatment adherence among patients attending primary health care clinics; The utility of the theory of planned behaviors. *South African Journal of Psychology, 36*(4), 699–714.

Kahn, J. A., Huang, B., Gillman, M. U., Field, A. E., Austin, S. B., & Colditz, G. A. (2008). Patterns & determinants of physical activity in US adolescents. *Journal of Adolescent Health, 42*(4), 369–377.

Kaiser Family Foundation. (2008). *Employer health benefits 2008 annual survey.* Retrieved from http://ehbs.kff.org/pfd/7790.pdf

Kaiser Family Foundation. (2023). *2023 employer health benefits survey.* Retrieved on June 27, 2024, from https://www.kff.org/health-costs/report/2023-employer-health-benefits-survey/

Kajetanowicz, A., & Kajetanowicz, A. (2016). Why parents refuse immunization? *Wiadomosci Lekarskie, 69*(3, Pt. 1), 346–351.

Kalichman, S. C., DiMarco, M., Austin, J., Luke, W., & DiFonzo, K. (2003). Stress, social support & HIV status disclosure to family and friends among HIV positive men and women. *International Journal of Behavioral Medicine, 26,* 315–332.

Kalin, M. F., & Zumoff, B. (1990). Sex hormones and coronary disease: A review of the clinical studies. *Steroids, 55,* 330–352.

Kampman, K. M. (2019). The treatment of cocaine use disorder. *Science Advances, 5*(10), eaax1532. doi: 10.1126/sciadv.aax1532

Kandel, D. B., Kessler, R. C., & Margulies, R. Z. (1978). Antecedents of adolescent initiation into stages of drug use: A developmental analysis. In D. B. Kandel (Ed.), *Longitudinal research on drug use: Empirical findings and methodological issues* (pp. 137–156). Washington, DC: Hemisphere Press.

Kandel, D. B., Simcha-Fagan, O., & Davies, M. (1986). Risk factors for delinquency and illicit drug use from adolescence to young adulthood. *Journal of Drug Issues, 16,* 67–90.

Kandel, D. B., Yamaguchi, K., & Chen, K. (1992). Stages of progression in drug involvement from adolescence to adulthood: Further evidence for the gateway theory. *Journal of Studies on Alcohol, 53,* 447–457.

Kang, M., Min, A., & Min, H. (2020). Gender convergence in alcohol consumption patterns: Findings from the Korea National Health and Nutrition Examination Survey 2007–2016. *International Journal of Environmental Research and Public Health, 17*(24), 9317. doi: 10.3390/ijerph17249317

Kann, L., McManus, T., Harris, W. A., Shanklin, S. L., Flint, K. H., Hawkins, J., . . . Zaza, S. (2016). Youth risk behavior surveillance – United States 2015. *MMWR Surveillance Summary, 65*(6), 1–174.

Kannel, W. B., Dawber, T. R., Friedman, G. D., Glennon, W. E., & McNamara, P. H. (1964). Risk factors in coronary heart disease. *Annals of Internal Medicine, 61*(5), 888–900.

Kapke, B. (2004). Yin & yang: Energy medicine. *Massage & Bodywork.*

Kaplan, H. B., Martin, S. S., & Robbins, C. (1984). Pathways to adolescent drug use: Self-derogation and adolescent drug use. *Journal of Health and Social Behavior, 25,* 270–285.

Karimy, M., Bastami, F., Sharifat, R., Heydarabadi, A. B., Hatamzadeh, N., Pakpour, A. H., . . . Araban, M. (2021). Factors related to preventive COVID-19 behaviors using health belief model among general population: A cross-sectional study in Iran. *BMC Public Health, 21,* 1934. doi: 10.1186/s12889-021-11983-3

Karlsson, M., Bergenheim, A., Larsson, M. E. H., Nordeman, L., van Tulder, M., & Bernhardsson, S. (2020). Effects of exercise therapy in patients with acute low back pain: A systematic review of systematic reviews. *BMC Systematic Reviews, 9,* 182. doi: 10.1186/s13643-020-01412-8

Katz, P. P. (1995). The impact of rheumatoid arthritis on life activities. *Arthritis Care & Research, 8*(4), 272–278.

Katz, P. P., & Yelin, E. H. (1994). Life activities of persons with rheumatoid arthritis with and without depressive symptoms. *Arthritis Care & Research, 7*(2), 69–77.

Kaur, S., Cohen, A., Dolor, R., Coffman, C. J., & Bastian, L. A. (2004). The impact of environmental tobacco smoke on women's risk of dying from heart disease: A meta-analysis. *Journal of Women's Health, 13*(8), 888–897.

Kawachi, I., Sparrow, D., Kubzansky, L. D., Spiro, A., Vokones, P. S., & Weiss, S. T. (1998). Prospective study of a self-report type-A scale & risk of coronary heart disease. *Circulation, 98,* 405–412.

Kawano, Y. (2008). Association of job-related stress factors with psychological and somatic symptoms among Japanese hospital nurses: Effects of departmental environment in acute care hospitals. *Journal of Occupational Health, 50*(1), 79–85.

Kawohl, W., & Nordt, C. (2020). COVID-19, unemployment, and suicide. *The Lancet, 7,* 389–390. doi: 10.1016/S2215-0366(20)30141-3

Keefe, F. J., Smith, S. J., Buffington, A. L. H., Gibson, J., Studts, J. L., & Caldwell, D. S. (2002). Recent advances and future directions in the biopsychosocial assessment and treatment of arthritis. *Journal of Consulting and Clinical Psychology, 70*, 640–655.

Kelley, E., Moy, E., Stryer, D., Burstin, H., & Clancy, C. (2005). The national healthcare quality and disparities reports: An overview. *Medical Care, 43*(3 suppl.), I3–I8.

Kelly, J. A., St Lawrence, J. S., Diaz, Y. E., Stevenson, L. Y., Hauth, A. C., Brasfield, T. L., . . . Andrew, M. E. (1991). HIV risk behavior reduction following intervention with key opinion leaders of population: An experimental analysis. *American Journal of Public Health, 81*(2), 168–171.

Kelly, Y., Zilanawala, A., Booker, C., & Sacker, A. (2019). Social media use and adolescent mental health: Findings from the UK Millennium Cohort Study. *The Lancet: eClinical Medicine, 6*, 59–68. doi: 10.1016/j.eclinm.2018.12.005

Kemp, E., Burton, S., Creyer, E. H., & Suter, T. A. (2007). When do nutrient content & nutrient content claims matter? Assessing consumer trade-offs between carbohydrates & fat. *Journal of Consumer Affairs, 41*, 47–73.

Kendro, W. (2008). Canadian disparities in access to healthcare. *Canadian Medical Association Journal, 179*(9), 892.

Kennedy, M. (2016). Lead-laced water in Flint: A step-by-step look at the makings of a crisis. *National Public Radio*. Retrieved August 2, 2023

Kenya, P. R., Gatiti, S., Muthami, L. N., Agwanda, R., Mwenesi, H. A., Katsivo, M. N., . . . van Andel, F. G. (1990). Oral rehydration therapy and social marketing in Kenya. *Social Science and Medicine, 31*, 979–987.

Kershaw, T. S., Mood, D. W., Newth, G., Ronis, D. L., Sanda, M. G., Vaishampayan, U., & Northouse, L. L. (2008). Longitudinal analysis of a model to predict quality of life in prostate cancer patients and their spouses. *Annals of Behavioral Medicine, 36*(2), 117–128.

Kessler, K. M. (1992). Syndrome X: The epicardial view. *Journal of the American College of Cardiology, 19*, 32–33.

Keyes, K. M., Grant, B. F., & Hasin, D. S. (2008). Evidence for a closing gender gap in alcohol use, abuse, and dependence in the United States population. *Drug and Alcohol Dependence, 93*(1–2), 21–29.

KFF. (2023). *2023 Employer Health Benefits Survey*. Retrieved February 28, 2024

KFF. (2024). *Health care costs: A primer*. Retrieved February 28, 2024

Khan, A., & Hussain, R. (2008). Violence against women in Pakistan: Perceptions and expressions of domestic violence. *Asian Studies Review, 32*(2), 239–253.

Khan, A., & Obhi, S. S. (2021). Don't sweat it! Neuroimaging studies of stress. In D. F. Ragin & J. P. Keenan (Eds.), *Handbook of research methods in health psychology* (pp. 184–197). New York, NY: Routledge/Taylor & Francis Group.

Khan, J. R., & Pearlon, L. I. (2006). Financial strain over the life course & health among older adults. *Journal of Health & Social Behavior, 47*(1), 17–31.

Khan, M. A. (2006). *The facts: Ankylosing spondylitis*. Oxford, UK: Oxford University Press.

Khan, M. A. (2023). HLA-B*27 and ankylosing spondylitis: 50 years of insights and discoveries. *Current Rheumatology Reports, 25*, 327–340. doi: 10.1007/s11926-023-01118-5

Khurana, V. G., Teo, C., Kundi, M., Hardell, L., & Carlberg, M. (2009). Cell phones and brain tumors: A review including the long-term epidemiological data. *Surgical Neurology, 72*, 205–214.

Kidd, B. L. (2006). Topical review: Osteoarthritis and joint pain. *Pain, 123*, 1–6. New York: Random House.

Kidder, T. (2003). *Mountains beyond mountains*. New York: Random House.

Kiecolt-Glaser, J.K., & Glaser, R. (1988). Psychological influences on immunity: Implications for AIDS. *American Psychologist, 43,* 892–898.

Kiecolt-Glaser, J.K., & Glaser, R. (1995). Psychoneuroimmunology and health consequences data & shared mechanisms. *Psychosomatic Medicine, 57,* 269–274.

Kiecolt-Glaser, J.K., Fisher, L.K., & Ogrocki, P. (1987). Marital quality, marital disruption, and immune function. *Psychosomatic Medicine, 49,* 13–33.

Kiecolt-Glaser, J.K., Gouin, J.P., & Hantsoo, L. (2009, September 12). Close relationship inflammation & health. *Neuroscience & Biobehavioral Review, 35*(1), 33–38.

Kiecolt-Glaser, J.K., Gouin, J.-P., & Hantsoo, L. (2010). Close relationships, inflammation, and Health. *Neuroscience & Biobehavioral Reviews, 35*(1), 33–38. doi: 10.1016/j.neubiorev.2009.09.003

Kiecolt-Glaser, J.K., & Newton, T.L. (2001). Marriage & health: His & hers. *Psychological Bulletin, 127,* 472–503.

Kiecolt-Glaser, J.K., Ricker, D., George, J., Messick, G., Speicher, C.E., Garner, W., & Glaser, R. (1984). Urinary cortisol levels, cellular immunocompetency & loneliness in psychiatric in-patients. *Psychosomatic Medicine, 46,* 15–23.

Kim, H., Neubert, J.K., San Miguel, A., Xu, K., Krishnaraju, R.K., Iadarola, M.J., . . . Dionne, R.A. (2004). Genetic influences on variability in human acute experimental pain sensitivity associated with gender, ethnicity & psychological temperament. *Pain, 109,* 488–496.

Kim, J., Han, J.Y., Shaw, B., McTavish, F., & Gustafso, D. (2010). The roles of social support and coping strategies in predicting breast cancer patients' emotional well-being: Testing mediation and moderation models. *Journal of Health Psychology, 15*(4), 543–552.

Kim, S., Koniak-Griffin, D., Fluskerund, J.H., & Guarnero, P.A. (2004). The impact of lay health advisors on cardiovascular health promotion: Using a community-based participatory approach. *Journal of Cardiovascular Nursing, 19*(3), 192–199.

Kim, Y.-R., Nakai, J.N., & Thomas, J.J. (2020). Introduction to a special issue on eating disorders in Asia. *International Journal of Eating Disorders, 54*(1), 3–6. doi: 10.1002/eat.23444

Kimball, C.P. (1981). *The biopsychosocial approach to the patient.* Baltimore: Williams & Wilkins.

King, E., DeSilva, M., Stein, A., & Patel, V. (2009). Interventions for improving the psychosocial well-being of children affected by HIV and AIDS. *Cochrane Database System Review, 15*(2), 733.

King, M.C., Marks, J.H., Mandell, J.B., & New York Breast Cancer Study Group. (2003). Breast and ovarian cancer risks due to inherited mutations in BRCA1 and BRCA2. *Science, 302,* 643–646.

Kirby, T. (2021). Global tuberculosis progress reversed by COVID-19 pandemic. *The Lancet: Respiratory Medicine, 9*(12), E118–E119. doi: 10.1016/S2213-2600(21)00496-3

Kirscht, J.P. (1977). Communication between patient and physician. *Annals of Internal Medicine, 86*(4), 499–500.

Kiwi, M., Hydén, L.-C., & Antelius, E. (2017). Deciding upon transition to residential care for persons living with dementia: Why do Iranian family caregivers living in Sweden cease caregiving at home? *Journal of Cross-Cultural Gerontology, 33,* 21–42. doi: 10.1007/s10823-017-9337-1

Klatsky, A.L. (2007). Alcohol cardiovascular diseases and diabetes mellitus. *Pharmacological Research, 55*(3), 237–247.

Klausen, M.K., Thomsen, M., Wortwein, G., & Fink-Jensen, A. (2021). The role of glucagon-like peptide 1 (GLP-1) in addictive disorders. *British Journal of Pharmacology, 179*(4), 625–641. doi: 10.1111/bph.15677

Klein, J.D., & St. Clair, S. (2000). Do candy cigarettes encourage young people to smoke? *British Medical Journal, 321,* 362–365.

Klein, J. D., Thomas, R. K., & Sutter, E. J. (2007). History of childhood candy cigarette use is associated with tobacco smoking by adults. *Preventive Medicine*, *45*(1), 26–30.

Klein, J. D., Wilson, K. M., & McNulty, M. (1999). Access to medical care for adolescents: Results from the 1997 Commonwealth Fund study of the health of adolescent girls. *Journal of Adolescent Health*, *25*, 120–130.

Klein, R. (2001). What's happening to Britain's national health service? *New England Journal of Medicine*, *345*(4), 305–308.

Knox, S. S., Hausdorff, J., & Markovitz, J. H. (2002). Reactivity as a predictor of subsequent blood pressure: Racial differences in the coronary artery risk development in young adults (CARDIA) study. *Hypertension*, *40*(6), 914–919.

Knussen, C., Tolson, D., Swan, I. R. C., Slott, D. J., & Brogan, C. A. (2005). Stress proliferation in caregivers: The relationship between caregiving stressors & deterioration in family relationships. *Psychology & Health*, *20*(2), 207–221.

Kochanek, K. D., Murphy, S. L., Jiaquan, B. S., & Tejada-Verz, B. (2016, June 30). National vital statistics report. *Deaths: Final Data for 2014*, *65*(4). Centers for Disease Control and Prevention.

Kochanek, K. D., Murphy, S. L., Xu, J., & Tejada-Vega, B. (2016). *Deaths: Final data for 2014* (National Vital Statistics report no. 65(4)). Hyattsville, MD: National Center for Health Statistics. Centers for Disease Control and Prevention.

Kochanek, K. D., Xu, J., Murphy, S. L., Miniño, A. M., & Kung, H. C. (2011). *Deaths: Preliminary data for 2009* (National Vital Statistics report no. 4). Hyattsville, MD: National Center for Health Statistics. Centers for Disease Control and Prevention.

Koh, K. B. (2011). *Stress and psychosomatic medicine*. Seoul, Korea: Ilchokak.

Koh, K. B., Lee, Y.-J., Beyn, K. M., Chu, S. H., Kim, D. M., & Won, Y. S. (2012). Effects of high and low stress on proinflammatory and antiinflammatory cytokines. *Psychophysiology*, *49*, 1290–1297.

Kohler, C. L., Grimley, D., & Reynolds, K. (1999). Theoretical approaches guiding the development and implementation of health promotion programs. In J. Raczynski & R. DiClemente (Eds.), *Handbook of health promotion and disease prevention* (pp. 23–44). New York: Kluwer Academic/Plenum Publishers.

Kolata, G., & Mueller, B. (2022, January 19). Halting progress and happy accidents: How mRNA vaccines were made. *International New York Times*. Retrieved April 20, 2023 from https://link.gale.com/apps/doc/A689825379/AONE?u=nysl_oweb&sid=googleScholar&xid=c95770d9

Kołodziej, J. (2016). Effects of stress on HIV infection progression. *HIV & AIDS Review*, *15*(1), 13–16. doi: 10.1016/j.hivar.2015.07.003

Komal, R., & Gurpreet, G. (2016). Loneliness in relation to social networking site usage among university students. *Indian Journal of Health & Well-Being*, *7*(5), 518–521.

Kombe Kombe, A. J., Li, B., Zahid, A., Mengist, H. M., Bounda, G. A., Zhou, Y., & Jin, T. (2021). Epidemiology and burden of human papillomavirus and related diseases, molecular pathogenesis, and vaccine evaluation. *Frontiers in Public Health*, *8*, 552028. doi: 10.3389/fpubh.2020.552028

Korotkin, B. D., Hoerger, M., Voorhees, S., Allen, C. O., Robinson, W. R., & Duberstein, P. R. (2019). Social support in cancer: How do patients want us to help? *Journal of Psychosocial Oncology*, *37*(6). doi: 10.1080/073473332.2019.1580331

Kosek, E., Cohen, M., Baron, R., Gebhart, G., Mico, J.-A., Rice, A., . . . Sluka, A. K. (2016). Do we need a third mechanistic descriptor for chronic pain states? *Pain*, *157*(7), 1382–1386. doi: 10.1097/j.pain.0000000000000507

Kostecka, B., Kordyńska, K. K., Murawiec, S., & Kucharska, K. (2019). Distorted body image in women and men suffering from anorexia nervosa – A literature review. *Archives of Psychiatry and Psychotherapy, 1,* 13–21. doi: 10.12740/APP/102833

Kotchick, B. A., Shaffer, A., Forehand, R., & Miller, K. S. (2001). Adolescent sexual risk behavior: A multi-system perspective. *Clinical Psychology Review, 21,* 493–519. doi: 10.1016/S0272-7358(99)00070-7

Kraft, P., & Kraft, B. (2023). Exploring the relationship between multiple dimensions of subjective socioeconomic status and self-reported physical and mental health: The mediating role of affect. *Frontiers in Psychology, 11.* Retrieved July 22, 2023, from www.frontiersin.org/articles/10.3389/fpubh.2023.1138367/full

Kramer, R. (2021). Social networks, depression, and stress. In D. F. Ragin & J. P. Keenan (Eds.), *Handbook of research methods in health psychology* (pp. 170–183). New York, NY: Routledge, Taylor & Francis Group.

Krammer, F., Smith, G. J. D., Fouchier, R. A. M., Peiris, M., Kedzierska, K., Doherty, P. C., . . . García-Sastre, A. (2018). Influenza. *Nature Reviews Disease Primers, 12*(1), 15–22.

Kranzler, H. R., & Soyka, M. (2018). Diagnosis and pharmacotherapy of alcohol use disorder: A review. *JAMA, 320*(8), 815–824. doi: 10.1001/jama.2018.11406

Krassner, M. (1986). Effective features of therapy from the healer's perspective: A study of *curanderismo*. *Smith College Studies in Social Work, 56,* 157–183.

Kraus, M. W., Adler, N., & Chen, T.-W. D. (2013). Is the association of subjective SES and self-rated health confounded by negative mood? An experimental approach. *Health Psychology, 32*(2), 138–145. doi: 10.1037/a0027343

Kraus, R., Patterson, M., & Lundmark, V. (1998). Internet paradox: A social technology that reduces social involvement and psychological well-being? *American Psychologist, 53,* 1017–1031.

Kreps, G. L. (2002). Consumer/provider communication research: A personal plea to address issues of ecological validity, relational, development, message diversity, and situational constraints. In D. F. Marks (Ed.), *The health psychology reader.* London: Sage Publications.

Kreps, G. L. (2018). Promoting patient comprehension of relevant health information. *Israel Journal of Health Policy Research, 7*(1), 56. doi: 10.1186/13584-018-0250-z

Kriss, J. L., Collins, S. R., Mahato, B., Gould, E., & Schoen, C. (2008). *Rite of passage: Why young adults become uninsured & how new policies can help. 2008 Update.* The Commonwealth Fund. Retrieved October 3, 2009, from www.commonwealthfund.org/Publications/Fund-Reports/2008/May/Rite-of-Passage – Why-Young-Adults-Become-Uninsured-and-How-New-Policies-Can-Help-2008-Update.aspx

Kropp, R. Y., & Halpern-Felsher, B. L. (2004). Adolescents' beliefs about the risks involved in smoking "light" cigarettes. *Pediatrics, 114*(4), 445–451.

Kross, E., Verduyn, P., Demiralp, E., Park, J., Lee, D. S., Lin, N., . . . Ybarra, O. (2013). Facebook use predicts decline in subjective well-being in young adults. *PLoS One, 8,* e698441.

Kublin, J. G., & Steketee, R. W. (2006). HIV infection and malaria: Understanding the interactions. *Journal of Infectious Diseases, 193*(1), 1–3.

Kuiper, N. A., & Nicholl, S. (2004). Thoughts of feeling better? Sense of humor & physical health. *International Journal of Humor Research, 14,* 37–66.

Kulak, J. A., & LaValley, S. (2018). Cigarette use and smoking beliefs among older Americans: Findings from a nationally representative survey. *Journal of Addictive Diseases, 37*(1–2), 46–54. doi: 10.1080/10550887.2018.1521255

Kulbok, P. A., & Cox, C. L. (2002). Dimensions of adolescent health behavior. *Journal of Adolescent Health, 31,* 294–400.

Kumpfer, K. L., & Turner, C. W. (1990–1991). The social ecology model of adolescent substance abuse: Implications for prevention. *International Journal of the Addictions, 25*, 435–463.

Kung, H.-C., Hoyert, D. L., Yu, J., & Murphy, S. L. (2008). Death: Final data for 2005. *National Vital Statistics Reports, 56*(10), 1–121. Centers for Disease Control and Prevention.

Kunz, J. R. M. (1982). *The American Medical Association family medical guide.* New York: Random House.

Kuo, P. X., Braungart-Rieker, J. M., Burke Lefever, J. E., Sarma, M. S., O'Neill, M., & Gettler, L. T. (2018). Fathers' cortisol and testosterone in the days around infants' births predict later paternal involvement. *Hormones and Behavior, 106*, 28–34. doi: 10.1016/j.yhbeh.2018.08.011

Kuoppala, J., Lamminpaa, A., & Husman, P. (2008). Work health promotion, job well-being & sickness absences: A systematic review and meta-analysis. *Journal of Occupational and Environmental Medicine, 50*(11), 1216–1227.

Kupper, N., & Denollet, J. (2007). Type D personality as a prognostic factor in heart disease. *Journal of Personality Assessment, 89*, 265–276.

Kurian, A. K., & Cardarelli, K. M. (2007). Racial and ethnic differences in cardiovascular disease risk factors: A systematic review. *Ethnic Diseases, 17*(1), 143–152.

Kwok, W., & Bhuvanakrishna, T. (2014). The relationship between ethnicity and the pain experience of cancer patients: A systematic review. *Indian Journal of Palliative Care, 20*(3), 194–200. doi: 10.4103/0973-1075.138391

Kyngas, H., Mikkonen, B., Nousianinen, E.-M., Rytilahti, M., Seppanes, P., Vaatlovaara, R., & Jamsa, T. (2001). Coping with the onset of cancer: Coping strategies and resources of young people with cancer. *European Journal of Cancer Care, 10*(1), 6–11.

Labbe, E., Schmidt, N., Babin, J., & Pharr, M. (2008). Coping with stress: The effectiveness of different types of music. *Applied Psychophysiology and Biofeedback, 32*(3–4), 163–168.

Lacey, J. H., & Dolan, B. M. (1988). Bulimia in British blacks and Asians: A catchment area study. *British Journal of Psychiatry, 152*, 73–79.

Lacey, M. (2009, April 29). From Edgar, 5, coughs heard around the world. *The New York Times*, p. A1 and A10.

Lai, H. T. M., Threapleton, D. E., Day, A. J., Williamson, G., Cade, J. E., & Burley, V. J. (2015). Fruit intake and cardiovascular disease mortality in the UK Women's Cohort Study. *European Journal of Epidemiology, 30*, 1035–1048. doi: 10.1007/s10654-015-0050-5

Laird, L. D., Curtis, C. E., & Morgan, J. R. (2017). Finding spirits in spirituality: What are we measuring in spirituality and health research? *Journal of Religion and Health, 56*, 1–20. doi: 10.1007/s10943-016-0316-6

Lalani, N. (2020). Meanings and interpretations of spirituality in nursing and Health. *Religions, 11*(9), 428. doi: 10.3390/rel11090428

Lallemant, M., Jourdain, G., Le Coeur, S., Mary, J. Y., Ngo-Giang-Huong, N., & Koetsawang, S. (2004). Single-dose perinatal nevirapine plus standard zidovudine to prevent mother-to-child transmission of HIV-1 in Thailand. *The New England Journal of Medicine, 351*, 217–228.

Lam, T. P. (2001). Strengths and weaknesses of traditional Chinese medicine and Western medicine in the eyes of some Hong Kong Chinese. *Journal of Epidemiological and Community Health, 55*, 762.

Landau, E. (2010). Studies show 'dark chapter' of medical research. *CNN.* Retrieved February 1, 2024, from www.cnn.com/2010/HEALTH/10/01/guatemala.syphilis.tuskegee/index.html

Lando, A. M., & Labiner-Wolfe, J. (2006). Helping consumers make more healthful food choices: Consumer views on modifying food labels and providing point-of-purchase nutritional information at quick-service restaurants. *Journal of Nutritional Education and Behavior, 39*(3), 157–163.

Landon, B. E., Reschovsky, J. D., Pham, H. H., Kitsantas, P., Wojtuskiak, J., & Hadley, J. (2009). Creating a parsimonious typology of physician financial incentives. *Health Services and Outcomes Research Methodology*, 9, 219–233. doi: 10.1007/s10742-010-0057-z

Lane, D. A., Langman, C. M., Lip, G. Y. H., & Nouwen, A. (2009). Illness perceptions, affective responses, health-related quality-of-life in patients with atrial fibrillation. *Journal of Psychosomatic Research*, 66(3), 211–220.

Lapate, R. C., Lee, H., Salomons, T. V., van Reekum, C. M., Greischar, L. L., & Davidson, R. J. (2011). Amygdalar function reflects common individual differences in emotion and pain regulation success. *Journal of Cognitive Neuroscience*, 24, 148–158.

Larson, H., Hartigan-Go, K., & de Figueiredo, A. (2019). Vaccine confidence plummets in the Philippines following dengue vaccine scare: Why it matters to pandemic preparedness. *Human Vaccines & Immunotherapeutics*, 15(3), 625–627. doi: 10.1080/21645515.2018.1522468

Lasselin, J., Alvarez-Salas, E., & Grigoleit, J.-S. (2016). Well-being and immune response: A multi-system perspective. *Current Opinion in Pharmacology*, 29, 34–41. doi: 10.1016/j.coph.2016.05.003

Lasser, K. E., Himmelstein, D. U., & Woolhandler, S. (2006). Access to care, health status & health disparities in the United States and Canada: Results of a cross-national population-based survey. *American Journal of Public Health*, 96(7), 1300–1307.

Lasser, K. E., Mintzer, I. L., Lambert, A., Cabral, H., & Bor, D. H. (2005). Missed appointment rates in primary care: The importance of site of care. *Journal of Health Care of the Poor and Underserved*, 16(3), 475–486.

Lau, J. S., Adams, S. H., Boscardin, W. J., & Irwin, C. E. (2014). Young adults' health care utilization and expenditures prior to the Affordable Care Act. *Journal of Adolescent Health*, 54(6), 663–671. doi: 10.1016/j.jadohealth.2014.03.001

Laurent, S., & Bautouyrie, P. (2007). Arterial stiffness: A new surrogate and end-point for cardiovascular disease? *Journal of Nephrology*, 20(suppl. 12), S45–S50.

LaVeist, T. A., & Nuru-Jeter, A. (2002). Is doctor-patient race concordance associated with greater satisfaction with care? *Journal of Health and Social Behavior*, 43(3), 296–306.

Lawrence, C. (2007). *Teens drive distracted*. CNN Transcript. Retrieved from www.Cnn.com/2007/ EDUCATION/01/25/transcript.fri/index.html#first

Lawrence, R. C., Helmick, C. G., Arnett, F. C., Deyo, R. A., Felson, D. T., Giannini, E. H., . . . Wolfe, F. (1998). Estimates of the prevalence of arthritis & selected musculoskeletal disorders in the United States. *Arthritis & Rheumatism*, 41(5), 778–799.

Lazarus, R. S., DeLonges, A., Folkman, S., & Gruen, R. (1985). Stress & adaptation outcomes: The problem of confounded measures. *American Psychologists*, 40(1), 770–779.

Lazarus, R. S., & Folkman, S. (1984a). Coping and adaptation. In W. D. Gentry (Ed.), *Handbook of behavioral medicine* (pp. 282–325). New York: Guilford Press.

Lazarus, R. S., & Folkman, S. (1984b). *Stress, appraisal and coping*. New York: Springer.

Lazarus, R. S., & Folkman, S. (1987). Transactional theory & research in emotions & coping. *European Journal of Personality*, 1, 141–169.

Lea, E. J., Crawford, D., & Worsley, A. (2006). Public views of the benefits and barriers to the consumption of a plant-based diet. *European Journal of Clinical Nutrition*, 60(7), 828–837.

Lechner, S. C., Carver, C. S., Antoni, M. H., Weaver, K. E., & Phillips, K. M. (2006). Curvilinear associations between benefit finding & psychosocial adjustment to breast cancer. *Journal of Consulting & Clinical Psychology*, 74(5), 828–840.

Lee, A. R. Y. B., Leong, I., Lao, G., Tan, A. W., Ho, R. C. M., Ho, C. S. H., & Chen, M. Z. (2023). Depression and anxiety in older adults with cancer: Systematic review and meta-summary of risks, protective and exacerbating factors. *General Hospital Psychiatry, 81*, 32–42.

Lee, I. M., & Paffenberger, R. S. (1992). Quetelet's index and risk of colon cancer in college alumni. *Journal of the National Cancer Institute, 84*, 1326–1331.

Lee, J., Pomeroy, E., & Bohman, T. (2007). Intimate partner violence & psychological health in a sample of Asian and Caucasian women: The roles of social support and caring. *Journal of Family Violence, 22*(8), 709–720.

Lee, L. V., & Foody, J. M. (2008). Cardiovascular disease in women. *Current Atherosclerosis Report, 10*(4), 295–302.

Lee, M. S., Kim, B. G., Huh, H. J., Ryu, H., Lee, H. S., & Chung, H. T. (2000). Effect of qi-training on blood pressure, heart rate & respiration rate. *Clinical Psychology, 20*, 173–176.

Lee, P., Le Saux, M., Siegel, R., Goyal, M., Chen, C., Ma, Y., & Meltzer, A. C. (2019). Racial and ethnic disparities in the management of acute pain in US emergency departments: Meta-analysis and systematic review. *American Journal of Emergency Medicine, 37*(9), 1770–1777. doi: 10.1016/j.ajem.2019.06.014

Lee, S. Y., Hwang, H., Hawkins, R., & Pingree, S. (2008). Interplay of negative emotion and health self-efficacy on the use of health information and its outcomes. *Communication Research, 35*(3), 358–381. doi: 10.1177/0093650208315962

Lees, B., Meredith, L. R., Kirkland, A. E., Bryant, B. E., & Squeglia, L. M. (2020). Effect of alcohol use on the adolescent brain and behavior. *Pharmacology Biochemistry and Behavior, 192*. doi: 10.1016/j.pbb.2020.172906

Leist, A. K. (2013). Social media use of older adults: A mini review. *Gerontology, 59*, 378–384.

Leisuk, T. (2008). The effects of preferred music listening on stress levels of air traffic controllers. *The Arts in Psychotherapy, 35*(1), 1–10.

LeMaster, P. J., Beub, J., Novins, D. K., & Manson, S. M. (2004). The prevalence of suicidal behaviors among Northern Plains American Indians. *Suicide & Life Threatening Behavior, 34*, 242.

Leonard, B. E. (2014). Impact of inflammation on neurotransmitter changes in major depression: An insight into the action of antidepressants. *Progress in Neuro-Psychopharmacology and Biological Psychiatry, 48*(3), 261–267.

Leonard, K. E., & Quigley, B. M. (2017). Thirty years of research show alcohol to be a cause of intimate partner violence: Future research needs to identify who to treat and how to treat them. *Drug and Alcohol Review, 36*, 7–9. doi: 10.1111/dar.12434

Lepore, S. T., Revenson, T. A., Weinberger, S. L., Weston, P., Pasquale, G., & Frisina, M. A. (2006). Effects of social stressors on cardiovascular reactivity in black and white women. *Annals of Behavioral Medicine, 31*(2), 120–127.

Lerchl, A., Klose, M., Grote, K., Wilhelm, A. F., Spathmann, O., Fiedler, T., . . . Clemens, M. (2015). Tumor promotion by exposure to radiofrequency electromagnetic fields below exposure limits for humans. *Biochemical and Biophysical Research Communications, 459*, 585–590. doi: 10.1016/j.bbrc.2015.02.151

Lerner, E. B., Jehle, D. H. V., & Janicke, D. M. (2000). Medical communication: Do our patients understand? *American Journal of Emergency Medicine, 18*, 764–766.

Leserman, J. (2008). Role of depression, stress and trauma in HIV disease progression. *Psychosomatic Medicine, 70*, 539–545.

Lesiuk, T. (2008). The effects of preferred music listening on stress levels of air traffic controllers. *The Arts in Psychotherapy, 35*(1), 1–10.

Levenson, R. W. (2019). Stress and Illness: A role for specific emotions. *Psychosomatic Medicine*, *81*(8), 720–730. doi: 10.1097/PSY.0000000000000736

Levine, P. B., McKnight, R., & Heep, S. (2011). How effective are public policies to increase health insurance coverage among young adults? *American Economic Journal: Economic Policy*, *3*(1), 129–156. doi: 10.1257/pol.3.1.129

Levinson, Z., Hulver, S., & Neuman, T. (2022). Hospital charity care: How it works and why it matters. *KFF*. Retrieved February 28, 2024

Levy, J. A., Shimabukuro, J., & Hollander, H. (1985). Isolation of AIDS-associated retrovirus from the cerebrospinal fluid and brain of patients with neurological symptoms. *Lancet*, *2*, 580–586.

Lewin, K. (1935). *A dynamic theory of personality*. London: McGraw-Hill.

Ley, P., & Spelman, M. S. (1965). Communications in an out-patient setting. *British Journal of Clinical Psychology*, *4*(2), 114–116.

Liberatos, P., Link, B. G., & Kelsey, J. L. (1988). The measurement of social class in epidemiology. *Epidemiologic Review*, *10*(1), 87–121.

Lima, S., Teixeira, L., Esteves, R., Ribeiro, F., Pereria, F., Teixeira, A., & Magalhães, C. (2020) Spirituality and quality of life in older adults: A path analysis model. *BMC Geriatrics*, *20*. Article No. 259. doi: 10.1186/s12877-020-01646-0

Lin, W., Hang, C. M., Yang, H. C., & Hung, M. H. (2011). Nutrition & health survey in Taiwan: The nutrition, knowledge, attitude & behavior of 19–64 years old adults. *Asia Pacific Journal of Clinical Nutrition*, *20*, 309–318.

Lindberg, L. D., & Kantor, L. M. (2022). Adolescents' receipt of sex education in a nationally representative sample, 2011–2019. *Journal of Adolescent Health*, *70*(2), 290–297. doi: 10.1016/j.jadohealth.2021.08.027

Lindberg, N. M., & Wellisch, B. (2001). Anxiety and compliance among women at risk for breast cancer. *Annals of Behavioral Medicine*, *23*, 298–303.

Lindegger, G., & Richter, L. (2000). Relationships between science and ethics in HIV/AIDS prevention trials. *South African Journal of Science*, *96*, 313–317.

Lindholm, L., Rehnsfeldt, A., Arman, M., & Hamrin, E. (2002). Significant other's experience of suffering when living with women with breast cancer. *Scandinavian Journal of Care Science (Special Issue: The Challenging Complexity of Cancer Care Research)*, *16*, 248–255.

Linton, S. J. (2000). A review of psychological risk factors in back and neck pain. *Spine*, *25*, 1148–1156.

Linzer, M., Bitton, A., Tu, S. P., Plews-Ogan, M., Horowitz, D., & Schwartz, M. (2015). The end of the 15–20 minute primary care visit. *Journal of General Internal Medicine*, *30*, 1584–1586. doi: 10.1007/s11606-015-3341-3

Lister, T., & McKenzie, D. (2021, December 2). How South African scientists discovered Omicron and set off a global chain reaction. *CNN*. Retrieved November 11, 2023

Little, H., Swinson, D. R., & Cruickshank, B. (1976). Upward subluxation of the axis in ankylosing spondylitis. *American Journal of Medicine*, *60*(2), 279–285.

Little, L. K. (Ed.). (2007). *Plague and the end of antiquity: The pandemic of 541–750*. New York: Cambridge University Press.

Littman, R. J., & Littman, M. L. (1973). Galena and the Antonine plague. *American Journal of Philology*, *94*, 254–255.

Liu, G., Hariri, S., Bradley, H., Gottlieb, S. L., Leichliter, J. S., & Markowitz, L. E. (2015). Trends and patterns of sexual behaviors among adolescents and adults aged 14 to 59 years, United States. *Sexually Transmitted Diseases*, *42*(1), 20–26. doi: 10.1097/OLQ.0000000000000231

Liu, R. V., & Chen, Z.-Y. (2006). The effects of marital conflict & disruption on depressive affect: A comparison between women in & out of poverty. *Social Science Quarterly*, 87, 250–271.

Livingston, I. L., Levine, D. M., & Moore, R. D. (1991). Social integration and Black intraracial variation in blood pressure. *Ethnicity & Disease*, 1, 135–149.

Lloyd-Jones, D. M., Huffman, M. D., Karmali, K. N., Sanghavi, D. M., Wright, J. S., Pelser, C., . . . Goff, D. C. (2017). Estimating longitudinal risks and benefits from cardiovascular preventive therapies among Medicare patients: The Million Hearts Longitudinal ASCVD Risk Assessment Tool: A special report from the American Heart Association and American College of Cardiology. *Circulation*, 135(13), e793–e813. doi: 10.1161/CIR.0000000000000467

Lock, J., & Fitzpatrick, K. K. (2009). Anorexia nervosa. *Clinical Evidence*, 10, 1011.

Locke, S. E., Kraus, L., & Lesserman, J. (1984). Life change stress, psychiatric symptoms, and natural killer cell activity. *Psychosomatic Medicine*, 46, 441–453.

Loeser, J. D. (2003). The decade of pain control and research. *American Pain Society Bulletin*, 13, 3.

Loewenson, R. (2007). Exploring equity and inclusion in the responses to AIDS. *AIDS Care*, 19(suppl. 1), S2–S11.

Lonn, S., Ahlbom, A., Hall, P., & Feychting, M. (2004). Mobile phone use and the risk of acoustic neuroma. *Epidemiology*, 15, 653–659.

Lopez, R. A. (2005). Use of alternative folk medicine by Mexican American women. *Journal of Immigrant Health*, 7(1), 23–31.

Lopez-Velez, M., Martinez-Martinez, E., & Del Valle-Rebes, C. (2003). The study of phenolic compounds as natural antioxidants in wine. *Critical Review of Food Science and Nutrition*, 43(3), 233–244.

Lord, K., Livingston, G., & Cooper, C. (2014). A systematic review of barriers and facilitators to and interventions for proxy decision-making by family carers of people with dementia. *International Psychogeriatrics*, 27(8), 1301–1312. doi: 10.1017/S1041610215000411

Lou, J.-H., & Chen, S.-H. (2009). Relationships among sexual knowledge, sexual attitudes, and safe sex behaviour among adolescents: A structural equation model. *International Journal of Nursing Studies*, 46(12), 1595–1603. doi: 10.1016/j.ijnurstu.2009.05.017

Lowe, R. A., Localio, A. R., Schwartz, D. F., Williams, S., Tuton, L. W., Maroney, S., . . . Feldman, H. I. (2005). Association between primary care practice characteristics and emergency department use in a Medicaid managed care organization. *Medical Care*, 43(8), 792–800.

Lowry, R., Holtzman, D., & Truman, B. (1994). Substance use and HIV-related sexual behaviors among US high school students: Are they related? *American Journal of Public Health*, 84, 1116–1120.

Lumish, H. S., Steinfield, H., Koval, C., Russo, D., Levinson, E., Wynn, J., . . . Chung, W. K. (2017). Impact of panel gene testing for hereditary breast and ovarian cancer in patients. *Journal of Genetic Counseling*, 26(5), 1116–1129.

Luna, E. (2003). Nurse-curanderas: Las que curan at the heart of Hispanic culture. *Journal of Holistic Nursing*, 21(4), 326–342.

Luszczynska, A., & Schwarzer, R. (2003). Planning and self-efficacy in the adoption and maintenance of breast self-examination: A longitudinal study of self-regulatory cognition. *Psychology & Health*, 18(1), 93–108.

Lwin, M. N., Serhal, L., Holroyd, C., & Edwards, C. J. (2020). Rheumatoid arthritis: The impact of mental health on disease: A narrative review. *Rheumatology and Therapy*, 7, 457–471. doi: 10.1007/s40744-020-00217-4

Lynch, H. T., Snyder, C. L., Shaw, T. G., Heinen, C. D., & Hitchins, M. P. (2015). Milestones of Lynch Syndrome 1895–2015. *Nature Reviews Cancer*, 15, 181–194. doi: 10.1038/nrc3878

Lynch, M. E., & Campbell, F. (2011). Cannabinoids for treatment of chronic noncancer pain, a systematic review of randomized trials. *British Journal of Clinical Pharmacology*, 72(5), 735–744.

Macharia, W. M., Shiroya, A., & Njeru, E. K. (1997). Knowledge, attitudes and beliefs of primary caretakers towards sickle cell anaemia in children. *East African Medical Journal*, 74(7), 416–419.

Madden, T. J., Ellen, P. S., & Ajzen, I. (1992). A comparison of the theory of planned behaviors and the theory of reasoned action. *Personality & Social Psychology Bulletin*, 18(1), 3–9.

Madison, A. A., Andridge, R., Shrout, M. R., Renna, M. E., Bennett, J. M., Jaremka, L. M., . . . Kiecolt-Glaser, J. K. (2022). Frequent interpersonal stress and inflammatory reactivity predict depressive-symptom increases: Two tests of the social-signal-transduction theory of depression. *Psychological Science*, 33(1), 152–164. doi: 10.1177/09567976211031225

Maes, M., Berk, M., Goehler, L., Song, C., Anderson, G., Galecki, P., & Leonard, B. (2012). Depression and sickness behavior are Janus-faced responses to shared inflammatory pathways. *BMC Medicine*, 20(10), 66.

Maes, M., Song, C., Lin, A., DeJongh, R., VanGastel, A., & Kenis, G. L. (1998). The effects of psychological stress on humans: Increased production of pro-inflammatory cytokines and a Th1-like response in stress-induced anxiety. *Cytokine*, 10, 313–318.

Mahajan, S., Caraballo, C., Lu, Y., Valero-Elizondo, J., Massey, D., Annapureddy, A. R., . . . Krumholz, H. M. (2021). Trends in differences in health status and health care access and affordability by race and ethnicity in the United States, 1999–2018. *JAMA*, 326(7), 637–648. doi: 10.1001/jama.2021.9907

Mahumud, R. A., Sahle, B. W., Owusu-Addo, E., Chen, W., Morton, R. L., & Renzaho, A. M. N. (2021). Association of dietary intake, physical activity, and sedentary behaviours with overweight and obesity among 282,213 adolescents in 89 low and middle income to high-income countries. *International Journal of Obesity*, 45, 2404–2418. doi: 10.1038/s41366-021-00908-0

Mahwasane, S. T., Middleton, L., & Boaduo, N. (2013). An ethnobotanical survey of indigenous knowledge on medicinal plants used by the traditional healers of the Lwamondo area, Limpopo province, South Africa. *South African Journal of Botany*, 88, 69–75. doi: 10.1016/j.sajb.2013.05.004

Mai, P. L., Sullivan-Hally, J., & Ursin, G. (2006). Activity and colon cancer risk among women in the California teachers study. *Cancer Epidemiology Biomarkers Prevention*, 16, 517–525.

Majeed, M., & Naseer, S. (2019). Is workplace bullying always perceived harmful? The cognitive appraisal theory of stress perspective. *Asian Pacific Journal of Human Resources*, 59(4), 616–644. doi: 10.1111/1744-7941.12244

Makenzius, M., & Larsson, M. (2013). Early onset of sexual intercourse is an indicator for hazardous lifestyle and problematic life situation. *Scandinavian Journal of Caring Sciences*, 27(1), 20–27. doi: 10.1111/j.1471-6712.2012.00989.x

Makwana, N. (2019). Disaster and its impact on mental health: A narrative review. *Journal of Family Medicine and Primary Care*, 8(10), 3090–3095. doi: 10.4103%2Fjfmpc.jfmpc_893_19

Malaria No More. (2010). *Learn the facts*. Retrieved July 6, 2010, from www.malarianomore.org/pages/the-solution

Malathi, A., & Damodaran, A. (1999). Stress due to exams in medical students-role of yoga. *Indian Journal of Physiological Pharmacology*, 43(2), 218–224.

Malcolm, C. E., Wong, K. K., & Elwood-Martin, R. (2008). Patient's perceptions of experiences of family medicine residents in the office. *Canadian Family Physician*, 54(4), 570–571.

Mallya, S., Reed, M., & Yang, L. (2019). A theoretical framework for using humor to reduce the effects of chronic stress on cognitive function in older adults: An integration of findings and methods from diverse areas of psychology. *Humor*, 32, 49–71.

Manary, M. J. (2005). *Local production and provision of ready-to-use therapeutic food for the treatment of severe child malnutrition* (Technical background paper). Geneva: WHO.

Manchikanti, L., Singh, V. M., Staats, P. S., Trescot, A. M. Prunskis, J., Knezevic, N. N., . . . Hirsch, J. A. (2022). Fourth wave of opioid (illicit drug) overdose deaths and diminishing access to prescription opioids and interventional techniques: Cause and effect. *Pain Physician, 25*, 97–124.

Manderson, L., & Kokanovic, R. (2009). "Worried all the time": Distress and the circumstances of everyday life among immigrant Australians with type 2 diabetes. *Chronic Illness, 5*(1), 21–32.

Manfredi, L., Accoto, A., Couyoumdjian, A., & Conversi, D. (2021). A systematic review of genetic polymorphisms associated with binge eating disorder. *Nutrients, 13*(3), 848. doi: 10.3390/nu13030848

Mangas-Sanjuan, C., & Jover, R. (2022). Familial colorectal cancer. *Best Practices & Research Clinical Gastroenterology, 58–59*. Retrieved March 16, 2023

Mangat, R., & Louie, T. (2023). Viral hemorrhagic fevers. In *StatPearls* [Internet]. Treasure Island, FL: StatPearls Publishing. Retrieved from www.ncbi.nlm.nih.gov/books/NBK560717/

Mangione, K. K., McCully, K., Gloviak, A., Lefebvre, I., Hoffman, M., & Craik, R. (1999). The effects of high-intensity and low-intensity cycle ergometry in older adults with knee osteoarthritis. *Journals of Gerontology: Biological Sciences and Medical Sciences, 59*, 86–93.

Manne, S. L., Ostroff, J., Rini, C., Fox, K., Goldstein, L., & Granna, G. (2004). The interpersonal process model of intimacy; the role of self-disclosure, partner-disclosure & partner responsiveness in interactions between breast cancer patients & their partners. *Journal of Family Psychology, 18*, 589–599.

Manne, S. L., Ostroff, J., Winkel, G., Grana, G., & Fox, K. (2005). Partner unsupportive responses, avoidant coping, and distress among women with early stage breast cancer: Patient and partner perspective. *Health Psychology, 24*(6), 635–641.

Manne, S. L., Taylor, K. L., Dougherty, J., & Kemeny, N. (1997). Supportive and negative responses in the partner relationship: Their association with psychological adjustment among individuals with cancer. *Journal of Behavioral Medicine, 20*, 101–125.

Maraboto, C., & Ferdinand, K. C. (2020). Update on hypertension in African-Americans. *Progress in Cardiovascular Diseases, 63*(1), 33–39. doi: 10.1016/j.pcad.2019.12.002

Marcus, R. F. (2008). Flight-seeking motivation in dating partners within an aggressive relationship. *Journal of Social Psychology, 148*(3), 261–276.

Markel, H., Gostin, L. O., & Fidler, D. P. (2007). Extensive drug-resistant tuberculosis: An isolation order, public health powers, and a global crisis. *JAMA, 298*(1), 83–86.

Marklund, M., Zheng, M., Veerman, J. L., & Wu, J. H. Y. (2020). Estimated health benefits, costs, and cost-effectiveness of eliminating industrial trans-fatty acids in Australia: A modelling study. *PLoS Medicine, 17*(11), e1003407. doi: 10.1371/journal.pmed.1003407

Markovitz, J. H., Matthews, K. A., Whooley, M., Lewis, C. E., & Greenlund, K. L. (2004). Increases in job strain are associated with incident hypertension in the CARDIA study. *Annals of Behavioral Medicine, 28*, 4–9.

Marks, D. (2002). Theories in health psychology. In D. Marks (Ed.), *The health psychology reader* (pp. 90–93). London, UK: Sage Publications.

Martin, R. A. (2001). Humor, laughter, and physical health methodological issues and research findings. *Psychological Bulletin, 127*(4), 504–519.

Martin, R. A. (2004). Sense of humor & physical health: Theoretical issues, recent findings & future directions. *International Journal of Humor Research, 14*, 1–19.

Martin, R. A. (2019). Humor. In M. W. Gallagher & S. J. Lopez (Eds.), *Positive psychological assessment: A handbook of models and measures* (pp. 305–316). American Psychological Association. doi: 10.1037/0000138-019

Martini, A., Lovell, D. J., Albani, S., Brunner, H. I., Hyrich, K. L., Thompson, S. D., & Ruperto, N. (2022). Juvenile idiopathic arthritis. *Nature Reviews Disease Primers*, 8. Article No. 5. doi: 10.1038/s41572-021-00332-8

Martinon, F., Krishnan, S., Lenzen, G., Magne, R., Gomard, E., Guillet, J.-G., . . . Meulien, P. (1993). Induction of virus-specific cytotoxic T lymphocytes in vivo by liposome-entrapped mRNA. *European Journal of Immunology*, 23(7), 1719–1922. doi: 10.1002/eji.1830230749

Martins, J. G., Guimarães, M. O., Jorge, K. O., de Paula Silva, C. J., Ferreira, R. C., Pordeus, I. A., . . . Zarzar, P. M. P. A. (2020). Binge drinking, alcohol outlet density and associated factors: A multilevel analysis among adolescents in Belo Horizonte, Minas Gerais State, Brazil. *Cadernos de Saude Publica*, 36(1). doi: 10.1590/0102-311X00052119

Martire, L. M., Schulz, R., Keefe, F. J., Starz, T. W., Osial, T. A., Jr., Dew, M. A., & Reynolds, C. F., III. (2003). Feasibility of a dyadic intervention for management of osteoarthritis: A pilot study with older patients and their spousal caregivers. *Aging & Mental Health*, 7(1), 53–60.

Marucha, P. T., Kiecolt-Glaser, J. K., & Favagehi, M. (1998). Mucosal wound healing is impaired by examination stress. *Psychosomatic Medicine*, 60, 362–365.

Marzuk, P. M., Tierney, H., & Tardiff, K. (1988). Increased risk of suicide in persons with AIDS. *Journal of American Medical Association*, 259, 1333–1337.

Masalu, J. R., & Astrom, A. N. (2003). The use of the theory of planned behavior to explore beliefs about sugar restriction. *American Journal of Health Behavior*, 27(1), 15–25.

Mason, J. W., Maher, J. T., Hartley, L. H., Mougey, E., Perlow, M. J., & Jones, L. G. (1976). Selectivity of corticosteroid & catecholamine response to various natural stimuli. In G. Serban (Ed.), *Psychopathology of human adaptation*. New York: Plenum Press.

Matarazzo, J. D. (1980). Behavioral health and behavioral medicine: Frontiers for a new health psychology. *American Psychologist*, 35, 807–817.

Mathers, C. D., Boerma, T., & Ma Fat, D. (2009). Global and regional causes of death. *British Medical Bulletin*, 92, 7–32.

Mathews, K. A., & Gump, B. B. (2002). Chronic work stress and marital dissolution increase risk of posttrial mortality in men from the multiple risk factor intervention trial. *Archives of Internal Medicine*, 162, 309–315.

Mathieu, E. (2023). How does age standardization make health metrics comparable? *Our World in Data*. Retrieved December 30, 2023

Mathieu, E., Ritchie, R., Rodés-Guirao, L., Appel, C., Giattino, C., Hasell, J., & Macdonald, J. (2020). *Coronavirus pandemic (COVID-19)* . Updated 2023. Retrieved April 2, 2023, from https://ourworldindata.org/coronavirus

Maul, J. S., Burt, R. W., & Cannon-Albright, L. A. (2007). A familial component to human rectal cancer, independent of colon cancer risk. *Clinical Gastroenterology & Hepatology*, 5(9), 1080–1084.

Mayer, J., & Salovey, P. (1997). *What is emotional intelligence?* New York: Basic Books.

Mayhew, D. R., Simpson, H. M., & Pak, A. (2003). Changes in collision rates among novice drivers during the first months of driving. *Accidents Annals of Prevention*, 35, 683–691.

Mayne, T. J. (1999). Negative effect and health: The importance of being earnest. *Cognition and Emotion*, 13(5), 601–635.

Mayo Clinic. (2022). *Herd immunity and COVID-19: What you need to know: Understand what's known about herd immunity and what it means for COVID-19*. Retrieved April 30, 2023

Mayo Clinic. (2006). *Heart disease: Sudden cardiac arrests*. Retrieved October 28, 2013, from http://www.mayoclinic.com/health/sudden-cardiac-arrest/DS00764/DSECTION=causes

Mayo Clinic. (2009). *Spinal cord injuries: Symptoms*. Retrieved November 27, 2009, from www.mayoclinic.com/health/spinal-cord-injury/DS00460/DSECTION=symptoms

Mayo Clinic. (2023a). *Diabetes*. Retrieved December 9, 2023

Mayo Clinic. (2023b). Pneumothorax – Symptoms and causes. Retrieved May 1, 2023

Mayo Clinic. (2024). *Fibromyalgia – Symptoms & causes*. Retrieved February 27, 2024

Mayo Foundation for Medical Education and Research. (2023). *3-D mammograms*. Retrieved March 29, 2023

McCloskey, W., Iwanicki, S., Lauterbach, D., Giammittorio, D. M., & Maxwell, K. (2015). Are Facebook friends helpful? Development of a Facebook-based measure of social support and examination of relationships among depression, quality of life and social support. *Cyberpsychology, Behavior & Social Networking*, *18*(9), 499–505.

McCrae, R. R., & Costa, P. T. (1987). Validation of the five-factor model of personality across instruments & observers. *Journal of Personality & Social Psychology*, *52*, 81–90.

McDermott, M. M., Spring, B., Tian, L., Treat-Jacobson, D., Ferrucci, L., Lloyd-Jones, D., . . . Rejeski, W. J. (2021). Effect of low-intensity vs high-intensity home-based walking exercise on walk distance in patients with peripheral artery disease: The LITE randomized clinical trial. *JAMA*, *325*(13), 1266–1276. doi: 10.1001/jama.2021.2536

McDonald, E. S., Oustimov, A., Weinstein, S. P., Synnestvedt, M. B., Schnall, M., & Conant, E. F. (2017). Effectiveness of digital breast tomosynthesis compared with digital mammography: Outcome analysis from 3 years of breast cancer screening. *The Journal of the American Medical Association: Oncology*, *2*(6), 737–743.

McDowell, I., & Newell, C. (1996). *Measuring health: A guide to rating scales and questionnaires* (2nd ed.). Oxford, UK: Oxford University Press.

McEvoy, C., & Hideg, G. (2017). *Global violent deaths: Time to decide*. Geneva: Small Arms Survey Graduate Institute of International and Development Studies.

McEvoy, O. (2023). Number of women's shelters in Europe. *Statista*. Retrieved January 12, 2024

McEwen, B. S. (2005). Stressed or stressed out: What is the difference? *Journal of Psychiatry & Neuroscience*, *30*(5), 315–318.

McEwen, B. S., & Winfield, J. C. (2003). The concept of allostasis in biology and biomedicine. *Hormones and Behavior*, *43*, 2–15.

McEwen, B. S., & Wingfield, J. C. (2007). Allostasis and allostatic load. In G. Fink (Ed.), *Encyclopedia of stress* (2nd ed., pp. 135–141). New York, NY: Academic Press.

McGinley, A. M. (2004). Health beliefs & women's rise of hormone replacement therapy. *Holistic Nursing Practices*, *18*(1), 18–25.

McGinnis, J. M., & Foege, W. H. (1993). Actual causes of death in the United States. *Journal of the American Medical Association*, *270*, 2207–2212.

McGraw, L. K., Turner, B. S., Stotts, N. A., & Dracup, K. A. (2008). A review of cardiovascular risk factors in US military personnel. *Journal of Cardiovascular Nursing*, *23*(4), 338–344.

McGuire, P. A. (1999). More psychologists are finding that discrete uses of humor promote healing in their patients. *American Psychological Association Monitor*, *30*, 1.

McKenna, M. T., & Hu, X. (2007). Recent trends in the incidence and morbidity associated with perinatal human immunodeficiency virus infection in the United States. *American Journal of Obstetrics and Gynecology*, *197*(3 suppl. 1), S10–S16.

McKenzie-Mohr, D. (2000). Fostering sustainable behavior through community-based social marketing. *American Psychologist*, *5*, 531–537.

McKeowan, T. (1988). *The origins of human disease*. Oxford, UK: Blackwell Press.

McKinley, J. B. (1975). Who is really ignorant – Physician or patient? *Journal of Health and Social Behavior, 16*, 3–11.

McLeroy, K. R., Bibeau, D., Steckler, A., & Glanz, K. (1988). An ecological perspective on health promotion programs. *Health Education Quarterly, 15*(4), 351–377.

McNamara, J. J., Molot, M. A., Stremple, J. F., & Cutting, R. T. (1971). Coronary artery disease in combat causalities in Vietnam. *JAMA, 216*(7), 1185–1187.

McPherson, S., Parent, S., Miguel, A., McDonell, M., & Roll, J. (2022). Contingency management is a powerful clinical tool for treating substance use: Research evidence and new practice guidelines for use. *Psychiatric Times, 39*, 9–11. Retrieved from researchgate.net

Means, R. K. (1975). *A history of health education in the United States*. Thorofare, NJ: Charles B. Slack.

Mechanic, D. (1972). Social psychological factors affecting the presentation of bodily complaints. *New England Journal of Medicine, 286*, 1132–1139.

Mechlin, B., Heymen, S., Edwards, C. L., & Girdler, S. S. (2010). Ethnic differences in cardiovascular-somatosensory interactions and in the central processing of noxious stimuli. *Psychophysiology, 48*(6), 762–773. doi: 10.1111/j.1469-8986.2010.01140.x

MedicalNewsToday. (2024). *Malaria vaccine rollout in Cameroon may lower death risk in children by 13%*. Retrieved February 4, 2024, from medicalnewstoday.com

Medicines Sans Frontières. (2017). *Malnutrition on the rise in Pibor*. Retrieved December 9, 2023

Mehler, P. S., Lasater, L., & Padillo, R. (2003). Obesity: Selected medical issues. *Eating Disorders, 11*, 317–330.

Mehra, P., & Mishra, A. (2021). Role of communication, influence, and satisfaction in patient recommendations of a physician. *Vikalpa, 46*(2), 99–111. doi: 10.1177/02560909211027090

Mehta, G., & Sheron, N. (2019). No safe level of alcohol consumption – Implications for global Health. *Journal of Hepatology, 70*(4), 587–589. doi: 10.1016/j.jhep.2018.12.021

Mehta, L. S., Watson, K. E., Barac, A., Beckie, T. M., Bittner, V., Cruz-Flores, S., . . . Volgman, A. S. (2018). Cardiovascular disease and breast cancer: Where these entities intersect: A scientific statement from the American Heart Association. *Circulation, 137*(8), e30–e66.

Meier, D., Emmons, C. A., Litke, A., Wallenstein, S., & Morrison, S. (2003). Characteristics of patients requesting and receiving physician assisted death. *Archives of Internal Medicine, 163*, 1537–1542.

Meijer, A., Conradi, H. J., Bos, E. H., Thombs, B. D., van Melle, J. P., & de Jonge, P. (2011). Prognostic association of depression following myocardial infarction with mortality and cardiovascular events: A meta-analysis of 25 years of research. *General Hospital Psychiatry, 33*(3), 203–216. doi: 10.1016/j.genhosppsych.2011.02.007

Meixner, L., Cohrdes, C., Schienkiewitz, A., & Mensink, G. B. M. (2020). Health-related quality of life in children and adolescents with overweight and obesity: Results from the German KIGGS survey. *BMC Public Health, 20*, 1722. doi: 10.1186/s12889-020-09834-8

Mejia, R., Perez, A., Pena, L., Kollath-Cattano, C., Morello, P., & Braun, S. (2017). Smoking in movies and adolescent smoking initiation: A longitudinal study among Argentinian adolescents. *Journal of Pediatrics, 180*, 222–228. doi: 10.1016/j.jpeds.2016.10.001

Mella, L. F. P., Bertolo, M. B., & Dalgalarrondo, P. (2010). Depressive symptoms in rheumatoid arthritis. *Brazilian Journal of Psychiatry, 32*(3). doi: 10.1590/S1516-44462010005000021

Mellor, D., McCabe, M., Ricciardelli, L., Yeow, J., Daliza, N., & Hapidzal, N. F. B. M. (2009). Sociocultural influences on body dissatisfaction and body change behaviors among Malaysian adolescents. *Body Image, 6*(2), 121–128.

Melzack, R. (1975). The McGill pain questionnaire: Major properties and scoring methods. *Pain, 1,* 277–299.

Melzack, R. (1993). Pain: Past, present and future. *Canadian Journal of Experimental Psychology, 47*(4), 615–629.

Melzack, R., & Wall, P. D. (1965). Pain mechanisms: A new theory. *Science, 150,* 971–979.

Melzack, R., & Wall, P. D. (Eds.). (2003). *Handbook of pain management.* Churchill: Livingston.

Mendes, P. M., Nobre, A. A., Griep, R. H., Guimaraes, J. M. N., Juvanhol, L. J., & Barreto, S. M. (2018). Association between perceived racial discrimination and hypertension: Findings from the ELSA-Brasil study. *Cadernos de Saúde Pública, 34*(2). doi: 10.1590/0102-311X00050317

Mende-Siedlecki, P., Lin, J., Ferron, S., Gibbons, C., Drain, A., & Goharzad, A. (2021). Seeing no pain: Assessing the generalizability of racial bias in pain perception. *Emotion, 21*(5), 932. doi: 10.1037/emo0000953

Menezes Succi, D. (2007). Mother-to-child transmission of HIV in Brazil during the years 2000 & 2001: Results of a multi-centric study. *Cadernos de Saude Publica, 23*(suppl. 3), S379–S389.

Mensah, G. A., Mokdad, A. H., Ford, E. S., Greenlund, K. J., & Croft, J. B. (2005). State of disparities in cardiovascular health in the United States. *Circulation, 111*(10), 1233–1241.

Mercurio, A., Aston, E. R., Claborn, K. R., Waye, K., & Rosen, R. K. (2019). Marijuana as a substitute for prescription medications: A qualitative study. *Substance Use & Misuse, 54*(11), 1894–1902. doi: 10.1080/10826084.2019.1618336

Merlin, A., Jager, J., & Schulenberger, J. E. (2008). Adolescent risk factors for adult alcohol use and abuse: Stability & change of predictive values across early and mid-adolescence. *Addiction, 103,* 84–99.

Merlis, M., Gould, D., & Mahato, B. (2006). *Rising out-of-pocket spending for medical care: A growing strain on family budgets.* The Commonwealth Fund. Retrieved October 28, 2013, from www.commonwealthfund.org/Publications/Fund-Reports/2006/Feb/Rising-Out-of-Pocket-Spending-for-Medical-Care-A-Growing-Strainon-Family-Budgets.aspx

Merritt, M. M., Bennett, G. G., Williams, R. B., Edwards, C. L., & Sollers, J. J. (2006). Perceived racism and cardiovascular reactivity and recovery to personally relevant stress. *Heath Psychology, 25*(3), 364–369.

Mervosh, S. (2022, July 31). Trained, armed and ready. To teach kindergarten. *The New York Times.* Retrieved June 19, 2023, from nytimes.com

Merzel, C., & D'Afflitti, J. (2003). Reconsidering community-based health promotion: Promise, performance and potential. *American Journal of Public Health, 93*(4), 557–580.

Messier, S. P., Loeser, R. F., Mitchell, M. N., Valle, G., Morgan, T., Rejesk, W. J., & Ettinger, W. H. (2000). Exercise and weight loss in obese older adults with knee osteoarthritis. *Journal of the American Geriatrics Society, 48,* 1062–1072.

Metcalfe, K. A., Poll, A., & Royer, R. (2009). Screening for founder mutations in BRCA1 & BRCA2 in unsolicited Jewish women. *Journal of Clinical Oncology, 28,* 387–391.

Metzer, W. S. (1989). The Caduceus and Aesculapian staff: Ancient Eastern origins and Western parallels. *Southern Medical Journal, 82,* 743–748.

Meyer, A. J., Nash, J. D., McAlister, A. L., Maccoby, N., & Farquhar, J. W. (1980). Skills training in cardiovascular health education campaign. *Journal of Consulting and Clinical Psychology, 48*(2), 129–142.

Mickalide, A. D. (1990). Sociocultural factors influencing weight among males. In A. Anderson (Ed.), *Males with eating disorders* (pp. 30–39). Philadelphia, PA: Brunner/Mazel.

Midwest HIDTA. (2021). *Marijuana legalization in the Midwest: The impacts.* Retrieved May 23, 2023, from Midwest-HIDTA-Marijuana-Impact-Report-Vol.-2.pdf (southdacola.com)

Migneault, J. P., Pallonen, U. E., & Velicer, W. F. (1997). Decisional balances and stages of change for adolescent drinking. *Addictive Behaviors, 22*(3), 339–351.

Miles, T. (2008). Neighborhood disorder, perceived safety and readiness to encourage use of local playgrounds. *American Journal of Preventive Medicine, 34*(4), 275–281.

Millbank, C., & Vira, B. (2022). Wildmeat consumption and zoonotic spillover: Contextualizing disease emergence and policy responses. *The Lancet: Planetary Health, 6*(5), E439–E448.

Miller, A. B., Sears, M. E., Morgan, L. L., David, D. L., Hardell, L., Oremus, M., & Soskolne, C. L. (2019). Risk to health and well-being from radio-frequency radiation emitted by cell phones and other wireless devices. *Frontiers in Public Health, 7,* 1–10, doi: 10.3389/fpubh.2019.00223

Miller, B. A., Maguin, E., & Downs, W. (1997). Alcohol, drugs and violence in children's lives. In M. Galanter (Ed.), *Recent developments in alcoholism: Vol 13, alcoholism and violence* (pp. 357–385). New York: Plenum.

Miller, L. H., & Su, X. (2011). Artemisinin: Discovery from the Chinese herbal garden. *Cell, 146*(6), 855–858. doi: 10.1016%2Fj.cell.2011.08.024

Miller, M. N., & Pumariega, A. J. (2001). Culture and eating disorders: A historical and cross-cultural review. *Psychiatry, 64*(2), 93–110.

Miller, W. R., & Thorensen, C. E. (2003). Spirituality, religion & health: An emerging research field. *American Psychologist, 58*(1), 24–35.

Mills, E. A. (2006). From the physical self to the social body: Expression & effects of HIV-related stigma in South Africa. *Journal of Community & Applied Social Psychology, 16*(6), 498–503.

Mills, P. R., Kessler, R. S., Cooper, J., & Sullivan, S. (2007). Impact of health promotion program on employee health risks and worker productivity. *American Journal of Health Promotion, 22*(1), 45–53.

Milne, S., Orbell, S., & Sherran, P. (2002). Combining motivational and volitional interventions to promote exercise participation: Protection motivation theory and implementation intentions. *British Journal of Health, 7,* 163–184.

Mince, S. E., & Stewart, D. E. (2007). Gender differences and depression in chronic pain conditions in a national epidemiological survey. *Psychosomatics, 48*(5), 394–399.

Minor, M., Stenstrom, C. H., Klepper, S. E., Hurley, M., & Ettinger, W. (2003). Work group recommendations: 2002 Exercise and physical activity conference. *Arthritis Care and Research, 49,* 453–454.

Mishra, S. I., DeForge, B., Barnet, S., Ntiri, S., & Grant, L. (2012). Social determinants of breast cancer screening in urban primary care practices: A community-engaged formative study. *Women's Health Issues, 22*(5), e429–e438. doi: 10.1016/j.whi.2012.06.004

Misra, V. H. (2001). Prehistoric human colonization of India. *Journal of Biosciences, 26*(4 suppl.), 491–531.

Mittleman, M. A., Lewis, R. A., & Maclure, M. (2001). Triggering myocardial infarction by marijuana. *Circulation, 103*(23), 2805–2809.

Mittleman, M. A., Maclure, M., Sherwood, J. B., Mulry, R. P., Tofler, G. H., Jacobs, S. C., . . . Muller, J. E. (1995). Triggering of acute myocardial infarction onset by episodes of anger: Determinants of myocardial infarction onset study investigators. *Circulation, 92,* 1720–1725.

Mizrachi, N. (2001). From causation to correlation: The story of psychosomatic medicine, 1939–1979. *Culture, Medicine & Psychiatry, 25,* 317–343.

MMWR. (1984). CDC update: Acquired Immunodeficiency Syndrome (AIDS), United States. *MMWR, 32,* 688–691.

MMWR. (2002). *Youth risk behavior surveillance – United States 2001, 51(SS04), 1–64.* Retrieved January 3, 2009, from www.cdc.gov/mmwr/preview/mmwrhtml/ss5104a1.htm

MMWR. (2004). Alcohol-attributable deaths & years of potential life lost – United States, 2001. *MMWR*, *43*(37), 866–870. Retrieved December 29, 2008, from www.cdc.gov/mmwr/preview/mmwrhtml/mm5337a2.htm?mobile=nocontent

MMWR. (2008a). HIV prevalence estimates – United States, 2006. *MMWR*, *57*(39), 1073–1076.

MMWR. (2008b). Smoking-attributable mortality, years of potential life lost & productivity losses, United States 2001–2004. *MMWR*, *57*(45), 1226–1228.

MMWR. (2008c). Subpopulation estimates from the HIV incidence surveillance system, United States 2006. *MMWR*, *57*(36), 985–989.

MMWR. (2011, June 3). HIV Surveillance – United States, 1981–2008. *MMWR*, *60*(21), 689–693.

MMWR. (2013). *Vital signs: Binge drinking among women & high school girls – United States 2011. MMWR*, *62*(1), 9–13.

MMWR. (2022). *Quick Stats: Age-adjusted rates of alcohol-induced deaths by urban-rural status – United States 2000–2020*. Retrieved May 18, 2023, from cdc.gov. doi: 10.15585/mmwr.mm7144a5

Moadei, A. B., & Harris, M. S. (2008). Cancer. In B. A. Boyer & M. I. Paharia (Eds.), *Comprehensive handbook of clinical health psychology*. Hoboken, NJ: John Wiley Sons.

Mobasseri, M., Shirmohammedi, M., Amiri, T., Vahed, N., Fard, H. H., & Ghojazaheh, M. (2020). Prevalence and incidence of type 1 diabetes in the world: A systematic review and meta-Analysis. *Health Promotion Perspectives*, *10*(2), 98–115. doi: 10.34172%2Fhpp.2020.18

Moen, A., Schistad, E. I., Rygh, L. J., Røe, C., & Gjerstad, J. (2014). Role of IL1A rs1800587, IL1B rs1143627 and IL1RN rs2234677 genotype regarding development of chronic lumbar radicular pain; a prospective one-year study. *PLoS One*, *9*(9), e107301. doi: 10.1371/journal.pone.0107301

Moerman, D. (1998). *Native American ethnobotany*. Portland, OR: Timber Press.

Mohebbi, Z., Dehkordi, S. F., Sharif, F., & Banitalebi, E. (2019). The effect of aerobic exercise on occupational stress of female nurses: A controlled clinical trial. *Investigación y Educación en Enfermería*, *37*(2). doi: 10.17533/udea.iee.v37n2e05

Moinuddin, A., Goel, A., Saini, S., Bajpai, A., & Misra, R. (2016). Alcohol consumption and gender: A critical review. *Journal of Psychology and Psychotherapy*, *6*(3), 267. doi: 10.4172/2161-0487.1000267

Mokdad, A. H., Marks, J. S., Stroup, D. F., & Gerberding, J. L. (2004). Actual causes of death in the United States. *Journal of the American Medical Association*, *291*, 1238–1245.

Mokdad, A. H., Serdula, M. K., Dietz, W. H., Bowman, B. A., Marks, J. S., & Koplan, J. P. (2000). The continuing epidemic of obesity in the United States. *Journal of the American Medical Association*, *282*, 1353–1358.

Molina, Y., Hohl, S. D., Ko, L. K., Rodriguez, E. A., Thompson, B., & Beresford, S. A. A. (2014). Understanding the patient-provider communication needs and experiences of Latina and non-Latina white women following an abnormal mammogram. *Journal of Cancer Education*, *29*, 781–789. doi: 10.1007/s13187-014-0654-6

Möller-Leimkühler, A. M. (2007). Gender differences in cardiovascular disease and comorbid depression. *Dialogues in Clinical Neuroscience*, *9*(1), 71–83. doi: 10.31887/DCNS.2007.9.1/ammoeller

Molnar, B. E., Gortmaker, S. C., Bull, F. C., & Buka, S. L. (2004). Unsafe to play? Neighborhood disorder and lack of safety predict reduced physical activity among children and adolescents. *American Journal of Health Promotion*, *18*(5), 378–386.

Monteleone, A. M., Pellegrino, F., Croatto, G., Carfagno, M., Hilbert, A., & Treasure, T. (2022). Treatment of eating disorders: A systematic meta-review of meta-analyses and network meta-analyses. *Neuroscience & Biobehavioral Reviews*, *142*, 104857. doi: 10.1016/j.neubiorev.2022.104857

Moore, A. A., Gould, R., Reuben, D. B., Greendale, G. A., Carter, M. K., & Zhou, Z. (2005). Longitudinal patterns and predictors of alcohol consumption in the United States. *American Journal of Public Health, 95*(3), 458–465.

Moore, K. W., de Waal Malefyt, R., Coffman, R. L., & O'Garra, A. (2001). Interleukin-10 and the interleukin-10 receptor. *Annual Review of Immunology, 19*(1), 683–765. doi: 10.1146/annurev. immunol.19.1.683

Moore, T. J., & Morris, T. (2021). *Shaping the habits of teen drivers*. National Bureau of Economic Research Working Papers. Retrieved October 20, 2023, from www.nber.org/papers/w28707

Morais, A. C. B., Stangarllin-Flori, L., Bertin, R. L., & Medelros, C. O. (2020). Consumers' knowledge and use of nutritional information on food labels [Conhecimento e uso de rotulos nutricionais por consumidores]. *Demetra: Food, Nutrition & Health, 15*. doi: 10.12957/demetra.2020.45847

Morales, A. L. (1998). *Remedios: Stories of earth and iron from the history of Puertorriquenas*. Boston: Beacon Press.

Morgaine, K. (2007). Domestic violence and human rights: Local challenges to a universal framework. *Journal of Sociology and Social Welfare, 34*(1), 109–129.

Morgan, K. K. (2022). *What is virus genome sequencing?* Retrieved December 22, 2023, from webmd.com

Morgenstern, M., Sargent, J. D., Engles, R. C. M. E., Scholte, R. H. J., Florek, E., Hunt, K., . . . Hanewinkel, R. (2013). Smoking in movies and adolescent smoking initiation: Longitudinal study in six European countries. *American Journal of Preventive Medicine, 44*(4), 339–344. doi: 10.1016/j.amepre.2012.11.037

Morris, T., Moore, M., & Morris, F. (2011). Stress and chronic illness: The case of diabetes. *Journal of Adult Development, 18*, 70–80. doi: 10.1007/s10804-010-9118-3

Mosbach, P., & Leventhal, H. (1988). Peer group identification and smoking: Implications for intervention. *Journal of Abnormal Psychology, 97*(2), 238–245.

Moscowitz, J. T., Epel, E. S., & Acree, M. (2008). Positive affect uniquely predicts lower risk of mortality in people with diabetes. *Health Psychology, 27*(1 suppl.), S73–S82.

Mosher, C. E., Duhamel, K. N., Egert, J., & Smith, M. Y. (2011). Self-efficacy for coping with cancer in a multiethnic sample of breast cancer patients: Associations with barriers to pain management and distress. *Clinical Journal of Pain, 26*(3), 227–34. doi: 10.1097/AJP.0b013e3181bed0e3

Moskowitz, J. T., Folkman, S., Colette, L., & Vittinghoff, E. (1996). Coping with mood: AIDS related caregiver bereavement. *Annals of Behavioral Medicine, 18*(1), 49–57.

Moslehi, R., Chu, W., Karlan, B., Fishman, D., Risch, H., Fields, A., . . . Narod, S. A. (2000). BRCA1 & BRCA2 mutation analysis of 208 Ashkenazi Jewish women with ovarian cancer. *American Journal of Human Genetics, 66*, 1259–1272.

Mozaffarin, D., Katan, M. B., Ascherio, A., Stampfer, M. J., & Willett, W. C. (2006). Trans fatty acids and cardiovascular disease. *New England Journal of Medicine, 354*, 1601–1613.

Msemburi, W., Karlinsky, A., Knutson, Aleshin-Guendel, S., Chatterji, S., & Wakefield, J. (2023). The WHO estimates of excess mortality associated with the COVID-19 pandemic. *Nature, 613*, 130–137. doi: 10.1038/s41586-022-05522-2

Mueller, I., & Tronick, E. (2019). Early life exposure to violence: Developmental consequences on brain and behavior. *Frontiers in Behavioral Neuroscience, 19*. doi: 10.3389/fnbeh.2019.00156

Mullen, K. D., McDermott, R. S., Gold, R. J., & Belcastro, P. A. (1996). *Connections for health* (4th ed.). Madison, WI: Brown & Benchmark.

Mulvey, K. L., Boswell, C., & Zheng, J. (2017). Causes and consequences of social exclusion and peer rejection among children and adolescents. *Report on Emotional & Behavioral Disorders in Youth, 17*(3), 71–75.

Mulvihill, B. A., Jackson, A. J., Mulvihill, F. X., Romaire, M., Gyaben, S., Telfair, J., & Caldwell, C. (2005). The impact of SCHIP enrollment on adolescent-provider communication. *Journal of Adolescent Health*, *37*(2), 94–102.

Munck, A., & Guyre, P. M. (1986). Glucocorticoid physiology, pharmacology & stress. *Advanced Experimental Medical Biology*, *196*, 81–96.

Munck, A., & Naray-Fejes-Toth, A. (1994). Glucocorticoids & stress: Permissive and suppressive actions. *Annals of the New York Academy of Science*, *746*, 115–130.

Munn, J. D., & Woznick, L. (2007). Single payer health care systems: The roles and responsibilities of the public and private sector. *Benefits Quarterly*, *23*(3), 7–17.

Muñoz, A., Kirby, A. J., Margolick, J. B., Visscher, B. R., Rinaldo, C. R., Kaslow, R. A., & Phair, J. P. (1995). Long-term survivors with HIV-1 infection: Incubation period and longitudinal patterns of CD4$^+$ lymphocytes. *Journal of Acquired Immune Deficiency Syndromes & Human Retrovirology*, *8*, 496–506.

Muscari Lin, E., Aikin, J. L., & Good, B. C. (1999). Premature menopause after cancer treatment. *Cancer Practice*, *7*(3), 114–121.

Muscat, J. E., Malkin, M. G., Shore, R. E., Thompson, S., Neugut, A. I., Stellmann, S. D., & Bruce, J. (2002). Handheld cellular phones and the risk of neuroma. *Neurology*, *58*, 1304–1306.

Muscat, J. E., Malkin, M. G., Thompson, S., Shore, R. E., Stellman, S. D., McRee, D., . . . Wynder, E. L. (2000). Handheld cellular telephone use and risk of brain cancer. *JAMA*, *284*, 3001–3007.

Myers, D. G. (2000). The funds, friends, and faith of happy people. *American Psychologists*, *55*(1), 56–67.

Mystakidou, K., Tsilika, E., Parpa, E., Hatzipli, I., Smyrnioti, M., Galanos, A., & Vlahos, L. (2008). Demographic and clinical predictions of spirituality in advanced cancer patients: A randomized control study. *Journal of Clinical Nursing*, *17*(13), 1779–1785.

Naar-King, S., Templin, T., & Wright, K. (2006). Psychosocial factors and medication adherence in HIV-positive youth. *AIDS Patient Care, STDS*, *20*, 44–47.

Naar-King, S., Wright, K., Parsons, J. T., Frey, M., Templin, T., & Ondersma, S. (2006). Transtheoretical model and condom use in HIV-positive youths. *Health Psychology*, *25*, 648–652. https://psycnet.apa.org/doi/10.1037/0278-6133.25.5.648

Naiyer, S., & Abbas, S. S. (2022). Effect of greenhouse gases on human health. In S. Sonwani & P. Saxena (Eds.), *Greenhouse gases: Sources, sinks and mitigation* (pp. 85–106). Singapore: Springer.

Nakajima, M., Sero, A., Jama, S., Habte, S., Taha, S., Habte, H., . . . al'Absi, M. (2023). Acculturation style is associated with stress and tobacco use among East African immigrants. *Journal of Psychoactive Drugs*, *55*(1), 112–121. doi: 10.1080/02791072.2022.2040659

Nakaya, N., Bidstrup, P. E., Saito-Nakaya, K., Frederiksen, K., Koskenvuo, M., Pukkala, E., . . . Johansen, C. (2010). Personality traits & cancer risk & survival based on Finnish & Swedish registry data. *American Journal of Epidemiology*, *172*, 377–385.

Namayandeh, S. M., Khazaei, Z, Najafi, M L, Goodarzi, E, & Moslem, A. (2020). Leukemia in children 0–14 statistics 2018: Incidence and mortality and human development index (HDI): GLOBOCAN sources and methods. *Asian Pacific Journal of Cancer Prevention*, *21*(5), 1487–1494.

National Academy of Medicine. (2022). *About the National Academy of Medicine*. Retrieved October 26, 2023, from https://nam.edu/about-the-nam/

National Academy on an Aging Society. (2000). *Heart disease: A disabling yet preventable condition* (No. 3). Washington, DC. Retrieved October 28, 2013, from www.agingsociety.org/agingsociety/publications/chronic/index.html

National Cancer Institute. (1996). *The FTC cigarette tests methods for determining tar, nicotine & carbon monoxide yields in US cigarettes: Report of the NCI Expert Committee.* Bethesda, MD: National Institutes of Health Publication No. 96–4028.

National Cancer Institute. (2001). *Risks associated with smoking cigarettes with low machine measured yields of tar and nicotine: Monograph 13.* Retrieved March 1, 2007, from www.cancer.gov/newscenter/qa/2001/monograph13qa

National Cancer Institute. (2007). *Screening mammograms: Questions and answers factsheet.* Retrieved January 23, 2010, from www.cancer.gov/cancertopics/types/breast

National Cancer Institute. (2010). *"Light" cigarettes and cancer risk.* Retrieved February 1, 2024.

National Cancer Institute. (2015). *Human papillomavirus (HPV) vaccine.* Retrieved June 18, 2022, from cancer.gov

National Cancer Institute. (2023). *Mammograms.* Retrieved March 29, 2023, from cancer.gov

National Cancer Institute. (n.d.-a). *What is cancer?* Retrieved January 28, 2023, from

National Cancer Institute. (n.d.-b). *Seer training modules: Cancer classification.* Retrieved February 9, 2023

National Cancer Institute. (n.d.-c). *What we know about electronic cigarettes.* Retrieved March 29, 2023

National Cancer Institute Staff. (2021). *Despite proven safety of HPV vaccines, more parents have concerns.* Cancer current blog of the National Cancer Institute, National Institutes of Health. Retrieved May 21, 2022, from cancer.gov

National Center for Chronic Disease Control & Prevention. (2014). *Health consequences of smoking - 50 years of progress: A report of the surgeon general.* Atlanta, GA: Centers for Disease Control.

National Center for Chronic Disease Prevention and Health Promotion. (2016). Introduction, conclusions, and historical background relative to E-cigarette. In *E-cigarette use among youth and young adults: A report of the surgeon general.* Atlanta, GA: CDC. Retrieved May 18, 2023, from nih.gov

National Center for Health Statistics. (2006). *Healthy United States in chartbook on trends in the health of Americans.* Retrieved August 7, 2009, from www.cdc.gov/nchs/data/hus/hus06.pdf

National Center for Health Statistics. (2021a). *New CDC/NCHS data confirm largest one-year increase in U.S. homicide rate in 2020.* Retrieved June 25, 2024, from https://www.cdc.gov/nchs/pressroom/nchs_press_releases/2021/202110.htm#:~:text=The%20new%20provisional%20data%20show,7.8%20per%20100%2C000%20in%202020

National Center for Health Statistics. (2021b). *Back, lower limb, and upper limb pain among U.S. adults, 2019.* NCHS Data Brief No. 415. Retrieved May 30, 2023, from https://www.cdc.gov

National Center for Health Statistics. (2022). *Health, United States, 2020–2021.* Retrieved May 20, 2023, from cdc.gov

National Conference of State Legislatures. (2006). *Childhood obesity 2006: Update & overview of policy options.* Retrieved October 28, 2013, from www.ncsl.org/research/health/childhood-obesity-2006-policyoptions-nutrition.aspx

National Health & Hospitals Reform Commission. (2009). A healthier future for all Australians: An overview of the final report of the National Health & Hospitals Reform Commission. *The Medical Journal of Australia, 191*(7), 383–387.

National Heart, Lung and Blood Institute. (1986). *Public perceptions of high blood pressure and sodium* (National Institute of Health Publication No. 86–2730). Bethesda, MD: National Heart, Lung and Blood Institute.

National Heart, Lung and Blood Institute. (2007). *Hemophilia*. Retrieved October 28, 2013, from http://www.nhlbi.nih.gov/health/health-topics/topics/hemophilia/

National Heart, Lung, and Blood Institute. (2008a). *Heart valve disease*. Retrieved October 10, 2008, from www.nhlbi.nih.gov/health/dci/Diseases/hvd/hvd_whatis.html

National Heart, Lung, and Blood Institute. (2008b). *High blood cholesterol*. Retrieved October 10, 2008, from www.nhlbi.nih.gov/health/dci/Diseases/Hbc/HBC_WhatIs.html

National Heart, Lung, and Blood Institute. (2008c). *NHLBI health information network e-Bulletin*. Retrieved February 15, 2010, from http://hp2010.nhlbihin.net/joinhin/news/HowToNWRD08.htm

National Heart, Lung and Blood Institute. (2009). *COPD*. Retrieved October 28, 2013, from www.nhlbi.nih.gov/health/public/lung/copd/what-is-copd/index.htm

National Hemophiliac Foundation. (2006). *HIV/AIDS*. Retrieved October 18, 2013, from www.hemophilia.org/NHFWeb/MainPgs/MainNHF.aspx?menuid=43&contentid=39

National Highway Traffic Safety Administration. (2005a). *Traffic safety facts: 2004 Data – speeding*. Washington, DC: National Highway Traffic Safety Administration, U.S. Department of Transportation Publication HS 809–915.

National Highway Traffic Safety Administration. (2005b). *Traffic safety facts 2005: Alcohol*. Washington, DC: National Highway Traffic Safety Administration, U.S. Department of Transportation. Retrieved from www.nhtsa.gov/Research/Human+Factors/Alcohol+Impairment

National Highway Traffic Safety Administration. (2006). *Traffic safety facts: Research notes*. Washington, DC: National Highway Traffic Safety Administration, U.S. Department of Transportation, NHTSA's National Center for Statistical Analysis.

National Highway Traffic Safety Administration. (2013). *2012 Motor vehicle crashes: Overview*. NHTSA Traffic Safety Facts: Research Notes. Retrieved October 30, 2016, from www.nhtsa.gov/About-NHTSA/Press-Releases/NHTSA-Data-Confirms-Traffic-Fatalities-Increased-In-2012

National Highway Traffic Safety Administration. (2021a). *Alcohol impaired driving*. Retrieved May 22, 2023, from https://www.nhtsa.gov/book/countermeasures-that-work/alcohol-impaired-driving#:~:text=In%202021%20there%20were%2013%2C384,Statistics%20and%20Analysis%2C%202023a)

National Highway Traffic Safety Administration. (2021b). *Traffic safety facts: Distracted driving in 2021*. Retrieved May 22, 2023, from https://www.dot.gov/

National Highway Traffic Safety Administration. (2022a). *Traffic safety facts: Young drivers*. Retrieved May 30, 2023, from dot.gov

National Highway Traffic Safety Administration. (2022b). *Traffic safety facts: Crash stats*. Retrieved May 30, 2023 https://crashstats.nhtsa.dot.gov/Api/Public/ViewPublication/813307

National Highway Traffic Safety Administration. (2023). *Traffic safety facts: 2021 data*. Retrieved June 25, 2024, from https://crashstats.nhtsa.dot.gov/Api/Public/ViewPublication/813492.pdf

National Indian Council on Aging. (2023). *American Indian suicide rate increases*. Retrieved June 12, 2023, from nicoa.org

National Institute of Alcohol Abuse and Alcoholism. (2023). *Alcohol-related emergencies and deaths in the United States*. Retrieved December 30, 2023, from nih.gov.

National Institute of Arthritis and Musculoskeletal and Skin Diseases. (2006). *Questions and answers about gout* (NIH Publications no. 07–5027). Washington, DC: U.S. Department of Health and Human Services.

National Institute of Arthritis and Musculoskeletal and Skin Diseases. (2009). *Juvenile arthritis*. Retrieved September 1, 2012 www.niams.nih.gov/health_info/juv_arthritis/juvenile_arthritis_ff.asp

National Institute of Arthritis and Musculoskeletal and Skin Diseases. (2021). *Juvenile idiopathic arthritis (JIA): Treatment & diagnosis.* Retrieved March 1, 2024, from nih.gov

National Institute of Arthritis and Musculoskeletal and Skin Diseases. (2023). *Osteoarthritis. What causes osteoarthritis, symptoms & more.* Retrieved February 28, 2024, from nih.gov

National Institute of Diabetes and Digestive and Kidney Diseases. (2017). *LiverTox: Clinical and research information on drug-induced liver injury.* Retrieved November 23, 2023, from nih.gov.

National Institute of Health. (2004). *Guidelines for the conduct of research involving human subjects at the Institutes of Health.* Washington, DC: U.S. Department of Health and Human Services, Public Health Services, 00–4783.

National Institute on Aging. (2022). *Parkinson's disease: Causes, symptoms, and treatments.* Retrieved November 5, 2023, from nih.gov.

National Institute on Alcohol Abuse and Alcoholism. (n.d.). *Understanding alcohol abuse disorder.* National Institute on Alcohol Abuse and Alcoholism (NIAAA). Retrieved January 9, 2024, from nih.gov

National Institutes of Health. *Number NIH07–5605.* Washington, DC: U.S. Department of Health and Human Services.

National Institutes of Health. (2022). *COVID-19 was third leading cause of death in the United States in both 2020 and 2021.* Retrieved April 22, 2023

National Public Radio. (2018). When you need a mammogram, should you get one in "3-D"? *NPR.* Retrieved March 29, 2023

National Public Radio. (2008). *Understanding Sen. Kennedy's cancer diagnosis.* Retrieved October 28, 2013, from www.npr.org/templates/story/story. php?storyId=90645054

National Safety Council. (2023). *Injury facts: Motor vehicle.* Retrieved January 11, 2024, from nsc.org

National Safety Council. (2024). *Deaths by demographics.* Retrieved February 10, 2024, from nsc.org

National Vital Statistics System. (2021). *Accidents or unintentional injuries. Mortality data 2021.* CDC Wonder. Retrieved May 18, 2023, from cdc.gov

Naylor, R., Baik, C., & Arkoudis, C. (2018). Identifying attrition risk based on the first year experience. *Higher Education Research & Development, 37*(2), 328–342. doi: 10.1080/07294360.2017.1370438

Nayor, M., Chernofsky, A., Spartano, N. L., Tanguay, M., Blodgett, J. B., Murthy, V. L. (2021). Physical activity and fitness in the community: The Framingham Heart Study, European Heart Journal, 42, 44, 4565–4575. doi: 10.1093/eurheartj/ehab580

NBC News. (2008). *NBC's Tim Russert dies of heart attack at 58.* Retrieved from www.msnbc.msn.com/id/25145431

NCSA. (2023, May). *Distracted driving in 2021.* Research Note. Report No. DOT HS 813 443.

Neiderreiter, L., Adolph, T. E., & Tilg, H. (2018). Food, microbiome, and colorectal cancer. *Digestive and Liver Disease, 50*(7), 647–652.

Nelson, M. C., Newmark-Strainer, D., Hannan, P. J., Sirard, J. R., & Story, M. (2006). Longitudinal and secular trends in physical activity and sedentary behavior during adolescence. *Pediatrics, 118*(6), 1627–1634.

Nelson, T. F., Naomi, T. S., Brewer, R. D., & Wechsler, H. (2005). The state sets the rate: The relationship among state-specific college binge drinking, state binge drinking rates, and selected state alcohol control policies. *American Journal of Public Health, 95*(3), 441–446.

Neria, Y. (2009). Posttraumatic stress disorder. *Psychotic Annals, 39*(6), 317–318.

Neuhausen, S., Gilewski, T., Norton, L., Tran, T., McGuire, P., & Swenson, J. (1996). Recurrent BRCA2 617delT mutations in Ashkenazi Jewish women affected by breast cancer. *Nature Genetics, 13,* 126–128.

New Zealand Government, Ministry of Health. (2022). *Immunization handbook: 22 varicella (chickenpox)*. Retrieved April 1, 2023.

Newlin, K., Knafl, K., & Melkus, G. (2002). African-American spirituality: A concept analysis. *Advances in Nursing Science*, 25(2), 57–70.

Newman, B., Mu, H., Butler, L. M., Millikan, R. C., Moorman, P. G., & King, M. C. (1998). Frequency of breast cancer attributable to BRCA1 in population-bases series of American women. *JAMA*, 279, 915–921.

NHLBI. (2023). *What is coronary heart disease*. Retrieved February 12, 2024.

NHLBI. (n.d.). *The Framingham Heart Study*. Retrieved July 1, 2023.

NHTSA. (2012a). *The effect of passengers on teen driver behavior*. Retrieved January 22, 2024, from www.nhtsa.gov/sites/nhtsa.gov/files/811613.pdf

NHTSA. (2012b). *Traffic safety facts 2010 data*. Retrieved June 28, 2013, from http://www-nrd.nhtsa.dot.gov/pubs/811625.pdf

NHTSA. (n.d.). *Understanding human behavior*. Retrieved January 20, 2024, from.

Nicita-Mauro, V., Maltese, G., Nicita-Mauro, C., & Basile, G. (2007). Vascular aging and the geriatric patient. *Minerva Cardioangiologica*, 55(4), 497–502.

Nickels, N., Kubicki, K., & Maestripieri, D. (2017). Sex differences in the effects of psychosocial stress on cooperative and prosocial behavior: Evidence for 'flight or fight' in males and 'tend and befriend' in females. *Adaptive Human Behavior and Physiology*, 3, 171–183. doi: 10.1007/s40750-017-0062-3

Nickol, M. E., & Kindrachuk, J. (2019). A year of terror and a century of reflection: Perspectives on the great influenza pandemic of 1918–1919. *BMC Infectious Diseases*, 19, 117. doi: 10.1186/s12879-019-3750-8

Nicolaidis, S. (2019). Environment and obesity. *Metabolism*, (100 Suppl.), 153942. doi: 10.1016/j.metabol.2019.07.006

NIDA. (2002). *Marijuana: Facts for teens*. Retrieved March 2008, from www.drugabuse.gov/MarijBroch/teenpg9–10.html

NIDA. (2006a). *NIDA InfoFacts: Crack and cocaine*. Retrieved March 2008, from http://nida.gov/info-Facts/Cocaine.html

NIDA. (2006b). *NIDA infofacts: Methamphetamine*. Retrieved from www.nida.nih.Gov/infofacts/methamphetamine.html

NIDA. (2011). *NIDA prescription drugs: Abuse and addiction*. Retrieved October 28, 2013, from http://www.drugabuse.gov/publications/research-reports/prescriptiondrugs

NIDA. (2012). *Heroin*. Retrieved May 20, 2013, from www.drugabuse.gov/drugs-abuse/heroin

NIDA. (2019). *Cannabis (marijuana) drugfacts*. Retrieved June 24, 2024, from www.nida.nih.gov/publications/drugfacts/cannabis-marijuana

NIDA. (2021). *Fentanyl drug facts*. Retrieved May 30, 2023, from View PDF (nih.gov)

Nikelly, A. G. (2005). Positive health outcomes of social interests. *Journal of Individual Psychology*, 61(4), 329–342.

Nilsson, U. (2009). Soothing music can increase oxytocin levels during bed rest and after open-heart surgery: A randomized control trial. *Journal of Clinical Nursing*, 18, 2153–2161.

Nipp, D., El-Jawahri, A., Moran, S. M., D'Arpino, S. M., Johnson, P. C., Lage, D. E., . . . Temel, J. S. (2017). The relationship between physical and psychological symptoms and health care utilization in hospitalized patients with advanced cancer. *Cancer*, 123(23), 4720–4727.

Nkansah-Amankra, S., & Minelli, M. (2016). "Gateway hypothesis" and early drug use: Additional findings from tracking a population-based sample of adolescents to adulthood. *Preventive Medicine*, 4, 134–141.

Noisy Hawk, J., & Trimble, J. E. (2019). Well-being considerations among selected North American Indian populations: Relationships, spirits, and connections. In C. Fleming & C. Manning (Eds.), *Routledge handbook of indigenous healing* (pp. 97–108). London: Taylor & Francis.

Nolen-Hoeksema, S., Larson, J., & Grayson. C. (1999). Explaining the gender difference in depressive symptoms. *Journal of Personality and Social Psychology*, 77, 1061–1072.

Noormohamed, S. E., Ferguson, K. J., Baghair, A., & Cohen, L. G. (1994). Students' knowledge base and attitudes on safer sex, condoms & AIDS: A study of three colleges of pharmacy. *American Journal of Pharmacological Education*, 58, 269–273.

Norem, J. K. (2001). Defensive pessimism, optimism & pessimism. In E. D. Chang (Ed.), *Optimism & pessimism: Theory research & practice* (pp. 77–100). Washington, DC: American Psychological Association Press.

Norring, C., & Sohlberg, S. (1988). Eating disorder inventory in Sweden: Description, cross-cultural comparison, and clinical utility. *Acta Psychiatrica Scandinavica*, 78, 567–575.

North American Menopause Society. (2017). The 2017 hormone therapy position statement of The North American Menopause Society. *Menopause*, 24(7), 728–753. doi: 10.1097/GME.0000000000000921

Northridge, M. E., & Sclar, E. (2003). A joint urban planning and public health framework: Contributions to health impact assessment. *American Journal of Public Health*, 93(1), 118–121.

Nosheen, H. (2009). Blacks face bone marrow donor shortage. *National Public Radio*. Retrieved July 20, 2010, from www.npr.org/templates/story/story.php?storyId=128173149

Notrica, D., Sayrs, L., Krishna, N., Davenport, K., Jamshidi, R., & McMahon, L. (2020). Impact of helmet laws on motorcycle crash mortality rates. *Journal of Trauma and Acute Care Surgery*, 89(5), 962–970. doi: 10.1097/TA.0000000000002861

Nuechterlein, K. H., Dawson, M. E., Gitlin, M., Ventura, J., Goldstein, M. J., Snyder, K. S., . . . Mintz, J. (1992). Developmental processes in schizophrenic disorders: Longitudinal studies of vulnerability and stress. *Schizophrenic Bulletin*, 18(3), 387–425.

Nunn, J. F. (1996). *Ancient Egyptian medicine*. Norman, Oklahoma: University of Oklahoma Press.

Nyhan, B., Reifler, J., Richey, S., & Freed, G. L. (2014). Effective messages in vaccine promotion: A randomized trial. *Pediatrics*, 133(4), e835–e842. doi: 10.1542/peds.2013-2365

Oates, J., Carpenter, D., Fisher, M., Goodson, S., Hannah, B., & Kwiatkowski, R. (2021). *BPS Code of Human Research Ethics*. Retrieved November 13, 2023, from inf180_2021.pdf (bps.org.uk)

Oetting, E. R., & Beauvis, R. (1987). Peer cluster theory, socialization characteristics, and adolescent drug use: A path analysis. *Journal of Counseling Psychology*, 34, 205–213.

Office for Human Research Protection. (2001). *Suspension letter to Johns Hopkins University Jul 19: 2*. Retrieved March 23, 2007, from www.hhs.gov/ohrp/detrm_letrs/jul01a.pdf

Ogata Jones, K., Denham, B. E., & Springston, T. K. (2006). Effects of mass and interpersonal communication on breast cancer screening: Advancing agenda-setting theory in a health context. *Journal of Applied Communication Research*, 34(1), 94–113.

Ogoma, S. O. (2020). Problem-focused coping controls burnout in medical students: The case of a selected medical school in Kenya. *Journal of Psychology and Behavioral Science*, 8(1), 69–79. doi: 10.15640/jpbs.v8n1a8

O'Halloran, J., Miller, G. C., & Britt, H. (2004). Defining chronic conditions for primary care in ICPC-2. *Family Practice*, 21(4), 381–386.

Olanrewaju, O., & Adeniyi, A. A. (2019). Examining the determinants of delayed access to primary healthcare in men. *Journal of Biology, Agriculture and Healthcare*, 9(14), 19–25. doi: 10.7176/JBAH

O'Leary, D. (2020). *Socioeconomic status, negative affect, and health*. Stanford University ProQuest Dissertations Publishing. Retrieved August 2, 2023, from www.proquest.com/docview/2432565580?pq-origsite=gscholar&fromopenview=true

Olivardia, R., Pope, H. G., Mangweth, B., & Hudson, J. I. (1995). Eating disorders in college men. *American Journal of Psychiatry, 152*, 1279–1285.

Oliver, G., & Wardle, J. (1999). Perceived effects of stress on food choice. *Physiology and Behavior, 66*, 511–515.

Olson, L. M., & Wahab, S. (2006). American Indian & suicide: A neglected area of research. *Trauma Violence Abuse, 7*, 19–33.

Omari, O., Wynaden, D., Al-Omari, H., & Khatatbeh, M. (2016). Coping strategies of Jordanian adolescents with cancer: An interpretative phenomenological analysis study. *Journal of Pediatric Hematology/Oncology Nursing, 34*(1). doi: 10.1177/1043454215622408

O'Neil, P. M., & Brown, J. D. (2005). Weighing the evidence: Benefits of regular weight monitoring for weight control. *Journal of Nutrition, Education & Behavior, 37*(6), 319–322.

Ong, L. M., deHess, J. C., Hoos, A. M., & Lammes, F. B. (1995). Doctor-patient communication: A review of the literature. *Social Science and Medicine, 40*(7), 903–918.

Orent, W. (2013). *Plague: The mysterious past & terrifying future of the world's most dangerous disease*. New York: Simon & Schuster.

Orji, C. C., Kanu, C. K., Adelodun, A. I., & Brown, C. M. (2020). Factors that influence mammography use for breast cancer screening among African American women. *Journal of the National Medical Association, 112*(6), 578–592. doi: 10.1016/j.jnma.2020.05.004

Orsal, O., Orsal, O., Alparslan, G. B., & Unsal, A. (2012). Evaluation of the relationship between quality of sleep & anxiety among university students. *HealthMed, 6*, 2244–2255.

OSHA. (1989, January 26). *Safety and health program management guidelines: Insurance of voluntary guidelines*. 54 Federal Regulations, 3904–3916.

Othman, C. N., & Farooqui, M. (2015). Traditional and complementary medicine. *Procedia – Social and Behavioral Sciences, 170*, 262–271.

Otwombe, K., Dietrich, J., Laher, F., Hornschuh, S., Nkala, B., Chimoyi, L., . . . Miller, C. L. (2015). Health-seeking behaviours by gender among adolescents in Soweto, South Africa. *Global Health Action, 8*, 1. doi: 10.3402/gha.v8.25670

Ouedraogo, A., Ouedraogo, T. L., Ouoba, D. E., & Sawagodo, J. P. (2000). The current situation with regard to nicotine addiction in Burkina Faso: Tobacco supply and data from the KAB-P survey of young people in Ouagadougou. *Sante, 10*(3), 177–181.

Ouyang, H. (2023, November 5). If childhood obesity is an "epidemic," how far should doctors go to treat it? Bariatric surgery at 16? *The New York Times Magazine*, pp. 24–33, 49.

Ozaki, T., & Asano, Y. (2016). Development of varicella vaccine in Japan and future prospects. *Vaccine, 34*(29), 3427–3433. doi: 10.1016/j.vaccine.2016.04.059

Paddock, C. (2019). Metabolic factors likely contribute to anorexia. *MedicalNewsToday*. Retrieved January 18, 2024, from medicalnewstoday.com

Paez, M. B., Luciano, C., & Gutierrez, O. (2007). Psychological treatment to cope with breast cancer: A comparative study between strategies of acceptance and cognitive control. *Psicooncologia, 4*(1), 75–95.

Paharia, M. I. (2008a). Insurance, managed care and integrated primary care. In B. A. Boyer & M. I. Paharia (Eds.), *Comprehensive handbook of clinical health psychology* (pp. 31–51). Hoboken, NJ: John Wiley & Sons.

Paharia, M.I. (2008b). Tobacco cessation. In B.A. Boyer & M.I. Paharia (Eds.), *Comprehensive handbook of clinical health psychology*. Hoboken, NJ: John Wiley & Sons.

Pain & Policy Studies Group. (2002). *Availability of opioid analgesics in Asia: Consumption trends, resources, recommendations*. Prepared for the 17th Study Programme for Overseas Experts on Drug Abuse & Narcotic Control, Tokyo, Japan.

Palmer, K.S. (1999). *A brief history: Universal health care efforts in the US*. Presentation to the Physicians for a National Health Program Meeting, Spring 1999. Retrieved June 23, 2013, from www.pnhp.org/facts/a-brief-history-universal-health-care-efforts-in-the-us

Palmgreen, P. (1984). Uses and gratifications: A theoretical perspective. In R.N. Bomstrom (Ed.), *Communication yearbook* (Vol. 8, pp. 61–72). Beverly Hills, CA: Sage Publication.

Palmieri, A., Fernandez, K.C., Cariolato, Y., Kleinbub, J.R., Salvatore, S., & Gross, J.J. (2022). Emotion regulation in psychodynamic and cognitive-behavioural therapy: An integrative perspective. *Clinical Neuropsychiatry*, 19(2), 103–113. doi: 10.36131%2Fcnfioritieditore20220204

Paltiel, A.D., Walensky, R.P., Schackman, B.R., Seage, G.R., III, Mercincavage, L.M., Weinstein, M.C., & Freedberg, K.A. (2005). Expanded HIV screening in the United States: Effect on clinical outcomes, HIV transmission and costs. *Annals of Internal Medicine*, 145(11), 797–806.

Pan, J., Barbeau, E.M., Levenstein, C., & Balbach, E.D. (2005). Smoke-free airlines and the role of organized labor: A case study. *American Journal of Public Health*, 195(3), 398–404.

Papaleontiou, L., Agaku, I.T., & Filippidis, F.T. (2020). Effects of exposure to tobacco and electronic cigarette advertisements on tobacco use: An analysis of the 2015 National Youth Tobacco Survey. *Journal of Adolescent Health*, 66(1), 64–71. doi: 10.1016/j.jadohealth.2019.05.022

Pape, J.W., Farmer, P., Koenig, S., Fitzgerald, D., Wright, P., & Johnson, W. (2008). The epidemiology of AIDS in Haiti refutes the claims of Gilbert et al. *PNAS*, 105(10), E13.

Parahoo, K., McDonough, S., McCaughan, E., Noyes, J., Semple, C., Halstead, E.J., . . . Dahm, P. (2013). Psychosocial interventions for men with prostate cancer. *Cochrane Database of Systematic Reviews*, (12). Article No.: CD008529. doi: 10.1002/14651858.CD008529.pub3. Retrieved from www.cochranelibrary.com

Pargament, K.I. (1997). *Theory, research & practice: The psychology of religion and coping*. New York: Guilford Press.

Park, J.H., Moon, J.H., Kim, H.J., Kong, M.H., & Oh, Y.H. (2020). Sedentary lifestyle: Overview of updated evidence of potential health risks. *Korean Journal of Family Medicine*, 41(6), 365–373. doi: 10.4082%2Fkjfm.20.0165

Park, N., Peterson, C., & Seligman, M.E.P. (2004). Strengths of character & well-being. *Journal of Social and Clinical Psychology*, 23(5), 603–619.

Park, S., Kim, H., & Kim, H. (2009). Relationship between parental alcohol abuse & social support, peer substance abuse risk & social support & substance use risk among South Korean adolescents. *Adolescence*, 44, 87–99.

Park, S.Y., Murphy, S.P., Sharmay, S., & Kolonel, L.N. (2005). Dietary intakes and health-related behaviors of Korean American women born in the USA & Korea: The multiethnic cohort study. *Public Health Nutrition*, 8(7), 904–911.

Parker, S., Hunter, T., Briley, C., Miracle, S., Hermann, J., Van Delinder, J., & Standridge, J. (2011). Formative assessment using social marketing principles to identify health & nutrition perspectives of Native American women living with the Chickasaw Nation boundaries in Oklahoma. *Journal of Nutrition Education & Behavior*, 43, 55–62.

Parker-Pope, T. (2008, June 3). Experts revive debate over cell phones and cancer. *The New York Times*.

Parkin, D. M., Bray, F., Ferlay, J., & Pisani, P. (2005). Global cancer statistics, 2002. *CA: A Cancer Journal for Clinicians*, *55*, 74–108.

Parks, S. H., & Pilisuk, M. (1991). Caregiver burden: Gender & the psychological cost of caregiving. *American Journal of Orthopsychiatry*, *61*(4), 501–509.

Parran, T. (1937). *Shadow on the land: Syphilis*. New York: Reynal & Hitchcock.

Partnership for Healthy Cities. (2023). *Osaka, Nairobi and New York City join the partnership!* Retrieved December 1, 2023, from cities4health.org.

Paschall, M. J., Grube, J. W., & Kypri, K. (2009). Alcohol control policies and alcohol consumption by youth: A multi-national study. *Addiction*, *104*(11), 1849–1855. doi: 10.1111/j.1360-0443.2009.02698

Pasteur, L., & Chamberland, R. (2002). Summary report of the experiments conducted at Pouille-le-Fort, near Melun, on the anthrax vaccination (T. Dasgupta, Trans.). *Yale Journal of Biology and Medicine*, *75*(1), 59–62.

Pate, J. E., Pumariega, A. J., Hester, C., & Gardner, D. (1992). Cross-cultural patterns in eating disorders: A review. *Journal of the American Academy of Child and Adolescent Psychiatry*, *31*, 802–809.

Patel, D. R., Philips, E. L., & Pratt, H. D. (1998). Eating disorders. *Indian Journal of Pediatrics*, *65*(4), 487–494.

Patel, M., Lee, A. D., Clemmons, N. S., Redd, S. B., Poser, S., Blog, D., . . . Gastañaduy, P. A. (2019). National update on measles cases and outbreaks – United States, January 1–October 1, 2019. *Morbidity and Mortality Weekly Report*, *68*(40), 893–896.

Patton, G. C., Sawyer, S. M., Santelli, J. S., Ross, D. A., Afifi, R., Allen, N. B., . . . Viner, R. M. (2016). Our future: A Lancet commission on adolescent health and wellbeing. *The Lancet*, *387*, 2423–2478.

Pawlyk, A. C., Morrison, A. R., Ross, R. J., & Brennan, F. X. (2008). Stress-induced changes in sleep in rodents: Model & mechanism. *Neuroscience & Biobehavioral Review*, *32*(1), 99–117.

Pazoki, R., Nabipour, I., Seyednezami, N., & Imami, S. R. (2007, August 23). Effects of a community-based health heart program in increasing healthy women's physical activity: A randomized controlled trial guided by community-based participatory research (CBPR). *BMC Public Health*, *7*, 216. doi:10.1186/1471-2458-7-216

PBS. (2023). Mass shooting in U.S. on a record pace in 2023 so far. *PBS NewsHour*. Retrieved June 1, 2023.

Pebley, K., Wang, X.-Q., Fahey, M. C., Patten, C. A., Mallawaarachchi, I., Talcott, G. W., . . . Little, M. A. (2023). Examination of tobacco-related messaging and tobacco use over time among U.S. military young adults. *Substance Use & Misuse*, *58*(1), 146–152. doi: 10.1080/10826084.2022.2151313

Pederson, L. L., & Lefcoe, N. M. (1987). Short- and long-term predictions of self-reported cigarette smoking in a cohort of later adolescents: Report of an 8-year follow-up of public school students. *Preventive Medicine*, *16*, 432–447.

Pell, J. P. (2003). The debate on public place defibrillators: Charged but shockingly ill informed. *Heart*, *89*, 1375–1376.

Pelland, L., Brosseau, L., Wells, G., MacLeay, L., Lambert, J., Lamothe, C., . . . Tugwell, P. (2004). Efficacy of strengthening exercises for osteoarthritis (part I): A meta-analysis. *Physical Therapy Review*, *9*, 77–108.

Pendry, B. (2001). *Stigma and HIV/AIDS in South Africa*. Presentation at the 21st United Nations General Assembly, Special Session on HIV/AIDS, June 2001.

Perez-Alvarez, M. (2016). The science of happiness: As felicious as it is fallacious. *Journal of Theoretical and Philosophical Psychology*, *36*(1), 1–19.

Perez-Pena, R. (2003, July 9). Obesity on rise in New York public schools. *The New York Times*.

Perpiñá-Galvañ, J., Orts-Beneito, N., Fernández-Alcántara, M., García-Sanjuán, S., García-Caro, M.P., & Cabañero-Martínez, M.J. (2019). Level of burden and health-related quality of life in caregivers of palliative care patients. *International Journal of Environmental Research and Public Health*, 16. doi: 10.3390/ijerph16234806

Perrin, K.M., & McDermott, R.J. (1997). The spiritual dimension of health: A review. *American Journal of Health Studies*, 13(2), 90–99.

Pesce, M., Speranza, L., Franceschelli, S., Ialenti, V., Iezzi, I., Patruno, A., . . . Grilli, A. (2013). Positive correlation between serum interleukin-1β and state anger in rugby athletes. *Aggressive Behavior*, 39(2), 141–148. doi: 10.1002/ab.21457

Peterson, C., & Seligman, M.E.P. (2004). *Character strengths & virtues: A handbook & classification*. New York: Oxford University Press.

Peterson, C.B., Thuras, P., Ackard, D.M., Mitchell, J.E., Berg, K., Sandager, N., . . . Crow, S.J. (2010). Personality dimensions in bulimia nervosa, binge eating disorder & obesity. *Comprehensive Psychiatry*, 51, 31–36.

Petersson, M., & Uvnas-Moberg, K. (2007). Effects of an acute stressor on blood pressure and heart rate in rats pretreated with intercerebroventricular oxytocin injections. *Psychoneuroendrocrinology*, 32, 959–965.

Peto, R., Darby, S., Deo, H., Silcocks, P., Whitley, E., & Doll, R. (2000). Smoking, smoking causation and lung cancer in the UK since 1950: Combination of national statistics with two case controlled studies. *British Medical Journal*, 321, 323–329.

Petraitis, J., Flay, B.R., & Miller, T.O. (1995). Reviewing theories of adolescent substance use: Organizing pieces in the puzzle. *Psychological Bulletin*, 117(1), 7–86.

Petrella, R.J., & Bartha, C. (2000). Home-based exercise therapy for older patients with knee osteoarthritis: A randomized clinical trial. *Journal of Rheumatology*, 27, 2215–2221.

Petridou, A., Siopi, A., & Mougios, V. (2019). Exercise in the management of obesity. *Metabolism*, 92, 163–169. doi: 10.1016/j.metabol.2018.10.009

Pfizer. (2023). *From basic health to herd immunity: What is the purpose of vaccines?* Retrieved April 30, 2023.

Pham, H.H., Landon, B.E., Reschovsky, J.D., Wu, B., & Schrag, D. (2009). Rapidity and modality of imaging for acute low back pain in elderly patients. *Archives of Internal Medicine*, 169(10), 972–981. doi: 10.1001/archinternmed.2009.78

Phillips, T. (2007). Everyone knew she was ill. The other girls, the model agencies . . . Don't believe it when they say they didn't. *The Guardian*. Retrieved May 28, 2009, from www.theguardian.com/lifeandstyle/2007/jan/14/fashion.features4

Philpott, D. (2009). An ethic of political reconciliation. *Ethics and International Affairs*, 23(4), 398–407.

Picket, G., & Hanlon, J.J. (1990). *Public health: Administration and practice* (9th ed.) St. Louis, MO: Times Mirror/Mosby.

Pietragalla, A., Arcieri, M., Marchetti, C., Scambia, G., & Fagotti, A. (2020). Ovarian cancer predisposition beyond BRCA1 and BRCA2 genes. *International Journal of Gynecologic Cancer*, 30(11). doi: 10.1136/ijgc-2020-001556

Pilevarzadeh, M., Amirshahi, M., Afsargharehbagh, R., Rafiemanesh, H., Hashemi, S.-H., & Balouchi, A. (2019). Global prevalence of depression among breast cancer patients: A systematic review and meta-analysis. *Breast Cancer Research & Treatment*, 176, 519–533.

Pingali, C., Yankey, D., Elam-Evans, L. D., Markowitz, L. E., Williams, C. L., Fredua, B., . . . Stokley, S. (2021). National, regional, state, and selected local area vaccination coverage among adolescents aged 13–17 years – United States, 2018. *Morbidity and Mortality Weekly Report*, 70, 1183–1190. doi: 10.15585/mmwr.mm7035a1external icon

Pinkerton, J. V. (2020). Hormone therapy for postmenopausal women. *The New England Journal of Medicine*, 382, 446–455. doi: 10.1056/NEJMcp1714787

Pinquart, M., & Sorensen, S. (2005). Caregiving distress and psychological health in caregivers. In K. V. Oxington (Ed.), *Psychology of stress* (pp. 165–206). New York, NY: Nova Biomedical Books.

Pischon, T., Lehmann, P. H., Boeing, H. Friedenreich, C., Norat, T., Tjønneland, A., . . . Riboli, E. (2006). Body size and risk of colon and rectal cancer in the European Prospective Investigation into Cancer and Nutrition (EPIC). *Journal of the National Cancer Institute*, 98, 920–931.

Pisetsky, D. S. (2007). Clinician's comment on the management of pain in arthritis. *Health Psychology*, 26(6), 657–659.

Pistrang, N., & Barker, C. (1995). The partner relationship in psychological response to breast cancer. *Social Science & Medicine*, 40, 789–797.

Pisu, M. G., Garau, A., Olla, P., Biggio, F., Utzeri, C., Dore, R., & Serra, M. (2013). Altered stress responsiveness and hypothalamic-pituitary-adrenal axis function in male rat offspring of socially isolated parents. *Journal of Neurochemistry*, 126(4), 493–502.

Pitt, T. M., Howard, A., HubkaRao, T., & Hagel, B. (2021). Identifying modifiable factors related to novice adolescent driver fault in motor vehicle collisions. *Traffic Injury Prevention*, 6, 437–442. doi: 10.1080/15389588.2021.1923700

Plaut, T. F., & Arons, B. S. (1994). President Clinton's proposal for health care reform: Key provisions and issues. *Hospital Community Psychiatry*, 45, 871–876.

Poage, E. D., Kitzenberger, K. E., & Olsen, J. (2004). Spirituality, contentment, and stress in recovering alcoholics. *Addictive Behaviors*, 29(9), 1857–1862.

Pope, H. G., Gruber, A. J., & Hudson, J. I. (2001). Neuropsychological performance in long-term cannabis users. *Archives of General Psychiatry*, 58(10), 909–915.

Portman, T. A. A., & Garrett, M. T. (2006). Native American healing traditions. *International Journal of Disability, Development and Education*, 53(4), 453–469.

Poss, J. E. (2001). Developing a new model for cross-cultural research: Synthesizing the health belief model and the theory of reasoned action. *Advances in Nursing Science*, 23(4), 1–15.

Post, F. L., Blustein, J., Gordon, E., & Neveloff, D. N. (1996). Pain: Ethics, culture, and informed consent to relief. *Journal of Law and Medical Ethics*, 24, 328–359.

Potter, C. W. (2001). A history of influenza. *Journal of Applied Microbiology*, 91, 572–579.

Potter, J. D. (1999). Colorectal cancer, molecules and populations. *Journal of the National Cancer Institute*, 91, 916.

Poudel, A., Gurung, B., & Khanal, G. P. (2020). Perceived social support and psychological wellbeing among Nepalese adolescents: The mediating role of self-esteem. *BMC Psychology*, 8(1), 43. doi: 10.1186/s40359-020-00409-1

Poulsen, L. H., Osler, M., Roberts, C., Becker, S. L., & Lauer, R. M. (2002) Exposure to teachers smoking and adolescent smoking behaviour: Analysis of cross sectional data from Denmark. *Tobacco Control*, 11, 246–251.

Prag, K. (2008). R. W. Hamilton, D. C. Baramki and the Lower Aqueduct at Bethlehem. *Palestine Exploration Quarterly*, 140(1), 27–38.

Prentice, J.C., & Pizer, S.D. (2007). Delayed access to care and mortality. *Health Services Research*, 42(2), 644–662.

Prentice-Hall, Inc. (1995–2002a). *Chapter review: The biological basis of behavior. The nervous system.* Retrieved February 25, 2010, from http://cwx.prenhall.com/bookbind/pubbooks/morris5/chapter2/custom1/deluxe-content.html

Prentice-Hall, Inc. (1995–2002b). *Chapter review: The biological basis of behavior. The sympathetic and parasympathetic systems.* Retrieved February 25, 2010, from http://cwx.prenhall.com/bookbind/pubbooks/morris5/chapter2/custom1/deluxe-content.html

Pressman, S.D., & Cohen, S. (2005). Does positive affect influence health? *Psychological Bulletin, 131*, 925–971.

Pressman, S.D., Cohen, S., Miller, G.E., Barkin, A., Rabin, B.S., & Treanor, J.J. (2005). Loneliness, social network size, and immune response to influenza vaccination in college freshmen. *Health Psychology, 24*, 297–306.

Prestwich, A., Conner, M., Baisley, W., Letman, J., & Molyneau, V. (2005). Individual and collaborative implementation intentions and the promotion of breast self-examination. *Psychology & Health, 20*(6), 743–760.

Price, A.J., Alvand, A., Troelsen, A., Katz, J.N., Hooper, G., Gray, A., . . . Beard, D. (2018). Knee replacement. *The Lancet, 392*(10158), 1672–1682. doi: 10.1016/S0140-6736(18)32344-4

Price, D.D. (2000). Psychological and neural mechanisms of the affective dimension of pain. *Science, 288*, 1769–1772.

Price, M.N., & Hyde, J.S. (2011). Perceived and observed maternal relationship quality predict sexual debut by age 15. *Journal of Youth and Adolescence, 40*, 1595–1606. doi: 10.1007/s10964-011-9641-y

Priebe, H.J. (2000). The aged cardiovascular risk patient. *British Journal of Anaesthesiology, 85*(5), 763–778.

Priebe, H.-J. (2016). Pharmacological modification of the perioperative stress response in noncardiac surgery. *Anaesthesiology, 30*(2), 171–189. doi: 10.1016/j.bpa.2016.03.001

Prince, R. (1983). Is anorexia nervosa a culture-bound syndrome? *Transcultural Psychiatric Research Review, 20*, 299–300.

Prochaska, J.O., & DiClemente, C.C. (1983). Stages and processes of self-change of smoking: Toward an integrative model of change. *Journal of Consulting and Clinical Psychology, 51*, 390–395.

Prochaska, J.O., Velicer, W.F., Rossi, J.S., Goldstein, M.G., Marcus, B.H., Rakowski, W., . . . Rossi, S.R. (1994). Stages of change and decisional balance for 12 problem behaviors. *Health Psychology, 13*, 39–46.

Public Broadcast Service. (1999). *The Kevorkian verdict: The law on assisted suicide.* Retrieved February 9, 2009, from www.pbs.org/wgbh/pages/frontline/kevorkian/law

Public Health Agency of Canada. (2009). *Heart disease and stroke in Canada 1997. Deaths from cardiovascular disease.* Retrieved from www.phac-aspc.gc.ca/publicat/2009/cvd-avc/index-eng.php

Public Health Agency of Canada. (2020). *Human papillomavirus (HPV).* Retrieved February 6, 2023, from Canada.ca

Public Health Law Center. (2009). *Restricting tobacco advertising.* Retrieved January 1, 2024, from publichealthlawcenter.org

Puhl, R.M., & Heuer, C.A. (2009). The stigma of obesity: A review and update. *Obesity, 17*, 941–964.

Puhl, R.M., & Latner, J.F.D. (2007). Stigma, obesity, and the health of the nation's children. *Psychological Bulletin, 13*, 557–580.

Puhl, R. M., Lessard, L. M., Himmelstein, M. S., & Foster, G. D. (2021). The roles of experienced and internalized weight stigma in healthcare experiences: Perspectives of adults engaged in weight management across six countries. *PLoS One, 16*(6), e0251566. doi: 10.1371/journal.pone.0251566

Pumariega, A. J. (1997). Body dissatisfaction among Hispanic and Asian-American girls. *Journal of Adolescent Health, 21*, 1.

Purdy, J. (2013). Chronic physical illness: A psychophysiological approach for chronic physical illness. *Yale Journal of Biology and Medicine, 86*(1), 15–28.

Putman, K. M., Lantz, J., Townsend, C. L., Gallegos, A. M., Potts, A. A., Roberts, R. C., . . . Foy, D. W. (2009). Exposure to violence, support needs, adjustment, and motivators among Guatemalan humanitarian aid workers. *American Journal of Community Psychology, 44*(1–2), 109–115.

Quah, S. R. (2003). Traditional healing systems and the ethos of science. *Social Science & Medicine, 57*, 1997–2012.

Ra, C. K., Pehlivan, N., Kim, H., Sussman, S., Unger, J. B., & Businelle, M. S. (2020). Smoking prevalence among Asian Americans: Associations with education, acculturation, and gender. *Preventive Medicine Reports, 30*, 102035. doi: 10.1016/j.pmedr.2022.102035

Rabin, B. S., Cohen, S., Ganguli, R., Lyle, D. T., & Cunnick, J. E. (1989). Bidirectional interaction between the central nervous system and immune system. *CRC Critical Reviews in Immunology, 9*(4), 279–312.

Radi, S., Lang, T., Lauwers-Cances, V., Diene, E., Chatellier, G., Larabi, L., . . . for the IHPAF Group. (2005). Job constraints and arterial hypertension: Different effects in men and women: The IHPAF II case control study. *Occupational and Environmental Medicine, 62*, 711–717.

Radu, A.-F., & Bungau, S. G. (2021). Management of rheumatoid arthritis: An overview. *Cells, 10*(11), 2857. doi: 10.3390/cells10112857

Radusin, M. (2012). The Spanish flu – Part II: The second and third wave. *Vojnosanitetski Pregled, 69*(10), 917–927.

Rafique, N., Al-Asoom, L. I., Latif, R., Al Sunni, A., & Wasi, S. (2019). Comparing levels of psychological stress and its inducing factors among medical students. *Journal of Taibah University Medical Sciences, 14*(6), 488–494. doi: 10.1016/j.jtumed.2019.11.002

Ragin, D. F., Griffing, S., Sage, R. E., Madry, L., Bingham, L., & Primm, B. J. (2000). Breaking the intergenerational cycle of violence: A social marketing approach to behavior change. In N. De Meillon (Ed.), *Creative rescue counselling and assistance for the children in our country: After conference proceedings*. University of South Africa (UNISA). Pretoria: Production Printers.

Ragin, D. F., Holohan, J. A., Ricci, E. M., Grant, C., & Richardson, L. D. (2005a). Shocking a community into action: A social marketing approach to cardiac arrests. *Journal of Health & Social Policy, 20*(2), 49–70.

Ragin, D. F., Hwang, U., Cydulka, R. K., Holson, D., Haley, L. L., Richards, C. F., . . . Emergency Medicine Patients' Access to Healthcare (EMPATH) Study Investigators. (2005b). Reasons for using the emergency department: Results of the EMPATH Study. *Academic Emergency Medicine, 12*(12), 1158–1166.

Ragin, D. F., Pilotti, M., Madry, L., Sage, R. E., Bingham, L. E., & Primm, B. J. (2002). Intergenerational substance abuse and domestic violence as familial risk factors for lifetime attempted suicide among battered women. *Journal of Interpersonal Violence, 17*(10), 1027–1045.

Ragin, D. F., Ricci, E. M., Rhodes, R., Holohan, J., Smirnoff, M., & Richardson, L. D. (2008). Defining the "community" in community consultation for emergency research: Findings from the community VOICES study. *Social Science & Medicine, 66*(6), 1379–1392.

Rahe, R. H., Mahan, J. L., & Arthur, R. J. (1970). Prediction of near-future health change from subject's preceding life change. *Journal of Psychosomatic Research, 14*(4), 401–406.

Rahimi, A., Anoosheh, M., Ahmadi, F., & Foroughan, F. (2013). Exploring spirituality in Iranian healthy elderly people: A qualitative content analysis. *Iranian Journal of Nursing and Midwifery Research*, *18*(2), 163–170.

Rahim-Williams, F. B., Riley, J. L., Herrera, D., Campbell, C. M., Hastie, B. A., & Fillingim, R. B. (2007). Ethnic identity predicts experimental pain sensitivity in African Americans and Hispanics. *Pain*, *129*, 177–184.

Raia-Barjat, T., Gannard, I., Virieux, D., Del Aguila-Berthelot, C., Nekaa, M., Chauvin, F., . . . Gagneux-Brunon, A. (2020). Health students' knowledge of sexually transmitted infections and risky behaviors before participation to the health promotion program. *Médecine et Maladies Infectieuses*, *50*(4), 368–371. doi: 10.1016/j.medmal.2020.01.015

Rakhkovskaya, L. M., & Warren, C. S. (2014). Ethnic identity, thin-ideal internalization, and eating pathology in ethnically diverse college women. *Body Image*, *11*(4), 438–445. doi: 10.1016/j.bodyim.2014.07.003

Ramagopalan, S. V., Knight, J. C., & Ebers, G. C. (2009). Multiple sclerosis and the major histocompatibility complex. *Current Opinion in Virology*, *22*(3), 219–225.

Ramchand, R., Ayer, L., & O'Connor, S. (2022). Unemployment, behavioral health, and suicide. *Health Affairs*. Retrieved from www.healthaffairs.org/do/10.1377/hpb20220302.274862/full/

Ranscombe, P. (2022). Vaccine voyages: Where science meets slavery. *The Lancet Infectious Diseases*, *22*(7), 956. doi: 10.1016/S1473-3099(22)00270-5

Ransom, S., Jacobson, P. B., Schmidt, J. E., & Andrykowski, M. A. (2005). Relationship of problem-focused coping strategies to changes in quality of life following treatment for early stage breast cancer. *Journal of Pain and Symptom Management*, *30*(3), 243–253.

Rao, N. D., & Shirts, B. H. (2023). Using species richness calculation to model the global profile of unsampled pathogenic variants: Examples from BRCA1 and BRCA2. *PLoS One*, *18*(2), e0278010. doi: 10.1371/journal.pone.0278010

Rao, R. D., & Cobleigh, M. A. (2012). Adjuvant endocrine therapy for breast cancer. *Oncology*, *26*(6), 541–547.

Rascombe, P. (2022). Vaccine voyages: Where science meets slavery. *The Lancet: Infectious Diseases*, *22*(7), 956. doi: 10.1016/S1473-3099(22)00270-5

Rasmussen, H. B., & Clausen, J. (2000). Genetic risk factors in multiple sclerosis and approaches to their identification. *Journal of Neurovirology*, (suppl. 2), S23–S27.

Rat, A.-C., Brignon, M., Beauvais, C., Beranger, M., Boujut, E., Cohen, J.-D., . . . Giraudet-Le Quintrec, J.-S. (2021). Patients and spouses coping with inflammatory arthritis: Impact of communication and spousal perceived social support and burden. *Joint Bone Spine*, *88*(3). doi: 10.1016/j.jbspin.2020.105125

Rathner, G., & Messner, K. (1993). Detection of eating disorders in a small rural town: An epidemiological study. *Psychological Medicine*, *23*, 175–184.

Raus, K., Mortier, E., & Eeckloo, K. (2022). Ethical reflections on Covid-19 vaccines. *Acta Clinica Belgica: An International Journal of Clinical and Laboratory Medicine*, *77*(3), 600–605. doi: 10.1080/17843286.2021.1925027

Ray, O. (2004). How the mind hurts and heals the body. *American Psychologist*, *59*, 29–40.

Reagan, L. J. (1997). Engendering the dread disease: Women, men and cancer. *American Journal of Public Health*, *87*(11), 1779–1787.

Rebane, K., Tuomi, A.-K., Kautiainen, H., Peltoniemi, S., Glerup, M., & Aalto, K. (2022). Abdominal pain in Finnish young adults with juvenile idiopathic arthritis. *Scandinavian Journal of Gastroenterology*, *57*(10), 1189–1194. doi: 10.1080/00365521.2022.2072691

Rebbeck, T. R., Friebel, T. M., Friedman, E., Hamann, U., Huo, D., Kwong, A., . . . Nathanson, K. L. (2018). Mutational spectrum in a worldwide study of 29,700 families with BRCA1 or BRCA2 mutations. *Human Mutation*, *39*(5), 593–620.

Redd, W. H., Montgomery, G. H., & DuHamel, K. N. (2001). Behavioral intervention for cancer treatment side effects. *Journal of the National Cancer Institute*, *93*(11), 810–823.

Redvers, N., & Blondin, B. (2020). Traditional indigenous medicine in North America: A scoping review. *PLoS One*, *15*(8), e0237531. doi: 10.1371/journal.pone.0237531

Reese, S. E., Dang, A., & Liddell, J. L. (2024). 'We'd just patch ourselves up': Preference for holistic approaches to healthcare and traditional medicine among members of a state-recognized tribe. *Journal of Holistic Nursing*, *42*, 34–48. doi: 10.1177/08980101231169867

Regan, G., Lee, R. E., Booth, K., & Reese-Smith, J. (2006). Obesogenic influences in public housing: A mixed-method analysis. *American Journal of Health Promotion*, *20*(4), 282–290.

Reich, J. A. (2021). Multiple ways of understanding vaccine hesitance and refusal. In D. F. Ragin & J. P. Keenan (Eds.), *Handbook of research methods in health psychology* (pp. 287–297). New York, NY: Routledge, Taylor & Francis Group.

Reich, J. F. (2020). Capitalizing on healthy lawyers: The business case for law firms to promote and prioritize lawyer well-being. *Villanova Law Review*, *65*, 361.

Reichert, K. L., Hole, K., Hamberger, A., Saelid, G., Edminson, P. D., Braestrup, C. B., Lingjaerde, O., Ledaal, P., & Orbeck, H. (1993). Biologically active peptide-containing fractions in schizophrenia and childhood autism. *Advances in Biochemical Psychopharmacology*, *28*, 627–643.

Reid, M. C., Papaleontiou, M., Ony, A., Buckman, R., Wethington, E., & Pillemer, K. (2008). Self-management strategies to reduce pain and improve function among older adults in community settings: A review of the evidence. *Pain Medicine*, *9*, 409–424.

Reid, T. L. B., & Smalls, C. (2004). Stress, spirituality and health promoting behaviors among African American college students. *Western Journal of Black Studies*, *28*(1), 283–291.

Reinhart, R. J. (2020, January 14). Fewer in U.S. continue to see vaccines as important. *Gallup*. Retrieved April 20, 2023, from gallup.com.

Republic of South Africa, Department of Health. (2022). *Update on Covid-19, 07 December 2022*. Retrieved June 12, 2023, from SA Corona Virus Online Portal.

Reschovsky, J. D., Hadley, J., & Landon, B. E. (2006). Compensation methods and physicians group structure on physician's perceived incentives to alter service to patients. *Health Services Research*, *41*(4 Pt. 1), 1200–1220.

Reschovsky, J. D., Rich, E. C., & Lake, T. K. (2015). Factors contributing to variations in physicians' use of evidence at the point of care: A conceptual model. *Journal of General Internal Medicine*, *30*(Suppl. 3), 555–561. doi: 10.1007/s11606-015-3366-7

Rethemiotaki, I. (2023). Global prevalence of cardiovascular diseases by gender and age during 2010–2019. *Archives of Medical Sciences: Atherosclerosis Disease*, *30*(8), e196–e205. doi: 10.5114/amsad/176654

Reyes-Gibby, C. C., Anderson, K. O., Shete, S., Bruera, E., & Yennurajalingam, S. (2012). Early referral to supportive care specialists for symptom burden in lung cancer patients: A comparison of non-Hispanic whites, Hispanics, and non-Hispanic blacks. *Cancer*, *118*(3), 856–863. doi: 10.1002/cncr.26312

RHO. (2008). *About cervical cancer. Preventing cervical cancer: Unprecedented opportunities for improving women's health*. Retrieved October 28, 2013, from www.rho.org/about-cervical-cancer.htm

Rice, S. M., Purcell, R. P., & McGorry, P. D. (2018). Adolescent and young adult male mental health: Transforming system failures into proactive models of engagement. *Journal of Adolescent Health*, *62*(3), S9–S17. doi: 10.1016/j.jadohealth.2017.07.024

Richards, H. M., Reid, M. E., & Watt, G. C. M. (2002). Socioeconomic variations in responses to chest pain: Qualitative study. *British Medical Journal, 324*(7349), 1308–1317.

Richardson, T. J., Lee, S. J., Berg-Weger, M., & Grossberg, G. T. (2013). Caregiver health: Health of caregivers of Alzheimer's and other dementia patients. *Current Psychiatry Reports, 15*, 367. doi: 10.1007/s11920-013-0367-2

Riddle, D. L., Jiranek, W. A., & Hayes, C. W. (2014). Use of a validated algorithm to judge the appropriateness of total knee arthroplasty in the United States: A multicenter longitudinal cohort study. *Arthritis & Rheumatology, 66*(8), 2134–2143. doi: 10.1002/art.38685

Ritvanen, T., Louhevaara, V., Helin, P., Halonen, T, & Hanninen, O. (2007). Effect of aerobic fitness on the physiological stress responses at work. *International Journal of Occupational Medicine & Environmental Health, 20*(1), 1–8.

Rix, K., Delgado, M. K., Ebert, J., McIntosh, C. W., Bocage, C., Xiong, R., . . . McDonald, C. (2022). 139 Measuring risky driving behaviors in adolescent drivers using a novel smartphone telematic app. *Injury Prevention, 28*(Suppl. 1), 50. doi: 10.1136/injuryprev-2022-SAVIR.128 6

Roberto, C. A., Larsen, P. D., Agnew, H., Baik, T., & Brownell, K. D. (2010). Evaluating the impact of menu labeling on food choices and intake. *American Journal of Public Health, 100*(2), 312–318.

Roberts, B. A. (2019). Legalized cannabis in Colorado emergency departments: A cautionary review of negative health and safety effects. *Western Journal of Emergency Medicine, 20*(4), 557–572.

Robinson, P. C., van der Linden, S., Khan, M. A., & Taylor, W. J. (2021). Axial spondylarthritis: Concept, construct, classification and implications for therapy. *Nature Reviews Rheumatology, 17*, 109–118. doi: 10.1038/s41584-020-00552-4

Robinson, T. N., Killen, J. D., Litt, I. F., Hammer, L. D., Wilson, D. M., Haydel, K. F., . . . Taylor, C. B. (1996). Ethnicity and body dissatisfaction: Are Hispanic and Asian girls at increased risk for eating disorders? *Journal of Adolescent Health, 19*, 384–393.

Roddy, E., Zhang, W., & Doherty, M. (2007). The changing epidemiology of gout. *National Clinical Practice of Rheumatology, 3*, 443–449.

Rodgers, R. F., Lombardo, C., Cerolini, S., Franko, D. L., Omori, M., Fuller-Tyszkiewicz, M., . . . Guillaume, S. (2020). The impact of the COVID-19 pandemic on eating disorder risk and symptoms. *International Journal of Eating Disorders, 53*(7), 1166–1170. doi: 10.1002/eat.23318

Rodrigues, J. M., Matos, L. C., Francisco, N., Dias, A., Azevedo, J., & Machado, J. (2021). Assessment of Qigong effects on anxiety of high-school students: A randomized controlled trial. *Advances in Mind-Body Medicine, 35*(3), 10–19.

Rodriguez, M. A., Bauer, H. M., Flores-Ortiz, Y., & Szkupinski-Quiroga, S. (1998). Factors affecting patient-physician communication for abused Latina and Asian immigrant women. *Journal of Family Practice, 47*(4).

Roger, V., Go, A. S., Lloyd-Jones, D. M., Benjamin, E. J., Berry, J. D., Borden, W. B., . . . Turner, M. B. (2012). Heart disease and stroke statistics – 2012 update: A report from the American Heart Association. *Circulation, 125*, e2–e220.

Rojas, I. G., Padgett, D. A., Sheridan, J. F., & Marucha, P. T. (2002). Stress-induced susceptibility to bacterial infection during cutaneous wound healing. *Brain, Behavior, and Immunity, 16*, 74–84.

Roman, N. V., Mthembu, T. G., & Hoosen, M. (2020). Spiritual care – 'A deeper immunity' – A response to Covid-19 pandemic. *African Journal of Primary Health Care and Family Medicine, 12*(1). Retrieved from https://hdl.handle.net/10520/EJC-1ead110600

Romero, L. M., Dickens, M. J., & Cyr, N. E. (2009). The reactive scope model: A new model integrating homeostasis, allostasis, and stress. *Hormones and Behavior, 55*, 375–389.

Rosamond, W., Flegal, K., Friday, G., Furie, K., Go, A., Greenlund, K., . . . Hong, Y. (2007). Heart disease and stroke statistics – 2007 update: A report from the American Heart Association Statistics Committee and Stroke Statistics Subcommittee. *Circulation*, *115*(5), e69–e171.

Rosen, S., Shephard, A., & Khan, J. A. (2018). US health care clinician's knowledge, attitudes, and practices regarding human papillomavirus vaccination: A qualitative systematic review. *Academic Pediatrics*, *18*(2 Suppl.), 553–565.

Rosenberg, L., Palmer, J. R., & Shapiro, S. (1990). Decline in the risk of myocardial infarction among women who stop smoking. *The New England Journal of Medicine*, *322*, 213–217.

Rosengren, A., Hawken, S., Ounpuu, S., Sliwa, K., Zubaid, M., Almahmeed, W. A., . . . Yusuf, S. (2004). Association of psychosocial risk factors with risk of acute myocardial infarction in 11,119 cases and 13,648 controls from 52 countries (the INTERHEART study): Case–control study. *The Lancet*, *364*, 953–962.

Rosenstock, I. M. (2005). Why people use health services. *The Milbank Quarterly*, *83*(4), 1–32.

Rosenstock, I. M., Strecher, V. S., & Becker, M. H. (1988). Social learning theory and the health belief model. *Health Education Quarterly*, *15*(2), 175–183.

Rosenthal, R., Hall, J. A., DiMatteo, M. R., Rogers, P. T., & Archer, D. (1979). *Sensitivity to nonverbal communication: The PONS test*. Baltimore, MD: Johns Hopkins University Press.

Ross, L., Kohler, C. L., Grimley, D. M., & Anderson-Lewis, C. (2007). The theory of reasoned action and intention to seek cancer information. *American Journal of Health Behavior*, *31*(2), 123–134.

Rossen, I., Hurlstone, M. J., Dunlop, P. D., & Lawrence, C. (2019). Accepters, fence sitters, or rejecters: Moral profiles of vaccination attitudes. *Social Science & Medicine*, *224*, 23–27. doi: 10.1016/j.socscimed.2019.01.038

Rovniak, L. S., Anderson, E. S., Winett, R. A., & Stephens, R. S. (2002). Social cognitive determinants of physical activity in young adults: A prospective structural equation analysis. *Annals of Behavioral Medicine*, *24*, 149–156.

Rubin, R. (2021). The price of success – How to evaluate COVID-19 vaccines when they're available outside of clinical trials. *Journal of the American Medical Association*, *325*(10), 918–921.

Rubin-Garcia, M., Martin, V., Vitelli-Storelli, F., Moreno, V., Aragones, N., Aradanaz, E., . . . Benavente, Y. (2022). Antecedentes familiars de primer grado como factor de riesgo en El cancer colorectal. *Gaceta Sanitaria*, *36*(4), 345–352.

Ruch, W., & Carrell, A. (1998). Trait cheerfulness and the sense of humor. *Personality and Individual Differences*, *24*, 551–558.

Rudd, R. A., Aleshire, N., Zibbel, J. E., & Gladden, M. (2016). Increases in drug and opioid overdose deaths – United States, 2000–2014. *Morbidity and Mortality Weekly Report*, *64*(50), 1378–1382. Retrieved November 9, 2016, from www.cdc.gov/mmwr/preview/mmwrhtml/mm6450a3.htm.

Ruehlman, L., Karoly, R., & Newton, C. (2005). Comparing the experiential and psychosocial dimensions of chronic pain in African Americans and Caucasians: Findings from a national community sample. *Pain Medicine*, *6*, 49–60.

Ruel, T., Penazzato, M., Zech, J. M., Archary, M., Cressey, T. R., Goga, A., . . . Abrams, E. J. (2023). Novel approaches to postnatal prophylaxis to eliminate vertical transmission of HIV. *Global Health: Science and Practice*, *11*, e2200401. doi: 10.9745/GHSP-D-22-00401

Russell, G. F. M. (1965). Metabolic aspects of anorexia nervosa. *Proceedings of the Royal Society of Medicine*, *58*, 811–814. Retrieved February 1, 2024, from procrsmed00191–0066.pdf (nih.gov)

Russell, S. T., Sinclair, K. O., Poteat, V. P., & Koenig, V. W. (2012). Adolescent health and harassment based on discriminatory bias. *American Journal of Public Health*, *102*(3), 493–495.

Rutledge, D. N. (1987). Factors related to women's practice of breast self-examination. *Nursing Research*, *36*, 117–121.

Ryan, R. M., & Deci, E. L. (2000). Self-determination theory and the facilitation of intrinsic motivation, social development, and well-being. *American Psychologist*, *55*(1), 68–78.

Sabet, K. (2021). Lessons learned in several states eight years after states legalized marijuana. *Current Opinion in Psychology*, *38*, 25–30.

Sacks, J., Helmick, C., Yao-Hun, L., Ilowite, N., & Bowyer, S. (2007). Prevalence of and annual ambulatory health care visits for pediatric arthritis and other rheumatologic conditions in the United States in 2001–2004. *Arthritis & Rheumatology*, *57*, 1439–1445.

Sadovnick, A. D., Baird, P. A., Ward, R. H., Opitz, J. M., & Reynolds, J. F. (1988). Multiple sclerosis: Updated risk for relatives. *American Journal of Medical Genetics*, *29*, 533–541.

Saeedi, P., Petersohn, I., Salpea, P., Malanda, B., Karuranga, S., Unwin, N., . . . Williams, R. (2019). Global and regional diabetes prevalence estimates for 2019 and projections for 2030 and 2045: Results from the International Diabetes Federation Diabetes Atlas, 9th edition. *Diabetes Research and Clinical Practice*, *157*. doi: 10.1016/j.diabres.2019.107843

Safaee, A., Moghimi-Dehkordi, B., Pourhoseingholi, M. A., Vahedi, M., Maserat, E., & Ghiasi, S. (2010). Risk of colorectal cancer in relatives: A case control study. *Indian Journal of Cancer*, *47*, 27–30.

Sagrestano, L. M., Rogers, A., & Service, A. (2008). HIV/AIDS. In B. A. Boyer & M. I. Paharia (Eds.), *Comprehensive handbook of clinical health psychology*. Hoboken, NJ: John Wiley & Sons.

Saha, S., Komaromy, M., Koepsell, T. D., & Bindman, A. B. (1999). Patient–physician racial concordance and the perceived quality and use of health care. *Archives of Internal Medicine*, *159*(9), 997–1004.

Saleem, T., Khalid, U., & Qidwai, W. (2009). Geriatric patient's expectations of their physicians: Findings from a tertiary care hospital in Pakistan. *BMC Health Services Research*, *13*(9), 205.

Salkind, N. J. (2006). *Exploring research* (6th ed.). Upper Saddle River, NJ: Prentice Hall.

Salleh, M. R. (2008). Life event, stress and illness. *Malaysian Journal of Medical Sciences*, *15*(4), 9–18.

Sallfors, C., Hallberg, L. R., & Fasth, A. (2003). Gender and age differences in pain, coping and health status among children with chronic arthritis. *Clinical and Experimental Rheumatology*, *21*(6), 785–793.

Sallis, J. F., Hovell, M. F., Hofstetter, C. R., Faucher, P., Elder, J. P., Blanchard, J., . . . Christenson, G. M. (1989). A multivariate study of determinants of vigorous exercise in a community sample. *Preventive Medicine*, *18*, 20–34.

Salmon, J. W. (Ed.). (2022). *Alternative medicines. Popular and policy perspectives*. New York, NY: Taylor & Francis.

Salovey, P., Rothman, A. J., Detweiler, J. B., & Steward, W. T. (2000). Emotional states and physical health. *American Psychologist*, *55*(1), 110–121.

Samwel, H. J. A., Kraaimaat, F. W., Crul, B. J. P., van Dongan, R. R., & Evers, A. W. M. (2009). Multidisciplinary allocation of pain treatment: Long-term outcome and correlates of cognitive-behavioral processes. *Journal of Musculoskeletal Pain*, *17*(1), 26–36.

Sanden, I., Larson, U. S., & Eriksson, C. (2000). An interview study of men discovering testicular cancer. *Cancer Nursing*, *23*(4), 304–309.

Sanders Thompson, V. L., Bazile, A., & Akbar, M. (2004). African American's perceptions of psychotherapy and psychotherapists. *Professional Psychology: Research and Practice*, *35*, 19–26.

Sandstrom, M., Wilen, J., Oftedal, G., & Hansson Mild, K. (2001). Mobile phone use and subjective symptoms. Comparison of symptoms experienced by users of analogue and digital mobile phones. *Occupational Medicine (London)*, *51*, 25–35.

San-Juan-Rodriguez, A., Piro, V. M., Good, C. B., Gellad, W. F., & Hernandez, I. (2021). Trends in list prices, net prices, and discounts of self-administered injectable tumor necrosis factor inhibitors. *Journal of Managed Care & Specialty Pharmacy*, 27(1), 112–117. doi: 10.18553/jmcp.2021.27.1.112

Sapolsky, R. (1998). The stress of Gulf War syndrome. *Nature*, 393, 308–309. doi: 10.1038/30606

Sapolsky, R. M. (2000). Social status and health in humans and other animals. *Annual Review of Anthropology*, 33, 393–418.

Sapolsky, R. M. (2004). *Why Zebras don't get ulcers* (3rd ed.). New York, NY: St. Martin's Griffin.

Sapolsky, R. M., Romero, L. M., & Munck, A. U. (2000). How do glucocorticoids influence stress responses? Integrating permissive, suppressive, stimulatory, and preparative actions. *Endocrine Reviews*, 21(1), 55–89.

Saraiya, M., Unger, E. R., Thompson, T. D., Lynch, C. F., Hernandez, B. Y., Lyu, C. W., . . . HPV Typing of Cancers Workgroup. (2015). US assessment of HPV types in cancers: Implications for current and 9-valent HPV vaccines. *Journal of the National Cancer Institute*, 107(6): djv086. doi: 10.1093%2Fjnci%2Fdjv086

Sargent, J. D., Dalton, M. A., Beach, M., Bernhardt, A., Pullin, D., & Stevens, M. (1997). Cigarette promotional items in public schools. *Archives of Pediatric & Adolescent Medicine*, 151(12), 1189–1196.

Saris, W. H., Blair, S. N., vanBaak, M. A., Eaton, S. B., Davis, P. S., & DiPeitro, L. (2003). How much physical activity is enough to prevent unhealthy weight gain? Outcome of the IASO 1st stock conference and consensus statement. *Obesity Reviews*, 4(2), 101–114.

Satienlerk, V., & Perawongmetha, A. (2022). Thailand massacre: Ex-cop kills 24 children in knife and gun rampage. *Reuters*. Retrieved June 3, 2023.

Saul, S. (2005, June 13). U.S. to review drug intended for one race. *The New York Times*.

Savage, L. (2007). Proposed human papillomavirus mandates rile health experts. *Journal of the National Cancer Institute*, 99(9), 665–666.

Savage, L. É., Tarabulsy, G. M., Pearson, J., Collin-Vézina, D., & Gagné, L.-M. (2019). Maternal history of childhood maltreatment and later parenting behavior: A meta-analysis. *Development and Psychopathology*, 31(1), 9–21. doi: 10.1017/S0954579418001542

Savulescu, J., & Spriggs, M. (2002). The hexamethorium asthma study and the death of a normal volunteer in research. *Journal of Medical Ethics*, 28, 3–4.

Sayed-Ahmed, M. (2016). Incidence history of West Nile virus in Africa and Middle East, with an emphasis on Egypt: A review. *Journal of Dairy, Veterinary & Animal Research*, 3(3), 101–104. doi: 10.15406/jdvar.2016.03.00080

SCDTSEA. (2015). *Funny seatbelt sayings*. Retrieved January 20, 2024, from scdtsea.org

Schaefer, J. D., Jang, S.-K., Vrieze, S., Iacono, W. G., McGue, M., & Wilson, S. (2021). Adolescent cannabis use and adult psychoticism: A longitudinal co-twin control analysis using data from two cohorts. *Journal of Abnormal Psychology*, 130(7), 691–701. doi: 10.1037/abn0000701

Schaefer, S., & Coleman, E. (1992). Shifts in meaning, purpose, and values following a diagnosis of human immunodeficiency virus (HIV) infection among gay men. *Journal of Psychology and Human Sexuality*, 5(1–2), 13–29.

Scherer, H. U., Häupl, T., & Burmester, G. R. (2020). The etiology of rheumatoid arthritis. Journal of Autoimminity, *110*. doi: 10.1016/j.jaut.2019.102400

Schliefer, S. J., Keller, S. E., & Meyerson, A. T. (1984). Lymphocyte function in major depressive disorder. *Archives of General Psychiatry*, 41(5), 484–486.

Schliefer, S. J., Keller, S. E., & Siris, S. G. (1985). Depression and immunity. *Archives of General Psychiatry*, *42*, 129–133.

Schmidt, T., Delorio, N. M., & McClure, K. B. (2006). The meaning of community consultation. *American Journal of Bioethics*, *6*, 30–32.

Schnall, P. L., Landsbergis, P. A., & Baker, D. (1990). The relationship between 'job strain,' workplace diastolic blood pressure, and left ventricular mass index. *JAMA*, *263*, 1929–1935.

Schneider, H., & Stein, J. (2001). Implementing AIDS policy in post-apartheid South Africa. *Social Science & Medicine*, *52*, 122–131.

Schneider, R. H., Staggers, F., Alexander, C. N., Sheppard, W., Rainforth, M., Kondwani, K., . . . King, C. G. (1995). A randomized controlled trial of stress reduction for hypertension in older African Americans. *Hypertension*, *26*, 820–827.

Schneiderman, N., & Siegel, S. D. (2012). Mental and physical health influence each other. In *The great ideas of clinical science* (pp. 359–376). Routledge/Taylor & Francis Group.

Schnoll, R. A., Knowles, J. C., & Harlow, L. (2002). Correlates of adjustment among cancer survivors. *Journal of Psychosocial Oncology*, *20*(1), 37–59.

Schoenborn, C. A., & Adams, P. F. (2002). *Alcohol use among adults: United States, 1997–1998*. Advanced Data from Vital and Health Statistics (Report No. 324). National Center for Health Statistics, CDC.

Schreiber, G. B., Robins, M., Striegel-Moore, R., Obarzanek, E., Morrison, J. A., & Wright, D. J. (1996). Weight modification efforts reported by black and white preadolescent girls: National Heart, Lung, and Blood Institute Growth and Health Study. *Pediatrics*, *98*, 3–70.

Schuchat, A., Houry, D., & Guy, G. P. (2017). New data on opioid use and prescribing in the United States. *JAMA*, *318*(5), 425–426. doi: 10.1001/jama.2017.8913

Schultz, A., & Northridge, M. E. (2004). Social determinants of health: Implications for environmental health promotion. *Health, Education & Behavior*, *31*(4), 455–471.

Schultz, A. M., Williams, D. R., Israel, B. A., & Lempert, L. B. (2002). Racial and spatial relations as fundamental determinants of health in Detroit. *Milbank Quarterly*, *80*(4), 677–707.

Schulz, R., Beach, S. R., Ives, D. G., Martire, L. M., Ariyo, A. A., & Kop, W. J. (2000). Association between depression and mortality in older adults: The Cardiovascular Health Study. *Archives of Internal Medicine*, *160*, 1761–1768.

Schulz, R., Martire, L. M., Beach, S. R., & Scheier, M. F. (2005). Depression and mortality in the elderly. In G. Miller & E. Chen (Eds.), *Current directions in health psychology*. Upper Saddle River, NJ: Prentice Hall.

Schutte, A. E., Ware, L. J., Huisman, H. W., Fourie, C. M. T., Greeff, M., Khumalo, T., & Wissing, M. P. (2014). Psychological distress and the development of hypertension over 5 years in black South Africans. *Journal of Clinical Hypertension*, *17*(2), 126–133. doi: 10.1111/jch.12455

Schüz, J., Morgan, G., Böhler, E., Kaatsch, P., & Michaelis, J. (2003). Atopic disease and childhood acute lymphoblastic leukemia. *International Journal of Cancer*, *105*, 255–260.

Schwartz, A. R., Gerin, W., Davidson, K. W., Pickering, T. G., Brosschot, J. F., Thayer, J. F., . . . Linden, W. (2003). Toward a causal model of cardiovascular responses to stress and the development of cardiovascular disease. *Psychosomatic Medicine*, *65*, 22–35.

Schwarzer, R., Schuz, B., Ziegelmann, J. P., Lippke, S., Luszczynska, A., & Scholz, U. (2007). Adoption and maintenance of four health behaviors: Theory-guided longitudinal studies on dental flossing, seat belt use, dietary behavior, and physical activity. *Annals of Behavioral Medicine*, *33*(2), 156–166.

Schwingshackl, L., Morse, J., & Hoffman, G. (2019). Mediterranean diet and health status: Active ingredients and pharmacological mechanisms. *British Journal of Pharmacology*, *177*(6), 1241–1257. doi: 10.1111/bph.14778

Science Museum Group. (2019). *Bubonic plague: The first pandemic.* Retrieved November 1, 2023, from https://www.sciencemuseum.org.uk/objects-and-stories/medicine/bubonic-plague-first-pandemic

Sclavo, M. (2001). Cardiovascular risk factors and prevention in women: Similarities and differences. *Italian Heart Journal Supplement, 2*(2), 125–141.

Scott, D. L., Berry, H., Capell, H., Coppock, J., Dayman, T., Doyle, D. V., . . . Wotjulewski, J. (2000). The long-term effects of non-steroidal anti-inflammatory drugs in osteoarthritis of the knee: A randomized placebo-controlled trial. *Rheumatology (Oxford), 39*(10), 1095–1101.

Scott, J., & Huskisson, E. C. (1976). Graphic representation of pain. *Pain, 2*(2), 175–184.

Scott, P. (2007). Chronic diseases: Another challenge for the developing world. *International Journal of Clinical Practice, 61*(9), 1422–1423.

Seaward, B. L. (1991). Spiritual well-being: A health education model. *Journal of Health Education, 22*(3), 166–169.

Segerstrom, S. C., & Miller, G. E. (2004). Psychological stress and the human immune system: A meta-analytic study of 30 years of inquiry. *Psychological Bulletin, 130*(4), 601–630.

Seligman, M. E. P. (2002). Positive psychology, positive prevention, and positive therapy. In C. R. Snyder & J. Shane (Eds.), *Handbook of positive psychology* (pp. 3–9). New York, NY: Oxford University Press.

Seligman, M. E. P. (2019). Positive psychology: A personal history. *Annual Review of Clinical Psychology, 15*, 1–23. Retrieved August 2, 2023, from annualreviews.org

Seligman, M. E. P., & Csikszentmihalyi, M. (2000). Positive psychology. *American Psychologist, 55*, 5–14.

Seligman, M. E. P., Park, N., & Peterson, C. (2004). The value in action (VIA) classification of character strength. *Ricechi di Psicologia, 27*(1), 63–78.

Seligman, M. E. P., Steen, T. A., Park, N., & Peterson, C. (2000). Positive psychology in progress. *American Psychologist, 60*(5), 410–421.

Selim, A. J., Fincke, G., Ren, X. S., Dego, R. A., Lee, A., Skinner, K., & Kazis, L. (2001). Racial differences in the use of lumbar spine radiographs: Results from the Veterans Health Study. *Spine, 26*, 1364–1369.

Sellick, S. M., & Crooks, D. L. (1999). Depression and cancer: An appraisal of the literature for prevalence, detection, and practice guideline development for psychological interventions. *Psychooncology, 8*, 315–333.

Selye, H. (1936). A syndrome produced by diverse nocuous agents. *Nature, 138*, 32.

Selye, H. (1946). The general adaptation syndrome and the diseases of adaptation. *Journal of Clinical Endocrinology, 6*(2), 117–231.

Selye, H. (1950). Stress and the general adaptation syndrome. *British Medical Journal, 1*(4667), 1383–1392.

Selye, H. (1975). *The stress of life.* New York, NY: McGraw-Hill.

Selye, H., & Fortier, C. (1950). Adaptive reaction to stress. *Psychosomatic Medicine, 12*(3), 149–157.

Seo, S. H., & Jang, Y. (2020). Cold-adapted live attenuated SARS-Cov-2 vaccine completely protects human ACE2 transgenic mice from SARS-Cov-2 infection. *Vaccines, 8*(4), 584. doi: 10.3390/vaccines8040584

Shang, C., Moss, A. C., & Chen, A. (2023). The expectancy-value theory: A meta-analysis of its application in physical education. *Journal of Sport and Health Science, 12*(1), 52–64. doi: 10.1016/j.jshs.2022.01.003

Sharma, S., Ferreira-Valente, A., de C. Williams, A. C., Abbott, J. H., Pais-Ribeiro, J., & Jensen, M. P. (2020). Group differences between countries and between languages in pain-related beliefs, coping, and catastrophizing in chronic pain: A systematic review. *Pain Medicine, 21*(9), 1847–1862. doi: 10.1093/pm/pnz373

Sharma, S., Malarcher, A. M., Giles, W. H., & Myers, G. (2004). Racial, ethnic and socioeconomic disparities in the clustering of cardiovascular disease risk factors. *Ethnic Diseases, 14*(1), 43–48.

Sharma, S., & Singh, L. (2018). Religion and well-being: The mediating role of positive virtues. *Journal of Religion and Health*, *58*(1), 19–31. doi: 10.1007/s10943-018-0559-5

Shattock, P., Kennedy, A., Powell, F., & Berney, T. P. (1991). Role of neuropeptides in autism and their relationships with classical neurotransmitters. *Brain Dysfunction*, *3*, 328–345.

Shattuck, E. C., & Muehlenbein, M. P. (2020). Religiosity/spirituality and physiological markers of health. *Journal of Religion and Health*, *59*, 1035–1054. doi: 10.1007/s10943-018-0663-6

Sheffield, D., Kirby, D. S., Biles, P. L., & Sheps, D. S. (1999). Comparison of perception of angina pectoris during exercise testing in African-Americans versus Caucasians. *The American Journal of Cardiology*, *83*, 106.

Sheikh, A. B., Nasrullah, A., Haq, A., Akhtar, A., Ghazanfar, H., Nasir, A., . . . Naqvi, S. W. (2017). The interplay of genetics and environmental factors in the development of obesity. *Cureus*, *9*(7), e1435. doi: 10.7759/cureus.1435

Sheikh, H., Brezar, A., Dzwonek, A., Yau, L., & Calder, L. A. (2018). Patient understanding of discharge instructions in the emergency department: Do different patients need different approaches? *International Journal of Emergency Medicine*, *11*(5). doi: 10.1186/s12245-018-0164-0

Sheldon, K. M., & King, L. (2001). Why positive psychology is necessary. *American Psychologist*, *56*, 216–217.

Sher, K. J. (1991). *Children of alcoholics*. Chicago, IL: University of Chicago Press.

Sher, L. (2005). Type D personality: The heart, stress and cortisol. *Quarterly Journal of Medicine*, *98*, 323–329.

Shiaw-Ling, W., Charron-Prochownik, D., Sereika, S. M., Siminerio, L., & Yookyung, K. (2006). Comparing three theories in predicting reproductive health behavioral intention in adolescent women with diabetes. *Pediatric Diabetes*, *7*(2), 108–115.

Shields, M., Tonmyr, L., Hovdestad, W. E., Gonzalez, A., & MacMillan, H. (2020). Exposure to family violence from childhood to adulthood. *BMC Public Health*, *20*, 1673. doi: 10.1186/s12889-020-09709-y

Shilts, R. (1987). *And the band played on: People, politics and the AIDS epidemic*. New York, NY: St. Martin Press.

Shimabukuro, T. T., Su, J. R., Marquez, P. L., Mba-Jones, A., Arana, J. E., & Cano, M. V. (2019). Safety of the 9-valent human papillomavirus vaccine. *Pediatrics*, *144*(6), e20191791. doi: 10.1542/peds.2019-1791

Shindo, N., & Briand, S. (2012). Influenza at the beginning of the 21st century. *Bulletin of the World Health Organization*, *90*(4), 247–247A.

Shmueli, L. (2021). Predicting intention to receive COVID-19 vaccine among the general population using the health belief model and the theory of planned behavior model. *BMC Public Health*, *21*, 804. doi: 10.1186/s12889-021-10816-7

Shuhata, M. H., Alhili, A., Al-Taee, M. M., Mohameed, D. A., & Ali, N. H. (2023). History of Egyptian medicine. *History of Medicine*, *8*, 12–21.

Sibbald, B. (2007). Graduated driver licensing in Canada: Slowly but surely. *Canadian Medical Association Journal*, *176*(6), 752.

Siddall, B., Ram, A., Jones, M. D., Booth, J., Perriman, D., & Summers, S. (2022). Short-term impact of combining pain neuroscience education with exercise for chronic musculoskeletal pain: A systematic review and meta-analysis. *Pain*, *163*(1), e20–e30. doi: 10.1097/j.pain.0000000000002308

Siddiqi, A., Zuberi, D., & Nguyen, Q. C. (2009). The role of health insurance in explaining immigrant versus non-immigrant disparities in access to health care: Comparing the United States to Canada. *Social Science & Medicine*, *69*(10), 1452–1459.

Sieper, J., Bruan, J., Rudewaleit, M., Boonen, A., & Zink, A. (2002). Ankylosing spondylitis: An overview. *Annals of Rheumatic Diseases*, *61*(suppl. 3), iii8–iii18.

Sighoko, D., Hunt, B. R., Irizarry, B., Watson, K., Ansell, D., & Murphy, A. M. (2018). Disparities in breast cancer mortality by age and geography in 10 racially diverse US cities. *Cancer Epidemiology, 53,* 178–183.

Silverman, A. B., Reinhertz, H., & Giaconia, R. M. (1996). The long-term sequelae of child and adolescent abuse: A longitudinal community study. *Child Abuse & Neglect, 20,* 709–723.

Simms, K. T., Hanley, S. J. B., Smith, M. A., Keane, A., & Canfell, K. (2020). Impact of HPV vaccine hesitancy on cervical cancer in Japan: A modelling study. *The Lancet: Public Health, 5*(4), e223–e234. doi: 10.1016/S2468-2667(20)30010-4

Simon, A. E., Chan, K. S., & Forrest, C. B. (2008). Assessment of children's health-related quality of life in the United States with a multidimensional index. *Pediatrics, 121*(1), e118–e126.

Simon, C., Kumar, S., & Kendrick, T. (2009). Cohort study of informal carers of first-time stroke survivors: Profiles of health and social changes in the first year of caregiving. *Social Science & Medicine, 69*(3), 404–410.

Simone, M., Emery, R. L., Hazzard, V. M., Eisenberg, M. E., Larson, N., & Neumark-Sztainer, D. (2021). Disordered eating in a population-based sample of young adults during the COVID-19 outbreak. *Eating Disorders, 54*(7), 1189–1201. doi: 10.1002/eat.23505

Simons, R. L., Murry, V., McLoyd, V., Lin, K., Cutrona, C., & Conger, R. D. (2002). Discrimination, crime, ethnic identity, and parenting as correlates of depressive symptoms among African American children: A multilevel analysis. *Developmental Psychopathology, 14,* 371–393.

Simonsen, L., Spreeuwenberg, P., Lustig, R., Taylor, R. J., Fleming, D. M., Kroneman, M., . . . Paget, W. J. (2013). Global mortality estimates for the 2009 influenza pandemic from the GLaMOR Project: A modeling study. *PLoS Medicine, 10*(11), e1001558. doi: 10.1371%2Fjournal.pmed.1001558

Simons-Morton, R., Lerner, N., & Singer, J. (2005). The observed effects of teenage passengers on the risky driving behavior of teenage drivers. *Accident Analysis & Prevention, 37,* 973–982.

Sims, K. D., Sims, M., Glover, L. M., Smit, E., & Odden, M. C. (2020). Perceived discrimination and trajectories of C-reactive protein: The Jackson Heart Study. *American Journal of Preventive Medicine, 58*(2), 199–207. doi: 10.1016/j.amepre.2019.09.019

Sin, N. L., Moskowitz, J. T., & Whooley, M. A. (2015). Positive affect and health behaviors across 5 years in patients with coronary heart disease: The Heart and Soul Study. *Psychosomatic Medicine, 77*(9), 1058–1066. doi: 10.1097%2FPSY.0000000000000238

Singleton, C. R., Winata, F., Parab, K. V., Adeyeme, O. S., & Aguiñaga, S. (2023). Violent crime, physical inactivity, and obesity: Examining spatial relationships by racial/ethnic composition of community residents. *Journal of Urban Health, 100,* 279–289. doi: 10.1007/s11524-023-00716-z

Size, M., Soyannwo, O. A., & Justins, D. M. (2007). Pain management in developing countries. *Anaesthesia, 62*(suppl. 1), 38–43.

Skaff, M. M., Mullan, J. T., Almeida, D. M., Hoffman, L., Masharani, U., Mohr, D., & Fisher, L. (2009). Daily negative mood affects fasting glucose in type 2 diabetes. *Health Psychology, 28*(3), 265–272.

Slack, P. (1989). The black death past and present. 2. Some historical problems. *Transactions of the Royal Society of Tropical Medicine and Hygiene, 83,* 461–463.

Slogrove, A. L., Esser, M. M., Cotton, M. F., Speert, D. P., Kollmann, T. R., Singer, J., Bettinger, J. A. (2017). A prospective cohort study of common childhood infections in South African HIV-exposed uninfected and HIV-unexposed infants. *Pediatric Infectious Disease Journal, 36*(2), e38–e44. doi: 10.1097/INF.0000000000001391

Smart, R., & Tsong, Y. (2014). Weight, body dissatisfaction, and disordered eating: Asian American women's perspectives. *Asian American Journal of Psychology, 5*(4), 344–352. doi: 10.1037/a0035599

Smetana, J. G., Campione-Barr, N., & Metzger, A. (2006). Adolescent development in interpersonal and societal contexts. *Annual Review of Psychology*, 57, 255–284. doi: 10.1146/annurev.psych.57.102904.190124

Smirnoff, M., Wilets, I., Ragin, D. F., Adams, R., Holohan, J., Rhodes, R., . . . Richardson, L. D. (2018). A paradigm for understanding trust and mistrust in medical research: The Community VOICES study. *American Journal of Bioethics: Empirical Bioethics*, 9(1), 39–47. doi: 10.1080/23294515.2018.1432718

Smith, A., & Cook-Cottone, C. (2011). A review of family therapy as an effective intervention for anorexia nervosa in adolescents. *Journal of Clinical Psychology in Medical Settings*, 18, 323–334.

Smith, E. R., Adams, S. A., Dos, I. P., Bottai, M., Fulton, J., & Herbert, J. R. (2008). Breast cancer survival among economically disadvantaged women: The influences of delayed diagnosis treatment on mortality. *Cancer Epidemiology Biomarkers & Prevention*, 17(10), 2882–2890.

Smith, M. J., Ellenberg, S. S., Bill, L. M., & Ruben, D. M. (2008). Media coverage of the measles-mumps-rubella vaccine and autism controversy and its relationship to MMR immunization rates in the United States. *Pediatrics*, 122(3), 684–685.

Smith, T. W., Glazer, K., Ruiz, J. M., & Gallo, L. C. (2004). Hostility, anger, aggressiveness, and coronary heart disease: An interpersonal perspective on personality, emotion, and health. *Journal of Personality*, 72(6), 1217–1270.

Smith, T. W., & Suls, J. (2004). Introduction to the special section on the future of health psychology. *Health Psychology*, 23(2), 115–118.

Sneed, R. S., & Cohen, S. (2014). Negative social interactions and incident hypertension among older adults. *Health Psychology*, 33, 554–565.

Snider, G. L. (1997). Tuberculosis then and now: A personal perspective in the last 50 years. *Annals of Internal Medicine*, 126, 237–243.

Snyder, A., Ribeiro Santiago, P. H., Sawyer, A., & Jamieson, L. (2023). A longitudinal mediation analysis of the effect of Aboriginal Australian mothers' experience of perceived racism on children's social and emotional well-being. *Australian Psychologist*, 58(5), 357–372. doi: 10.1080/00050067.2023.2198077

Sobo, E. J. (2015). Social cultivation of vaccine refusal and delay among Waldorf (Steiner) school parents. *Medical Anthropology Quarterly*, 29, 381–399. doi: 10.1111/maq.12214

Sobralske, M. (2006). Machismo sustains health and illness beliefs of Mexican American men. *Journal of the American Academy of Nurse Practitioners*, 18(8), 348–350.

Solana, L., Pirrotta, E., Ingravalle, V., & Fayella, P. (2009). The family physician and the psychologists in the office together: A response to fragmentation. *Mental Health in Family Medicine*, 6(22), 91–98.

Solmi, M., Collantoni, E., Meneguzzo, P., Tenconi, E., & Favaro, A. (2018). Network analysis of specific psychopathology and psychiatric symptoms in patients with anorexia nervosa. *European Eating Disorders Review*, 27(1), 24–33. doi: 10.1002/erv.2633

Solmi, M., Monaco, F., Højlund, M., Monteleone, A. M., Trott, M., Firth, J., . . . Correll, C. U. (2024). Outcomes in people with eating disorders: A transdiagnostic and disorder-specific systematic review, meta-analysis and multivariable meta-regression analysis. *World Psychiatry*, 23(1), 124–138. doi: 10.1002/wps.21182

Solomon, G. F. (1987). Psychoneuroimmunology: Interactions between central nervous system and immune system. *Journal of Neuroscience Research*, 18, 1–9.

Solomon, G. F., & Moos, R. H. (1964). Emotions, immunity and disease: A speculative theoretical integration. *Archives of General Psychiatry*, 11, 657–674.

Solovieva, S., Leino-Arjas, P., Saarela, J., Luoma, K., Raininko, R., & Riihimaki, H. (2004). Possible association of interleukin 1 gene locus polymorphisms with lower back pain. *Pain*, 109, 8–19.

Sonel, A. F., Good, C. B., Mulgund, J., Roe, M. T., Gibler, W. B., Smith, C. C., . . . CRUSADE Investigators. (2005). Racial variations in treatment and outcomes of black and white patients with high-risk non-ST-elevation acute coronary syndrome. *Circulation, 111*, 1225–1232.

Song, C., Luchtman, D., Kang, Z., Tam, E. M., Yatham, L. N., Su, K.-P., & Lam, R. W. (2015). Enhanced inflammatory and T-helper-1 type responses but suppressed lymphocyte proliferation in patients with seasonal affective disorder and treated by light therapy. *Journal of Affective Disorders, 185*, 90–96.

Sothern, M. S. (2004). Obesity prevention in children: Physical activity and nutrition. *Nutrition, 20*(7–8), 704–708.

South African AIDS Vaccine Initiative. (2007). *Ethical issues: HIV/AIDS vaccine ethics group*. Retrieved July 1, 2007, from www.saavi.org.za/haveg/htm.

Sparrenberger, F., Cichelero, F. T., Ascoli, A. M., Fonseca, F. P., Weiss, G., Berawanger, O., . . . Fuchs, F. D. (2008). Does psychosocial stress cause hypertension? A systematic review of observational studies. *Journal of Human Hypertension, 23*(1), 12–19.

Spiegel, D., Bloom, J. R., Kraemer, H. C., & Gottheil, E. (1989). Effects of psychosocial treatment on survival of patients with metastatic breast cancer. *The Lancet, 2*, 888–891.

Spiegel, D., Bloom, J. R., & Yalom, I. (1981). Group support for patients with metastatic cancer. *Archives of General Psychiatry, 38*, 527–531.

Spiegel, D., Butler, L. D., Giese-Davis, J., Koopman, C., Miller, E., DiMiceli, S., . . . Kraemer, H. C. (2007). Effects of supportive-expressive group therapy on survival of patients with metastatic breast cancer. *Cancer, 110*(5), 1130–1138.

Spiegel, D., & Giese-Davis, J. (2003). Depression and cancer: Mechanisms and disease progression. *Biological Psychiatry, 54*, 527–531.

Spitalnick, J. S., DiClemente, R. J., Wingood, G. M., Crosby, R. A., Milhausen, R. R., Sales, J. M., . . . Younge, S. N. (2007). Brief report: Sexual sensation seeking and its relationship to risky sexual behaviors among African-American adolescent females. *Journal of Adolescence, 30*, 165–173.

Splansky, G. L., Corey, D., Yang, Q., Atwood, L. D., Cupples, L. A., Benjamin, E. J., . . . Levy, D. (2007). The Third Generation Cohort of the National Heart, Lung, and Blood Institute's Framingham Heart Study: Design, recruitment, and initial examination. *American Journal of Epidemiology, 165*(11), 1328–1335.

Spruill, T. M. (2010). Chronic psychosocial stress and hypertension. *Current Hypertension Reports, 12*, 10–16. doi: 10.1007/s11906-009-0084-8

Stahl, S. (2008). Health: Juvenile rheumatoid arthritis. *CBS The CW Philly 57*. Retrieved August 30, 2009, from http://cbs3.com/health/Health.Alert.Stephanie.2.788670.html

Stallings, J., Flemming, A. S., Corter, C., Worthman, C., & Steiner, M. (2001). The effects of infant cries and odors on sympathy, cortisol, and autonomic responses in new mothers and nonpostpartum women. *Parenting: Science and Practice, 1*, 71–100.

Stämpfli, M., & Anderson, G. (2009). How cigarette smoke skews immune responses to promote infection, lung disease and cancer. *Nature Reviews Immunology, 9*, 377–384. doi: 10.1038/nri2530

Stanislawski, K. (2019). The Coping Circumplex Model: An integrative model of the structure of coping with stress. *Frontiers in Psychology, 10*. doi: 10.3389/fpsyg.2019.00694

Stanley, M. (2008). HPV vaccines: Are they the answer? *British Medical Bulletin, 88*(1), 59–74.

Stanley, R. O., & Burrows, G. D. (2008). Psychogenic heart disease, stress and the heart: A historical perspective. *Stress and Health, 24*, 181–187.

Stanojević, P., Lajunen, T., Jakšić, D., Jovanović, D., & Matović, B. (2022). Effectiveness of implementing a Graduated Driver Licensing (GDL) law among young Serbian drivers. *Journal of Safety Research, 83*, 339–348.

Stanton, B., Fang, X., Li, X., Feigelman, S., Gallbraith, J., & Ricardo, I. (1997). Evolution of risk behaviors over 2 years among a cohort of urban African American adolescents. *Archives of Pediatric & Adolescent Medicine, 151,* 398–406.

Starr, P. (1982). Transformation of defeat: The changing objectives of national health insurance, 1915– 1980. *American Journal of Public Health, 72,* 78–88.

Steadman, M., Bush, J. K., Thygerson, S. M., & Barnes, M. D. (2014). Graduated driver licensing provisions: An analysis of state policies and what works. *Traffic Injury Prevention, 15*(4), 343–348. doi: 10.1080/15389588.2013.822493

Steben, M., Norris, T., & McFayden, A. (n.d). HPV? Spread facts, not fear! *HPV Global Action.* Retrieved October 26, 2022.

Steca, P., D'Addario, M., Magrin, M. E., Miglioretti, M., Monzani, D., Pancani, L., . . . Greco, A. (2016). A type A and type D combined personality typology in essential hypertension and acute coronary syndrome patients: Associations with demographic, psychological, clinical, and lifestyle indicators. *PLoS One.* doi: 10.1371/journal.pone.0161840

Stelander, L. T., Høye, A., Bramness, J. G., Selbaek, G., Lunde, L.-H., Wynn, R., & Grønli, O. K. (2021). The changing alcohol drinking patterns among older adults show that women are closing the gender gap in more frequent drinking: The Tromsø study, 1994–2016. *Substance Abuse Treatment, Prevention & Policy, 16*(1), 45. doi: 10.1186/s13011-021-00376-9

Steptoe, A., Wikman, A., Molloy, G. J., Messerli-Bürgy, N., & Kaski, J. C. (2013). Inflammation and symptoms of depression and anxiety in patients with acute coronary heart disease. *Brain, Behavior, and Immunity, 31,* 183–188. doi: 10.1016/j.bbi.2012.09.002

Steptoe, A., Willemsen, G., Owen, N., Flower, L., & Mohamed-Ali, V. (2001). Acute mental stress elicits delayed increases in circulating inflammatory cytokine levels. *Clinical Science, 101,* 185–192.

Sternhell, P. S., & Corr, M. J. (2002). Psychiatric morbidity and adherence to antiretroviral medication in patients with HIV/AIDS. Australian & New Zealand Journal of Psychiatry, 36, 528–533.

Stetler, H. C., Grenade, T. C., Nunez, C. A., Meza, R., Terrell, S., Amador, L., & George, J. R. (1997). Field evaluation of rapid HIV serologic tests for screening and confirming HIV-1 infection in Honduras. *AIDS, 11*(3), 369–375.

Stevens, G. D., Mistry, R., Zuckerman, B., & Halfon, N. (2005). The patient–provider relationship: Does race/ethnicity concordance or discordance influence parent reports of the receipt of high quality basic pediatric preventive services? *Journal of Urban Health, 82*(4), 560–574.

Stewart, A. J., & Delvin, P. M. (2006). The history of the smallpox vaccine. *Journal of Infection, 52*(5), 329–334. doi: 10.1016/j.jinf.2005.07.021

St. John, D. J. B., McDermott, F. T., & Hopper, L. J. (1993). Cancer-risk in relatives of patients with common colorectal cancer. *Annals of Internal Medicine, 118,* 785–790.

Stoffel, E. M., & Murphy, C. C. (2020). Epidemiology and mechanisms of the increasing incidences of colon and rectal cancers in young adults. *Gastroenterology, 158*(2), 341–353. doi: 10.1053/j. gastro.2019.07.055

Stokols, D. (1996). Translating social ecological theory into guidelines for community health promotion. *American Journal of Health Promotion, 10*(4), 282–298.

Stolenberg, S. G., & Mueller, B. (2023, February 28). *Amid politically fraught debate, a split persists on a virus origin. The New York Times,* p. 6.

Stolzenberg, L., D'Alessio, S. J., & Flexon, J. L. (2019). The impact of violent crime on obesity. *Social Sciences, 8*(12), 329. doi: 10.3390/socsci8120329

Stone, L. J., & Clements, J. A. (2009). The effects of nursing home placement on the perceived levels of caregiver burden. *Journal of Gerontological Social Work*, *52*(3), 193–214. doi: 10.1080/01634370802609163

Storey, A. E., Walsh, C. J., Quinton, R. L., & Wynne-Edwards, K. E. (2000). Hormonal correlates of paternal responsiveness in new and expectant fathers. *Evolution and Human Behavior*, *21*, 79–95.

Strating, M., Schuur, W., & Suurmeijer, T. (2006). Contribution of partner support in self-management of rheumatoid arthritis patients: An application of the theory of planned behavior. *Journal of Behavioral Medicine*, *29*(1), 51–60.

Streltzer, J. (1983). Psychiatric aspects of oncology: A review of past research. *Hospital Community Psychiatry*, *34*, 716–729.

Strickland, O. L., Giger, J. N., Nelson, M. A., & Davis, C. M. (2007). The relationships among stress, coping, social support, and weight class in premenopausal African American women at risk for coronary heart disease. *Journal of Cardiovascular Nursing*, *22*(4), 272–278.

Stringer, H. (2024). Psychologists are innovating to tackle substance use. *Monitor on Psychology*, *55*(1), 68–71.

Stringo, I. A., Simmons, A. N., Matthews, S. C., Craig, A. D., & Paulus, M. P. (2008). Increased bias revealed using experimental graded heat stimuli in young depressed adults: Evidence of "emotional allodynia." *Psychosomatic Medicine*, *70*, 338–344.

Strode, A., Slack, C. M., & Mushariwa, M. (2005). HIV vaccine research: South Africa's ethical and legal framework and its ability to promote the welfare of trial participants. *South African Medical Journal*, *95*(8), 598–601.

Strong, K., Mathers, C., Leeder, S., & Beaglehole, R. (2005). Preventing chronic diseases: How many lives can we save? *The Lancet*, *366*(9496), 1578–1582.

Strzelak, A., Ratajczak, A., Adamiec, A., & Feleszko, W. (2018). Tobacco smoke induces and alters immune responses in the lung triggering inflammation, allergy, asthma and other lung diseases: A mechanistic review. *International Journal of Environmental Research and Public Health*, *15*, 1033. doi: 10.3390/ijerph15051033

Substance Abuse and Mental Health Services Administration. (2005). *Results from the 2004 National Survey on Drug Use and Health: National findings*. Office of Applied Studies, NSDUH Series H-28, DHHS Publication No. SMA 05-4062. Rockville, MD: Author.

Suh, M. J., Lee, C. H., Kim, Y. S., Lee, H. R., Park, C. J., & Yoo, S. J. (2000). *Adult nursing* (4th ed.). Seoul: Soo Moon Publications.

Sullivan, A. D., Hedberg, K., & Flemming, D. W. (2000). Legalized physician assisted suicide in Oregon: The second year. *The New England Journal of Medicine*, *342*(8), 598–604.

Summerfield, D. (2001). The invention of post-traumatic stress disorder and the social usefulness of a psychiatric category. *British Medical Journal*, *322*, 95–98.

Sun, H., Huang, H., Ji, S., Chen, X., Xu, Y., Zhu, F., & Wu, J. (2019).The efficacy of cognitive behavioral therapy to treat depression and anxiety and improve quality of life among early-stage breast cancer patients. *Integrative Cancer Therapies*, *18*. doi: 10.1177/1534735419829573

Sun, K. S., Cheng, Y. H., Wun, Y. T., & Lam, T. P. (2017). Choices between Chinese and Western medicine in Hong Kong – Interactions of institutional environment, health beliefs and treatment outcomes. *Complementary Therapies in Clinical Practice*, *28*, 70–74. doi: 10.1016/j.ctcp.2017.05.012

Sundararajan, L. (2005). Happiness donut: A Confucian critique of positive psychology. *Journal of Theoretical and Philosophical Psychology*, *25*(1), 35–60.

Sung, H., Ferlay, J., Siegel, R. L., Laversanne, M., Soeerjomataran, I., Jemal, A., & Bray, F. (2021). Global cancer statistics 2020: GLOBOCAM estimates of incidences and mortality worldwide for 36 cancers in 185 countries. *CA: A Cancer Journal for Clinicians*, *71*, 209–249. doi: 10.3322/caac.21660

Sury, L., Burns, K., & Brodaty, H. (2013). Moving in: Adjustment of people living with dementia going into a nursing home and their families. *International Psychogeriatrics*, *25*(6), 867–876. doi: 10.1017/S1041610213000057

Suter, T., & Burton, S. (1996). An examination of correlates and effects associated with a concise measure of consumer nutrition knowledge. *Family and Consumer Sciences Research Journal*, *25*(2), 117–136.

Svaldi, J., Caffier, D., & Tuschen-Caffier, B. (2010). Emotion suppression but not re-appraisal increases desire to binge in women with binge eating disorder. *Psychotherapy and Psychosomatics*, *79*(3), 188–190.

Swardh, E., Biguet, G., & Opava, C. H. (2008). Views on exercise maintenance variations among patients with rheumatoid arthritis. *Physical Therapy*, *88*(9), 1049–1060.

Sweeting, H., Walker, L., MacLean, A., Patterson, C., Räisänen, U., & Hunt, K. (2015). Prevalence of eating disorders in males: A review of rates reported in academic research and UK mass media. *International Journal of Men's Health*, *14*(2). doi: 10.3149/jmh.1402.86

Szabo, S. (1998). Hans Selye and the development of the stress concept. *Annals of the New York Academy of Sciences*, *30*(851), 19–27.

Szkody, E., Stearns, M., Stanhope, L., & McKinney, C. (2020). Stress-buffering role of social support during COVID-19. *Family Process*, *60*(3), 1002–1015. doi: 10.1111/famp.12618

Tafur, M. M., Crowe, T. K., & Torres, S. E. (2009). A review of curanderismo and healing practices among Mexicans and Mexican Americans. *Occupational Therapy International*, *16*(1), 82–88.

Takeshita, J., Wang, S., Loren, A. W., Mitra, N., Schults, J., Shin, D. B., & Sawinkski, D. L. (2020). Association of racial/ethnic and gender concordance between patients and physicians with patient experience ratings. *JAMA Network Open*, *3*(11), e2024583. doi: 10.1001/jamanetworkopen.2020.24583

Talumaa, B., Brown, A., Batterham, R. L., & Kalea, A. Z. (2022). Effective strategies in ending weight stigma in healthcare. *Obesity Reviews*, *23*(10), e13494. doi: 10.1111/obr.13494

Tan, S. A., Tan, L. G., Lukman, S. T., & Berk, L. S. (2007). Humor, as an adjunct therapy in cardiac rehabilitation, attenuates catecholamines and myocardial infarction recurrence. *Advances in Mind-Body Medicine*, *22*, 8–12.

Tan, S. Y., & Berman, E. (2008). Robert Koch (1843–1910): Father of microbiology and Nobel laureate. *Singapore Journal of Medicine*, *49*(11), 854–855.

Tandon, P. S., Wright, J., Zhou, C., Rogers, C. B., & Christiakis, D. A. (2010). Nutrition menu labels may lead to lower-calorie restaurant meal choices for children. *Pediatrics*, *25*(2), 244–248.

Tanser, F., Varnighausen, T., Grapsa, E., Zaidi, T., & Newell, M. L. (2013). High coverage of ART associated with decline in risk of HIV acquisition in rural Kwa-Zulu-Natal, South Africa. *Science*, *339*, 966–971.

Taplin, S. H., Ichikawa, L., & Yood, M. U. (2004). Reason for late-stage breast cancer: Absence of screening or detection, or breakdown in follow-up? *Journal of the National Cancer Institute*, *96*, 1518–1527.

Tatrow, K., & Montgomery, G. H. (2006). Cognitive behavioral therapy techniques for distress and pain in breast cancer patients: A meta-analysis. *Journal of Behavioral Medicine*, *29*(1), 17–27.

Taubenberger, J. K., & Morens, D. M. (2006). 1918 influenza: The mother of all pandemics. *Emerging Infectious Diseases*, *12*(1), 15–22.

Tavernise, S. (2021, May 6). Vaccine skepticism was viewed as a knowledge problem. It's actually about gut beliefs. *The New York Times*.

Taylor, J., & Turner, R. J. (2001). A longitudinal study of the role and significance of mattering to others for depressive symptoms. *Journal of Health and Social Behavior, 42*, 310–325.

Taylor, S. E. (1989). *Positive illusions: Creative self-deception and the healthy mind.* New York, NY: Basic Books.

Taylor, S. E., Kemeny, M. E., Reed, G. M., Bower, J. E., & Gruenewald, T. L. (2000). Psychological resources, positive illusions, and health. *American Psychologist, 55*(1), 99–109. https://psycnet.apa.org/doi/10.1037/0003-066X.55.1.99

Taylor, S. E., Klein, L., Lewis, B., Gruenewald, T., Gurung, R., & Updegraff, J. (2000). Biobehavioral responses to stress in females: Tend-and-befriend, not fight-or-flight. *Psychological Review, 107*, 411–429.

Taylor, S. E., & Master, S. L. (2011). Social responses to stress: The tend-and-befriend model. In R. Contrada & A. Baum (Eds.), *The handbook of stress science: Biology, psychology, and health* (pp. 101–110). New York, NY: Springer.

Teasdale, C. A., Marais, B. J., & Abrams, E. J. (2011). HIV: Prevention of mother-to-child transmission. *BMJ, Clinical Evidence, 1*, 909.

Tedesco, A., D'Agostino, D., Soriente, I., Amato, P., Piccoli, R., & Sabatini, P. (2009). A new strategy for the early diagnosis of rheumatoid arthritis: A combined approach. *Autoimmunity Reviews, 8*(3), 233–237.

Tefft, B. C., Williams, A. F., & Grabowski, J. G. (2012). *Teen driver risk in relation to age and number of passengers.* Technical report. Washington, DC: AAA Foundation for Traffic Safety.

Tekur, P., Singphon, C., Nagendra, H. R., & Raghuram, N. (2008). Effect of short-term intensive yoga program on pain, functional disability, spinal flexibility in chronic low back pain: A randomized control study. *Journal of Alternative and Complementary Medicine, 14*, 637–644.

Temcheff, C. E., Serebin, L. A., Martin-Storey, A., Stack, D. M., Hodgins, S., & Lendingham, J. (2008). Continuity and pathways from aggression in childhood to family violence in adulthood: A 30-year longitudinal study. *Journal of Family Violence, 23*(4), 231–242.

Temple, N. J. (2020). Front-of-package food labels: A narrative review. *Appetite, 144*. doi: 10.1016/j.appet.2019.104485

Temple, N. J., & Fraser, J. (2014). Food labels: A critical assessment. *Nutrition, 30*(3), 257–260. doi: 10.1016/j.nut.2013.06.012

Tenney, E., Poole, J., & Diener, E. (2016). Subjective well-being and organizational performance. In A. Brief & B. M. Staw (Eds.), *Research in organizational behavior.* Greenwich, CT: JAI Press.

Teoh, D. G. K. (2019). The power of social media for HPV vaccination: Not fake news! *American Society of Clinical Oncology, 39*, doi: 10.1200/EDBK_239363

Terjestam, Y., Jouper, J., & Johannson, C. (2010). Effects of scheduled Qigong exercise on pupils' well-being, self-image, distress and stress. *Journal of Alternative and Complementary Medicine, 18*(9), 939–944.

Testai, F. D., Gorelick, P. B., Aparicio, H. J., Filbey, F. M., Gonzalez, R., Gottesman, R. F., . . . Song, S. Y. (2022). Use of marijuana: Effect on brain health: A scientific statement from the American Heart Association. *Stroke, 53*(4), e176–e187. doi: 10.1161/STR.0000000000000396

Teusch, C. (2003). Patient–doctor communication. *Medical Clinics of North America, 87*(5).

Thaler, A., Gupta, A., & Cohen, S. P. (2011). Cannabinoids for pain management. *Advances in Psychosomatic Medicine, 30*, 125–138.

Thaler, R. H., & Sunstein, C. A. (2009). *Nudge: Improving decisions about health, wealth, and happiness.* London: Penguin Books, Ltd.

The Belmont Report. (1979). Ethical principles and guidelines for the protection of human subjects of research. *Federal Register, 44*(76).

The Carter Center. (2016a). *Guinea worm case totals*. Retrieved December 27, 2016, from www. cartercenter.org/health/guinea_worm/case-totals.html

The Carter Center. (2016b). *Guinea worm case totals*. Retrieved October 23, 2016, from www.cartercenter. org/health/guinea_worm/case-totals.html

The Carter Center. (2023). *Guinea worm disease reaches all-time low: Only 13* human cases reported in 2022*. Retrieved April 13, 2023, from cartercenter.org

The World Bank. (2023). *The world by income and region*. Retrieved June 20, 2023, from https:// datatopics.worldbank.org/world-development-indicators/the-world-by-income-and-region.html

Thom, D., Hall, M.A., & Paulson, L.G. (2004). Measuring patient's trust in physicians when assessing quality of care. *Health Affairs, 23*, 124–132.

Thom, T., Hause, N., Rosamond, U., Howard, V.J., Rumsfeld, J., & Manolio, T. (2006). Heart disease and stroke statistics: 2006 update: A report from the American Heart Association Statistics Committee and Stroke Statistics Sub-Committee. *Circulation, 113*, e85–e151.

Thomas, M., Hariharan, M., Rana, S., Swain, S., & Andrew, A. (2014). Medical jargons as hindrance in doctor–patient communication. *Psychological Studies, 59*, 394–400. doi: 10.1007/s12646-014-0262-x

Thomas, S.H., & Quinn, S.C. (1991). The Tuskegee Syphilis Study, 1932 to 1297: Implications for HIV education and AIDS risk education programs in the black community. *American Journal of Public Health, 81*(1), 1498–1505.

Thombs, B.D., Bass, E.B., Ford, D.E., Stewart, K.J., Tsilidis, K.K., Patel, U., . . . Ziegelstein, R.C. (2006). Prevalence of depression in survivors of acute myocardial infarction: Review of the evidence. *Journal of General Internal Medicine, 21*, 30–38. doi: 10.1111/j.1525-1497.2005.00269.x

Thompson, B., & Kinne, S. (1990). Social change theory: Applications to community health. In N. Bracht (Ed.), *Health promotion at the community level* (pp. 45–65). Newbury Park, CA: Sage.

Thompson, W., & Hickey, J. (2005). *Society in focus*. Boston, MA: Allen & Bacon.

Thomson, A., Vallee-Tourangeau, G., & Suggs, L.S. (2018). Strategies to increase vaccine acceptance and uptake: From behavioral insights to context-specific, culturally-appropriate, evidence-based communications and interventions. *Vaccine, 36*(44), 6457–6458. doi: 10.1016/j.vaccine.2018.08.031

Thorlacius, S., Struewing, J.P., Hartge, P., Olafsdottir, G.H., Sigvaldason, H., Tryggvadottir, L., . . . Eyfjörd, J.E. (1998). Population-based study risk of breast cancer in carriers of BRCA2 mutation. *The Lancet, 352*, 1337–1339.

Thun, M.J., Carter, B.D., Feskanich, D., Freedman, N.D., Prentice, R., Lopez, A.D., . . . Gapstur, S.M. (2013). 50-Year trends in smoking-related mortality in the United States. *The New England Journal of Medicine, 368*, 351–364.

Thune-Boyle, I.C.V., Stygall, J., Keshtgar, M.R.S., Davidson, T.I., & Newman, S.P. (2013). Religious/ spiritual coping resources and their relationship with adjustment in patients newly diagnosed with breast cancer in UK. *Psycho-Oncology, 22*(3), 646–658.

Tian, N., Goovaertz, P., Zhan, F.B., & Wilson, J.G. (2010). Identification of racial disparities in breast cancer mortality: Does scale matter? *International Journal of Health Geographics, 9*, 35–48.

Tickle, J.J., Sargent, J.D., Dalton, M.A., Beach, M.L., & Heatherton, T.F. (2001). Favorite movie stars, their tobacco use in contemporary movies, and its association with adolescent smoking. *Tobacco Control, 10*, 16–22.

Tilbrook, H.E., Cox, H., Hewitt, C.E., Kang'ombe, A.R., Chuang, L.H., Jayakody, S., . . . Torgerson, D.J. (2011). Yoga for chronic low back pain. *Annals of Internal Medicine, 155*, 569–578.

Tisdall, S. (1993, December 30). US admits years of atomic radiation tests on people. *The Guardian*, p. 11.

Tobiyama, A. J. (2019). Stress and obesity. *Annual Review of Psychology*, 70, 703–718. doi: 10.1146/annurev-psych-010418-102936

Todd, C. S., Mountvarner, G., & Lichenstein, R. (2005). Unintended pregnancy risk in an emergency department population. *Contraception*, 71(1), 35–39.

Todd, K. H., Lee, T., & Hoffman, J. R. (1994). The effects of ethnicity on physician estimates of pain in patients with isolated extremity trauma. *Journal of the American Medical Association*, 271, 925–978.

Todd, K. H., Samaroo, N., & Hoffman, J. R. (1993). Ethnicity as a risk factor for inadequate emergency department analgesics. *Journal of the American Medical Association*, 269, 1537–1539.

Tomlinson, M. F., Brown, M., & Hoaken, P. N. S. (2016). Recreational drug use and human aggressive behavior: A comprehensive review since 2003. *Aggression and Violent Behavior*, 27, 9–29. doi: 10.1016/j.avb.2016.02.004

Tongue, J. R., Epps, H. R., & Forese, L. L. (2005). Communication skills for patient-centered care: Research-based, easily learned techniques for medical interviews that benefit orthopaedic surgeons and their patients. *The Journal of Bone & Joint Surgery*, 87(3), 652–658.

Torkington, S. (2022). The global fight against polio is not over. *World Economic Forum*. Retrieved April 20, 2023, from weforum.org

Torres, E., & Sawyer, T. (2005). *Curanderismo: A life in Mexican folk healing*. Albuquerque, NM: University of New Mexico Press.

Torvik, F. A., Rosenström, T. H., Gustavson, K., Ystrom, E., Kendler, K. S., Bramness, J. G., . . . Reichborn-Kjennerud, T. (2019). Explaining the association between anxiety disorders and alcohol use disorder: A twin study. *Depression and Anxiety*, 36(6), 522–532. doi: 10.1002/da.22886

Tournoud, M., Ecochard, R., Kuhn, L., & Coutsoudis, A. (2008). Diversity of risk of mother-to-child HIV-1 transmission according to feeding practices, CD4 cell count, and haemoglobin concentrations in a South African cohort. *Tropical Medicine & International Health*, 13(3), 310–318.

Toye, F. M., Barlow, J., Wright, C., & Lamb, S. E. (2006). Personal meanings in the construction of need for total knee replacement surgery. *Social Science & Medicine*, 63, 43–53.

Traill, W. B., Chambers, S. A., & Butler, L. (2012). Attitudinal and demographic determinants of diet quality and implications for policy targeting. *Journal of Human Nutrition and Dietetics*, 25, 87–94.

Tran, S. T., Koven, M. L., Castro, A. S., Goya Arce, A. B., & Carter, J. S. (2020) Sociodemographic and environmental factors are associated with adolescents' pain and longitudinal health outcomes. *Journal of Pain*, 21(1–2), 170–181. doi: 10.1016/j.jpain.2019.06.007

Treur, J. L., Demontis, D., Smith, G. D., Sallis, H., Richardson, T. G., Wiers, R. W., . . . Munafò, M. R. (2021). Investigating causality between liability to ADHD and substance use, and liability to substance use and ADHD risk, using Mendelian randomization. *Addiction Biology*, 26(1), e12849. doi: 10.1111/adb.12849

Trimble, J. E. (2021). "The circling spirits call us home": Marginal methods, the Shaman, and relational approaches to healing research. In D. F. Ragin & J. P. Keenan (Eds.), *Handbook of research methods in health psychology*. New York, NY: Routledge/Taylor & Francis Group.

Trinidad, D. R., Unger, J. P., Chih-Ping, C., & Anderson, J. C. (2005). Emotional intelligence and acculturation to the United States: Interactions on the perceived social consequences of smoking in early adolescence. *Substance Use & Misuse*, 40(11), 1697–1706.

Trotter, J. L., & Allen, N. E. (2009). The good, the bad and the ugly: Domestic violence survivors' experience with their informal social networks. *American Journal of Community Psychology*, 43(3–4), 221–231.

Trotter, R. T. (2001). Curanderismo: A picture of Mexican-American folk healing. *Journal of Alternative and Complementary Medicine*, *7*(2), 129–131.

Trouvin, A.-P., & Perrot, S. (2019). New concepts of pain. *Best Practices & Research Clinical Rheumatology*, *33*(3). doi: 10.1016/j.berh.2019.04.007

Trudel, X., Brisson, C., Gilbert-Ouimet, M., Vézina, M., Talbot, D., & Milot, A. (2019). Long working hours and the prevalence of masked and sustained hypertension. *Hypertension*, *72*(2), 535–538. doi: 10.1161/HYPERTENSIONAHA.119.12926

Truelove, V., Freeman, J., & Davey, J. (2019). "You can't be deterred by stuff you don't know about": Identifying factors that influence graduated driver licensing rule compliance. *Safety Science*, *111*, 313–323. doi: 10.1016/j.ssci.2018.09.007

Truman, B. I., Gooch, B. F., Sulemana, I., Gift, H. C., Horowitz, A. M., Evans, C. A., . . . Task Force on Community Preventive Services. (2002). Reviews on evidence on interventions to prevent dental caries, oral and pharyngeal cancers, and sports-related craniofacial injuries. *American Journal of Preventive Medicine*, *23*(1S), 21–54.

Tryggvadottir, L., Tulinius, H., Eyfjord, J. E., & Sigurvinsson, T. (2001). Breastfeeding & reduced risk of breast cancer in an Icelandic cohort study. *American Journal of Epidemiology*, *154*(1), 37–42.

Tsai, Y. F. (2007). Gender differences in pain and depressive tendency among Chinese elders with knee osteoarthritis. *Pain*, *130*(1–2), 1881–1894.

Tsang, A., Von Korff, M., Lee, S., Alonso, J., Karan, E., Angermeyer, M. C., . . . Watanabe, M. (2008). Common chronic pain conditions in developed and developing countries: Gender and age differences and comorbidity with depression-anxiety disorders. *Journal of Pain*, *9*, 883–891.

Tsang, H., Cheung, L., & Lak, D. (2002). Qigong as a psychosocial intervention for depressed elderly with chronic physical illnesses. *International Journal of Geriatric Psychiatry*, *17*, 1146–1154.

Tsiros, M. D., Sinn, N., Coates, A. M., Howe, P. R. C., & Buckley, J. D. (2008). Treatment of adolescent overweight and obesity. *European Journal of Pediatrics*, *167*(1), 9–16.

Tucker, J. S., Ellickson, P. L., & Klein, D. J. (2002). Five year prospective study of risk factors for daily smoking among early nonsmokers and experimenters. *Journal of Applied Social Psychology*, *32*, 1588–1603.

Tugwell, B. D., Lee, L. E., Gillette, H., Lorber, E. M., Hedberg, K., & Cieslak, P. R. (2004). Chickenpox outbreak in a highly vaccinated school population. *Pediatrics*, *113*(3), 455–459.

Tullis, L. M., Dupont, R., Frost-Pineda, K., & Gold, M. S. (2003). Marijuana and tobacco: A major connection? *Journal of Addictive Diseases*, *22*(3), 51–62.

Tumushabe, J. (2006). *The politics of HIV/AIDS in Uganda*. Social Policy & Development Programme Paper Number 28. Geneva: United Nations Research Institute for Social Development.

Tung, E. L., Wroblewski, K. E., Boyd, K., Makelarski, J. A., Peek, M. E., & Lindau, S. T. (2018). Police-recorded crime and disparities in obesity and blood pressure status in Chicago. *Journal of the American Heart Association*, *7*(7). doi: 10.1161/JAHA.117.008030

Tunio, M. A., Raf, M., & Hashmi, A. (2011). Hereditary nonpolyposis colorectal cancer in Pakistan: Results of a pilot study. *Pakistan Journal of Medical Sciences*, *27*, 339–343.

Tunks, E. R. (2008). Chronic pain and the psychiatrist. *The Canadian Journal of Psychiatry*, *53*(4), 211–212.

Turk, D. C., Swanson, K. S., & Tunks, E. R. (2008). Psychological approaches in the treatment of chronic pain patients – When pills, scalpels and needles are not enough. *The Canadian Journal of Psychiatry*, *53*(4), 213–223.

Tuskegee Syphilis Study Legacy Committee. (1996, May 20). *Bad blood: Final report of the Tuskegee Syphilis Study Legacy Committee*. Retrieved October 28, 2013, from http://exhibits.hsl.virginia.edu/badblood/report/

Twenge, J. M., & Campbell, W. K. (2019). Media use is linked to lower psychological well-being: Evidence from three datasets. *Psychiatric Quarterly, 90,* 311–331. doi: 10.1007/s11126-019-09630-7

UCLA Integrated Substance Abuse Program. (2006). *Methamphetamine: Overview.* Retrieved from http://www.methamphetamine.org/html/overview.html

Uhrhammer, N., & Bignos, Y. J. (2008). Report of a family segregating mutations in both the APC and MSH2 genes: Juvenile onset of colorectal cancer in a double heterozygote. *International Journal of Colorectal Disease, 23*(11), 1131–1135.

Uitterhoeve, R. J., Vernooy, M., Litjens, M., Potting, K., Bensing, J., De Mulder, P., & van Achterberg, T. (2004). Psychosocial interventions for patients with advance cancer: A systematic review of the literature. *British Journal of Cancer, 91,* 1050–1062.

Ukraine Ministry of Health. (2000). *HIV/AIDS epidemic in Ukraine: Social and demographic aspects.* New York, NY: United Nations Development Program.

Ulmer, R. G., Preusser, D. F., Williams, A. F., Ferguson, S. A., & Farmer, C. M. (2000). Effect of Florida's graduated licensing program on the crashes of teenage drivers. *Accident Analysis & Prevention, 32,* 527–532.

UNAIDS. (2001). *Condom social marketing: Selected case studies.* Best Practice Collection. Geneva: Author.

UNAIDS. (2004). *Ukraine: Epidemiological fact sheets on HIV/AIDS and sexually transmitted infections.* Geneva: World Health Organization Press.

UNAIDS. (2008a). *2008 report on the global AIDS epidemic.* Geneva: Author.

UNAIDS. (2008b). *2008 report on the global AIDS epidemic.* Executive Summary. Retrieved from www.unaids.org/en/dataanalysis/knowyourepidemic/epidemiologypublications/2008reportontheglobalaidsepidemic/

UNAIDS. (2010). *Global campaign against HIV/AIDS.* Retrieved June 9, 2010, from www.unaids.org/

UNAIDS. (2023). *Fact sheet 2022: Global HIV statistics.* Retrieved April 8, 2023, from unaids.org

Unal, B., Critchley, J., & Capewell, S. (2005). Modelling the decline in CHD deaths in England and Wales, 1981–2000: Comparing contributions from primary and secondary prevention. *British Medical Journal, 331,* 614–615.

UNICEF. (2001a). *Official summary. The state of the world's children 2001.* New York, NY: Author.

UNICEF. (2001b, January 29–February 2). Chapter 3: Organizational arrangements for the preparatory process and the special session. Update on reviews and appraisals. In *Report of the Preparatory Committee for the Special Session of the General Assembly on Children.* New York.

UNICEF. (2002a). *Young people and HIV/AIDS: Opportunity in crisis.* Geneva: UNICEF, UNAIDS, and WHO.

UNICEF. (2002b). *Young people and HIV/AIDS: A UNICEF fact sheet.* New York, NY: Author.

UNICEF. (2004). *HIV/AIDS menaces progress in Ukraine.* Retrieved February 1, 2007, from http://www.unicef.org/media/media_20869.html

UNICEF. (2008). *UNICEF nominee Paul Farmer receives CDC foundation hero award.* Retrieved February 23, 2009, from www.unicef.org/infobycountry/usa_45896.html

U.N. International Drug Control Programme. (1997). *World drug report.* New York, NY: Oxford University Press.

United Nations. (2007). *World population prospects: The 2006 revision highlights.* Working Paper No esa/p/wp.202. New York, NY: United Nations Department of Economic and Social Affairs, Population Division. Retrieved December 12, 2009, from www.un.org/esa/population/publications/wpp2006/WPP2006_Highlights_rev.pdf

United Nations. (2010, July). *Population and vital statistics report.* Statistical Papers. Series A. Vol. LXII.

United Nations. (2011, January). *Population and vital statistics report.* Statistical Papers. Series A. Vol. LXIII.

United Nations. (2016). *Population and vital statistics report.* Technical note, Table 3: Live births, deaths, and infant death rates, latest year available. Retrieved from unstats.un.org/unsd/demographic/products/vitstats/

United Nations. (n.d.). *Climate action.* Retrieved February 8, 2024, from www.un.org/en/climatechange/paris-agreement

University of Arkansas, Division of Agriculture. (2007). *Natural resources. Uses of other tree species.* Retrieved June 26, 2008, from www.arnatural.org/wildfoods/uses_Trees.htm

University of Bristol. (2012). *Researchers identify which sensory nerve cells contribute to chronic nerve pain.* Retrieved August 21, 2012, from www.bris. ac.uk/news/2012/8709.html

University of California, Agricultural and Natural Resources. (2007). *UC Study: Teen drivers distracted by passengers 'fooling around".* News and Information Outreach, Governmental and External Relations. Retrieved February 1, 2008, from http://news.ucanr.org/newsstorymain.cfm?story=1049

University of Minnesota. (2008). *Sarcomas.* Masonic Cancer Center, University of Minnesota. Retrieved October 20, 2008, from www.umphysicians.org/cancercare/cancerinformation/bone-soft-tissue-cancers/soft-tissue-sarcomas/.

University of Oxford. (2022). *Vaccine knowledge: Global vaccine schedules.* Retrieved November 20, 2023, from ox.ac.uk

UN News. (2023). *Global homicides hit record high in 2021 as post-lockdown stress set in.* Retrieved January 3, 2024.

UNODC. (2021). *World drug report.* Retrieved May 30, 2023, from WDR21_Booklet_1_takeaways.pdf (unodc.org)

UN Women. (2021). *Violence against women: Prevalence estimates 2021.* Retrieved from WHO-SRH-21.6-eng.pdf

Urberg, K.A., Degirmencioglu, S.M., & Pilgrim, C. (1997). Close friends and group influences on adolescent cigarette smoking and alcohol use. *Developmental Psychology, 33*(5), 834–844.

Uritsky, T., McPherson, M.L., & Prudel, F. (2011). Assessment of hospice health professionals' knowledge, views, and experience with medical marijuana. *Journal of Palliative Medicine, 14*, 1291–1295.

U.S. Department of Health and Human Services. (n.d.). *Office for Human Research Protections.* Retrieved November 1, 2023, from HHS.gov.

U.S. Cancer Statistics Working Group. (2009). *United States cancer statistics: 1999–2009: Incidence and mortality web-based report.* Atlanta, GA: U.S. Department of Health and Human Services, Centers for Disease Control and Prevention, and National Cancer Institute. Retrieved from www.cdc.gov/uscs

U.S. Census Bureau. (2007). *Current population survey, 2006 and 2007 annual social and economic supplements.* Retrieved October 28, 2013, from www.census.gov/hhes/www/poverty/data/incpovhlth/2006/index.html

U.S. Census Bureau. (2012a). *Health insurance: Highlights 2011.* Retrieved January 27, 2013, from http://www.census.gov/hhes/www/hlthins/data/incpovhlth/2011/highlights.html

U.S. Census Bureau. (2012b). *Statistical abstracts of the U.S.* Retrieved January 28, 2013, from www.census.gov/compendia/statab/2012/tables/12s0312.pdf

U.S. Census Bureau. (2023). *Health insurance coverage in the United States: 2022.* Retrieved February 28, 2024, from census.gov

U.S. Congress AIDS PAC. (2007). *Ryan White comprehensive AIDS resource emergency act of 1990.* Retrieved June 24, 2024, from https://www.congress.gov/bill/101st-congress/senate-bill/2240

U.S. Department of Agriculture. (2020). *Dietary guidelines for Americans, 2020–2025* (9th ed.). Retrieved from DietaryGuidelines.gov

U.S. Department of Transportation. (2015). *Graduated drivers license systems.* Retrieved June 1, 2023.

U.S. Department of Health and Human Services. (1994). *Preventing tobacco use among young people: A report of the surgeon general.* Washington, DC: USGPO.

U.S. Department of Health and Human Services. (2000). *Reducing tobacco use: A report of the surgeon general.* Atlanta, GA: U.S. Department of Health and Human Services, Centers for Disease Control and Prevention, National Center for Chronic Disease Prevention and Health Promotion, and Office of Smoking and Health.

U.S. Department of Health and Human Services. (2011). *Healthy people 2020.* Washington, DC: Government Printing Office.

U.S. Department of Health and Human Services. (2013). *Key features of the Affordable Care Act by year.* Retrieved June 2, 2013, from www.hhs.gov/healthcare/facts/timeline/timeline-text.html

U.S. Department of Justice, Office on Violence Against Women. (2023). *Domestic violence.* Retrieved January 12, 2024, from justice.gov

U.S. Environmental Protection Agency. (2007). *Asthma: Indoor environmental asthma triggers: Cockroaches and pets.* Retrieved December 17, 2007, from www.epa.gov/asthma/pests.html

U.S. Environmental Protection Agency. (2022). *Superfund: National priorities list (NPL).* Retrieved June 23, 2024, from https://web.archive.org/web/20220907204242/https://www.epa.gov/superfund/superfund-national-priorities-list-npl

U.S. Food and Drug Administration. (2005). *FDA News. FDA approves BiDil heart failure drug for black patients.* Retrieved October 28, 2013, from www.fda.gov/downloads/drugs/guidancecomplianceregulatoryinformation/guidances/ucm332181.pdf

U.S. Food and Drug Administration. (2007). *Expanded access and expedited approvals of new therapies related to HIV/AIDS.* Retrieved June 1, 2007, from www.fda.gov/forconsumers/byaudience/forpatientadvocates/hivandaidsactivities/ucm134331.htm.

U.S. National Library of Medicine & National Institutes of Health. (2009). *MedlinePlus. Arthritis in hip.* Retrieved December 12, 2009, from www.nlm.nih.gov/medlineplus/ency/imagepages/19678.htm

U.S. National Library of Medicine & National Institutes of Health. (2010). *MedlinePlus. Knee joint.* Retrieved January 30, 2010, from www.nlm.nih.gov/medlineplus/ency/imagepages/19309.htm

USEPA. (n.d.). *Greenhouse gas emissions.* Retrieved February 8, 2024, from chicago.gov.

Vahedian-Shahroodi, M., Tehrani, H., Robat-Sarpooshi, D., Gholian – Aval, M., Jafari, A., & Alizadeh-Siuki, H. (2021). The impact of health education on nutritional behaviors in female students: An application of health belief model. *International Journal of Health Promotion and Education, 59*(2), 70–82. doi: 10.1080/14635240.2019.1696219

Valentine, N., Verdes-Tennant, E., & Bonsel, G. (2015). Health systems' responsiveness and reporting behaviour: Multilevel analysis of the influence of individual-level factors in 64 countries. *Social Science & Medicine, 138,* 152–160. doi: 10.1016/j.socscimed.2015.04.022

Valenzuela, T.D., Roe, D.J., Nichol, G., Clark, L.L., Spaite, D.W., & Hardman, R.G. (2000). Outcomes of rapid defibrillation by security officers after cardiac arrests in casinos. *The New England Journal of Medicine, 343*(17), 1206–1209.

Valkenburg, P. M., & Peter, J. (2007). Online communication and adolescent well-being: Testing the stimulation versus the displacement hypothesis. *Journal of Computer-Mediated Communication, 12*(4), 1169–1182. doi: 10.1111/j.1083-6101.2007.00368.x

Vallerand, A. H., Hasenau, S., Templin, T., & Collins-Bohler, D. (2005). Disparities between black and white patients with cancer pain: The effects of perception of control over pain. *Pain Medicine, 6,* 242–250.

Vallerand, A. H., Riley-Doucet, C., Hasenau, S., & Templin, T. (2003). *Cancer related pain in the outpatient clinic population.* Paper presented at the 7th National Conference on Cancer Nursing Research. San Diego, CA: Oncology Nursing Society.

Vallöf, D., Kalafateli, A. L., & Jerlhag, E. (2020). Long-term treatment with a glucagon-like peptide-1 receptor agonist reduces ethanol intake in male and female rats. *Translational Psychiatry, 10,* 238. doi: 10.1038/s41398-020-00923-1

vanBeurden, E., Zask, A., Brooks, L., & Dight, R. (2005). Heavy episodic drinking and sensation seeking in adolescents as predictors of harmful driving and celebrating behaviors: Implications for prevention. *Journal of Adolescent Health, 37,* 37–43.

van Dam, K. (2020). Individual stress prevention through qigong. *International Journal of Environmental Research and Public Health, 17*(19), 7342. doi: 10.3390/ijerph17197342

Van de Bongard, D., Reitz, E., Sandfort, T., & Deković, M. (2015). A meta-analysis of the relations between three types of peer norms and adolescent sexual behavior. *Personality and Social Psychology Review, 19*(3), 203–234. doi: 10.1177/1088868314544223

van der Linden, S. L., Clarke, C. E., & Mailbach, E. W. (2015). Highlighting consensus among medical scientists increases public support for vaccines: Evidence from a randomized experiment. *BMC Public Health, 15,* 1207. doi: 10.1186/s12889-015-2541-4

van der Mei, I. A., Ponsonby, A. L., & Dwyer, T. (2003). Past exposure to sun, skin phenotype, and risk of multiple sclerosis: Case-control study. *British Medical Journal, 327,* 311–316.

VanDervanter, N. L., Messeri, P., Middlestadt, S. E., Bleakley, A., Merzel, C. R., & Hogben, M. (2005). A community-based intervention designed to increase preventive health care seeking among adolescents: The Gonorrhea Community Action Project. *American Journal of Public Health, 95,* 331–337.

van der Valk, E. S., Savas, M., & van Rossum, E. F. C. (2018). Stress and obesity: Are there more susceptible individuals? *Current Obesity Reports, 7,* 193–203. doi: 10.1007/s13679-018-0306-y

van der Wal, C. V., & Kok, R. N. (2019). Laughter-inducing therapies: Systematic review and meta-analysis. *Social Science & Medicine, 232,* 473–488. doi: 10.1016/j.socscimed.2019.02.018

VanderWeele, T. J., Yu, J. U., Cozier, Y. C., Wise, L., Argentieri, M. A., Rosenberg, L., . . . Shields, A. E. (2017). Attendance at religious services, prayer, religious coping, and religious/spiritual identity as predictors of all-cause mortality in the Black Women's Health Study. *American Journal of Epidemiology, 185*(7), 515–522. doi: 10.1093/aje/kww179. Erratum in: *American Journal of Epidemiology* (2017), *186*(4), 501.

Van geertruyden, J. P., & D'Alessandro, U. (2007). Malaria and HIV: A silent alliance. *Trends in Parasitology, 23*(10), 465–467.

van Oosterhout, R. E. M., de Boer, A. R., Maas, A. H. E. M., Rutten, F. H., Bots, M. L., & Peters, S. A. E. (2020). Sex differences in symptom presentation in acute coronary syndromes: A systematic review and meta-analysis. *JAMA, 9,* e014733. doi: 10.1161/JAHA.119.014733

vanRyzin, M. J., Fosco, G. M., & Dishion, T. J. (2012). Family and peer predictors of substance use from early adolescence to early adulthood: An 11-year prospective analysis. *Addictive Behaviors, 37,* 1314–1324.

Vanthomme, K., Rosskamp, M., De Schutter, H., & Vandenheede, H. (2022). Colorectal incidence and survival inequalities among labour immigrants in Belgium during 2004–2013. *Scientific Reports, 12*, 15727. doi: 10.1038/s41598-022-19322-1

van Wyk, B.-E. (2008). A review of the Khoi-San and Cape Dutch medical ethnobotany. *Journal of Ethnopharmacology, 119*, 331–341.

Varela, F. H., Pinto, L. A., & Scotta, M. C. (2019). Global impact of varicella vaccination programs. *Human Vaccines & Immunotherapeutics, 15*(3), 645–657. doi: 10.1080/21645515.2018.1546525

Vargas, L. A., & Koss-Chioino, J. D. (Eds.). (1992). *Working with culture: Psycho-therapeutic interventions with ethnic minority children and adolescents.* San Francisco, CA: Jossey-Bass.

Vasan, R. S., Pan, S., Xanthakis, V., Beiser, A., Larson, M. G., Seshadri, S., & Mitchell, G. F. (2022). Arterial stiffness and long-term risk of health Outcomes: The Framingham Heart Study. *Hypertension, 79*(5), 1049–1056.

Vázquez-Alonzo, C. A., Guzman-Feliciano, M. F., De la Cruz-Luna, A. G., & García-Ortiz, L. (2023). Etiology of bulimia nervosa: A literature review. *Revista Enfermería de la Universidad CUSUR*

Vecino-Ortiz, A. I., Nagarajan, M., Elaraby, S., Guzman-Tordecilla, D. N., Paichadze, N., & Hyder, A. A. (2022). Saving lives through road safety risk factor interventions: Global and national estimates. *The Lancet, 400*, 237–250.

Veenis, J. F., Brunner-La Rocca, H.-P., Linssen, G. C., Geerlings, P. R., Van Gent, M. W. F., Aksoy, I., . . . Brugts, J. J. (2019). Age differences in contemporary treatment of patients with chronic heart failure and reduced ejection fraction. *European Journal of Preventive Cardiology, 26*(13), 1399–1407. doi: 10.1177/2047487319835042

Vickers, A. (2000). Why aromatherapy works (even if it doesn't) and why we need less research. *British Journal of General Practice, 50*(455), 444–445.

Vijayan, V., Naeem, F., & Veesenmeyer, A. F. (2021). Management of infants born to mothers with HIV infection. *American Family Physician, 104*(1), 58–62.

Villa, A., Patton, L. L., Giuliana, A. R., Estrich, C. G., Pahlke, S. C., O'Brien, K. K., et al. (2020). Summary of the evidence on the safety, efficacy & effectiveness of human papillomavirus vaccine: Umbrella review of systematic review. *Journal of American Dental Association, 151*(4), 245–254.

Villavicencio, L., Svencara, A. M., Kelley-Baker, T., & Tefft, B. C. (2022). Passenger presence and the relative risk of teen driver death. *Journal of Adolescent Health, 70*(5), 757–762. doi: 10.1016/j.jadohealth.2021.10.038

Virginia Tech Transportation Institute. (2016). *New VTTI study results continue to highlight the dangers of distracted driving.* Retrieved October 28, 2016, from www.vtti.vt.edu/featured/?p=193

Vitaliano, P. P., Zhang, J., & Scanlon, J. M. (2003). Is caregiving hazardous to one's physical health? A meta-analysis. *Psychological Bulletin, 129*(6), 946–972.

Vogel, B., Acevedo, M., Appelman, Y., Merz, C. N. B., Chieffo, A., Figtree, G. A., . . . Mehran, R. (2021). The Lancet Women and Cardiovascular Disease Commission: Reducing the global burden by 2030. *The Lancet, 397*(10292), 2385–2438. doi: 10.1016/S0140-6736(21)00684-X

Vogels, T., van der Vliet, R., Danz, M., Hopman-Rock, M., & Visser, A. (1993). Young people and sex: Behavior and health risks in Dutch school students. *International Journal of Adolescent Medicine and Health, 2*, 137–147.

Vouri, H. (1987). Patient satisfaction: An attribute or indicator of the quality of care? *Quality Review Bulletin, 13*, 106–108.

Vouri, H. (1991). Patient satisfaction: Does it matter? *Quality Assurance Health Care, 3*, 183–189.

Wachholtz, A. B., & Pargament, K. I. (2008). Migraines and meditation: Does spirituality matter? *Journal of Behavioral Medicine, 31*(4), 351–366.

Wade, D. T., & Halligan, P. W. (2004). Do biomedical models of illness make for good healthcare systems? *British Medical Journal, 329*, 1398–1491.

Wagemakers, A., Corstjens, R., Koelen, M., Vaandrager, L., van't Reit, H., & Dijkshoor, H. (2008). Participatory approaches to promote healthy lifestyles among Turkish and Moroccan women in Amsterdam. *Promotion and Education, 15*(4), 17–23.

Wakefield, A. J., Murch, S. H., Anthony, A., Linnell, J., Casson, D. M., Malik, M., . . . Walker-Smith, J. A. (1998). Ileal-lymphoid-nodular hyperplasia, non-specific colitis, and pervasive developmental disorder in children. *The Lancet, 351*(9103), 637–641.

Walda, I. C., Tabak, C., Smit, H. A., Rasanen, L., Fidanza, F., Menotti, A., . . . Kromhout, D. (2002). Diet and 20-year chronic obstructive pulmonary disease mortality in middle-aged men from three European countries. *European Journal of Clinical Nutrition, 56*(7), 638–643.

Walker, N., Parag, V., Wong, S. F., Youdan, B., Broughton, B., Bullen, C., & Beaglehole, R. (2020). Use of e-cigarettes and smoked tobacco in youth aged 14–15 years in New Zealand: Findings from repeated cross-sectional studies (2014–2019). *The Lancet, 5*(4), e204–e212. doi: 10.1016/S2468-2667(19)30241-5

Wallace, J. M., Yamaguchi, R., Bachman, J. G., O'Malley, P. M., Schulenberg, J. E., & Johnston, L. D. (2007). Religiosity and adolescent substance use: The role of individual and contextual influences. *Social Problems, 54*(2), 308–327.

Wallis, D. J., & Hetherington, M. M. (2004). Stress and eating: The effects of ego-threat and cognitive demand on food intake in restrained and emotional eaters. *Appetite, 43*, 39–46.

Walloe, L. (2008). Medieval and modern bubonic plague: Some clinical continuities. *Medical History*, (suppl. 27), 59–73.

Walsh, B. T. (1997). Eating disorders. In A. Tasman, J. Kay, & J. A. Lieberman (Eds.), *Psychiatry* (Vol. 2, pp. 1202–1216). London: John Wiley & Sons.

Walsh, S., O'Neill, A., Hannigan, A., & Harmon, D. (2019). Patient-rated physician empathy and patient satisfaction during pain clinic consultations. *Irish Journal of Medical Science, 188*, 1379–1384. doi: 10.1007/s11845-019-01999-5

Walsh, S. R., Manuel, J. C., & Avis, N. E. (2005). The impact of breast cancer on younger women's relationships with their partner and children. *Families, Systems, & Health, 23*, 80–93.

Walter, H. J., Vaughan, R. D., Gladis, M. M., Ragin, D. F., Kasen, S., & Cohall, A. T. (1992). Factors associated with AIDS risk behaviors among high school students in an AIDS epicenter. *American Journal of Public Health, 82*(4), 528–532.

Walter, H. J., Vaughan, R. D., Gladis, M. M., Ragin, D. F., Kasen, S., & Cohall, A. T. (1993). Factors associated with AIDS-related behavioral intentions among high school students in an AIDS epicenter. *Health Education Quarterly, 20*(3), 409–420.

Walter, H. J., Vaughan, R. D., Ragin, D. F., Cohall, A. T., & Kasen, S. (1994). Prevalence and correlates of AIDS-related behavioral intentions among urban minority high school students. *AIDS Education and Prevention, 6*(4), 339–350.

Walters, J. H. (1978). Influenza 1918: The contemporary perspective. *Bulletin of the New York Academy of Medicine, 54*, 855–864. www.ncbi.nlm.nih.gov/pmc/articles/PMC1807529/pdf/bullnyacadmed00134-0037.pdf

Walters, K. L., Johnson-Jennings, M., Stroud, S., Rasmus, S., Charles, B., John, S., . . . Boulafentis, J. (2020). Growing from our roots: Strategies for developing culturally grounded health promotion interventions in American Indian, Alaska Native, and Native Hawaiian communities. *Prevention Science*, *21*(Suppl. 1), 54–64. doi: 10.1007/s11121-018-0952-z

Wang, M., Gong, W., Sun, D., Pei, P., Lv, J., Yu, C., & Yu, M. (2023). Associations between experience of stressful life events and cancer prevalence in China: Results from the China Kadoorie Biobank study. *BMC Cancer, 23*, 1142. doi: 10.1186/s12885-023-11659-8

Wang, S. X., Wang, Z. H., Cheng, X. T., Li, J., Sang, Z. P., Zhang, X. D., . . . Wang, Z. Q. (2007). Arsenic and fluoride exposure in drinking water: Children's IQ and growth in Shanyin county, Shanxi province, China. *Environmental Health Perspectives, 115*(4), 643–647.

Wang, Y., & Beydoun, M. A. (2007). The obesity epidemic in the United States – Gender, age, socioeconomics, racial/ethnic, and geographic characteristics: A systematic review and meta-regression analysis. *Epidemiology Review, 29*, 6–28.

Ward, A., & Mann, T. (2000). Don't mind if I do: Disinhibited eating under cognitive load. *Journal of Personality and Social Psychology, 78*, 753–763.

Ward, C. L., Martin, E., & Distiller, G. B. (2007). Factors affecting resilience in children exposed to violence. *South African Journal of Psychology, 37*(1), 165–187.

Wardle, J. (1995). Cholesterol and psychological well-being. *Journal of Psychosomatic Research, 39*(5), 549–562.

Wardle, J., Hasse, A. M., Steptoe, A., Nillapun, M., Jonwutiewes, K., & Bellisle, F. (2004). Gender differences in food choice: The contribution of health beliefs and dieting. *Annals of Behavioral Medicine, 27*, 107–116.

Ware, J. E., & Sherbourne, C. D. (1992). The MOS 36-item short-form health survey (SF-36). I. Conceptual framework and item selection. *Medical Care, 30*, 473–483.

Warner, E., Foulkes, W., Goodwin, P., Meschino, W., Blondel, J., Paterson, C., . . . Narod, S. (1999). Prevalence and penetrance of BRCA1 and BRCA2 gene mutation in unselected Ashkenazi Jewish women with breast cancer. *Journal of the National Cancer Institute, 91*(14), 1241–1247.

Wartik, N. (2003, August 26). Rising obesity in children prompts call to action. *The New York Times*, p. 5.

Washam, C. (2005). Targeting teens and adolescents for HPV vaccine could draw fire. *Journal of the National Cancer Institute, 97*(14), 1030.

Watson, H. J., Yilmaz, Z., Thornton, L. M., Hubel, C., Coleman, J. R. I., Gaspar, H. A., . . . Bulik, C. M. (2019). Genome-wide association study identifies eight risk loci and implicates metabo-psychiatric origins for anorexia nervosa. *Nature Genetics, 51*, 1207–1214. doi: 10.1038/s41588-019-0439-2

Watson, W. E., Minzenmayer, T., & Bobler, M. (2006). Type-A personality characteristics and the effects on individual and team academic performance. *Journal of Applied Social Psychology, 36*(5), 1110–1128.

Weaver, S. R., Rendeiro, C., McGettrick, H. M., Philip, A., & Lucas, S. J. E. (2021). Fine wine or sour grapes? A systematic review and meta-analysis of the impact of red wine polyphenols on vascular health. *European Journal of Nutrition, 60*, 1–28. doi: 10.1007/s00394-020-02247-8

Weiner, K. A. (2003). 2001–2010: The decade of pain control and research. *The Pain Practitioner*, Spring. Retrieved July 20, 2010, from www.aapainmanage.org/literature/PainPrac/V13N1_Weiner_DecadeOfPainControl.pdf

Weir, H. K., Thun, M. J., Hankey, B. F., Reis, L. A. G., Howe, H. L., Wingo, P. A., . . . Edwards, B. K. (2003). Special article: Annual report to the nation on the status of cancer, 1975–2000, featuring the uses of surveillance data for cancer prevention and control. *Journal of the National Cancer Institute, 95*(17), 1276–1299.

Weir, L. A., Elelson, D., & Brand, D. A. (2006). Parents' perception of neighborhood safety and children's physical activity. *Preventive Medicine, 43*(3), 212–217.

Weisberg, J.N., & Keefe, F.J. (1999). Personality, individual differences, and psychopathology in chronic pain. In R.J. Gatchel & D.C. Turk (Eds.), *Psychosocial factors in pain: Critical perspectives* (pp. 56–73). New York, NY: Guilford.

Weiss, N.S. (2003). Breast cancer mortality in relation to clinical breast examination and breast self-examination. *The Breast Journal, 9*, 586–589.

Welch, E., Jangmo, A., Thornton, L.M., Norring, C., von Hausswolff-Juhlin, Y., Herman, B.K., . . . Bulik, C.M. (2016). Treatment-seeking patients with binge-eating disorder in the Swedish national registers: Clinical course and psychiatric comorbidity. *BMC Psychiatry, 16*, 163. doi: 10.1186/s12888-016-0840-7

Wells, B.I., & Horn, J.W. (1992). Stage at diagnosis in breast cancer: Race and socioeconomic factors. *American Journal of Public Health, 82*, 1383–1385.

Wendt, C., & Margolin, S. (2019). Identifying breast cancer-susceptibility genes: A review of the genetic background in familial breast cancer. *Acta Oncologica, 58*(2), 135–146.

Weng, H.C. (2008). Does the physician's emotional intelligence matter? Impacts of the physician's relationship and satisfaction. *Health Care Management Review, 33*(4), 280–288.

Wetherell, M.A., Byrne-Davis, L., Dieppe, P., Donovan, J., Brookes, S., Byron, M., . . . Miles, J. (2005). Effects of emotional disclosure on psychological and physiological outcomes in patients with rheumatoid arthritis: An exploratory home-based study. *Journal of Health Psychology, 10*, 277–285.

Whirledge, S., & Cidlowski, J.A. (2010). Glucocorticoids, stress, and fertility. *Minerva Endocrinology, 35*(2), 109–125.

Whisman, M.A., & Sbarra, D.A. (2012). Marital adjustment and interleukin-6 (IL-6). *Journal of Family Psychology, 26*(2), 290–295.

Whitfield, C.L. (2003). *The truth about depression: Choices for healing*. Deerfield Beach, FL: Health Communications.

Whitfield, C.L., Anda, R.F., Dube, S.R., & Felitti, V.J. (2003). Violent childhood experiences and the risk of intimate partner violence in adults. *Journal of Interpersonal Violence, 18*(2), 166–185.

Whittle, J., Conigliaro, J., Good, C.B., & Lofgren, R.P. (1993). Racial differences in the use of invasive cardiovascular procedures in the Department of Veterans Affairs medical system. *The New England Journal of Medicine, 329*, 621–627.

WHO Ebola Response Team. (2016). Ebola virus disease among male and female persons in West Africa. *The New England Journal of Medicine, 374*, 96–98. doi: 10.1056/NEJMc1510305

Wiet, S. (2009). *Care for the caregivers: Information, simplification, peace of mind and time*. Retrieved June 2, 2009, from www.strengthforcaring.com/manual/about-you-the-caregiver-role/care-for-the-caregiverinformation-simplification-peace-of-mind-and-time/

Wijnen, J.T., Brochet, R.M., vanEijk, R., Jagmohan-Changun, S., Middledor, P.A., Tops, C.M., . . . Vasen, H.F.A. (2008). Chromosome 8q23.3 and 11q23.1 variants modify colorectal cancer risk in Lynch syndrome. *Gastroenterology, 136*, 131–137.

Wilkinson, R.G. (1996). *Unhealthy societies: The afflictions of inequality*. London: Routledge.

Willi, J., & Grossman, S. (1983). Epidemiology of anorexia nervosa in a defined region of Switzerland. *American Journal of Psychiatry, 140*, 564–567.

Williams, A.F. (2003). Teenage drivers: Patterns of risk. *Journal of Safety Research, 34*, 5–15.

Williams, A.F. (2017). Graduated driver licensing (GDL) in the United States in 2016: A literature review and commentary. *Journal of Safety Research, 63*, 29–41. doi: 10.1016/j.jsr.2017.08.01

Williams, D.M., Anderson, E.S., & Winett, R.A. (2005). A review of the outcome expectancy construct in physical activity research. *Annals of Behavioral Medicine, 29*(1), 70–79.

Williams, D. R., & Neighbors, H. (2001). Racism, discrimination and hypertension: Evidence and needed research. *Ethnicity and Disease, 11*, 800–816.

Williams, J. E., Paton, C. C., Siegler, I. C., Eignebrodt, M. L., Neito, F. J., & Tyroler, H. A. (2000). Anger proneness predicts coronary heart disease risk. *Circulation, 101*, 2034–2039.

Williams, R., & Williams, V. (1993). *Anger kills*. New York, NY: Random House.

Wills, T. A., Sargent, J. D., Stoolmiller, M., Gibbons, F. X., Worth, K. A., & Cin, S. (2007). Movie exposure to smoking cues and adolescent smoking onset for mediation through peer affiliations. *Health Psychology, 26*(6), 769–776.

Wilson, D. J. (2005). *Living with polio: The epidemic and its survivors*. Chicago, IL: University of Chicago Press.

Wilson, F. A., & Stimpson, J. P. (2010). Trends in fatalities for distracted driving in the United States: 1999–2008. *American Journal of Public Health, 100*(11), 2213–2219.

Wilson, K. M., & Klein, J. D. (2000). Adolescents who use the emergency department as their usual source of care. *Archives of Pediatric & Adolescent Medicine, 154*, 361–365.

Wilson, S. J., Bailey, B. E., Malarkey, W. B., & Kiecolt-Glaser, J. K. (2021). Linking marital support to aging-related biomarkers: Both age and marital quality matter. *The Journals of Gerontology: Series B, 76*(2), 273–282. doi: 10.1093/geronb/gbz106

Win, A. K., Jenkins, M. A., Dowty, J. G., Antoniou, A. C., Lee, A., Giles, G. G., . . . MacInnis, R. J. (2017). Prevalence and penetrance of major genes and polygenes for colorectal cancer. *Cancer Epidemiology, Biomarkers & Prevention, 26*, 404–412.

Winkleby, M. A., Robinson, T. N., Sundquist, J., & Kraemer, H. C. (1999). Ethnic variations in cardiovascular disease risk factors among children and young adults. *Journal of the American Medical Association, 281*(11), 1006–1013.

Wipfli, H., & Samit, J. M. (2016). One hundred years in the making: The global tobacco epidemic. *Annual Review of Public Health, 37*, 149–166.

Wippold, G. M., Frary, S. G., Garcia, K. A., & Wilson, D. K. (2023). Implementing barbershop-based health-promotion interventions for Black men: A systematic scoping review. *Health Psychology, 42*(7), 435. doi: 10.1037/hea0001294

Wirth, O., & Sigurdsson, S. O. (2008). When workplace safety depends on behavior change: Topics for behavioral safety. *Journal of Safety Research, 39*, 589–598.

Wirtz, P. H., von Kanel, R., Emini, L., Suter, T., Fontana, A., & Ehlert, U. (2007). Variations in anticipatory cognitive stress appraisal and differential proinflammatory cytokine expression in response to acute stress. *Brain, Behavior, and Immunity, 21*, 851–859.

Withers, A., Zuniga, K., & Van Sell, S. L. (2017). Spirituality: Concept analysis. *International Journal of Nursing & Clinical Practices, 4*, 234–239. doi: 10.15344/2394-4978/2017/234

Wold, S. J., Brown, C. M., Chastain, C. E., Griffis, M. D., & Wingate, J. (2008). Going the extra mile: Beyond health teaching to political involvement. *Nursing Forum, 43*(4), 171–176.

Wollast, R., Schmitz, M., Bigot, A., & Luminet, O. (2021). The theory of planned behavior during the COVID-19 pandemic: A comparison of health behaviors between Belgian and French residents. *PLoS One, 16*(11), e0258320. doi: 10.1371/journal.pone.0258320

Wong, W. C. W., Lee, A., Wong, S. Y. S., Wu, A. C., & Robinson, N. (2006). Strengths, weaknesses, and development of traditional medicine in the health system of Hong Kong: Through the eyes of future Western doctors. *Journal of Alternative and Complementary Medicine, 12*(2), 185–189.

Wood, F. C. (1924, April). Must women die of cancer? *Women Citizen, 11*, 24.

Wood, W., & Neal, D. T. (2016). Healthy through habit: Interventions for initiating & maintaining health behavior change. *Behavioral Science & Policy, 2*(1), 71–83. doi: 10.1177/237946151600200109

Woodgate, J., & Brawley, L. R. (2008). Self-efficacy for exercise in cardiac rehabilitation: Review and recommendation. *Journal of Health Psychology, 13*(3), 366–387.

Wooster, R., Bignell, G., Lancaster, J., Swift, S., Seal, S., & Mangion, J. (1995). Identification of the breast cancer susceptibility gene BRCA2. *Nature, 378,* 789–792.

World Bank. (2013). *Data: How we classify countries.* Retrieved June 27, 2013, from http://data.worldbank.org/about/country-classifications

World Health Organization. (1948). Constitution of the World Health Organization. *Chronicle of the World Health Organization, 1.*

World Health Organization. (1992). *World Health Organization basic documents* (39th ed.). Geneva: Author.

World Health Organization. (1999). *Dracunculiasis or Guinea worm.* CEE Documentation Center. Geneva: Author.

World Health Organization. (2000). *Guide to drug abuse epidemiology.* Geneva: Department of Mental Health and Substance Dependence, Noncommunicable Diseases and Mental Health Cluster, and World Health Organization.

World Health Organization. (2002a). *Strategic approaches to the prevention of HIV infections in infants.* Report of a WHO meeting, Morges, Switzerland, 20–22 March 2002. Retrieved May 20, 2013, from www.who.int/hiv/pub/mtct/en/StrategicApproachesE.pdf

World Health Organization. (2002b). *The World Health Report 2002: Reducing risks, promoting healthy lives.* Geneva: Author.

World Health Organization. (2003). *Traditional medicine.* Fact sheet No. 134. Retrieved from www.who.int/mediacentre/factsheets/fs134/en/

World Health Organization. (2004a). *Malaria and HIV interactions and their implications for public health policy: Report of a technical consultation.* Geneva: Author.

World Health Organization. (2004b). *World Health Organization supports global effort to relieve chronic pain.* Retrieved January 16, 2013, from www.who.int/mediacentre/news/releases/2004/pr70/en/index.html

World Health Organization. (2005a). *Facing the facts #3. Chronic diseases in low and middle income countries.* Geneva: Author.

World Health Organization (Roll Back Malaria Department). (2005b). *Malaria.* Geneva: Author.

World Health Organization. (2005c). *Preventing chronic diseases: A vital investment.* Geneva: Author.

World Health Organization. (2005d). *A systematic approach to developing and implementing mental health legislation.* Report of a regional meeting of experts, New Delhi, India, 6–8 December 2004. WHO Project ICP MNH 001. New Delhi: Author.

World Health Organization. (2005e). *HIV/AIDS antiretroviral newsletter, No. 11.* Manila: Author.

World Health Organization. (2006a). *Cholera.* Retrieved November 1, 2006, from www.who.int/mediacentre/factsheets/fs107/en/

World Health Organization. (2006b). *Measles.* Retrieved November 1, 2006, from www.who.int/mediacentre/factsheets/fs286/en/

World Health Organization. (2006c). *WHO research agenda for radio frequency fields.* Retrieved January 13, 2013, from www.who.int/peh-emf/research/rf_research_agenda_2006.pdf

World Health Organization. (2006d). *Guidelines for the early detection and screening of breast cancer* (O. M. N. Khatib & A. Modjtabai, Eds.). EMRO Technical Publication Series 30. Retrieved March 29, 2023, from who.int

World Health Organization. (2007a). *Malaria*. Fact sheet no. 94. Retrieved October 31, 2007, from www. who.int/mediacentre/factsheets/fs094/en/print.html

World Health Organization. (2007b). *Tuberculosis*. Fact sheet No. 104. Retrieved April 30, 2007, from www.who.int/mediacentre/factsheets/fs104/en/index.html

World Health Organization. (2008a). *Cancer*. Fact sheet No. 297. Retrieved from www.who.int/mediacentre/factsheets/fs297/en/

World Health Organization. (2008b). *Cardiovascular disease: Fact sheet*. Retrieved July 10, 2008, from www.who.int/cardiovascular_diseases/en

World Health Organization. (2008c). *Cholera*. Fact sheet No. 107. Retrieved December 27, 2016, from www.who.int/mediacentre/factsheets/fs107/en/

World Health Organization. (2008d). *Global tuberculosis control: Surveillance, planning, finance*. Geneva: Author.

World Health Organization. (2009a). *About dracunculiasis*. Retrieved April 29, 2009, from www.who.int/dracunculiasis/disease/en/

World Health Organization. (2009b). *Malnutrition*. Retrieved October 28, 2013, from http://www.who.int/maternal_child_adolescent/topics/child/malnutrition/en/

World Health Organization. (2009c). *Pandemic influenza preparedness and response: A WHO guidance document*. Retrieved February 23, 2010, from https://www.ncbi.nlm.nih.gov/books/NBK143061/figure/ch4.f1/?report=objectonly

World Health Organization. (2009d). *Wild poliovirus 2008*. Retrieved August 9, 2009, from www.who.int/vaccines-surveillance/graphies/htmls/global_polio_03.html

World Health Organization. (2010a). *Influenza A (H1N1): Update 42*. Retrieved June 2, 2010, from www.who.int/csr/don/2009_06_01a/en/

World Health Organization. (2010b). *Suicide prevention*. SUPRE Publication, World Health Organization. Retrieved February 24, 2010, from www.who.int/mental_health/prevention/suicide/suicideprevent/en/

World Health Organization. (2010c). *About WHO*. Retrieved July 9, 2010, from www.who.int/about/en

World Health Organization. (2011a). *Electromagnetic fields and public health: Mobile phones*. Fact sheet No. 196. Retrieved January 12, 2013, from www.who.int/mediacentre/factsheets/fs193/en/

World Health Organization. (2011b, May 5). *Implementation of the International Health Regulations (2005)*. Report of the Review Committee on the functioning of the International Health Regulations (2005) in relation to pandemic (H1N1) 2009. Sixty-fourth World Health Assembly Provisional Agenda Item 13.2. Retrieved October 23, 2016, from www.who.int/ihr/review_committee/en/

World Health Organization. (2011c). *Global HIV/AIDS response: Epidemic update and health sector progress towards universal access*. Progress Report 2011. Geneva: Author.

World Health Organization. (2011d). *Top 10 causes of death*. Fact sheet No. 310. Retrieved January 12, 2013, from www.who.int/mediacentre/factsheets/fs310/en/

World Health Organization. (2011e). *Guidelines for drinking-water quality* (4th ed.). Retrieved August 2, 2023, from 9789241548151_eng.pdf

World Health Organization. (2012). *WHO guidelines on the pharmacological treatment of persistent pain in children with medical illnesses*. Geneva: Author.

World Health Organization. (2014). *Varicella and herpes zoster vaccines: WHO position paper*. Retrieved April 20, 2023, from WER8925_265–287.PDF (who.int)

World Health Organization. (2015). *Biodiversity and health*. Retrieved September 7, 2023, from who.int

World Health Organization. (2016a). *Cumulative number of confirmed human cases for avian influenza A(H5N1) reported to WHO.* Retrieved October 22, 2016, from www.who.int/influenza/human_animal_interface/H5N1_cumulative_table_archives/en/

World Health Organization. (2016b). *Ebola situation report.* Retrieved October 22, 2016, from http://www.who.int/csr/disease/ebola/situation-reports/archive/en/

World Health Organization. (2016c). *Global tuberculosis report.* Retrieved October 23, 2016, from www.who.int/tb/publications/global_report/en/

World Health Organization. (2016d). *Mental health: Suicide data.* Retrieved October 30, 2016, from www.who.int/mental_health/prevention/suicide/suicideprevent/en/

World Health Organization. (2017). *WHO report on the global tobacco epidemic 2017, monitoring tobacco use and prevention policies.* Geneva: Author. Retrieved March 24, 2023, from 9789241512824-eng.pdf (who.int)

World Health Organization. (2018a). *Alcohol: Global status report on alcohol and health, 2018.* Geneva. Retrieved June 24, 2024, from https://iris.who.int/bitstream/handle/10665/274603/9789241565639-eng.pdf

World Health Organization. (2018b). *Asbestos: Elimination of asbestos-related diseases.* Retrieved March 23, 2023, from who.int

World Health Organization. (2019a). *The WHO special initiative for mental health (2019–2023): Universal health coverage for mental health.* Retrieved December 9, 2023, from WHO-MSD-19.1-eng.pdf

World Health Organization. (2019b). *WHO global report on traditional and complementary medicine.* Geneva: Author.

World Health Organization. (2021a). *WHO report on the global tobacco epidemic: Addressing new and emerging products.* Geneva: Author.

World Health Organization. (2021b). *Obesity and overweight.* Retrieved June 12, 2023, from who.int

World Health Organization. (2021c, January 14–February 10). *WHO-convened global study of origins of SARS-CoV-2: China Part.* Joint WHO – China study. Joint report.

World Health Organization. (2022a). *Global Health Observatory Data Repository.* Retrieved May 19, 2023, from who.int

World Health Organization. (2022b). *Key facts – Traffic accidents.* Retrieved January 11, 2024, from who.int

World Health Organization (Global Market Study). (2022c). *Market information for access to vaccines: Global Market Study HPV.* Retrieved September 22, 2022, from https://www.who-hpv-vaccine-global-market-study-april-2022.pdf

World Health Organization. (2022d). *Cancer: Key facts.* Retrieved February 2, 2023, from who.int

World Health Organization. (2022e). *World health statistics 2022: Monitoring health for the SDGs, sustainable development goals.* Geneva: Author.

World Health Organization. (2022f). *Tobacco.* Retrieved December 5, 2023, from who.int.

World Health Organization. (2023a). *Multiple sclerosis: Key facts.* Retrieved November 1, 2023, from who.int.

World Health Organization. (2023b). *Emergency dashboard: Global South Africa.* Retrieved June 14, 2023, from https://covid19.who.int/region/afro/country/za

World Health Organization. (2023c). *The top 10 causes of death.* Retrieved March 7, 2023, from who.int

World Health Organization. (2023d). *WHO statement regarding cluster of pneumonia cases in Wuhan, China.* Retrieved November 12, 2023, from.

World Health Organization. (2023e). *The true death toll of COVID-19: Estimating global excess mortality.* Retrieved from who.int

World Health Organization. (2023f). *Smallpox.* Retrieved December 1, 2023, from who.int

World Health Organization. (2023g). *Global tuberculosis report 2021. 2.1 TB incidence.* Retrieved April 18, 2023, from www.who.int/publications/digital/global-tuberculosis-report-2021/tb-disease-burden/incidence

World Health Organization. (2023h). *Measles: Fact sheet.* Retrieved April 18, 2023, from who.int.

World Health Organization. (2023i). *Emergencies: Measles emergencies in the European region.* Retrieved November, 11, 2023, from who.int

World Health Organization. (2023j). *Vision statement.* Retrieved December 1, 2023, from who.int

World Health Organization. (2023k). *Who we are.* Retrieved December 1, 2023, from.

World Health Organization. (2023l, June 17). *Launch of the WHO world mental health report: Transforming mental health for all.* Department of Mental Health and Substance Use. Retrieved December 1, 2023, from.

World Health Organization. (2023m). *Disease Outbreak News 2009 – Netherlands.* Retrieved December 9, 2023, from who.int

World Health Organization. (2023n). *History of the smallpox vaccine.* Retrieved December 1, 2023, from who.int

World Health Organization. (2023o). *Q&A: How Belize eliminated malaria.* Retrieved November 23, 2023, from who.int

World Health Organization. (2023p). *WHO prequalifies a second malaria vaccine, a significant milestone in prevention of the disease.* Retrieved January 2, 2024, from.

World Health Organization. (2023q). *Traditional medicine has a long history of contributing to conventional medicine and continues to hold promise.* Retrieved November 7, 2023, from who.int

World Health Organization. (2023r). *The global health observatory: Cause-specific mortality 2000–2019.* Retrieved February 23, 2023, from who.int

World Health Organization. (2023s). *WHO coronavirus (COVID-19) dashboard.* Retrieved April 14, 2023, from.

World Health Organization. (2023t). World Cancer Day: Know the facts – tobacco and alcohol both cause cancer. Retrieved March 24, 2023, from who.int

World Health Organization. (2023u, October 3). *Cumulative number of confirmed human cases for avian influenza A(H5N1) reported to WHO, 2003–2023, 2023.* Retrieved November 11, 2023, from.

World Health Organization. (2023v). *Alcohol: Fact sheet.* Retrieved December 29, 2023, from who.int

World Health Organization. (2023w). *Global cancer rates could increase by 50% to 15 million by 2020.* Retrieved February 23, 2023, from who.int

World Health Organization. (2023x). *Timeline: WHO's COVID-19 response.* Retrieved March 31, 2023, from.

World Health Organization. (2024a). *Cannabis.* Alcohol, Drugs and Addictive Behaviours Unit. Retrieved January 4, 2024, from who.int

World Health Organization. (2024b). *Tobacco.* Retrieved February 10, 2024, from https://www.who.int.

World Health Organization. (2024c). *Top 10 causes of death.* Retrieved February 10, 2024, from https://www.who.int

World Medical Association. (2000). *The Declaration of Helsinki: Ethical principles for medical research involving human subjects.* Geneva: World Health Organization. Retrieved January 15, 2007, from www.wma.net/en/30publications/10policies/b3/

World Population Review. (2023a). *School shootings by country 2023.* Retrieved June 16, 2023, from worldpopulationreview.com

World Population Review. (2023b). *Countries with universal health care in 2023*. Retrieved August 1, 2023, from worldpopulationreview.com

World Site Atlas. Retrieved February 24, 2010, from www.sitesatlas.com/Maps/Maps/714.gif

World Trade Organization. (2023). Chapter 2: The policy context for action on innovation and access. In *Promoting access to medical technologies and innovation intersections between public health, intellectual property and trade*. Retrieved November 7, 2023, from wto.org

Worley, K. D., Walsh, S., & Lewis, K. (2004). An examination of parenting experiences in male perpetrators of domestic violence: A qualitative study. *Psychology and Psychotherapy*, 77(Pt. 1), 35–54.

Worosz, M., & Wilson, N. L. W. (2012). A cautionary tale of purity, labeling and product literacy in the gluten-free market. *Journal of Consumer Affairs*, 46, 288–332.

Wu, G., Hu, Z., & Zheng, J. (2019). Role stress, job burnout, and job performance in construction project managers: The moderating role of career calling. *International Journal of Environmental Research and Public Health*, 16(13), 2394. doi: 10.3390/ijerph16132394

Wu, S., Yan, S., Marsiglia, F. F., & Perron, B. (2020). Patterns and social determinants of substance use among Arizona youth: A latent class analysis approach. *Children and Youth Services Review*, 110, 104769. doi: 10.1016/j.childyouth.2020.104769

Wu, X., Guo, T., Zhang, C., Hong, T.-Y., Cheng, C.-M., Wei, P., . . . Luo, J. (2021). From "Aha!" to "Haha!" using humor to cope with negative stimuli. *Cerebral Cortex*, 31(4), 2238–2250. doi: 10.1093/cercor/bhaa357

Xi, Y., & Xu, P. (2021). Global colorectal cancer burden in 2020 and projections to 2040. *Translational Oncology*, 14(10).

Xia, S., Zhang, Y., Wang, Y., Wang, H., Yang, Y., Yao, G. F., & Tan, W. (2021). Safety and immunogenicity of an inactivated SARS-CoV-2 vaccine, BBIBP-CorV: A randomised, double-blind, placebo-controlled, phase 1/2 trial. *The Lancet: Infectious Diseases*, 21(1), 39–51. doi: 10.1016/S1473-3099(20)30831-8

Xu, C., Xu, Y., Xu, S., Zhang, Q., Liu, X., & Shao, Y. (2020). Cognitive reappraisal and the association between perceived stress and anxiety symptoms in COVID-19 isolated people. *Frontiers in Psychology*, 11. doi: 10.3389/fpsyt.2020.00858

Xuan, Z., Blanchette, J. G., Nelson, T. F., Nguyen, T. H., Hadland, S. E., Oussayef, N. L., . . . Naimi, T. S. (2015). Youth drinking in the United States: Relationships with alcohol policies and adult drinking. *Pediatrics*, 136(1), 18–27. doi: 10.1542%2Fpeds.2015-0537

Yager, J. (1988). The treatment of eating disorders. *Journal of Clinical Psychiatry*, (49 Suppl.), 18–25.

Yale Medicine. (2024). *Fact sheet: E-cigarette, or vaping product, use associated lung oInjury (EVALI)*. Retrieved June 24, 2024, from www.yalemedicine.org/conditions/evali

Yanez, N. D., Weiss, N. S., Romand, J.-A., & Treggiari, M. M. (2020). COVID-19 mortality risk for older men and women. *BMC Public Health*, 20, 1742. doi: 10.1186/s12889-020-09826-8

Yang, E. J., Chung, H. K., Kim, W. Y., Bianchi, L., & Song, W. O. (2007). Chronic diseases and dietary changes in relation to Korean Americans length of residence in the United States. *Journal of the American Dietetic Association*, 107(6), 942–950.

Ye, X., Wang, Y., Zou, Y., Tu, J., Tang, W., Yu, R., . . . Huang, P. (2023). Associations of socioeconomic status with infectious diseases mediated by lifestyle, environmental pollution and chronic comorbidities: A comprehensive evaluation based on UK Biobank. *Infectious Diseases of Poverty*, 12. Article No. 5. doi: 10.1186/s40249-023-01056-5

Yellow Horse Brave Heart, M. (2003). The historical trauma response among natives and its relationship with substance abuse: A Lakota illustration. *Journal of Psychoactive Drugs*, 35, 7–13.

Yentür, S. B., Ataş, N., Öztürk, M. A., & Oskay, D. (2021). Comparison of the effectiveness of Pilates exercises, aerobic exercises, and Pilates with aerobic exercises in patients with rheumatoid arthritis. *Irish Journal of Medical Science*, *190*, 1027–1034. doi: 10.1007/s11845-020-02412-2

Yeo, I. S. (2003). The concept of disease in Galen. *Uisahak*, *12*(1), 54–65.

Young, L. (2015, February 11). "We failed" in presentation of HPV vaccine story, Star publisher says. *Global News*. Retrieved February 1, 2023, from https://globalnews.ca/news/1825017/toronto-star-did-not-give-proper-weight-to-science-in-hpv-vaccine-article-public-editor/

Young, Y., Alharthy, A., & Hosler, A. S. (2021). Transformation of Saudi Arabia's health system and its impact on population health: What can the USA learn? *Saudi Journal of Health Systems Research*, *1*(3), 93–102. doi: 10.1159/000517488

Yousaf, O., Grunfeld, E. A., & Hunter, M. S. (2013). A systematic review of the factors associated with delays in medical and psychological help-seeking among men. *Health Psychology Review*, *9*(2), 264–276. doi: 10.1080/17437199.2013.840954

Yu, H., & Hemminki, K. (2020). Genetic epidemiology of colorectal cancers and associated cancers. *Mutagenesis*, *35*(3), 207–219. doi: 10.1093/mutage/gez022

Yu, J., & Williford, W. R. (1992). The age of alcohol onset and alcohol, cigarette and marijuana use patterns: An analysis of drug use progression of young adults in New York State. *The International Journal of the Addictions*, *279*(11), 1313–1323.

Yu, T. S., Wong, S. L., Lloyd, O. L., & Wong, T. W. (1995). Ischemic heart disease. Trends in mortality in Hong Kong 1970–1989. *Journal of Epidemiology Community Health*, *49*(1), 16–21.

Yuan, H., Ma, Q., Ye, L., & Piao, G. (2016). The traditional medicine and modern medicine from natural products. *Molecules*, *21*(5), 559. doi: 10.3390/molecules21050559

Zanella, M. T., Kohlmann, O., & Ribeiro, A. B. (2001). Treatment of obesity hypertension and diabetes syndrome. *Hypertension*, *38*, 705–708.

Zellner, D. A., Loaiza, S., Gonzalez, Z., Pita, J., Morales, J., Pecora, D., & Wolf, A. (2006). Food selection changes under stress. *Physiology & Behavior*, *87*, 789–793.

Zellner, D. A., Saito, S., & Gonzalez, J. (2007). The effect of stress on men's food selection. *Appetite*, *49*, 696–699.

Zhang, H. J. (2004). Through gendered lens: Explaining Chinese caregivers' task performance and care reward. *Journal of Women & Aging*, *16*(1), 123–142.

Zhang, J., & Dulawa, S. C. (2021). The utility of animal models for studying the metabo-psychiatric origins of anorexia nervosa. *Frontiers in Psychiatry*, *12*, 711181. doi: 10.3389/fpsyt.2021.711181

Zhang, J.-M., & An, J. (2007). Cytokines, inflammation and pain. *International Anesthesiology Clinics*, *45*(2), 27–37.

Zhang, S., Peng, L., Li, Q., Zhao, J., Xu, D., Zhao, J., . . . Zeng, X. (2022). Spectrum of spondyloarthritis among Chinese populations. *Current Rheumatology Reports*, *24*, 247–258. doi: 10.1007/s11926-022-01079-1

Zhang, Z. F., Morgenstern, H., & Spitz, M. R. (1999). Marijuana use and increased risk of squamous cell carcinoma of the head and neck. *Cancer Epidemiology, Biomarkers & Prevention*, *8*(12), 1071–1078.

Zheng, W., McLerran, D. F., Rolland, B. A., Zu, F., Boffetta, P., He, J., . . . Potter, J. D. (2014). Burden of total and cause-specific mortality related to tobacco smoking among adults aged >45 years in Asia: A pooled analysis of 21 cohorts. *PLoS Medicine*, *11*(4), e1001631. doi: 10.1371/journal.pmed.1001631

Zhong, Y., Wang, J., & Nichols, S. (2020). Social support and depressive symptoms among family caregivers of older people with disabilities in four provinces of urban China: The mediating role of caregiver burden. *BMC Geriatrics*, *20*. Article No. 3. doi: 10.1186/s12877-019-1403-9

Zhou, B., Zang, R., Zhang, M., Song, P., Liu, L., Bie, F., . . . Gao, S. (2022). Worldwide burden and epidemiological trends of tracheal, bronchus, and lung cancer: A population-based study. *eBioMedicine*, *78*. doi: 10.1016/j.ebiom.2022.103951

Zhou, K. (2009). The history of medical insurance in the United States. *Yale Journal of Medicine & Law: An Undergraduate Publication*, *6*, 38–39.

Zickler, P. (2007). Methamphetamine evokes and subverts brain protective responses. *NIDA Notes: Research Trends and News from the National Institute on Drug Abuse*, *20*(6), 8–9.

Zimbardo, P. G. (1973). On the ethics of intervention in human psychological research: With special reference to the Stanford prison experiment. *Cognition*, *2*(2), 243–256.

Zimbardo, P. G. (2007). Revisiting the Stanford prison experiment: A lesson in the power of situation. *Chronicle of Higher Education*, *53*(30), B6–B7.

Zimmer, Z., Fraser, K., Grol-Prokopczyk, H., & Zajacova, A. (2022).

Zimmerman, L., Darnell, D. A., Rhew, I. C., Lee, C. M., & Kaysen, D. (2015). Resilience in community: A social ecological development model for young adult sexual minority women. *American Journal of Community Psychology*, *55*, 179–190. doi: 10.1007/s10464-015-9702-6

Ziv, A., Boulet, J. R., & Slap, G. B. (1999). Utilization of physicians' offices by adolescents in US. *Pediatrics*, *104*, 35–42.

Zubieta, J. K., Smith, Y. R., Bueller, J. A., Xu, Y., Kilbourn, M. R., Jewett, D. M., . . . Stohler, C. S. (2001). Regional mu opioid receptor regulation of sensory and affective dimensions of pain. *Science*, *293*, 311–315.

Zuckerman, S., & Shen, Y. C. (2004). Characteristics of occasional and frequent emergency department users: Do insurance coverage and access to care matter? *Medical Care*, *42*, 176–182.

Zulauf, C. A., Sprich, S. E., Safren, S. A., & Wilens, T. E. (2014). The complicated relationship between attention deficit/hyperactivity disorder and substance use disorders. *Current Psychiatry Reports*, *16*, 436. doi: 10.1007/s11920-013-0436-6

Zunkel, G. (2002). Relational coping process: Couples' response to a diagnosis of early stage breast cancer. *Journal of Psychosocial Oncology*, *20*, 39–55.

Zuskin, E., Lipozencic, J., Pucarin-Cvetkovic, J., Mustajbegovic, J., Schachter, N., Mucic-Pucic, B., & Neralic-Meniga, I. (2008). Ancient medicine: A review. *Acta Dermatovenerological Croatica: ADC*, *16*(3), 149–157.

Index

Note: Page numbers in *italics* indicate figures, **bold** indicate tables in the text, and page numbers in ***bold italics*** indicate boxes.